ANESTHESIA

ANESTHESIA

SECRETS

BRIAN M. KEECH, MD
Associate Professor of Anesthesiology
University of Colorado School of Medicine
Aurora, Colorado
Pediatric Anesthesiologist
Denver Health Medical Center
Denver, Colorado

RYAN D. LATERZA, MD
Assistant Professor of Anesthesiology
University of Colorado School of Medicine
Aurora, Colorado
Critical Care Anesthesiologist
Denver Health Medical Center
Denver, Colorado

ELSEVIER

Elsevier
1600 John F. Kennedy Blvd.
Ste 1800
Philadelphia, PA 19103-2899

Notices

Knowledge and best practice in this field are constantly changing. As new research and experience broaden our
understanding, changes in research methods, professional practices, or medical treatment may become necessary.

Practitioners and researchers must always rely on their own experience and knowledge in evaluating and using any
information, methods, compounds, or experiments described herein. In using such information or methods they should
be mindful of their own safety and the safety of others, including parties for whom they have a professional responsibility.

With respect to any drug or pharmaceutical products identified, readers are advised to check the most current information
provided (i) on procedures featured or (ii) by the manufacturer of each product to be administered, to verify the
recommended dose or formula, the method and duration of administration, and contraindications. It is the responsibility
of practitioners, relying on their own experience and knowledge of their patients, to make diagnoses, to determine dosages
and the best treatment for each individual patient, and to take all appropriate safety precautions.

To the fullest extent of the law, neither the Publisher nor the authors, contributors, or editors, assume any liability for any
injury and/or damage to persons or property as a matter of products liability, negligence or otherwise, or from any use or
operation of any methods, products, instructions, or ideas contained in the material herein.

Library of Congress Control Number: 2020931443

Content Strategist: Marybeth Thiel
Director, Content Development: Ellen Wurm-Cutter
Sr. Content Development Specialist: Kathleen Nahm
Publishing Services Manager: Deepthi Unni
Project Manager: Radjan Lourde Selvanadin
Designer: Bridget Hoette
Marketing Manager: Kathleen Patton

Printed in India

Last digit is the print number: 9 8 7 6 5 4 3

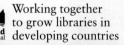

Working together
to grow libraries in
developing countries

www.elsevier.com • www.bookaid.org

To my wife Molly, thank you for all your love and support, and to my Mom, Dad, and brother Jeff for always being there for me. I am so grateful for you. And to my niece Harlow, my nephews John and Rory, and my godsons Mateusz and Isaac, may your lives be filled with peace and love.

Brian M. Keech

To my grandmother Shirley and grandfather Dennis, thank you for all your love, encouragement, and support. To my mother, father, and the rest of my family, thank you as well for all your love, encouragement, and support. I also want to thank Dr. Glenn Gravlee and Dr. Adam Levine for their mentorship, guidance, and inspiration.

Ryan D. Laterza

CONTENTS

6   ANESTHESIA AND SELECT PATIENT POPULATIONS

CONTRIBUTORS

David Abts, MD
Anesthesiologist
Department of Anesthesiology, Denver Health
  Medical Center
Denver, CO
Assistant Professor
Department of Anesthesiology, University of Colorado
  School of Medicine
Aurora, CO

Megan L. Albertz, MD
Assistant Professor
Department of Anesthesiology, Children's Hospital Colorado
Aurora, CO

Sama Ansari, MD
Resident Physician
Department of Anesthesiology, Mount Sinai Morningside
  and Mount Sinai West
New York, NY

Nicole Arboleda, MD
Pediatric Anesthesiologist
Department of Anesthesiology, Denver Health
  Medical Center
Denver, CO
Assistant Professor
Department of Anesthesiology, University of Colorado
  School of Medicine
Aurora, CO

Sona S. Arora, MD
Assistant Professor
Department of Anesthesiology
Emory University

Charles J. Bengson, MD
Critical Care Anesthesiology Fellow
Department of Anesthesiology and Perioperative Medicine,
  Oregon Health and Science University
Portland, OR

Bethany Benish, MD
Assistant Professor of Anesthesiology
Department of Anesthesiology, University of Colorado
  School of Medicine
Aurora, CO
Attending Anesthesiologist
Department of Anesthesiology, Denver Health
  Medical Center
Denver, CO

Andrew Bowman, MD
Resident Physician
Department of Anesthesiology, Emory University
Atlanta, GA

Jason C. Brainard, MD
Associate Professor
Department of Anesthesiology, University of Colorado
  School of Medicine
Aurora, CO

Khalil Chaibi, MD
Chief Resident
Reanimation Medico-Chirurgicale
Avicenne University Hospital, Bobigny
France

Mark Chandler, MD
Associate Professor of Anesthesiology
Department of Anesthesiology, University of Colorado
  School of Medicine
Aurora, CO
Associate Director
Department of Anesthesiology, Denver Health and Hospital
  Authority
Denver, CO

Christopher L. Ciarallo, MD, FAAP
Associate Professor
Department of Anesthesiology, University of Colorado
  School of Medicine
Aurora, CO
Director of Pediatric Anesthesiology
Department of Anesthesiology, Denver Health Medical
  Center
Denver, CO
Pediatric Anesthesiologist
Department of Anesthesiology, Children's Hospital Colorado
Aurora, CO

Colin Coulson, MSNA, CRNA
Instructor
Department of Anesthesiology, University of Colorado
  School of Medicine
Aurora, CO
Certified Registered Nurse Anesthetist
Department of Anesthesiology, University of Colorado
  Hospital
Aurora, CO

Christopher P. Davis, MD
Regional Anesthesiology Fellow
Department of Anesthesiology, Washington University
  in St. Louis
St. Louis, MO

Jeffrey Davis, MD
Assistant Professor
Department of Anesthesiology and Perioperative Medicine,
  Oregon Health and Science University
Portland, OR

Samuel DeMaria, Jr, MD
Professor
Department of Anesthesiology, Perioperative and Pain
  Medicine, Icahn School of Medicine at Mount Sinai
New York, NY

David J. Douin, MD
Senior Instructor
Department of Anesthesiology, University of Colorado
  School of Medicine
Aurora, CO

Mitchell Fingerman, MD
Division Chief and Fellowship Director
Regional and Ambulatory Division, Department
  of Anesthesiology,
Washington University School of Medicine
St. Louis, MO

Philip Fung, MD
Assistant Professor
Internal Medicine, Denver Health Medical Center/University
  of Colorado School of Medicine
Denver, CO

Paul Garcia, MD
Associate Professor
Department of Anesthesiology, Columbia University Medical
  Center
New York, NY
Director of Neuroanesthesia Division
Department of Anesthesiology, Columbia University
  Medical Center
New York, NY

Stephane Gaudry, MD, PhD
Professor
Reanimation Medico-Chirurgicale
Avicenne Univeristy Hospital
Bobigny, France

Erin Gibbons, MD
Assistant Professor
Department of Anesthesiology, Washington University
  in St Louis
St Louis, MO

Samuel Gilliland, MD
Assistant Professor
Department of Anesthesiology, University of Colorado
  School of Medicine
Aurora, CO

Andrew Goldberg, MD
Assistant Professor
Department of Anesthesiology, Perioperative and Pain
  Medicine, Icahn School of Medicine at Mount Sinai
New York, NY

Thomas R. Gruffi, MD
Assistant Professor
Department of Anesthesiology, Mount Sinai Morningside
  and Mount Sinai West
New York, NY

Ryan Guffey, MD
Assistant Professor
Department of Anesthesia, Washington University
St Louis, MO

Thomas Gulvezan, MD, MBA
Resident Physician
Department of Anesthesiology, University of Colorado
  School of Medicine
Aurora, CO

Monica Hoagland, MD
Assistant Professor
Department of Anesthesiology, Children's Hospital
  Colorado
Aurora, CO

Eugene Hsu, MD, MBA
Adjunct Lecturer
Clinical Excellence Research Center, Stanford University
  School of Medicine
Stanford, CA

Richard Ing, MBBCh, FCA(SA)
Professor
Department of Anesthesiology, University of Colorado,
  Children's Hospital
Aurora, CO

Daniel J. Janik, MD, FASA
Professor of Clinical Anesthesiology
Department of Anesthesiology, University of Colorado
  School of Medicine
Aurora, CO
Director of Intraoperative Neuromonitoring
Department of Anesthesiology, University of Colorado
  School of Medicine,
Aurora, CO
Vice Chair for Faculty Affairs
Department of Anesthesiology, University of Colorado
  School of Medicine
Aurora, CO

Alma N. Juels, MD
Assistant Professor
Department of Anesthesiology, University of Colorado
  School of Medicine
Aurora, CO
Attending Physician
Department of Anesthesiology, Denver Health Medical
  Center
Denver, CO

Rachel Kacmar, MD
Associate Professor
Department of Anesthesiology, University of Colorado
  School of Medicine
Aurora, CO
Obstetric Anesthesia Fellowship Director
Department of Anesthesiology, University of Colorado
  School of Medicine
Aurora, CO

Mark Kearns, MD
Assistant Professor
Division of Pulmonary and Critical Care, Denver Health
  Medical Center
Denver, CO

Brian M. Keech, MD
Pediatric Anesthesiologist
Department of Anesthesiology, Denver Health
  Medical Center
Denver, CO
Associate Professor
Department of Anesthesiology, University of Colorado
  School of Medicine
Aurora, CO
Medical Director
Ambulatory Surgery, Department of Anesthesiology, Denver
  Health Medical Center
Denver, CO

Michael Kim, DO
Assistant Professor
Department of Anesthesiology and Critical Care, Keck
  School of Medicine of USC
Los Angeles, CA

Martin Krause, MD
Assistant Professor
Department of Anesthesiology, University of Colorado
  School of Medicine
Aurora, CO

Alison Krishna, MD
Assistant Professor
Department of Anesthesiology, Mount Sinai Morningside
  and Mount Sinai West
New York, NY

Peiman Lahsaei, MD
Assistant Professor
Department of Anesthesiology and Pain Management,
  UT Southwestern
Dallas, TX

Ryan D. Laterza, MD
Assistant Professor
Department of Anesthesiology, University of Colorado
  School of Medicine
Aurora, CO
Critical Care Anesthesiologist
Department of Anesthesiology Denver Health
  Medical Center
Denver, CO

Ryan A. Lawless, MD, FACS
Staff Surgeon
Department of Surgery, Denver Health Medical Center
Denver, CO
Assistant Professor of Surgery
Department of Surgery, University of Colorado
Aurora, CO

Marshall Lee, MD
Assistant Professor
Department of Anesthesiology and Perioperative Medicine,
  Oregon Health and Science University
Portland, OR

Adam I. Levine, MD
Professor
Department of Anesthesiology, Perioperative and Pain
  Medicine, Icahn School of Medicine at Mount Sinai
New York, NY
Professor
Department of Otolaryngology, Icahn School of Medicine at
  Mount Sinai
New York, NY
Professor
Department of Pharmacological Sciences, Icahn School of
  Medicine at Mount Sinai
New York, NY

Justin N. Lipper, MD
Assistant Professor
Department of Anesthesiology, Mount Sinai Morningside
  and Mount Sinai West
New York, NY

Benjamin Lippert, DO, FAAP
Pediatric Anesthesiologist
Department of Anesthesiology, Denver Health Medical
  Center
Denver, CO
Assistant Professor
Department of Anesthesiology, University of Colorado
  School of Medicine
Aurora, CO

Ross Martini, MD
Assistant Professor
Department of Anesthesiology and Perioperative Medicine,
  Oregon Health and Science University
Portland, OR

S. Andrew McCullough, MD
Assistant Professor of Clinical Medicine
Division of Cardiology, Department of Medicine, Weill
  Cornell Medicine
New York, NY

Brennan McGill, MD
Resident Physician
Department of Anesthesiology, University of Colorado
  School of Medicine
Aurora, CO

Howard J. Miller, MD
Director of Service
Department of Anesthesiology, Denver Health
  Medical Center
Denver, CO
Associate Professor
Department of Anesthesiology, University of Colorado
  School of Medicine
Aurora, CO
Medical Director
Perioperative Services, Denver Health Medical Center
Denver, CO

Joanna Miller, MD
Instructor
Department of Anesthesiology, Perioperative and Pain
  Medicine, Icahn School of Medicine at Mount Sinai
New York, NY

Thomas B. Moore, MSNA
Certified Registered Nurse Anesthetist
Department of Anesthesiology, Denver Health
  Medical Center
Denver, CO

Joseph Morabito, DO
Fellow
Cardiothoracic Anesthesiology, University of Colorado
  Hospital
Aurora, CO

Aaron Murray, MD
Assistant Professor
Department of Anesthesiology, University of Colorado
  School of Medicine
Aurora, CO
Anesthesiologist
Department of Anesthesiology, Denver Health
  Medical Center
Denver, CO

Manchula Navaratnam, MBChB
Clinical Associate Professor
Department of Anesthesiology, Preoperative and Pain,
  Medicine, Stanford Children's Hospital
Palo Alto, CA

Jessica L. Nelson, MD
Critical Care Fellow
Department of Anesthesiology, University of Colorado
  School of Medicine
Aurora, CO

Katelyn O'Connor, MD
Chief Resident
Department of Anesthesiology, Perioperative and Pain
  Medicine
Icahn School of Medicine at Mount Sinai
New York, NY

Anthony M. Oliva, MD, PhD
Assistant Professor
Department of Anesthesiology, University of Colorado
  School of Medicine
Aurora, CO

Joanna Olsen, MD, PhD
Assistant Professor
Department of Anesthesiology and Perioperative Medicine,
  Oregon Health and Science University
Portland, OR

Abimbola Onayemi, MSc, MD
Resident
Department of Anesthesiology, Mount Sinai Morningside
  and Mount Sinai West
New York, NY

Jason Papazian, MD
Assistant Professor
Department of Anesthesiology, University of Colorado
  School of Medicine
Aurora, CO

Raj Parekh, MD
Assistant Professor of Anesthesiology
Department of Anesthesiology, Mount Sinai Morningside
  and Mount Sinai West
New York, NY

Chang H. Park, MD
Assistant Professor
Department of Anesthesiology, Perioperative and Pain
  Medicine, Icahn School of Medicine at Mount Sinai
New York, NY

Thomas Phillips, MD
Resident
Department of Anesthesiology and Perioperative Medicine,
  Oregon Health and Science University
Portland, OR

Deepa Ramadurai, MD
Chief Resident Physician
Internal Medicine Residency Training Program,
  University of Colorado
Aurora, CO

Brittany Reardon, MD
Resident Physician
Department of Anesthesiology, Mount Sinai Morningside
  and Mount Sinai West
New York, NY

Matthew J. Roberts, MA, BM, BCh, DMCC FRCA
Attending Anesthesiologist
Department of Anesthesiology, Denver Health
  Medical Center
Denver, CO
Associate Professor
Department of Anesthesiology, University of Colorado
  School of Medicine
Aurora, CO

Robert G. Saldana, BA
Stanford University
Stanford, CA

Nick Schiavoni, MD
Resident Physician
Department of Anesthesiology, University of Colorado
  School of Medicine
Aurora, CO

Dominique Schiffer, MD
Doctor
Department of Anesthesiology, University of Colorado
  School of Medicine
Aurora, CO

Joseph Schoenfeldt, MD
Regional Anesthesiology Fellow
Department of Anesthesiology, Washington University
  in St. Louis
St. Louis, MO

Lawrence I. Schwartz, MD
Associate Professor
Department of Anesthesiology, Children's Hospital
  Colorado, University of Colorado
Aurora, CO

Thomas Scupp, MD
Fellow in Anesthesia Critical Care
Department of Anesthesiology, University of Colorado
  School of Medicine
Aurora, CO

David Shapiro, MD
Assistant Professor
Department of Anesthesiology, Perioperative and Pain
  Medicine, Icahn School of Medicine at Mount Sinai
New York, NY

Alan J. Sim, MD
Assistant Professor
Department of Anesthesiology, Perioperative and Pain
  Medicine, Icahn School of Medicine at Mount Sinai
New York, NY

Robert H. Slover, MD
Director of Pediatrics
The Barbara Davis Center for Diabetes, University of
  Colorado Denver
Aurora, CO
Professor of Pediatrics
University of Colorado Denver
Aurora, CO

Robin Slover, MD
Medical Director Pain Consultation Service
Department of Anesthesiology, Children's Hospital
  Colorado
Aurora, CO
Associate Professor
Department of Anesthesiology, University of Colorado
  School of Medicine
Aurora, CO

Natalie K. Smith, MD
Assistant Professor
Department of Anesthesiology, Perioperative and Pain
  Medicine, Icahn School of Medicine at Mount Sinai
New York, NY

William B. Somerset, DO
Assistant Professor of Anesthesiology
Department of Anesthesiology, Denver Health Medical
  Center
Denver, CO
Assistant Professor Anesthesiology
Department of Anesthesiology, University of Colorado
  School of Medicine
Aurora, CO

Tanaya Sparkle, MBBS
Assistant Professor of Anesthesiology
Department of Anesthesiology - Cardiac Anesthesia,
  University of Toledo College of Medicine and Life
  Sciences
Toledo, OH

Stephen Spindel, MD
Cardiothoracic Surgeon
Cardiothoracic Surgery, Ochsner Medical Center
New Orleans, LA

Lee D. Stein, MD
Pediatric Anesthesiologist
Department of Anesthesiology, Denver Health
  Medical Center
Denver, CO
Assistant Professor
Department of Anesthesiology, University of Colorado
  School of Medicine
Aurora, CO

Marc E. Stone, MD
Professor
Department of Anesthesiology, Perioperative and Pain
  Medicine, Icahn School of Medicine at Mount Sinai
New York, NY

Program Director, Fellowship in Cardiothoracic
Department of Anesthesiology, Perioperative and Pain
  Medicine, Icahn School of Medicine at Mount Sinai
New York, NY

Annmarie Toma, MD
Resident Physician
Department of Anesthesiology, Mount Sinai Morningside
  and Mount Sinai West
New York, NY

Tim T. Tran, MD
Assistant Professor
Department of Anesthesiology, University of Colorado
  School of Medicine
Aurora, CO

Mark D. Twite, MB, BChir, FRCP
Director of Pediatric Cardiac Anesthesia
Department of Anesthesiology
Children's Hospital Colorado and University of Colorado
Denver, CO

Mahesh Vaidyanathan, MD, MBA
Assistant Professor
Department of Anesthesiology, Northwestern University
Chicago, IL

Scott Vogel, DO
Assistant Professor
Department of Anesthesiology, University of Colorado
  School of Medicine
Aurora, CO

Johannes von Alvensleben, MD
Pediatric Electrophysiologist
Pediatric Cardiology, Children's Hospital Colorado
Aurora, CO

John A. Vullo, MD
Assistant Professor
Department of Anesthesiology, Perioperative and
  Pain Medicine, Icahn School of Medicine at
  Mount Sinai
New York, NY
Assistant Professor
Institute for Critical Care Medicine, Icahn School of Medicine
  at Mount Sinai
New York, NY

Nathaen Weitzel, MD
Associate Professor
Department of Anesthesiology, University of Colorado
  School of Medicine
Aurora, CO

Barbara Wilkey, MD
Assistant Professor
Department of Anesthesiology, University of Colorado
  School of Medicine
Aurora, CO

Katie Yang, MD
Fellow Physician
Department of Anesthesiology, Washington University
  in St. Louis
St. Louis, MI

PREFACE

Thank you for selecting *Anesthesia Secrets* sixth edition as your study aide. Although this edition shares the concise style and presentation of general anesthesia topics found in previous editions, its content and layout have been significantly revised. This edition introduces several new chapters emphasizing such topics as the history and scope of anesthesia practice, cardiac physiology and the electrocardiogram, volume status assessment, perioperative ethics, regional anesthesia, and perioperative ultrasound. Our primary goal is to provide an appropriate breadth and depth of pertinent anesthesia topics that can be integrated into the practice of medicine in general. We hope that the content of this book excites you as much as us and ultimately contributes to your decision to enter our esteemed profession.

We would like to express our sincere appreciation to all the authors of this sixth edition. We also wish to acknowledge the previous edition's chapter authors for their important contributions. Each new edition of *Anesthesia Secrets* builds on the foundation set forth in the previous edition. Finally, we would like to offer our profound gratitude to the late Dr. James C. Duke for his extraordinary dedication to the *Anesthesia Secrets* series, including almost 20 years as the principal editor of all prior editions.

Brian M. Keech, MD

Ryan D. Laterza, MD

TOP 100 SECRETS

Brian M. Keech, MD, Ryan D. Laterza, MD

1. Opioid side effects include respiratory depression, nausea and vomiting, pruritus, cough suppression, urinary retention, and biliary tract spasm. Some opioids may induce histamine release and cause hives, bronchospasm, and hypotension.
2. One-lung ventilation (OLV) can be achieved with double-lumen endotracheal tubes (DLTs), bronchial blockers, and standard single-lumen endotracheal tubes (ETTs), each of which has advantages and disadvantages.
3. Anesthesia awareness is most likely to occur in situations where minimal anesthetic is administered, often because of hemodynamical instability, such as during cardiopulmonary bypass, trauma, and in obstetrics. Symptoms of awareness can be nonspecific, and the use of neuromuscular blockade increases the risk of unrecognized awareness.
4. Methohexital is the most common induction agent for electroconvulsive therapy because it has minimal anticonvulsant properties, has a rapid onset with a short duration of action, and has low cardiac toxicity.
5. Common indications for permanent pacemaker placement are the following: symptomatic bradycardia that is not reversible, second-degree type II heart block, and third-degree heart block.
6. Pacemaker code positions I, II, and III define the chamber in which pacing occurs, the chamber in which sensing occurs, and the mode of the response to the sensed or triggered event, respectively. Asynchronous pacing modes are most commonly used for temporary pacing or to allow for the safe use of surgical electrocautery during surgery.
7. Chronic alcohol use leads to delayed gastric emptying and relaxation of the lower esophageal sphincter, the risk of which increase the risk of aspiration.
8. The fetal circulation is a parallel circulation containing three shunts (i.e., ductus venosus, foramen ovale, and ductus arteriosus) that function to deliver the most highly oxygenated fetal blood from the placenta to the developing heart and brain.
9. The ductus venosus shunts oxygenated blood from the placenta in the umbilical vein through the liver to the right atrium. This blood is then shunted through the foramen ovale to the left side of the heart and into the ascending aorta. In the presence of high pulmonary vascular resistance (e.g., low arterial partial oxygen pressure [PaO_2] from atelectasis, amniotic fluid filled lungs), blood returning to the right atria and ventricle is shunted from the main pulmonary artery through the ductus arteriosus to the descending aorta. This blood then preferentially flows by a lower systemic vascular resistance pathway back to the placenta for reoxygenation via the umbilical artery.
10. The newborn heart is less compliant, develops less contractile force, and is less responsive to inotropic support than mature hearts. Myocardial maturation is generally complete by 6 to 12 months of age.
11. Efficient oxygen transport relies on the ability of hemoglobin to reversibly load oxygen in the lungs and unload it peripherally, and the sigmoid shape of the oxyhemoglobin dissociation curve is a graphic representation of this capability. The oxyhemoglobin dissociation curve describes the relationship between oxygen tension, or PaO_2, and binding (percent oxygen saturation of hemoglobin).
12. In the lungs, where oxygen tension is high, hemoglobin will nearly fully saturate under normal circumstances. As oxygenated blood moves through the peripheral tissues, and oxygen tension begins to lower, oxygen will be released at an accelerating rate from hemoglobin to maintain the necessary oxygen tension needed for adequate oxygen diffusion from blood to the cells of the periphery.
13. The American College of Cardiology/American Heart Association guidelines are the gold standard for directing appropriate cardiac testing before noncardiac procedures. In general, additional cardiac evaluation and testing is not necessary for the following: patients with moderate or excellent functional capacity (metabolic equivalents [METs] $\geq$4), patients undergoing emergent surgical operations, or patients undergoing low-risk surgical operations (e.g., eye surgery).
14. The ability to climb two or three flights of stairs (METs $\geq$4), without significant symptoms (angina, dyspnea), is considered evidence of adequate functional capacity. Such patients can generally undergo high-risk surgical operations without further cardiac testing.
15. Ketamine is the best induction agent for hypovolemic trauma patients. It is also a good agent for patients with active bronchospastic disease (e.g., asthma). Elevated intracranial pressure (ICP) has traditionally thought to be a contraindication to ketamine; however, recent studies suggest it may be safe in this patient population and may even lower ICP.
16. Propofol is generally regarded as safe for use in adult patients with documented egg allergies, but it should be avoided in children with known anaphylaxis to eggs.
17. Local anesthetic agents are classified as either esters or amides. The two classes differ primarily in their allergic potential and method of biotransformation. Lipid solubility, pKa, and protein binding determine their potency, onset, and duration of action, respectively.

1

18. Local anesthetic–induced central nervous system (CNS) toxicity manifests with excitation, followed by seizures, then loss of consciousness. Cardiac toxicity generally occurs after CNS toxicity and includes hypotension, conduction blockade, dysrhythmias, and cardiac arrest. Bupivacaine has the highest risk of producing severe cardiac dysrhythmias and cardiovascular arrest. Local anesthetic toxicity is treated with lipid emulsion therapy (i.e., Intralipid 20%).

19. Adequate oxygenation, controlled postoperative pain, and resolved postoperative nausea and vomiting (PONV) are requirements for postanesthesia care unit discharge.

20. With the exception of spinal anesthesia in multiple sclerosis, neither general nor regional anesthesia exacerbates the course of most degenerative neurological diseases and neuropathies. Many patients afflicted with these conditions are at aspiration risk secondary to bulbar muscle weakness.

21. Careful attention to glucose control before, during, and after surgery is important to reduce the risk of wound infection, promote rapid wound healing, avoid metabolic complications, and shorten hospital stay. The goal for insulin management during most surgical operations is to maintain glucose between 90 and 180 mg/dL.

22. Patients with diabetes have a high incidence of coronary artery disease, with an atypical or silent presentation. Maintaining adequate coronary perfusion pressure, controlling heart rate, continuous electrocardiogram observation, and a high index of suspicion during periods of refractory hypotension are key considerations.

23. Chronic exogenous glucocorticoid therapy should not be discontinued abruptly. Doing so may precipitate acute adrenocortical insufficiency.

24. The shoulder is primarily supplied by the axillary nerve inferiorly and the suprascapular nerve superiorly, both of which can be anesthetized by an interscalene block. Complications of the interscalene block includes the following: ipsilateral phrenic nerve block, resulting in hemidiaphragmatic paralysis, Horner syndrome, unilateral recurrent laryngeal nerve paralysis, pneumothorax, inadvertent neuraxial injection, and accidental intravascular injection.

25. Regional anesthesia is beneficial for patients in whom general anesthesia should be avoided or in whom pain may be difficult to control. For example, patients with severe cardiopulmonary disease, obstructive sleep apnea, PONV, chronic pain, and substance abuse.

26. Age-related physiological changes include left ventricular hypertrophy, increased reliance on preload for cardiac output, decreased venous compliance, increased closing capacity, decreased glomerular filtration rate, decreased hepatic function, and increased risk for postoperative delirium.

27. Malignant hyperthermia (MH) is a hypermetabolic disorder that presents in the perioperative period after exposure to triggering agents, such as volatile agents or succinylcholine. The sine qua non of MH is an unexplained rise in end-tidal carbon dioxide and rigidity in a patient with unexplained tachycardia. Temperature rise is a late feature.

28. Neonates, infants, and small children may be difficult to intubate because they have a more anterior larynx, relatively large tongues, and a long, floppy epiglottis. In addition, they desaturate more rapidly than adults because of increased oxygen consumption and decreased functional residual capacity (FRC).

29. The fundamental reason to give intravenous fluids is to increase stroke volume. Dynamic indices (e.g., arterial line variability) use the Frank-Starling law to predict volume responsiveness (i.e., hypovolemia) and are much more accurate than other modalities (static indices, such as central venous pressure, physical examination, imaging studies, etc.) in assessing for hypovolemia.

30. Point-of-care ultrasound has a variety of roles in the perioperative setting, including global assessment of left ventricular and right ventricular cardiac function, evaluation of volume status/responsiveness, and pulmonary evaluation, including identification of pneumothorax, hemidiaphragm paresis, pleural effusions, or consolidations.

31. Transesophageal or transthoracic echocardiography should be considered in any case where the nature of the procedure or the patient's underlying known or suspected cardiovascular pathology might result in hemodynamic, pulmonary, or neurological instability or compromise.

32. Patients with reactive airway disease (i.e., asthma, chronic obstructive pulmonary disease) require thorough preoperative preparation, including inhaled β-agonist therapy and possibly steroids. An actively wheezing patient is never a good candidate for an elective surgical procedure.

33. *All that wheezes is not asthma.* Also consider mechanical airway obstruction, congestive failure, allergic reaction, pulmonary embolus, pneumothorax, aspiration, and endobronchial intubation.

34. Lung protection ventilation strategies should be viewed as harm reduction ventilation strategies and applied to all mechanically ventilated patients, not just those with acute respiratory distress syndrome (ARDS).

35. Initial management of trauma patients focuses on the ABCs: airway, breathing, and circulation. Once the airway is secure, placement of multiple large bore intravenous catheters for hypovolemic resuscitation is a priority.

36. Trauma-induced coagulopathy is an independent predictor of transfusion, multiorgan failure, and mortality. Correction of coagulopathy is one of the primary goals of acute trauma management. Early ratio-driven transfusion of 1:1:1 red blood cell: plasma: platelet should be used, until viscoelastic hemostatic assays (thromboelastography [TEG] or rotational thromboelastometry [ROTEM]) are available for goal-directed hemostatic resuscitation.

37. Depolarizing agents include succinylcholine and nondepolarizing agents include steroidal agents (vecuronium and rocuronium) and benzylisoquinolinium agents (atracurium and cisatracurium). A *phase I block* is seen with depolarizing agents and a *phase II block* with nondepolarizing neuromuscular blocking agents.

38. The best practice to ensure termination of the relaxant effect from neuromuscular blocking agents are to dose them sparingly and to allow enough time for normal metabolism to occur.

39. It is best practice to administer reversal agents to all patients receiving nondepolarizing neuromuscular blocking agents, unless there is documented evidence that the T4:T1 is greater than 0.9. If for some reason a patient is not recovering from neuromuscular blockade, they should remain intubated on supported ventilation, until they can demonstrate return of strength.

40. Cardiotoxicity because of hyperkalemia should be immediately treated with intravenous calcium chloride or calcium gluconate.

41. Patients who receive high volumes of fluid, especially normal saline, often develop hyperchloremia and a nonanion gap metabolic acidosis.

42. Minimum alveolar concentration (MAC) is defined as the minimum alveolar concentration of inhaled anesthetic required to prevent movement in 50% of patients in response to surgical incision.

43. The MAC of inhaled anesthetics is decreased by old age or prematurity, hyponatremia, hypothermia, opioids, barbiturates, α_2 blockers, calcium channel blockers, acute alcohol intoxication, and pregnancy. It is increased by hyperthermia, chronic alcoholism, hypernatremia, and acute intoxication with CNS stimulants (e.g., amphetamine).

44. Because of its rapid egress into air-filled spaces, nitrous oxide should not be used in the setting of pneumothorax, bowel obstruction or pneumocephalus, or during middle ear or ophthalmological surgery.

45. The lung is heterogeneous and characterized by regional ventilation/perfusion ($\dot{V}/\dot{Q}$) mismatch, resulting in dead space (zone one) and shunt (zone three).

46. Causes of hypoxemia include the following: low inspired oxygen, alveolar hypoventilation, $\dot{V}/\dot{Q}$ mismatch, right-left shunt, and impaired oxygen diffusion.

47. No single pulmonary function test measurement absolutely contraindicates surgery. Factors, such as physical examination, arterial blood gases, and coexisting medical problems must be considered in determining suitability for surgery.

48. The output of traditional vaporizers depends on the proportion of fresh gas that bypasses the vaporizing chamber compared with the proportion that passes through the vaporizing chamber. The exception, however, is desflurane, whereby the vaporizer actively injects vapor into the fresh gas stream.

49. Severe anaphylaxis generally presents as hypotension followed by bronchospasm. Rash and edema are late findings and may not be clinically apparent on presentation. Epinephrine, volume resuscitation, and cardiopulmonary resuscitation are the mainstay treatments.

50. Patients require close monitoring with the potential for aggressive fluid resuscitation and vasopressor support in the setting of neuraxial anesthesia (i.e., spinal or epidural anesthesia) because of the onset of a dense sympathectomy.

51. Epidural anesthesia is segmental (i.e., it has an upper and a lower level). The block is most intense near the site of catheter or needle insertion and diminishes with distance.

52. Bicarbonate supplementation is only indicated in the presence of a severe metabolic acidosis pH under 7.20.

53. Possessing medical decision-making capacity entails the following: (1) understanding the proposed treatment, (2) appreciating the severity of the situation, (3) using reason in the decision-making process, and (4) being able to communicate their decision to the care team.

54. Do-not-resuscitate (DNR) orders are generally suspended in the perioperative period because of the temporary and reversible nature of anesthesia, leading to respiratory failure and/or hemodynamic instability.

55. Phenylephrine is a direct α_1 adrenergic agonist, whereas ephedrine is an indirect $\alpha_1 = \beta_1$ adrenergic agonist.

56. Intravenous epinephrine and norepinephrine have a short half-life ($\sim$90 seconds). Because of the short half-life of these agents, they are generally administered by continuous infusion or by frequent rebolusing (e.g., every 3–5 minutes, in the setting of advanced cardiac life support).

57. Recall blood pressure is the product of cardiac output and resistance; therefore excessive use of vasopressor to normalize the blood pressure does not ensure normal cardiac output.

58. Nicardipine is a selective arterial vasodilator. It is one of the few calcium channel blockers that has no negative inotropic effects.

59. Glycopyrrolate is often preferred over atropine in the perioperative setting. Because glycopyrrolate does not cross the blood-brain barrier, it is associated with little to no sedation compared with atropine.

60. Nitroglycerin vasodilates veins more than arteries; the converse is true for nitroprusside.

61. Laparoscopic surgery decreases pulmonary compliance, venous return, cardiac output and pH because of elevated arterial partial pressure of carbon dioxide ($PaCO_2$).

62. Sympathetic nerves originate from the spinal cord at T1–L2.

63. Patients with high spinal cord injuries (T6 and above) are at risk for autonomic dysreflexia, a condition associated with excessive sympathetic response to painful stimuli below the level of the lesion.

64. The primary determinants of myocardial oxygen demand are increases in afterload (wall tension) and heart rate.

65. Renin-angiotensin system antagonists (angiotensin-converting enzyme inhibitors and angiotensin receptor blockers), if continued on the day of surgery, can cause profound refractory hypotension that usually responds best to vasopressin administration.

66. Obesity decreases pulmonary compliance, decreasing FRC, and is associated with increased oxygen consumption because of the larger body habitus.

67. Patients with obesity should be placed in the ramp position before the induction of anesthesia.

68. Ramp positioning can improve pulmonary mechanics (increase pulmonary compliance and increase FRC) and reduce the incidence of hypoxemia on induction.

69. Sustained end-tidal CO_2 detection should be used to confirm proper ETT placement on intubation.
70. In the absence of $\dot{V}/\dot{Q}$ abnormalities, end-tidal CO_2 is approximately 3 to 5 mm Hg less than $PaCO_2$.
71. Abrupt decreases in cardiac output will cause a "drop in end-tidal CO_2."
72. Normal body temperature is 37°C, hypothermia is less than 36°C, and hyperthermia is greater than 38°C.
73. The recurrent laryngeal nerve, a branch of the vagus nerve, innervates the glottis and trachea.
74. The superior laryngeal nerve, a branch from the vagus nerve, innervates the base of tongue, arytenoids, and posterior surface of the epiglottis.
75. Risk factors for difficult intubation include the following: history of head and neck cancer and/or radiation, history of known difficult intubation from prior anesthetics, obesity, pregnancy, airway trauma, poor mouth opening, decreased neck range of motion, inability to bite upper lip, decreased thyroid mental distance, short neck, and large neck circumference.
76. The sniffing position facilitates alignment of airway axes, allowing direct visualization of the glottis with direct laryngoscopy.
77. The sniffing position can be achieved with head extension and neck flexion. In general, the patient is said to be in proper sniffing position when the ear and sternal notch are aligned.
78. Rapid sequence induction and intubation (also known as *RSI*) with cricoid pressure and a fast-acting neuromuscular blocking agent (e.g., succinylcholine) is the gold standard for patients at high-risk for aspiration who need to be intubated.
79. The Macintosh blade is placed anterior to the epiglottis in the vallecula, while the Miller blade is placed posterior and directly lifts the epiglottis.
80. Patients with risk factors for difficult intubation, especially head and neck cancer and/or radiation, are strong candidates for awake intubation.
81. Multiple attempts in instrumenting the airway may cause significant airway trauma, eventually causing an iatrogenic "can't intubate, can't ventilate" situation.
82. Complications of central venous catheterization include pneumothorax, arterial injury, bleeding, thoracic duct injury, air embolus, deep venous thrombosis, and infection.
83. The Seldinger technique involves placing a guidewire into a vein, which facilitates the exchange of catheters over the guidewire into the vein.
84. Quantitative nerve monitoring to assess neuromuscular blockade and adequate reversal (by measuring the T4:T1 ratio) is strongly encouraged.
85. There are two types of aspiration: aspiration pneumonitis and aspiration pneumonia. The former is primarily irritative and obstructive in pathology, whereas the latter is primarily infectious.
86. The model of end-stage liver disease (MELD) score predicts 90-day mortality and is used to prioritize recipients for organ transplant.
87. Hypoxia, hypercarbia, or acidosis can increase pulmonary vascular resistance.
88. Patients must be completely anticoagulated before cardiopulmonary bypass is initiated; otherwise, a dire thrombotic complication may occur.
89. Low-flow (<1 L/min) anesthetic techniques with sevoflurane is safe in humans and better for the environment compared with using higher flows or other commonly used inhalational agents (i.e., desflurane, nitrous oxide).
90. Mechanical ventilation settings for patients with ARDS includes tidal volume at 6 mL/kg of ideal body weight and limiting plateau pressures to less than 30 cm H_2O.
91. Pain assessment should not rely solely on numeric pain scores but should include functional impairment and treatment goals (e.g., breathe or sleep without pain). Pain is a symptom not a vital sign.
92. Postoperative vision loss can occur with spine surgery.
93. The Cushing reflex is the classic triad of systemic hypertension, bradycardia, and irregular respiration. It implies medullary ischemia and is often because of brainstem compression because of brain herniation.
94. Physiological alterations in pregnancy include an increase in cardiac output, heart rate, plasma volume, minute ventilation, and oxygen consumption; decreases in systemic vascular resistance and FRC; dilutional anemia; and a hypercoagulable state.
95. Spinal anesthesia for cesarean delivery produces a reliable and dense sensory and motor block, is relatively easy to perform, has a rapid onset, and carries no risk of local anesthetic toxicity.
96. The risk of epidural hematoma as a complication of neuraxial techniques is extremely low when the platelet count is greater than 70,000 mm^{-3}.
97. Uterine atony is the most common cause of postpartum hemorrhage and often results in substantial blood loss.
98. When emergency blood transfusion is necessary, use O negative blood and switch to type-specific blood, as soon as available.
99. Transfusion-associated circulatory overload (TACO) causes hydrostatic pulmonary edema (too much volume) whereas transfusion-related acute ling injury (TRALI) causes nonhydrostatic pulmonary edema (inflammatory response).
100. Recipient human leukocyte antigen (HLA) antibodies against donor neutrophils causes febrile, nonhemolytic transfusion reactions, whereas donor HLA antibodies against recipient neutrophils causes TRALI.

INTRODUCTION TO ANESTHESIA

Ryan D. Laterza, MD, Brian M. Keech, MD, Mark Chandler, MD, Matthew J. Roberts, MA, BM, BCh, DMCC FRCA

1. **Where did the term "anesthesia" come from?**
   Oliver Wendell Holmes, Sr. (1809–1894), the legendary physician, poet and polymath, suggested the term *anesthesia* in a now famous letter (although sadly, lost to historical archivists) after the public demonstration of ether in 1846. Holmes is said to have derived the term from Greek where "an" means "without," and "aesthesis" means "sensation."

2. **What were the earliest anesthetics?**
   Efforts to prevent pain associated with surgery likely date back to the earliest efforts at performing surgical procedures. Sumerians isolated opium from poppy as early as 4000 BCE, Chinese physicians in the Shang Dynasty used acupuncture to relieve surgical pain as early as 1600 BCE, and India's Sushruta used cannabis vapors to sedate surgical patients as early as 600 BCE. However, alcohol, virtually ubiquitous in all ancient cultures in one form or another, was probably the most universally used anesthetic and dates back well before recorded history.

3. **When and by whom was inhalation anesthesia discovered?**
   Interestingly, this simple question is without a simple answer. Nitrous oxide (N_2O) was first synthesized in 1772 by Joseph Priestly (1733–1804), and its analgesic qualities were first described in 1800 by Humphry Davy (1778–1829) in *Researches, Chemical and Philosophical*, where he coined the phrase "laughing gas." But the first use of nitrous oxide as an anesthetic is usually attributed to dentist Horace Wells (1815–1848), who experimented with nitrous oxide as early as December 1844, to diminish the pain of dental extraction. Unfortunately, his attempt to publicly demonstrate the effectiveness of nitrous oxide anesthesia in dental procedures in January 1845 at Harvard Medical School met with limited success, and thus won him few converts.

   With its ability to render full unconsciousness and insensibility, most historians recognize the introduction of ether as the true birth of anesthesia, but when and by whom this discovery was made remains controversial. Crawford Long (1815–1878), a physician working in Jefferson, Georgia, successfully used ether anesthesia to remove a tumor from the neck of a patient on March 30, 1842 (now known as *Doctor's Day*). Despite using ether anesthesia in a number of subsequent cases, Long did not publish his findings until 1849 in the *Southern Medical and Surgical Journal*. Meanwhile, William T. G. Morton (1819–1868), a dentist from Massachusetts, successfully demonstrated the use of ether anesthesia in a well-attended and publicized exhibition at Harvard Medical School in the Bullfinch Auditorium (since renamed the *Ether Dome*) on October 16, 1846 (now known as *Ether Day*). This momentous occasion was captured in *The First Operation under Ether* by Robert C. Hinckley (1853–1941), one of the most recognized paintings in all of medical history.

   In addition to Wells, Long and Morton, a well-known and accomplished scientist and physician, Charles T. Jackson (1805–1880), competed for public recognition as the discoverer of anesthesia. Although Jackson certainly played a role in training Morton (as did Wells), his claim was disputed by his three rivals.

   At present, history does not recognize any single person as the uncontested discoverer of anesthesia.

4. **When did the modern anesthetic vaporizer come about?**
   The means of administering volatile anesthetics date back to their first public demonstration, when Morton used his personally designed "Morton Inhaler," essentially a hollow glass sphere with a mouthpiece and a second opening to entrain fresh air, to administer ether. From that beginning, both ether and chloroform would see various means of administration, from the very simple rags and cloth-cones, to devices, such as the "Chisolm Inhaler," a small dual-piped nasal apparatus designed by a Confederate surgeon during the Civil war to preserve the South's limited supply of chloroform. But modern vaporizers, with a more precise means of delivering volatile agents, were first recognized in the 1930s and beyond, with the decline of ether and the introduction of more modern anesthetics, such as cyclopropane, trichloroethylene, and halothane.

5. **When were intravenous anesthetics developed?**
   In 1656 in a room in Wadham College, Oxford, Sir Christopher Wren (1632–1723), Professor of Astronomy and later architect of St Paul's Cathedral in London, used an animal bladder and a goose quill to inject a mix of opium and wine into a dog and produced sleep. Similar experiments were performed over the following decade but for reasons that remain obscure, the leap to human intravenous anesthesia was not made. Two centuries later in the 1850s, a decade after the introduction of ether, Nikolai Pirogov (1810–1881), who was professor of surgery at the Military Medico-Surgical Academy in St. Petersburg, postulated that, to be effective, ether must gain access to the blood

and thence the nervous system and therefore inhalation might be only one of possible routes for administration. In experiments on dogs, he introduced ether into veins and arteries but, as he found this to be invariably fatal, he abandoned this approach.

6. Why were intravenous anesthetics developed?

The early 1900s saw a renewed interest in intravenous anesthesia, in part to address the problem of surgery to the head and face, where surgeon and anesthetist were sharing the same space. Hedonal, a derivative of urethane, and intravenous ether were first used clinically in Germany and the United Kingdom. The latter, administered as a 5% solution, resulted in a smoother induction than inhaled ether, and was noted to produce less nausea and pulmonary irritation upon awakening. The next major breakthrough was the introduction of barbiturates. Thiopental was first used in 1934 by Ralph Waters (1883–1979) at the University of Wisconsin-Madison, and by John S. Lundy (1894–1973) and Ralph M. Tovell (1901–1967) at the Mayo Clinic. Thiopental received some negative and, in retrospect, undeserved publicity when a civilian surgeon treating casualties at Pearl Harbor claimed that the drug killed in greater numbers than did the Japanese. Despite this, thiopental remained one of the most important drugs in the anesthetist's armamentarium until the introduction of propofol in the late 1980s. Propofol with its smooth induction and recovery characteristics, in addition to a relatively short half-life, seemed tailor-made for continuous intravenous anesthesia, especially in conjunction with the newer short-acting opiates, sufentanil and remifentanil. These characteristics, combined with syringe drivers controlled by pharmacokinetic computer models, have led to the development of target-controlled anesthesia, which is widely used outside of the United States.

7. Who were the key players in the development of local anesthesia?

In 1853 Alexander Wood (1817–1884), a Scottish physician, and Charles G. Pravaz (1791–1853), a French physician, developed an early form of the hypodermic needle. This hollow needle which, when attached to a syringe, allowed the injection of hypodermic morphine for the relief of pain near the site of injection. Of note, Dr. Wood's wife died of an overdose of morphine using one of her husband's syringes.

Meanwhile, coca leaves, which had been used by South American natives as a stimulant (and probably as a topical anesthetic as well) for centuries, was brought to Europe and the extracted cocaine was investigated in Germany for possible medical applications. Sigmund Freud (1856–1939) was studying cocaine as a possible treatment for morphine addiction and noticed, as had others, its numbing effect on the tongue. He shared this with his friend Carl Koller (1857–1944) who went on to introduce the use of cocaine as a local anesthetic for eye surgery in 1884.

8. Who were the key players in the development of regional anesthesia?

William Halstead (1852–1922), a New York surgeon, recognized the possibilities for using cocaine to block major nerves and introduced the brachial plexus block, among others. By 1886 Halstead was a cocaine addict, as was Sigmund Freud, and was hospitalized and treated with morphine, which he remained addicted to for the rest of his life. He later became the first Professor and Chief of Surgery at John Hopkins.

Heinrich I. Quincke (1842–1922) introduced lumbar puncture in 1891 as a diagnostic tool and August Bier (1861–1949) performed the first true spinal anesthetic for surgery using cocaine in 1898. After a few experiments with the technique on patients, Bier and his assistant, Dr. Hildebrand, decided to investigate further on each other. Hildebrand successfully accessed Bier's subarachnoid space but could not attach the syringe to the needle and much cerebrospinal fluid was lost; the attempt was abandoned. Bier then successfully performed the block on Hildebrand, assessing the adequacy of the block by applying heavy blows to the shins, burning cigars to the skin, plucking pubic hairs, and inserting needles to the femur. They celebrated their success with wine and cigars. In the morning Hildebrand had very painful shins and Bier suffered a spinal headache for 9 days.

9. What is meant by the term "balanced anesthesia"?

After the introduction of the inhaled drugs ether and chloroform in the mid-19th century, most anesthetics involved the administration of a single active drug; polypharmacy was widely regarded as a bad thing. There were exceptions, such as the combination of alcohol, chloroform, and ether (A.C.E.) by George Harley (1829–1896) in the 1880s and the introduction of the nitrous oxide and ether combination by Joseph Clover (1825–1882) in 1876. By the end of the 19th century, the technology existed to allow the delivery of nitrous oxide (gas), oxygen, and ether (i.e., GOE) in combination. This GOE combination became the mainstay of anesthesia for much of the first half of the 20th century, with ether later being substituted by halothane and other volatile anesthetics.

Morphine, administered subcutaneously after induction, was introduced as an adjunct to inhalational anesthesia in the 1860s, and in 1869 Claude Bernard (1813–1878) investigated the use of morphine as a premedication, finding that this resulted in a smoother induction and the need for less chloroform. He termed this technique *mixed anesthesia*.

George W. Crile (1864–1943), an American Surgeon, in his theory of anoci-association suggested the use of local anesthesia to block the afferent signals from the surgical site in combination with general anesthesia. He claimed that this would decrease the depth of general anesthesia required and therefore lessen any untoward effects.

John S. Lundy (1894–1973), an American anesthesiologist, in 1926 went on to further develop this concept, comparing anesthesia with a balanced meal: "It is proposed that anesthesia in this case be produced by the combination effects of a moderate amount of preliminary hypnotic, a moderate amount of local anesthetic, a moderate amount of nitrous oxide or ethylene, and an amount of ether sufficient to obtain the desired result. It is assumed that this person will have very little untoward effect from any one of the anesthetics here used, but that when combined they will usually produce satisfactory anesthesia."

G. Jackson Rees (1918–2001) and T. Cecil Gray (1913–2008) of Liverpool, United Kingdom in the 1950s proposed the concept of the triad of anesthesia consisting of narcosis, analgesia (or reflex suppression) and relaxation. They suggested targeting these separate components with different drugs, thereby avoiding deep and dangerous levels of general anesthesia.

10. **When were muscle relaxants introduced?**
Muscle relaxation had traditionally been effected by the use of deep inhalational and/or regional anesthesia. This changed in 1942 when Harold Griffith (1896–1985) of Montreal first used curare as a component of anesthetic for appendectomy. Curare has its origins as an arrow poison used by South American Indians and was known in Europe since the 17th century. Experiments in the early 19th century demonstrated that it was possible to keep an animal, poisoned with curare, alive by artificial respiration. In 1857 Claude Bernard (1813–1878) demonstrated that the poison acted at the neuromuscular junction. Early clinical uses were as a relaxant in the treatment of tetanus and, in the late 1930s, in metrazol-induced convulsive therapy, the forerunner of electroconvulsive therapy. After the introduction of curare into anesthetic practice, it was primarily used in North America with the intention of enhancing the muscle relaxation produced by the anesthetic to facilitate surgery. Respiratory suppression was regarded as a side effect to be managed and the technique was heavily criticized. In the United Kingdom, the situation was different. In Liverpool, Cecil Gray and John Halton (1903–1968) developed the Liverpool technique, where larger doses of curare were used to intentionally paralyze, while using positive pressure ventilation, an intravenous induction with thiopental, and a nitrous oxide oxygen mixture for maintenance of anesthesia. Gray and Halton concluded in their 1946 paper with a "grave and insistent warning to the inexperienced that we are dealing with one of the most potent poisons known."

11. **What is the modern scope of practice for anesthesiology?**
The scope of practice for anesthesiology is broad and includes perioperative care (before, during, and after surgery), acute and chronic pain management, hospice and palliative care, critical care, obstetrics, cardiothoracic surgery, echocardiography, pediatrics, and sleep medicine. Although the general practice of anesthesia may touch on a variety of these fields, most require advanced subspecialty training (i.e., fellowship) to practice within that subspecialty.

12. **How does the scope of practice for anesthesiology vary around the world?**
The practice of anesthesiology varies considerably around the world. In most countries outside of the United States, critical care medicine is often integrated within anesthesia training. The scope of anesthesiology in these jurisdictions not only extends outside of the operating room into the intensive care unit but may also extend outside of the hospital. For example, in several European countries (e.g., France, Germany, Belgium), the allowing advanced on-scene treatment, such as the initiation of extracorporeal membrane oxygenation for cardiac arrest.

13. **What is the role of resuscitation in the practice of anesthesiology?**
Resuscitation is fundamental to the practice of anesthesiology so much so that the title "anesthesiology" in many countries is arguably better termed *reanimation* to describe the management, mechanical ventilation, cardiopulmonary bypass, echocardiography, arterial resuscitating "shock physiology" whether iatrogenic (e.g., general anesthesia or high spinal) or from acute illness (e.g., hemorrhagic or cardiogenic shock).

In the United States, the role of resuscitation and anesthesiology is best exemplified by the anesthesiologist, Peter Safar (1924–2003), who is credited as the "father of cardiopulmonary resuscitation (CPR)" and created the first intensive care unit and the first critical care medicine training program in the United States. Dr. Safar was a 3-time nominee for the Nobel Prize in medicine and founding chair for the Department of Anesthesiology and Critical Care Medicine at the University of Pittsburgh.

14. **Define general anesthesia and the different levels of sedation.**
See Table 1.1.

15. **What is the difference between monitored anesthesia care (MAC) and moderate sedation?**
Moderate or conscious sedation (see Table 1.1) describes the depth of anesthesia which may be delivered by the physician who is also performing a therapeutic or diagnostic procedure. In contrast, MAC is when an anesthesiologist or anesthesia provider participates in the procedure, which may range from no sedation and simply cardiopulmonary support to deep sedation or general anesthesia, depending upon what is necessary for patient safety and comfort. An important distinguishing aspect of MAC is that the clinician must have the ability to convert to general anesthesia, deliver acute clinical interventions to treat physiologic derangements to sustain life, and to provide patient comfort and safety during the procedure.

16. **Is general anesthesia the same as physiologic sleep?**
Anesthesiologists and anesthesia providers often explain to patients that they are "going to sleep" as a gentle way to describe induction and maintenance of general anesthesia. However, this could not be further from the truth. Physiologic sleep is an arousable state characterized by cycling between rapid eye movement (REM) and non-REM stages, each with distinct electroencephalogram (EEG) patterns. General anesthesia, however, is more accurately characterized as a medically induced coma; it is an unarousable state with coma-like EEG findings (high amplitude, low frequency signals). Moreover, general anesthesia functionally approximates brain death because it results in

Table 1.1 Continuum of Depth of Sedation: Definition of General Anesthesia and Levels of Sedation/Analgesia

	MINIMAL SEDATION ANXIOLYSIS	MODERATE SEDATION/ ANALGESIA ("CONSCIOUS SEDATION")	DEEP SEDATION/ ANALGESIA	GENERAL ANESTHESIA
Responsiveness	Normal response to verbal stimulation	Purposeful[a] response to verbal or tactile stimulation	Purposeful[a] response following repeated or painful stimulation	Unarousable even with painful stimulus
Airway	Unaffected	No intervention required	Intervention may be required	Intervention often required
Spontaneous ventilation	Unaffected	Adequate	May be inadequate	Frequently inadequate
Cardiovascular function	Unaffected	Usually maintained	Usually maintained	May be impaired

[a]Reflex withdrawal from a painful stimulus is not considered a purposeful response.
Adopted from the ASA Continuum of Depth of Sedation: Definition of General Anesthesia and Levels of Sedation/Analgesia. Committee of Origin: Quality Management and Departmental Administration. (Approved by the ASA House of Delegates on October 13, 1999, and last amended on October 15, 2014).

the following: unresponsiveness to nociceptive stimuli; absence of corneal, gag, and oculocephalic reflexes; absence of spontaneous ventilation; hemodynamic instability; loss of thermoregulatory reflexes; and, at large enough doses, an isoelectric EEG. Furthermore, emergence from general anesthesia approximates caudal to rostral progression of brain stem recovery: (1) spontaneous respiratory ventilation and hemodynamic stability indicate activation of the cardiopulmonary centers in the medulla; (2) return of gag and corneal reflex, swallowing, and grimacing indicate return of cranial nerves; and (3) ability to follow commands indicates return of cortical function. In summary, although "general anesthesia" is frequently associated with "sleep" it is more accurate to describe this state as a medically induced coma that clinically resembles brain death.

17. What is the classical triad of anesthesia?
    The classical triad of anesthesia includes hypnosis/amnesia, analgesia, and muscle relaxation. Although this can be realized with a single anesthetic agent (e.g., ether), it often requires dangerously high doses to be effective. As a result, the concept of "balanced anesthesia" developed, whereby each component of the triad could be realized by balancing various agents to improve safety and limit harm. In practice, this is often accomplished by using inhaled or intravenous anesthetics for hypnosis and amnesia, opioids for analgesia, and neuromuscular blocking agents for muscle relaxation.

18. What is the perioperative surgical home?
    The American Society of Anesthesiology (ASA) defines the perioperative surgical home (PSH) as "a patient-centric, team-based model of care that emphasizes value, patient satisfaction, and reduced cost." The goal is to deliver coordinated, interdisciplinary care that spans the entire perioperative period. This often involves a preanesthesia care clinic whereby patients are seen weeks or months in advance for preparation and medical optimization (often termed *prehabilitation*). The PSH also extends into the postoperative domain, such as the intensive care unit or the surgical floor. The PSH involves coordinating care with multiple specialties, including nursing, pharmacy, nutrition, physical therapy, hospitalist medicine, intensivists, and surgeons throughout various phases of care to facilitate high-quality, high-value, evidence-based care.

    It is important to appreciate the critical role anesthesiologists play in the PSH. For example, a medically complex patient with chronic pain undergoing a major surgical operation could be seen in the preoperative anesthesia clinic to coordinate care with several anesthesiologists within the same department, such as a general anesthesiologist, a pain physician, and a critical care anesthesiologist. In the immediate perioperative period, the general anesthesiologist would care for the patient during surgery. They would then transfer care to a critical care anesthesiologist in the intensive care unit. Thereafter, the pain physician could help manage postoperative acute on chronic pain.

Although implementation of the PSH will vary by setting, the role of the anesthesiologist is to coordinate interdisciplinary care, minimize disruption, and facilitate delivery of high-quality, evidence-based care, all with an eye on maximizing value.

19. **What is enhanced recovery after surgery?**
Enhanced recovery after surgery (ERAS) are evidence-based protocols that establish pathways for specific surgical operations to optimize outcomes and minimize cost. ERAS protocols were originally implemented for patients undergoing colorectal operations, demonstrating favorable outcomes and reducing costs. ERAS protocols are implemented throughout all phases of care, including preoperatively and postoperatively. These protocols involve several aspects of care ranging from optimizing the patient's nutritional status just before surgery (e.g., oral carbohydrate drinks up to 2 hours before surgery) to antibiotic selection and fluid management intraoperatively. Postoperatively, they include guidelines for evidence-based practice regarding glucose control, early ambulation, early enteral nutrition, early removal of central lines and urinary catheters, and early extubation.

20. **What is the difference between the PSH and ERAS?**
ERAS protocols are often operation or surgery specific, whereas the PSH is more patient specific. The PSH focuses on the patient, their medical history, and optimizing care between different care teams as patients transition from the pre-, intra-, and postoperative domain. The PSH often incorporates ERAS protocols; however, its focus is more on interdisciplinary coordination of care throughout the patient's entire surgical experience. The main benefit of ERAS protocols and the PSH are to improve outcomes and reduce costs.

21. **Define value-driven care.**
To ensure the economic sustainability of health care, it is vital to embrace value driven care defined as the following:

$$Value = \frac{Quality\ of\ Care}{Costs\ of\ Care}$$

It is important to appreciate that "quality" in healthcare ranges broadly, from improving outcomes (e.g., decreased surgical site infections) to improving the patient's experience and respecting their goals of care. For example, a patient with a terminal illness may define quality of care as pain control, life with dignity, and dying at home rather than the prolongation of life by an extra few weeks or months in the intensive care unit.
Both ERAS and the PSH embrace the concept of value driven care by improving outcomes and reducing costs.

22. **What are some of the seminal articles published in the history of anesthesiology?**
Anesthesiology and its techniques have been at the center of some of the most important advances ever produced in the field of medicine. Listed subsequently, are a few of the seminal articles published in our proud specialty:
- Bigelow HJ. Insensibility during surgical operations produced by inhalation. Boston Med Surg J 1846;35:309–317. Discussing the discovery and application of anesthesia, this article is widely regarded as the most important ever published in the New England Journal of Medicine.
- Koller C. On the use of cocaine for producing anaesthesia on the eye. Lancet 1884;124:990–992. Discussing the anesthetic properties of cocaine, this article describes using the compound as a local anesthetic for surgery, thus obviating the need for general anesthesia and its attendant risks in certain circumstances.
- Cushing H. On routine determinations of arterial tension in operating room and clinic. Boston Med Surg J 1903;148:250–256. Dr. Harvey Cushing, then a fourth year medical student, after developing the first anesthesia record featuring heart rate and respirations, added blood pressure determination using the Riva-Rocci mercury-sphygmomanometer, thus quantifying systolic blood pressure for the first time.
- Simpson JY. Notes on the use of the inhalation of sulphuric ether in the practice of midwifery. Monthly J Med Sci 1847;7:721–728. Discusses the first use of anesthesia for the attenuation of labor pain in a parturient with cephalopelvic disproportion. Notably, this was controversial at the time because of religious concerns about God's admonition to women that pain was to be a natural and expected part of childbirth (Genesis 3:16).
- Anand KJ, Hickey PR. Pain and its effects in the human neonate and fetus. N Engl J Med 1987;317:1321–1329. This review changed the perioperative care of the neonate more than any other scientific contribution, resulting in the idea that humane considerations should apply as forcefully to the care of neonates and young infants as they do to children and adults in similar painful situations.
- Griffith HR, Johnson GE. The use of Curare in general anesthesia. Anesthesiology 1942;3:418–420. This article details the first use of Curare for the supplementation of general anesthesia. Of note, this was done without institutional research approval or personal clinical experience with the drug.
- Severinghaus JW, Bradley AF. Electrodes for blood PO_2 and PCO_2 determination. J Appl Physiol 1958;13:515–520. Describes the first modern blood gas analysis apparatus.
- Safar P, Brown TC, Holtey WJ, et al. Ventilation and circulation with closed-chest cardiac massage in man. JAMA 1961;176:57457-6. Describes the importance of ventilation in addition to chest compressions, thus laying the foundation for modern CPR: A (airway), B (breathing), C (circulation).

KEY POINTS: INTRODUCTION OF ANESTHESIA

1. The term *anesthesia* is derived from Greek where "an" means "without," and "aesthesis" means "sensation."
2. William T. G. Morton was an American dentist who first publicly demonstrated the use of inhaled ether as a surgical anesthetic at Harvard Medical School in an operating amphitheater, now known as the *Ether Dome*, on October 16, 1846.
3. Thiopental, introduced in 1934, was one of the most widely used intravenous induction agents until the advent of propofol in the late 1980s.
4. Cocaine was the first local anesthetic used in clinical practice.
5. Dr. Quincke introduced lumbar puncture in 1891 and Dr. Bier performed the first spinal anesthetic for surgery using cocaine in 1898.
6. An important distinguishing aspect of MAC compared with "conscious sedation" is that the clinician must have the ability to convert to general anesthesia, deliver acute clinical interventions to treat physiologic derangements to sustain life, and to provide patient comfort and safety during the procedure.
7. MAC defines the availability of a particular skillset not the level of sedation.
8. Emergence from general anesthesia approximates caudal to rostral progression of brain stem recovery in the following order: (1) recovery of cardiopulmonary centers in the medulla, (2) recovery of cranial nerves (swallowing, gag reflex, etc.), (3) recovery of cortical function (i.e., ability to follow commands).
9. The classical triad of anesthesia includes hypnosis/amnesia, analgesia, and muscle relaxation.
10. Balanced anesthesia uses a separate agent for each arm of the classic triad of anesthesia to minimize the side effect or risks of each agent. This is often accomplished by using an inhaled or intravenous anesthetic for hypnosis/amnesia, opioids for analgesia, and neuromuscular blocking agents for muscle relaxation.
11. The PSH and ERAS are methods to deliver interdisciplinary, patient-centric care using evidence-based medicine that optimizes outcomes, increases patient satisfaction, and minimizes costs to deliver value drive care.
12. Value driven care is defined as the ratio of "quality of care"/"costs of care."
13. Anesthesiologists have significantly contributed to the science and practice of medicine in numerous ways by developing anesthetic techniques that allow surgery to be performed that would otherwise not be possible, development of the first arterial blood gas machine, development of advanced airway management techniques, including endotracheal intubation, and the development of positive pressure mechanical ventilation, critical care medicine, and modern CPR: Airway, Breathing, Circulation.

SUGGESTED READINGS

Barasch P, Bieterman K, Hersey D. Game changers: the 20 most important anesthesia articles ever published. Anesth Analg. 2015;120 (3):663–770.

Brown EN, Lydic R, Schiff ND. General anesthesia, sleep, and coma. N Engl J Med. 2010;363(27):2638–2650.

Davy H. Researches, Chemical and Philosophical; Chiefly Concerning Nitrous Oxide or dephilogisticated Nitrous Air, and Its Respiration. Bristol: Biggs and Cottle; 1800.

History of Anesthesia Timeline. Available at https://www.woodlibrarymuseum.org/history-of-anesthesia/#4000bce

Porter ME. What is value in health care? N Engl J Med. 2010;363(26):2477–2481.

Preistly J. Experiments and Observations on Different Kinds of Air; 1776.

Whalen FX. Inhaled anesthetics: an historical overview. Best Pract Res Clin Anaesthesiol. 2005;19(3):323–330.

Zuck D. The development of the anaesthetic vaporizer. Anaesthesia. 1988;43(9):773–775.

CHAPTER 2

PRE-OPERATIVE EVALUATION

William B. Somerset, DO, Thomas Gulvezan, MD, MBA

QUESTION/ANSWERS

1. **What are the goals of the preoperative evaluation?**
   The preoperative evaluation consists of gathering necessary information about the patient and formulating an appropriate anesthetic plan. The overall objective is to make sure the patient is medically optimized when time permits to limit perioperative risks.

2. **Discuss what needs to happen before commencing anesthetic care?**
   Before the delivery of anesthetic care, the following should occur:
   - Review of medical record and determination of American Society of Anesthesiologists (ASA) status
   - Physical examination, which at a minimum includes an evaluation of the airway, heart, and lungs
   - Discuss medical conditions, allergies, previous anesthetics, family history of problems with anesthesia, and nothing by mouth (NPO) status
   - Review available pertinent medical records and order additional tests and consults if necessary

3. **Why is it important to ask about previous anesthetic complications?**
   A patient's previous anesthetic experience may provide valuable information, which could change anesthetic management. For example, patients who have had a family history of malignant hyperthermia or fevers under anesthesia should receive a nontriggering anesthetic (see Chapter 45 for more information). Patients with history of postoperative nausea and vomiting (PONV) may benefit from preoperative medications, regional anesthesia and/or a total intravenous anesthetic technique. Also, patients with known difficult airways are often informed of this after receiving prior anesthetics and may recall the need to tell future clinicians when prompted.

4. **What are the features of informed consent?**
   The person giving consent must have the capacity to make an informed decision. The patient must be informed on the risks, benefits and options, in language they clearly understand. Translators should be offered and all attempts to respect cultural differences should be made. Lastly, the patient must be allowed to make a voluntary decision without coercion.

5. **How does one manage a patient with a DNR order presenting for surgery?**
   Patients with do not resuscitate (DNR) orders require a discussion before surgery, including which interventions and resuscitation options may be used during surgery. Because the administration of anesthesia involves interventions potentially viewed as resuscitative efforts (e.g., endotracheal intubation, blood product administration, vasopressor administration), it is imperative to clarify what interventions are available to the clinician. Many times DNR resuscitative orders are placed on temporary hold during the perioperative period; however patients should not be forced to rescind these orders. This is best accomplished with a discussion involving the patient, family members, and/or legal representatives.

6. **Discuss the physical status classification of the American Society of Anesthesiologists.**
   The ASA classification system is a 1 to 6 grading system quantitating a patient's physical status immediately before a procedure. It is does not predict operative risk.
   - Class 1: A normal healthy patient (e.g., a healthy, nonsmoker)
   - Class 2: A patient with mild systemic disease (e.g., controlled hypertension, smoker, obesity, etc.)
   - Class 3: A patient with severe systemic disease (e.g., compensated congested heart failure [CHF], chronic obstructive pulmonary disease [COPD], morbid obesity)
   - Class 4: A patient with severe systemic disease that is a constant threat to life (e.g., uncompensated CHF or COPD)
   - Class 5: A moribund patient who is not expected to survive without the operation (e.g., severe head injury, massive trauma)
   - Class 6: A declared brain-dead patient whose organs are being removed for donor purposes
     The addition of "E" denotes an Emergency surgery. An emergency is defined as existing when any delay in treatment would significantly increase the threat of death and/or loss of body part.

7. **What are clinical risk calculators?**
   Clinical calculators attempt to quantify perioperative risk by entering patient and surgery specific information. Two commonly used risk calculators are the RCRI and the American College of Surgeons NSQIP risk prediction calculators.

The RCRI calculator is a series of Yes/No questions which include the following: (1) high-risk surgery, (2) history of ischemic heart disease, (3) history of CHF, (4) history of cerebrovascular disease, (5) preoperative treatment with insulin, (6) preoperative creatinine greater than 2 mg/dL. Answering "Yes" to any questions 1 to 6 increases the risk of a major cardiac event during surgery.

The NSQIP risk model identifies five underlying factors as predictors of perioperative myocardial infarction or cardiac arrest, including: (1) type of surgery, (2) dependent functional status, (3) abnormal creatinine, (4) ASA functional status, and (5) increased age. A calculator was developed for this model which includes approximately 20 questions and produces a composite risk score.

8. **What are the preoperative fasting (NPO) guidelines for healthy patients undergoing elective procedures?**
   - Clear liquids—2 hours
   - Breast milk—4 hours
   - Infant formula, nonhuman milk, nonclear liquids—6 hours
   - Light meal—6 hours
   - Full meal, fried or fat-rich foods—6 to 8 hours

9. **Are NPO guidelines always be followed?**
   Emergency cases should proceed regardless of NPO status. For urgent cases, a discussion regarding the risk of waiting versus the risk of proceeding to surgery with a full stomach should occur. For nonemergent, nonurgent elective cases, it is considered best practice to honor the current NPO guidelines.

10. **What is ERAS?**
    ERAS stands for enhanced recovery after surgery. It is a protocol-driven multimodal perioperative treatment plan designed to achieve early recovery after surgical procedures. Key components of ERAS protocols include preoperative counselling, optimization of nutrition, standardized analgesic and anesthetic regimens, minimization of opioids, and early mobilization.

11. **How is ERAS changing traditional NPO guidelines?**
    ERAS' focus on preoperative optimization of nutrition is causing anesthesiologists to reexamine the practice of prolonged NPO time periods before surgery. Although no clear guidelines have been presented, many institutions are liberalizing the time during which patients may have clear liquids in the preoperative setting. Some even encourage the use of carbohydrate drinks preoperatively to enhance recovery.

12. **What is the perioperative surgical home (PSH)?**
    The PSH model of care is an integrated interdisciplinary team approach to perioperative care. The goal is to deliver more efficient care, and to decrease resource utilization and complications, thus resulting in better outcomes.

13. **What routine preoperative tests which should be done before surgery?**
    Routine laboratory testing of asymptomatic patients is not recommended. Selective laboratory tests should be obtained to guide decision making in perioperative period based on a patients' history, physical examination, and planned procedure.

14. **Should one obtain a baseline hemoglobin? Coagulation studies? Electrolytes?**
    - Blood typing/crossing should be done in patients where there is a reasonable likelihood of needing a transfusion. This can be secondary to preexisting anemia or a procedure with high expected blood loss.
    - Routine hemoglobin testing is not indicated. Considerations for testing should include the invasiveness of procedure, coexisting diseases, extremes of age, dyspnea, history of anemia or bleeding, and medication history.
    - Coagulation studies should be considered for patients with history of a bleeding diathesis, liver or kidney dysfunction, or in those who are on anticoagulant medications.
    - Routine serum chemistry testing is not indicated unless the patient's history (e.g., kidney disease/diuretic use) would increase the likelihood of an abnormal test value. Also it may be considered in high-risk patients to better quantify preoperative risk as serum creatinine is sometimes used in risk calculators.

15. **Should a pregnancy test be performed before all procedures?**
    All female patients of reproductive age should at least be offered a pregnancy test before receiving an anesthetic. Many institutions have policies in place to test all females of reproductive age. In general, elective procedures are deferred until after delivery. The second trimester is regarded as the safest time for procedures because organogenesis has occurred and the risk of spontaneous abortion or preterm labor is lower.

    Note that pregnant women should never be denied indicated procedures regardless of trimester and none of the commonly used anesthetic agents have been definitively shown to be teratogenic. If the decision to operate on a woman with a viable aged fetus (usually 24 weeks) is made, then plans for expedient delivery and/or cesarean section, along with subsequent care of the infant and mother, must be in place.

16. **At what age should patients have an electrocardiogram?**
    The 2014 ACC/AHA guideline gives a IIa recommendation that preoperative resting 12-lead electrocardiogram is reasonable for patients with known coronary artery disease, significant arrhythmia, peripheral arterial disease,

cerebrovascular disease, or other significant structural heart disease. This recommendation is excepted for those undergoing low-risk surgery.

In general, if a patient is having an invasive procedure, where large amounts of blood loss are expected, where postoperative organ dysfunction may occur, and having baseline laboratory tests would be helpful, or if the formal quantification of preoperative risk is desired (see later), then preoperative laboratory tests are reasonable. The routine ordering of tests on all patients regardless of clinical status is not appropriate.

17. **What is a MET? Why is it important?**
MET is an abbreviation for metabolic equivalent, with one MET approximating the amount of oxygen consumed in resting basal state (about 3.5 mL/kg/min). The 2014 ACC/AHA guidelines, on preoperative cardiac testing, recommend no further testing for patients who can perform more than 4 METS (e.g., climb two flights of stairs, walk four blocks). In general, patients who can perform more than 4 METS have a low risk for postoperative complications, whereas patients with less functional capacity have a higher risk for postoperative complications.

18. **Describe the recommended approach to the perioperative cardiac evaluation of patients scheduled for noncardiac surgery.**
The 2014 ACC/AHA guideline presents an algorithmic approach to perioperative cardiac evaluation in patients undergoing noncardiac surgery. It requires an assessment of a patient's cardiac risks before surgery, taking into account the urgency of surgery, the presence of active cardiac conditions, the invasiveness of the planned surgery, the patient's functional status, and the presence of clinical risk factors for ischemic heart disease. Taken together, this algorithm underscores the importance of a history focused on cardiac issues for all surgical patients.

19. **What are the named clinical risk factors in the 2014 ACC/AHA guideline on Perioperative Cardiovascular Evaluation and Management of Patients Undergoing Noncardiac Surgery?**
   - Coronary artery disease
   - Cerebrovascular disease
   - Heart failure
   - Cardiomyopathy
   - Valvular heart disease
   - Arrhythmias and conduction disorders
   - Pulmonary vascular disease
   - Adult congenital heart disease

20. **Summarize the 2016 AHA/ACC guidelines for patients presenting for surgery after cardiac stent placement.**
Patients who are status post (s/p) cardiac stent placement are frequently on oral antithrombotic agents to prevent stent thrombosis and subsequent major adverse cardiovascular events (MACE). Of note, the risk of MACE is heightened in the perioperative period, thus making the cessation of antithrombotic agents risky. When a patient with recent stent placement presents for surgery, it is important to know what type of stent was placed, as well as the timing of the intervention. The common cardiac interventions include balloon angioplasty, coronary stenting with either a BMS or DES, and/or coronary artery bypass grafting surgery. The summary of these guidelines are as follows:
   - Elective noncardiac surgery should be delayed 30 days after BMS implantation and optimally 6 months after DES implantation.
   - For patients treated with dual antiplatelet therapy (DAPT) after coronary stent implantation, undergoing a surgical procedure that mandates the discontinuation of P2Y12 inhibitor therapy, it is recommended that aspirin be continued if possible and the P2Y12 platelet receptor inhibitor be restarted as soon as possible after surgery.
   - When noncardiac surgery is required in patients currently taking a P2Y12 inhibitor, a consensus decision among treating clinicians regarding the relative risks of surgery and continuation/discontinuation of antiplatelet therapy is advised.
   - Elective noncardiac surgery may be considered 3 months after DES implantation in patients in whom P2Y12 inhibitor therapy will need to be discontinued, if the risk of further delay of surgery is greater than the expected risks of stent thrombosis.
   - Elective noncardiac surgery should not be performed within 30 days of BMS implantation or within 3 months of DES implantation if it requires the discontinuation of DAPT.
   - Patients with DES for more than 6 months may stop DAPT and proceed with surgery.

21. **What are the preoperative considerations for patients with pacemakers and/or AICDs?**
A patient with a pacemaker (PM) and/or implantable cardioverter-defibrillator (ICD) requires preoperative consultation involving cardiology, the institutional ICD team, or the manufacturer, in addition to the anesthesiologist and surgeon. Important details of the assessment include type of device, manufacturer, model number, settings, current function, and response to magnet placement over the device.

If the patient is pacer dependent and electromagnetic interference is anticipated (e.g., electrosurgery unit), the PM or combination PM/ICD should be reprogrammed to an asynchronous mode to avoid the possibility of bradycardia and/or asystole. ICDs should have antitachycardia therapy suspended before EMI exposure.

Magnets can be applied over the PM or ICD to temporarily reprogram the device, and the clinician should confirm a specific device's response to magnet placement before surgery. When a magnet is applied, most PMs will reprogram to an ansyncronous pacing mode, and most ICDs will deactivate antitachycardia therapy.

22. **Why is it important to inquire about preoperative steroid use?**
Patients on chronic steroid therapy are at risk for adrenal insufficiency, which can present as unexplained hypotension in the perioperative period. These patients may need to be treated with stress dose steroids. In general, patients on steroids for less than 3 weeks or receiving an AM dose of 5 mg prednisone (or equivalence) daily do not need supplemental therapy.

23. **How are beta blockers managed in high-risk patients perioperatively?**
Beta blockers should be continued in patients undergoing surgery who are currently taking them. Initiating beta blockers perioperatively in patients who are at high risk for myocardial ischemia or who have multiple cardiac risk factors is occasionally done as well.

24. **What is the concern for patients on an ACEi and ARBs?**
Patients on ACEi and ARBs are prone to experiencing intraoperative hypotension. For this reason, many institutions will instruct patients to refrain from taking these drugs on the day of surgery. However, it is noteworthy that these medications have been shown to be beneficial, and definitive guidelines on stopping these drugs is currently lacking. It is important to be aware of the risk of periprocedural hypotension and to be prepared to treat it in patients who have taken these medications.

25. **Discuss the preoperative considerations for patients taking antithrombotic agents.**
Antithrombotic drugs can be divided into two main classes: antiplatelet and anticoagulant. Antiplatelet drugs include cyclooxygenase inhibitors, adenosine diphosphate receptor inhibitors, phosphodiesterase inhibitors, and glycoprotein IIb-IIIa inhibitors. Anticoagulant drugs include antithrombin III activators, heparin-like and direct factor Xa inhibitors, direct thrombin inhibitors, and vitamin K antagonists.

Antithrombotic drugs have varied durations of action depending on their individual half-lives. Generally there are not specific recommendations regarding when to stop each drug before surgery. The American Society of Regional Anesthesia does have guidelines for stopping antithrombotic medications before neuraxial procedures, and these represent a more conservative approach than what is generally needed for surgery. It is important to remember that thrombotic events are a major source of perioperative morbidity and mortality, and that the management of these medications perioperatively is an important decision that should occur after careful consideration of the risks and benefits among all clinicians involved in the patient's care.

Drug	Mechanism	Half-Life	Time to Stop Before Neuraxial Procedure
Aspirin	COX inhibition	20 min	Continue
Clopidogrel	ADP receptor inhibitor	7 hours	5–7 days
Prasugrel	ADP receptor inhibitor	7 hours	7–10 days
Ticlopidine	ADP receptor inhibitor	4 days	10 days
Ticagrelor	ADP receptor inhibitor	8 hours	5–7 days
Cilostazol	PDE inhibitor	12 hours	2 days
Abciximab	GP IIb–IIIa inhibitor	30 min	24–48 hours
Eptifibatide	GP IIb–IIIa inhibitor	2.5 hours	4–8 hours
Tirofiban	GP IIb–IIIa inhibitor	2 hours	4–8 hours
Heparin	IIa >Xa inhibition	1.5 hours	4–12 hours
Low-molecular-weight heparin	Xa >IIa inhibition	4.5 hours	12–24 hours
Fondaparinux	Xa >IIa inhibition	20 hours	
Rivaroxaban	Direct Xa inhibition	9 hours	72 hours
Apixaban	Direct Xa inhibition	12 hours	72 hours
Bivalrudin	IIa inhibitor	25 min	
Hirudin	IIa inhibitor	1.5 hours	
Argatroban	IIa inhibitor	45 min	
Dabigatran	IIa inhibitor	12 hours	5 days
Warfarin	Vitamin K antagonism	2–4 days	5 days

ADP, Adenosine diphosphate; *COX*, cyclooxygenase; *GP*, glycoprotein; *PDE*, phosphodiesterase.

26. **What are the considerations for anticoagulated patients who present for urgent or emergent procedures? What agents are able to be emergently reversed?**
Clinicians occasionally need to reverse a patient's anticoagulant therapy for urgent or emergency procedures. Reversal of anticoagulation should be reserved for anticipated severe life-threatening bleeding, as once a

patient's anticoagulation is reversed, the risk of perioperative thrombotic complications increases.
Three common agents that can be rapidly reversed are:

1) Warfarin is a vitamin K antagonist with a prolonged clinical effect. With warfarin reversal, timing is important. For semi-urgent reversal, warfarin should be held and vitamin K given. Immediate reversal can be facilitated with prothrombin complex concentrates (PCCs) or plasma products (e.g., fresh frozen plasma).
2) Dabigatran functions as an oral direct thrombin inhibitor, and can be reversed with idarucizumab.
3) Rivaroxaban, apixaban, and edoxaban function as oral direct factor Xa inhibitors, and can be reversed with andexanet alfa. PCCs have been used to reverse direct factor Xa inhibitors for life-threatening bleeding, but supporting evidence is lacking.

27. How would perioperative anticoagulant management occur in a high-risk patient on warfarin therapy who presents for an elective procedure, whose surgeon is requesting it reversed using low-molecular-weight heparin (LMWH)?

As an example, warfarin could be stopped 5 days before the procedure and bridging therapy could then commence with LMWH. The patient could be given a therapeutic dose of LMWH starting the first day after warfarin was held. It would then be stopped 24 hours before surgery. On postoperative day 1, warfarin would be resumed and LMWH resumed for 48 to 72 hours. This approach would enable the patient to experience a brief window during which their risk of bleeding is reduced, while minimizing the time that they are at elevated risk for a experiencing a thrombotic event. Note, these types of decisions regarding anticoagulation management usually require multidisciplinary input.

28. How are herbal medications and supplements managed in the perioperative period?

Traditionally, all herbal medications and supplements are held for a week before surgery. Note that these products are not regulated by the US Food and Drug Administration, and exact doses, effects, and drug-interactions are not well known. Some clinically relevant (and commonly tested) side effects of herbal supplements include:

- Increased bleeding seen with ginger, gingko, and garlic, via interference with platelet function
- Induction of P450 system by St. John's wort, potentially increasing metabolism (decreasing efficacy) of a variety of medications

In general, procedures should not be delayed if a patient presents on herbal medications.

29. Discuss the preoperative considerations for chronic pain patients, including the management of those patients taking methadone, buprenorphine, and Suboxone.

Opioid dependent patients, in general, should take their daily maintenance dose of opioids before surgery. Patients with transdermal fentanyl patches should continue wearing these throughout the perioperative period when feasible, with special consideration taken to avoid damaging or applying heat to the patches during the perioperative period. Patients taking methadone or buprenorphine, typically as maintenance therapy for opioid addiction, should take these medications before surgery. Buprenorphine is a partial mu opioid receptor agonist/antagonist at the kappa opioid receptor, thus potentially reducing the efficacy of other opioids. Of note, in addition to instructing patients to continue their buprenorphine, clinicians should maximize the use of nonopioids for analgesia when appropriate. Also perioperative use of opioid antagonists, such as naloxone and naltrexone, can precipitate withdrawal symptoms in opioid dependent patients, and should be avoided in the perioperative period.

For patients taking combination buprenorphine and naloxone (trade name Suboxone) for opioid dependency, there is not a clear perioperative management strategy. Providers should coordinate with the patient's prescribing clinician. For minor procedures, with low levels of postoperative pain, frequently the patient may continue Suboxone and the perioperative team needs to be aware that the patient may have increased analgesic requirements. For procedures with expected high levels of postoperative pain, the Suboxone will often be discontinued preoperatively and resumed after the procedure, so as not to diminish the effects of opioid analgesics during this time period.

30. Discuss the benefits of perioperative smoking cessation.

According to American College of Surgeons, quitting smoking 4 to 6 weeks before an operation, and staying smoke-free 4 weeks after, can decrease the rate of wound complications by up to 50%. The ASA recommends patients abstain from smoking for as long as possible before and after surgery, but even quitting for only a brief period is still beneficial. Of note, there is no data to support the common belief that quitting too close could have negative effects by increasing coughing or airway irritability.

31. What are the risk factors for postoperative pulmonary complications?

COPD, age over 50 years, CHF, current cigarette use, pulmonary hypertension, poor general health status, low preoperative oxygen saturation, emergency surgery, upper abdominal and thoracic surgery, and current respiratory infections.

32. Are there ways to predict postoperative respiratory complications?

A few different risk calculators can be used to quantify pulmonary risk and may be useful for high-risk patients. These include the ARISCAT risk index (from the Assess Risk in Surgical Patients in Catalonia Trial, 2010), the Arozullah respiratory failure index, the Gupta calculator for postoperative respiratory failure, and the Gupta calculator for postoperative pneumonia.

33. **List the goals of premedication.**

Premedications are given before procedure to minimize the likelihood of nausea, pain, hemodynamic instability, anxiety, aspiration and pruritus, and to decrease postoperative narcotic requirements. Commonly used premedications and their doses are listed in Table 2.1.

Factors to consider regarding premedication include:

- Patient age, allergies, and physical status
- Preprocedural levels of anxiety and pain
- History of PONV or motion sickness
- History of alcohol, and/or drug abuse
- Full stomach and risk of aspiration
- Suspected postoperative pain levels

34. **Is it safe to give oral (PO) medications before surgery?**

Yes, but with some notable exceptions. Patients who are at high risk for aspiration (e.g., bowel obstruction) or who are having specific gastrointestinal procedures (e.g., gastric bypass) generally should not receive PO medications before surgery. Apart from these situations, administering oral medications, with minimal water preoperatively, is usually acceptable. Most patients should continue their prescribed medications on the day of surgery, including their pain medications.

Table 2.1 Commonly Used Preoperative Medications

PURPOSE/ CLASS	EXAMPLE MEDICATION	DOSE/NOTES
Anxiolytic	Midazolam	Titrate to effect: Adult IV usually 1–2 mg, Pediatric PO 0.25–0.5 mg/kg (max 20 mg) IV Initial: 0.05–0.1 mg/kg. May have antiemetic effects. Usually avoided in elderly and debilitated patients
Antiemetic	Transdermal scopolamine	0.2 mg transdermal patch. Given slow onset of action ideally applied at least 2 hours before procedure
Analgesic	Gabapentin	300–1200 mg given PO before surgery for analgesic and potential antiemetic affects, when combined with opioids may increase risk of respiratory depression
Analgesic/opioids	Fentanyl	Adult: 25–100 mcg, monitor for respiratory depression
	Morphine	Adult: 2–10 mg, monitor for respiratory depression
Analgesic	Acetaminophen	Available PO and IV, Adult PO dose 325–1000 mg
Analgesic/COX2	Celecoxib	Adult PO 200 mg, may have opioid sparing effects
Analgesic/NSAIDs	Ketorolac	Adult IV 10–30 mg, may be contraindicated in certain surgeries
	Ibuprofen	Adult PO 200–800 mg PO, may be contraindicated in certain surgeries
Gastrointestinal stimulants	Metoclopramide	May be considered in patients at risk for aspiration, not recommended for routine use
H2 receptor antagonist	Famotidine, ranitidine	May be considered in patients at risk for aspiration, not recommended for routine use
Antacids	Sodium citrate, sodium bicarbonate	Only use nonparticulate antacids, may be considered in patients at risk for aspiration, not recommended for routine use
Anticholinergic Antisialagogue	Glycopyrrolate	Glycopyrrolate 0.1–0.2 mg IV, mainly used for drying of airway secretions. For info on anticholinergic medications to prevent bradycardia please see pediatric chapter

COX2, Cyclooxygenase 2; *IV*, intravenous; *PO*, oral; *NSAID*, nonsteroidal antiinflammatory drug.

KEY POINTS

1. The goal of the preoperative evaluation is to gather necessary information, perform a focused physical examination and formulate an appropriate anesthetic plan in an attempt to minimize perioperative risk.
2. Common medical management issues encountered during the preanesthetic evaluation include antihypertensive therapy with angiotensin converting enzyme inhibitor (ACEi)/angiotensin receptor blockers (ARBs), anticoagulant therapy, diabetes, steroid use, chronic pain, and pacemaker/automated implantable cardioverter defibrillators (AICDs).
3. The most current American Heart Association (AHA)/American College of Cardiology (ACC) guidelines (2016) are the gold standard for directing appropriate cardiac testing before noncardiac procedures. In general, for nonemergency low-risk surgery and people with moderate functional capacity do not need additional cardiac evaluation.
4. Clinical risk calculators may be used to quantify perioperative risk. Two commonly used calculators are the revised cardiac risk index (RCRI) and the national surgery quality improvement program (NSQIP).
5. Routine preoperative laboratory testing of asymptomatic patients is not recommended. Selective laboratory tests should be obtained to guide decision making in the perioperative period based on the patients' history, physical examination, and planned procedure.
6. Elective noncardiac surgery should be delayed 30 days after bare metal stent (BMS) implantation and optimally 6 months after drug eluting stent (DES) implantation.

Suggested Readings

2014 ACC/AHA Guideline on Perioperative Cardiovascular Evaluation and Management of Patients Undergoing Noncardiac Surgery. Circulation. 2014;130:e278–e333.

2016 ACC/AHA Guideline. Focused Update on Duration of Dual Antiplatelet Therapy in Patients With Coronary Artery Disease: A Report of the American College of Cardiology/American Heart Association Task Force on Clinical Practice Guidelines.

ASA Practice Advisory for the perioperative management of patients with cardiac implantable electronic devices: pacemakers and implantable cardioverter-defibrillators. Anesthesiology. 2011;114.

Duggan EW, Carlson K, Umpierrez GE, Perioperative hyperglycemia management. Anesthesiology. 2017;126:547–560.

Horlocker TT, Vandermeulen E, Kopp SN, et al. Regional anesthesia in the patient receiving antithrombotic or thrombolytic therapy: American Society of Regional Anesthesia and Pain Medicine Evidence-Based Guidelines. REG Anesth Pain Med. 2018;43(3):263–309.

Practice Advisory for Preanesthesia Evaluation: an updated report by the American Society of Anesthesiologists Task Force on Preanesthesia Evaluation. Anesthesiology. 2012;116(3):522–538.

CHAPTER 3

AIRWAY MANAGEMENT

Joanna Miller, MD, David Shapiro, MD, Andrew Goldberg, MD

1. **Describe the anatomy of the upper and lower airway.**
   The upper airway consists of the nose, mouth, pharynx, larynx, and the lower airway, the tracheobronchial tree. The two openings to the upper airway (nose and mouth) are separated anteriorly by the palate and connected posteriorly by the pharynx. The pharynx connects the nose and mouth to the larynx and esophagus. A cartilaginous structure at the base of the tongue, known as the *epiglottis*, protects the opening of the larynx, known as the *glottis*, against aspiration with swallowing (Fig. 3.1).

   Below the epiglottis lies the larynx, commonly known as the *voice box*. The larynx is a cartilaginous structure that houses and protects the vocal folds, which enable phonation. The inferior border of the larynx is defined by the cricoid cartilage, which is the only complete cartilaginous ring of the tracheobronchial tree. Below the cricoid cartilage is the lower airway, which contains the trachea and mainstem bronchi, which lead to the left and right lungs.

2. **Describe the sensory innervation of the upper and lower airway.**
   The mucous membranes of the nasal passages are innervated by the ophthalmic division of the trigeminal nerve (V1) anteriorly, and the maxillary division of the trigeminal nerve (V2) posteriorly. The palatine nerves (consisting of V1 and V2) supply the soft and hard palate separating the oral and nasal passages. The lingual nerve (the mandibular branch of trigeminal nerve) and the glossopharyngeal nerve provide sensation to the anterior two-thirds and posterior one-third of the tongue, respectively. The glossopharyngeal nerve also provides sensory innervation to the tonsils, pharyngeal roof, and parts of the soft palate. Branches of the vagus nerve provide sensory innervation to the upper airway below the epiglottis. The superior laryngeal nerve provides sensory innervation between the epiglottis and larynx, whereas the recurrent laryngeal nerve provides sensory innervation between the larynx and trachea.

3. **What components of the patient history are important in airway evaluation during the preoperative assessment?**
   Because airway management complications remain the single most common cause of morbidity and mortality attributable to anesthesia, a proper and thorough assessment of a patient's airway is a key component of the preoperative workup. Previous anesthetic records, if available, can provide information about airway management problems in the past, including mask ventilation, intubation, and special airway techniques or equipment required for successful airway management. It is also important to ask the patient about prior anesthetics, as this may provide important information that could alert the practitioner to have additional personnel or airway management equipment immediately available. In addition, during the history, it is important to inquire about previous medical interventions or trauma that may have implications on airway management such as: (1) cervical spine injury or surgery, (2) history of tracheostomy, (3) head and neck surgery, (4) head and neck radiation treatment, (5) congenital craniofacial abnormalities, and (6) predisposition to atlantoaxial instability (e.g., rheumatoid arthritis, achondroplasia, Down syndrome).

4. **What components of the physical examination are important in airway evaluation during the preoperative assessment?**
   A proper physical examination of the airway should begin with a general inspection of the patient's physical appearance. Important things to note include morbid obesity, frailty, and mental status. This should be followed by gross inspection of the face and neck for anything suggestive of a difficult airway. Several features that are suggestive of a potentially difficult intubation include: (1) short neck, (2) inability to fully flex and/or extend the neck, (3) large neck circumference (>42 cm), (4) evidence of prior operations (especially tracheostomy), and (5) abnormal neck masses (including but not limited to tumor, goiter, hematoma, abscess, or edema). Next, attention should be paid to the mouth. Concerning features include small mouth opening (interincisor distance <3 cm), large tongue, micrognathia or undersized jaw, short thyromental distance (<3 finger breadths), Mallampati score of III or IV, and inability to bite the upper lip.

   It is also important to examine the patient's dentition. Teeth that are chipped, missing, or loose should be documented. If the case is elective, and there is high risk for tooth dislodgement, it may be prudent to have the patient see a dentist for extraction before the case. Dental appliances that are loose or easily removable should be removed before anesthesia, as they can impede airway management or pose an aspiration risk. If the patient is edentulous, direct laryngoscopy and intubation may be easier, but mask ventilation may prove more challenging.

5. **What are the predictors of difficult mask ventilation?**
   Although there is much focus on the predictors of a difficult intubation, the ability to effectively mask ventilate a patient is equally or perhaps more important. For example, if a patient is found to be difficult to intubate, the ability to

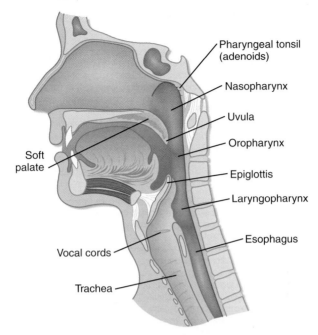

Fig. 3.1 Anatomy of the airway.

mask ventilate helps temporize the situation, while other airway management equipment and providers are summoned. If the patient is both a difficult intubation and mask ventilation (i.e., can't intubate, can't ventilate [CICV]/oxygenate), this is an emergency because the patient can desaturate, and without a means to oxygenate the patient, he or she is at risk for cardiac arrest and anoxic brain injury.

The reported incidence of difficult mask ventilation in the adult general population is 5%. There are five key patient factors that are considered independent risk factors for difficult mask ventilation: (1) presence of a beard, (2) lack of teeth, (3) obstructive sleep apnea or snoring history, (4) age over 55 years, and (5) obesity.

6. What is the Mallampati classification?
The Mallampati classification system is a scoring system used to predict the difficulty of intubation when combined with other features of the airway examination that are suggestive of a difficult intubation (Fig. 3.2). A score of III or IV means the patient is at higher risk of being a difficult intubation. To assess Mallampati classification, a patient must be sitting upright with the head neutral, mouth open, tongue protruded, and not phonating. A score of I to IV is assigned based on which structures are visible:
   I. Tonsillar pillars, uvula, and soft palate
   II. Base of uvula and soft palate
   III. Soft palate only
   IV. Hard palate only

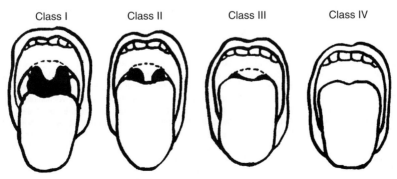

Fig. 3.2 Mallampati classification of the oropharynx.

7. **What are the general indications for endotracheal intubation? How does this apply to general anesthesia?**

There are three main indications to intubate a patient:
1) Inability to protect airway (e.g., altered mental status)
2) Hypercapnic respiratory failure (e.g., chronic obstructive respiratory disease)
3) Hypoxemic respiratory failure (e.g., acute respiratory distress syndrome)

Hemodynamic instability is also an indication for intubation, particularly in the setting of cardiac arrest, but this is primarily because of altered mental status caused by hypotension, which may lead to aspiration (inability to protect airway) and/or upper airway obstruction leading to hypoventilation.

Patients under general anesthesia are primarily intubated for airway protection to prevent aspiration. Although general anesthetic agents and opioids suppress respiratory drive and can cause hypercapnic respiratory failure, this unto itself is not an absolute indication for endotracheal intubation, as mask ventilation or placement of a supraglottic airway can treat temporary hypercapnic respiratory from general anesthesia in short surgical operations (i.e., 1–2 hours). In summary, patients under general anesthesia are primarily intubated for airway protection and secondarily because of hypercapnic respiratory failure.

8. **What equipment should I have available when planning to intubate a patient?**

One must ensure that the necessary medications and equipment (including backup devices), are available, accessible, and in working order. It is also critically important to have awareness of who is available for assistance and how those individuals can be contacted in the event of an emergency.

Medications that will be used for the induction of anesthesia should be drawn up in preparation for endotracheal intubation. In addition, emergency medications, including vasopressors for hemodynamic management and short acting paralytics (i.e., succinylcholine), should readily be available.

The patient should be attached to standard American Society of Anesthesiologists monitors (i.e., blood pressure, pulse oximeter, electrocardiogram) before induction of anesthesia and end-tidal CO_2 ($ETCO_2$) monitoring and a stethoscope should be available to confirm correct endotracheal tube placement, following intubation. A ventilator or anesthesia machine should also be available, but importantly, a standard bag-valve-mask (Ambu bag) should be immediately available to allow for mask ventilation if intubation proves difficult and to serve as backup in case of ventilator machine failure.

Specific airway management equipment should include:
- Appropriately fitting mask
- Direct laryngoscope, video laryngoscope, or flexible intubating scope
- Endotracheal tube (in multiple sizes)
- Lubricant
- Oral and/or nasal airways
- Adhesive tape
- Tongue depressor
- Suction
- Supraglottic airway (e.g., laryngeal mask airway [LMA])
- Bag-valve-mask device
- Oxygen source

9. **What is the purpose of preoxygenation before the induction of anesthesia?**

The goal of preoxygenation before induction of anesthesia is to increase the safe apnea time before intubation. Safe apnea time is defined as the duration of time after cessation of breathing or ventilation, until arterial oxygen levels begin to decrease below a critical value (i.e., pulse oximetry [SpO_2] <90%). Because of the steep slope of the oxygen-hemoglobin dissociation curve, oxygen desaturation will quickly drop below this critical value. During preoxygenation, when the patient inhales 100% oxygen (rather than 21% oxygen contained in room air), he or she is removing nitrogen from the lungs (a process known as *denitrogenation*) and filling the functional residual capacity (FRC) of the lungs with 100% oxygen. FRC is formally defined as the summation of expiratory reserve volume and residual volume and is the resting lung volume in an apneic patient, following induction of anesthesia. When the FRC is full of 100% O_2, safe apnea time is increased roughly fivefold compared with a patient breathing room air (100% is roughly 5 times > 21%).

10. **What techniques can be used to effectively mask ventilate a patient?**

Mask ventilation is a skill that is easy to learn but takes practice to master. To successfully mask ventilate, pay careful attention to ensure the mask overlies both the oral and nasal openings to allow for an adequate seal between the mask and patient's face. This enables the provider to generate positive pressure for ventilation. Without this seal, the anesthesia reservoir bag may not inflate, and it is difficult to deliver positive pressure breaths.

The provider may use the left hand only (most common technique) or two hands (in more challenging airways) to hold the mask and apply it to the patient's face. Subsequently, the provider should lift the patient's face into the mask by thrusting the mandible forward, using the third, fourth, and fifth fingers (resembles the shape of an "E"). Mandibular protrusion pulls the tongue and epiglottis anteriorly to promote airway patency. Next, the first and second fingers should press the mask to the face (resembles the shape of a "C") to create a seal. It is often helpful to extend the head as well, which straightens the upper airway reducing turbulent flow.

11. **What is a rapid sequence induction of anesthesia and intubation?**

Rapid sequence induction of anesthesia and intubation (RSII), more commonly referred to as *rapid sequence induction (RSI)*, is an established method to rapidly secure an airway with an endotracheal tube in a patient who is at increased risk of aspiration. RSI frequently involves the following components:

1) Rapid injection of anesthetic agents and a rapid onset paralytic (i.e., succinylcholine or double dose rocuronium)
2) Avoidance of mask ventilation and immediate laryngoscopy and intubation, following induction
3) An assistant to provide cricoid pressure (CP) to block gastric contents from moving up the esophagus, into the pharynx, and into the tracheobronchial tree
4) Avoidance of other medications before induction of anesthesia that can precipitate aspiration, such as benzodiazepines or opioids

Although the avoidance of aspiration is the primary indication for RSI, preventing hypoxia is paramount. In general, it is important to avoid mask ventilation when performing an RSI to minimize gastric insufflation, which can also increase the risk of aspiration itself. However, if necessary, mask ventilation can be performed if hypoxemia ensues and the provider is unable to intubate ideally with CP being applied (modified RSI).

12. **What patients are at risk of aspiration?**

RSI is used to minimize the risk of aspiration in several clinical situations, including:

- Emergent intubation in acutely ill patients or in patients whose nothing-by-mouth status cannot be confirmed
- Pregnancy
- Acute intraabdominal process, particularly small or large bowel obstruction but also should be considered in appendicitis or cholecystitis
- Delayed gastric emptying (i.e., trauma, alcohol or opioid use, end-stage renal disease, poorly controlled diabetics)
- Active or recent vomiting
- Patients who have not adequately fasted (>8 hours for food and >2 hours for clear liquids)
- Severe gastroesophageal reflux disease

13. **What is cricoid pressure? Does it work?**

CP involves applying pressure to the cricoid cartilage to minimize the risk of aspiration when performing an RSI. It is thought to work by compressing the esophagus; however, one magnetic resonance imaging study showed that it compresses the hypopharynx and not the esophagus per se. The efficacy of CP is debated, particularly as CP can worsen the view on laryngoscopy. It is in the author's opinion to recommend CP, as it can easily be aborted if it interferes with intubation. CP is generally applied before induction of anesthesia and released following confirmation of $ETCO_2$, after successful intubation.

14. **What is sniffing position?**

Sniffing position is a method to align the upper and lower airway axes to facilitate direct laryngoscopy, allowing for a direct line of site to the glottic opening hence the term *direct laryngoscopy*. This involves cervical flexion and atlantooccipital extension or more simply put, "head extension and neck flexion" (Fig. 3.3). The patient is said to be in sniffing position if an imaginary line from the external auditory meatus to the sternal notch is parallel to the floor.

Relative contraindications to sniffing position include atlantoaxial instability (e.g., Down syndrome, rheumatoid arthritis) or unstable cervical spine (e.g., trauma patient presenting with a cervical collar in situ). Sniffing position should be avoided in this patient population, with strong consideration for flexible scope intubation or video laryngoscopy to facilitate indirect laryngoscopy. However, if hypoxemia ensues on induction airway triumphs cervical spine and sniffing position is acceptable in dire situations.

15. **How is direct laryngoscopy performed?**

Direct laryngoscopy can be performed using a variety of different blades. The two most common laryngoscope blades are the Macintosh (curved) and Miller (straight). Laryngoscope blades are available in various sizes that are chosen based on the patient's size and anatomy but in general most patients can be intubated with a Macintosh 3 or Miller 2 blade.

Following induction of anesthesia, the mouth should be opened, as wide as possible, using the "scissor" technique to introduce the blade into the mouth. The laryngoscope should be held gripping the handle as low down as possible to provide maximal control. After the blade is advanced into the mouth, the provider should place their right hand under the patient's head to extend the head and, if necessary, lift the head off the table (which flexes the neck) to facilitate sniffing position. The right hand can be used to align the airway axes so the glottic opening can be directly visualized, thus allowing the provider to use less force with their left hand holding the laryngoscope blade. Note, sniffing can also be realized using pillows or blankets to flex the neck before induction; however, sometimes this leads to excessive or inadequate neck flexion.

When using the Macintosh blade, the laryngoscope is advanced slowly into the mouth and down the tongue, while identifying relevant anatomy. Once the tip of the blade is in the vallecula (groove between the base of tongue and epiglottis), the provider lifts the blade upward and to the back corner of the room at a 45-degree angle.

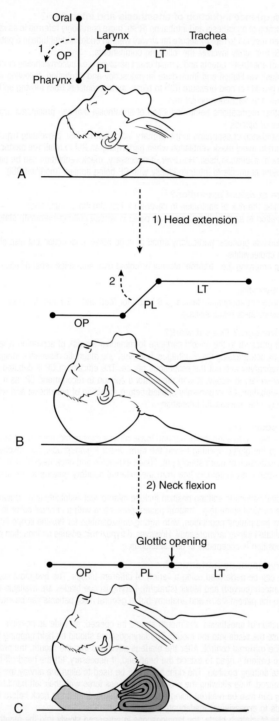

Fig. 3.3 Schematic diagram demonstrating "sniffing position" for direct laryngoscopy. (A) Successful direct laryngoscopy to visualize the glottic opening requires alignment of the oral-pharyngeal (*OP*), pharyngeal-laryngeal (*PL*), and laryngeal-tracheal (*LT*) axes. (B) Head extension using the provider's right hand aligns the OP axis. (C) Neck flexion using the provider's right hand to lift the head off the table will align the PL axes so that the OP, PL, and LT axes are all aligned, allowing direct visualization of the glottis. Note, neck flexion can also be facilitated using pillows or blankets placed under the patient's head.

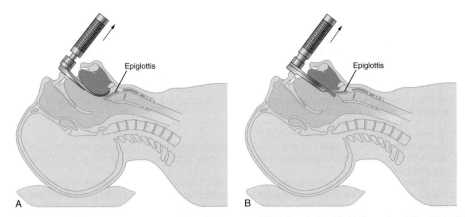

Fig. 3.4 Schematic diagram depicting the proper position of the laryngoscope blade for exposure of the glottic opening. (A) The distal end of the curved blade is advanced into the vallecula (space between the base of the tongue and the epiglottis). (B) The distal end of the straight blade is advanced beneath the epiglottis. Regardless of blade design, forward and upward movement exerted along the axis of the laryngoscopy handle, as denoted by the *arrows*, serves to elevate the epiglottis and expose the glottic opening. (From Klinger K, Infosino A. Airway management. In: Manuel PC, Miller RD, eds. Basics of Anesthesia. 7th ed. Philadelphia: Elsevier; 2018:252.)

This transmits a force to the hyoepiglottic ligament (see Fig. 3.1), which lifts the epiglottis off the posterior pharynx revealing the glottic opening. During laryngoscopy with the Miller blade, the tip of the blade is placed just posterior to the epiglottis. The epiglottis is then lifted to reveal the glottic opening (Fig. 3.4). External manipulation of the larynx may be helpful to improve visualization with both blades. Glottic structures will be revealed in this order: (1) posterior arytenoids, (2) glottic opening, and (3) vocal cords.

16. **What is the classification system used to describe the view on laryngoscopy?**
    The quality of the view of the glottic structures is described by the Cormack-Lehane classification system:
    1:    Full view of glottis
    2a: Partial view of glottis
    2b: Only posterior glottis or posterior arytenoids seen
    3:    Only epiglottis seen (none of glottis)
    4:    Neither glottis nor epiglottis seen

17. **When is it appropriate to choose direct laryngoscopy (Macintosh or Miller blade) versus indirect laryngoscopy (video laryngoscope or flexible intubating scope)?**
    It is generally appropriate to proceed with direct laryngoscopy following induction of anesthesia in patients who have no history, risk factors, or evidence on examination consistent with a difficult airway. In patients in whom it is impossible to achieve sniffing position because of limited cervical range of motion or a desire to maintain cervical spine stability, indirect laryngoscopy can aid in visualization of the glottic structures.
    Indirect laryngoscopy is generally used to facilitate endotracheal intubation in patients with a challenging airway or in clinical situations where cervical spine movement should be minimized. The flexible intubating scope, also referred to as the *fiberoptic bronchoscope*, is considered the gold standard to manage difficult airways, particularly in patients with a history of head and neck surgery, cancer, and/or radiation. Benefits of flexible scope intubation include complete visualization of the airway during intubation, confirmation of tube placement in the trachea, limited need for manipulating the cervical spine, and less potential for airway and dental trauma.

18. **How is a flexible scope intubation performed?**
    There are several steps in performing a flexible scope (fiberoptic) intubation. As with any procedure, it is imperative that the anesthesia provider ensure that all necessary equipment is available and in working order, including the flexible scope itself and backup equipment. Flexible scope intubation is most commonly performed with the patient supine (although it can be performed in almost any position). It can be achieved via both orotracheal and nasotracheal routes. An antisialagogue (i.e., glycopyrrolate) may be given preemptively to minimize secretions that may obstruct the lens of the scope. The flexible scope is advanced into the oropharynx (or nasopharynx) and slight anterior deflection can bring the vocal cords into view. The scope is then advanced between the cords and into the trachea where the tracheal rings can be identified anteriorly. The scope is further advanced so the carina can be identified, at which point the endotracheal tube is advanced off the scope into the airway. After the endotracheal tube is placed in the trachea, the scope is withdrawn with care to ensure that the tube remains in place.

19. What are indications for an awake intubation?

Flexible scope intubation can be performed with the patient "awake" or "asleep". If the clinician has a suspicion that a patient may be difficult to mask ventilate and intubate, the patient is strong candidate for an awake intubation. A key factor in determining if a patient needs an "awake" versus an "asleep" intubation is if the patient is likely easy to mask ventilate. All the factors of difficult mask ventilation and intubation (listed in previous questions) should be considered. An awake intubation preserves oropharyngeal muscle tone, airway reflexes, and the ability to ventilate spontaneously. It does not require cervical spine manipulation. In addition, it may permit the clinician to minimize hemodynamic changes during induction as minimal induction medications are needed, once the endotracheal tube is properly placed.

20. How is an awake intubation performed?

Flexible scope intubation in awake patients is well tolerated provided the airway is properly tropicalized with local anesthetic. Lidocaine is the first-choice local anesthetic in airway topicalization and has a long safety record with a high degree of success.

Reviewing the concepts behind airway topicalization for an awake intubation is a great way to review airway anatomy and its innervation. The glossopharyngeal nerve provides sensory innervation to the posterior one-third of the tongue, tonsils, soft palate, and pharynx up to the level of the epiglottis. To block this nerve, local anesthetic may be aerosolized into the oropharynx or applied via cotton swabs. Branches of the vagus nerve (superior laryngeal and recurrent laryngeal) provide sensory innervation to the airway below the epiglottis. The superior laryngeal nerve provides sensory innervation between the epiglottis and larynx. The superior laryngeal nerve block can be achieved by injecting local anesthetic lateral to the superior cornu of the hyoid bone bilaterally. The recurrent laryngeal nerve provides sensory innervation below the vocal cords. Block of this nerve is accomplished via transtracheal injection of local anesthetic. To achieve this, the cricothyroid membrane is identified, and a needle is advanced, until air is aspirated into the syringe attached to the needle, at which point local anesthetic is injected. Coughing induced by this block spreads the local anesthetic throughout the airway.

21. Is it ok to give sedation to facilitate an "awake" intubation?

Airway topicalization and blocks are sometimes combined with sedation; however, it cannot be emphasized enough that the whole point of an "awake" intubation is that the patient needs to remain "awake" because of concerns of managing a difficult airway if the patient were to be sedated. Knowing the airway anatomy, its innervation, and clinical competence in performing airway topicalization, related blocks, and using the flexible scope will reduce the need to sedate a patient to perform an "awake" intubation.

22. We have talked about endotracheal intubation, but what other methods can be used for airway management?

Supraglottic airways (e.g., laryngeal mask airway) are devices that are inserted into the pharynx above the glottis to facilitate ventilation. They are less invasive than an endotracheal tube and more secure than a facemask. They are versatile and can be used for both spontaneous (negative pressure) and mechanical (positive pressure) ventilation. They do not require the use of neuromuscular blockade for placement, which is another advantage. Disadvantages include the lack of protection from laryngospasm or aspiration of gastric contents. They are generally used in healthy patients undergoing short operations (i.e., 1–2 hours), but can also be used as a rescue device in patients who are difficult to intubate or as a conduit to facilitate flexible scope intubation.

23. What criteria do you use to determine if a patient is safe for extubation at the end of surgery?

Developing a plan for extubation is as important, if not more so, than a plan for intubation. In general, the criteria for extubation are the converse for the criteria to intubate. A patient is considered safe to extubate if: (1) they are awake and can protect their airway, (2) are not in hypoxemic respiratory failure, (3) are not in hypercapnic respiratory failure (this includes residual paralysis, overdose of opioids, or airway edema), and (4) are hemodynamically stable. In general, this can be realized by ensuring the patient is awake and alert with stable vital signs, can follow commands, has an adequate tidal volume and a normal respiratory rate (i.e., rapid shallow breathing index criteria <105), and can protect his or her own airway (exhibiting airway reflexes, such as gagging on the endotracheal tube). In addition, it is important to ensure adequate reversal of neuromuscular blockade via quantitative twitch monitoring as residual paralysis following extubation can lead to hypercapnic respiratory failure and failure to protect their airway.

Preparation for extubation should include placement of an oropharyngeal airway, preoxygenation with a fraction of inspired oxygen of 100%, and suctioning of the oropharynx. In patients at high risk for aspiration, precautionary steps may include decompression of the stomach with an orogastric tube and placement of the patient in the head up position.

24. Why is it important to place an oropharyngeal airway in the patient's mouth before emergence and extubation?

Oropharyngeal airways serve three important purposes on extubation. First, the device displaces the tongue off the posterior oropharynx and palate, thereby preventing obstruction of the upper airway and impedance of gas flow during respiration. This is because patients emerging from anesthesia may not have adequate airway tone because of residual anesthetic or residual paralysis and therefore may be prone to upper airway obstruction, particularly in patients with a history of obstructive sleep apnea.

Second, should respiratory support become necessary after extubation, a properly placed oral airway can serve as a conduit to maintain airway patency facilitating mask ventilation. Finally, the oral airway can be used as a bite block to prevent the development of negative pressure pulmonary edema, which can occur if the patient were to bite down on the endotracheal tube and attempt to inspire a large tidal volume.

25. **Which patients are at risk for "can't intubate, can't ventilate"? How does one manage this situation?**

A CICV situation is also referred to as *can't intubate, can't oxygenate* (CICO) to emphasize that hypoxemia and not hypercapnia is the main problem because hypoxemia is the most frequent cause of death or complications in these situations. Furthermore, oxygenation does not necessarily require ventilation and other modalities, such as apneic oxygenation with high-flow nasal cannula, can be used to prevent this dreaded situation. Although a CICV situation may occur de novo without any apparent risk factors, a frequent cause is iatrogenic from airway trauma because of multiple laryngoscopy attempts. In these situations, a provider is often initially able to mask ventilate; however, multiple direct laryngoscopy attempts may cause significant airway trauma (bleeding and edema) and the ability to mask ventilate is lost. Other specific risk factors include head and neck cancer, especially in patients who have received head and neck radiation treatment and in patients presenting with severe head and neck trauma (e.g., self-inflected gunshot wound to head/face). Most of these situations can be avoided or successfully managed by taking the following steps:

1) Have a low threshold to perform an awake flexible scope intubation in patients with known risk factors on history or by examination (e.g., head and neck cancer and/or radiation treatment)
2) Minimize laryngoscopy attempts ($<$2–3 attempts) and use the provider's right hand to help align the airway axes so the blade can be gently held with the left hand to minimize airway trauma
3) Give paralytics if awaking the patient from anesthesia is not an option
4) Call for help early (surgeons and other anesthesia providers)
5) Perform a surgical cricothyroidotomy early (needle cricothyroidotomy is less favorable and has been shown to have a high failure rate). Remember, a patient should never die from a CICV with a virgin neck
See Fig. 3.5 for Difficult Intubation Guidelines.

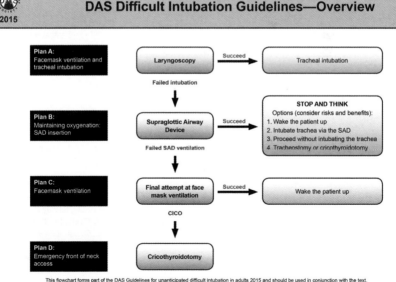

Fig. 3.5 Difficult Airway Society (*DAS*) difficult intubation algorithm. *CICO,* Can't intubate, can't oxygenate; *SAD,* supraglottic airway device. Note, other algorithms exist, such as the ASA 2013 difficulty airway algorithm. Practitioners should be aware and mindful of the clinical guidelines that pertain to the jurisdiction for which they practice. (From Frerk C, Mitchell VS, McNarry AF, et al. Difficult Airway Society 2015 guidelines for management of unanticipated difficult intubation in adults. Br J Anaesth. 2015;115(6):827–848.)

KEY POINTS: AIRWAY MANAGEMENT

1. Risk factors for difficult intubation include the following: history of head and neck cancer and/or radiation, history of known difficult intubation from prior anesthetics, obesity, pregnancy, airway trauma, poor mouth opening, decreased neck range of motion, inability to bite upper lip, decreased thyroid mental distance, short neck, and large neck circumference.
2. Sniffing position facilitates alignment of airway axes allowing direct visualization of the glottis with direct laryngoscopy.
3. Sniffing position can be achieved with head extension and neck flexion.
4. RSI often involves CP and a short, rapid acting paralytic to facilitate rapid intubation following induction of anesthesia. RSI is indicated in patients with a high risk of aspiration.
5. Risk factors for aspiration include pregnancy, acute intraabdominal pathology (e.g., small bowel obstruction), delayed gastric emptying (e.g., diabetes, trauma, chronic opioid use), and emergent intubations (e.g., stroke, respiratory failure).
6. The Macintosh blade is placed anterior to the epiglottis in the vallecula, whereas the Miller blade is placed posterior and directly lifts the epiglottis.
7. Indirect laryngoscopy includes the flexible intubating scope or video laryngoscope.
8. Patients with risk factors for difficult intubation, especially head and neck cancer and/or radiation, are strong candidates for awake intubation.
9. Multiple attempts in instrumenting the airway may cause significant airway trauma eventually causing an iatrogenic "can't intubate, can't ventilate" situation.
10. Limit direct laryngoscopy attempts to less than 2 or 3 attempts and then attempt other approaches (i.e., video laryngoscopy, flexible scope intubation, LMA, or if waking the patient is not an option, surgical cricothyroidotomy, while mask ventilating).

SUGGESTED READINGS

Apfelbaum JL, Hagberg CA, Caplan RA, et al. Practice guidelines for management of the difficult airway: an updated report by the American Society of Anesthesiologists Task Force on Management of the Difficult Airway. Anesthesiology. 2013;118(2):251–270.

Fourth National Audit Project of the Royal College of Anaesthetists and Difficult Airway Society. In: Cook TM, Woodall N, Frerk C, eds. Major Complications of Airway Management in the United Kingdom. Report and Findings. London: Royal College of Anaesthetists.

Frerk C, Mitchell VS, McNarry AF, et al. Difficult Airway Society 2015 guidelines for management of unanticipated difficult intubation in adults. Br J Anaesth. 2015;115(6):827–848.

Hagberg CA, Artime CA. Airway management in the adult. In: Miller RD, ed. Miller's Anesthesia. 8th ed. Philadelphia, Elsevier Saunders; 2015:1647–1683.

CHAPTER 4

AUTONOMIC NERVOUS SYSTEM

Brian M. Keech, MD

1. **Describe the autonomic nervous system.**
   The autonomic nervous system (ANS) is a network of nerves and ganglia that provide involuntary (i.e., unconscious) control of the physiological actions that maintain internal homeostasis and respond to stress. The ANS innervates structures within the cardiovascular, pulmonary, endocrine, exocrine, gastrointestinal (GI), genitourinary, skeletal muscle, and central nervous systems (CNS) and can influence metabolism and thermal regulation.
   The ANS consist of three components: sympathetic nervous systemic (SNS), parasympathetic nervous system (PNS), and enteric nervous system (ENS). The ENS governs the function of the GI tract, is the largest component of the ANS, and can function independent of the CNS. The SNS produces widespread effects, whereas the PNS tends to produce more localized, discrete effects. The SNS and PNS generally have opposing effects on most organs. At rest, the PNS predominates (i.e., rest-and-digest), whereas in stressful situations, the SNS predominates (i.e., fight-or-flight).

2. **What is the origin of the terms *sympathetic* and *parasympathetic*?**
   The origin of the term *sympathetic* (nervous system) comes from the Greek word "sympathy," which can be traced to the Greek physician and scientist, Claudius Galen (129–210 CE). Galen described the nervous system as the framework which facilitates a physiologic "sympathy," coordinating synergistic interactions among various organ systems. Parasympathetic (nervous system) comes from the Greek word "para" + "sympathy," where "para" denotes the meaning of "near, alongside, contrary, or against."

3. **Review the anatomy of the sympathetic nervous system.**
   Preganglionic sympathetic neurons originate from the intermediolateral columns in the spinal cord (T1–L2). These myelinated fibers exit via the ventral root of the spinal nerve, travel into the sympathetic chain, and synapse with three types of ganglia (Fig. 4.1):
   1) *Paravertebral sympathetic ganglia*—A chain of paired ganglia located lateral to the vertebral column (i.e., paravertebral), which runs from the skull to the coccyx forming the sympathetic trunk.
   2) *Prevertebral sympathetic ganglia*—Unpaired ganglia that are located anterior to the vertebral column (i.e., prevertebral).
   3) *Adrenal medulla*—A modified ganglia located within the adrenal gland. Although other ganglia function as relay stations with long postganglionic fibers that innervate specific organs, the adrenal medulla directly secretes catecholamines into the venous blood stream.
   Preganglionic sympathetic neurons may ascend or descend the sympathetic chain multiple levels and a single preganglionic fiber may synapse with multiple ganglia. On average, one preganglionic sympathetic fiber synapses with approximately 20 ganglia. Whereas most preganglionic sympathetic fibers that enter the sympathetic trunk ultimately synapse with paravertebral sympathetic ganglia, some will not and instead continue through the sympathetic trunk and synapse with other ganglia (e.g., prevertebral ganglia or adrenal medulla). Preganglionic sympathetic fibers release acetylcholine at their synapse to stimulate nicotinic cholinergic postganglionic neurons (or chromaffin cells of the adrenal medulla).
   Postganglionic adrenergic neurons synapse at target organs and release norepinephrine (NE, and epinephrine in the adrenal medulla), except in the case of sweat glands, where acetylcholine is released (Fig. 4.2).

4. **List examples of specific sympathetic ganglia that are often used as a target for interventional pain management.**
   Stellate ganglia—Paired paravertebral sympathetic ganglia formed as a fusion of the inferior cervical ganglia and the first thoracic ganglia from the sympathetic trunk. They are located at the level of C7, anteromedial to the vertebral artery, and posterior to the carotid, internal jugular, and phrenic nerve. They provide most of the sympathetic innervation to the head, neck, and upper extremities. It is a common target for a nerve block to treat complex pain disorders, such as complex regional pain syndrome of the upper extremity.
   Celiac plexus—A collection of prevertebral sympathetic ganglia located anterior to the aorta in the retroperitoneal space. It provides sensory and sympathetic outflow to the stomach, liver, spleen, pancreas, kidney, and GI tract up to the splenic flexure. It is a common target for a nerve block to treat complex abdominal pain disorders, such as pain from pancreatic cancer.

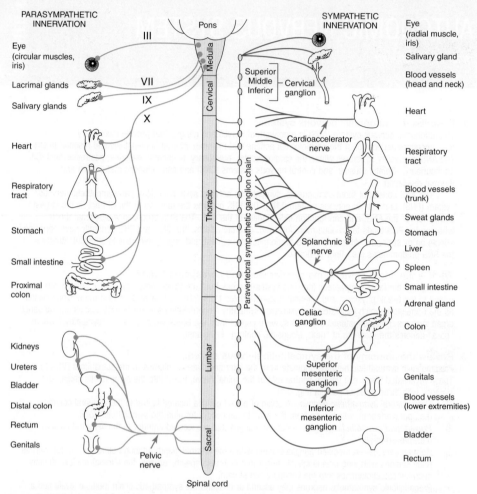

Fig. 4.1 Schema of the autonomic nervous system depicting the functional innervation of peripheral effector organs and the anatomic origin of peripheral autonomic nerves from the spinal cord. (From Bylund DB. Introduction to the autonomic nervous system. In: Wecker L, Crespo L, Dunaway G, et al, eds. Brody's Human Pharmacology: Molecular to Clinical. ed 5. Philadelphia: Mosby; 2010:95.)

5. **Describe the anatomy and function of the parasympathetic nervous system.**
   Preganglionic parasympathetic neurons originate from cranial nerves III, VII, IX, and X and sacral segments 2 to 4 (see Fig. 4.1). Of these, the vagus nerve accommodates approximately 75% of PNS traffic. Preganglionic parasympathetic neurons, as opposed to preganglionic sympathetic neurons, synapse with postganglionic neurons close to the target end-organ facilitating fine, discrete physiological effect. Both preganglionic and postganglionic parasympathetic neurons release acetylcholine; these cholinergic receptors are subclassified as either nicotinic or muscarinic. The response to cholinergic stimulation is summarized in Table 4.1.

6. **What are the adrenergic receptors and what is their response to agonism?**
   There are alpha-1 (α_1), alpha-2 (α_2), beta-1 (β_1), and beta-2 (β_2) adrenergic receptors. The α_1, β_1, and β_2 receptors are postsynaptic and are stimulated by the neurotransmitter NE. The α_2 receptors are presynaptic and are also stimulated by NE. Stimulation of α_2 receptors inhibits the presynaptic release of NE, reducing overall sympathetic response. Molecular pharmacologists have further subdivided these receptors, but this is beyond the scope of this discussion. The response to receptor activation at different sites is described in Table 4.1.

7. **What are catecholamines? Which occur naturally? Which are synthetic?**
   Catecholamines are monoamines that stimulate adrenergic nerve terminals. NE, epinephrine, and dopamine are naturally occurring catecholamines, whereas dobutamine and isoproterenol are synthetic catecholamines.

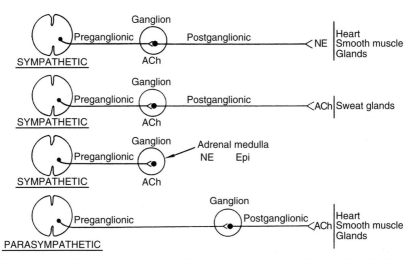

Fig. 4.2 Neuronal anatomy of the autonomic nervous system with respective neurotransmitters. *ACh,* Acetylcholine; *Epi,* epinephrine; *NE,* norepinephrine. (From Glick DB. The autonomic nervous system. In: Miller RD, ed. Miller's Anesthesia. 8th ed. Philadelphia: Elsevier Saunders; 2015:347.)

Table 4.1 End-Organ Effects of Autonomic Stimulation

ORGAN	ADRENERGIC RESPONSE	RECEPTOR	CHOLINERGIC RESPONSE	RECEPTOR
Cardiac (chronotropy)	Increased	β_1	Decreased	M_2
Cardiac (inotropy)	Increased	β_1		
Veins	Vasoconstriction	α_1		
Arteries (most)	Vasoconstriction	α_1		
Arteries (skeletal muscle)	Vasodilation	β_2		
Lung	Bronchodilation	β_2	Bronchoconstriction	M_3
Uterus	Relaxation	β_2	Contraction	M_3
Gastrointestinal tract	Relaxation	α_2	Contraction	M_3
Pupil	Dilation (mydriasis)	α_1	Constriction (miosis)	M_3
Kidney (renin secretion)	Increased	β_1		
Bladder (detrusor muscle)	Relaxation	β_2	Contraction	M_3
Pancreas (insulin release)	Decreased	α_2		
Fat cells (lipolysis)	Increased	β_1		
Liver (glycogenolysis)	Increased	α_1, β_2		
Salivary glands (secretion)	Increased/Decreased	α_1/α_2	Increased	M_3
Sweat glands (secretion)	Increased	M_3		

8. **Review the synthesis of dopamine, norepinephrine, and epinephrine.**
   The amino acid tyrosine is actively transported into the adrenergic presynaptic nerve terminal cytoplasm, where it is converted to dopamine by two enzymatic reactions: hydroxylation of tyrosine by tyrosine hydroxylase to L-DOPA and subsequent decarboxylation by aromatic L-amino acid decarboxylase to dopamine. Dopamine is transported into storage vesicles, where it is hydroxylated by dopamine β-hydroxylase to NE. Epinephrine is synthesized in the adrenal medulla from NE, through methylation by phenylethanolamine *N*-methyltransferase.

9. How are catecholamines metabolized?

Although NE is primarily removed from the synaptic junction by reuptake into the presynaptic nerve terminal, a small amount enters the circulation and undergoes metabolism. Catecholamines are metabolized in the blood, liver, and kidney by the enzymes monoamine oxidase and catecholamine O-methyltransferase. The important metabolites of epinephrine and NE are metanephrine and normetanephrine, respectively.

10. Why is it important to know the metabolites of epinephrine and norepinephrine?

Because the half-life of catecholamines is ultrashort ($t_{1/2} \approx 2$ minutes), it is difficult to directly measure catecholamines when diagnosing catecholamine secreting tumors, such as a pheochromocytoma. The catecholamine metabolites, metanephrine and normetanephrine, have a much longer half-life ($t_{1/2} \approx 1$–2 hours) and are often measured to diagnose pheochromocytoma. Catecholamine metabolites can be measured directly from the plasma or from a 24-hour urine sample.

11. What enzyme metabolizes acetylcholine?

Acetylcholine (ACh) is rapidly metabolized to choline and acetate by acetylcholinesterase (AChE), an enzyme located within the junctional cleft.

12. What problems could result from acethylcholine accumulation in the junctional cleft?

Inhibition of AChE, such as with neuromuscular blocking reversal agents (e.g., neostigmine) will result in accumulation of ACh, causing the following side effects: bradycardia, salivation, lacrimation, urination, defecation, and emesis. In general, these side effects can be mitigated with anticholinergic agents, such as glycopyrrolate. However, excessive accumulation may result in cholinergic crisis, causing severe bradycardia, bronchoconstriction, blindness, and muscular paralysis in addition to the aforementioned. The latter more severe side effects may be seen with pesticides (e.g., organophosphates) or in chemical warfare (e.g., Sarin gas).

13. How should cholinergic crisis be treated?

Cholinergic crisis should be treated with atropine and intubation for respiratory support. Atropine will antagonize muscarinic receptors located within the cleft at parasympathetic innervated organs; however, it will not antagonize nicotinic receptors located within the neuromuscular junction. Paralysis caused by cholinergic crisis requires intubation and respiratory support, until the offending agents abates.

14. What are the indications for using β-adrenergic antagonists?

β-Adrenergic antagonists, commonly called *β blockers*, are antagonists at β_1 and β_2 receptors. β blockers are a common treatment for hypertension, angina, and dysrhythmias. Perioperative β blockade is essential in patients with coronary artery disease, and the use of these medications has been shown to reduce death after myocardial infarction.

15. Review the mechanism of action for β antagonists and their side effects.

β_1 and β_2 antagonism decreases the activation of adenylate cyclase, resulting in decreased production of cyclic adenosine monophosphate (cAMP). β blockers may be cardioselective (relatively selective β_1-antagonist properties), or noncardioselective. β_1-Blockade produces negative chronotropic and inotropic effects, decreasing heart rate, contractility, cardiac output, and myocardial oxygen requirement. β_1-Blockers also inhibit renin secretion, thereby reducing fluid retention and angiotensin II. Because volatile anesthetics also depress myocardial contractility, intraoperative hypotension may result with perioperative β-blocker administration. Abrupt withdrawal of these medications is not recommended because receptor upregulation can lead to hypertension, tachycardia, and myocardial ischemia. Because of their benefits in ischemic heart disease, patients receiving β-blocker therapy should continue their usual regimen the day of surgery.

β blockers interfere with the translocation of potassium ions across the cellular membrane and can cause hyperkalemia. β blockers may also decrease signs of hypoglycemia (i.e., tachycardia and tremor); thus it should be used with caution in diabetic insulin-dependent patients.

16. Review the effects of β_2 antagonism.

For our purposes, β_2 receptors are located on vascular and bronchial smooth muscle. β_2-Blockade produces peripheral vasoconstriction, bronchoconstriction, and inhibits insulin release and glycogenolysis. Because of this, selective β_1 blockers should be used in patients with peripheral vascular disease, chronic obstructive pulmonary disease, or reactive airway disease because of concerns for vascular and bronchial constriction, respectively.

17. Can β blockade be used to attenuate the surgical stress response?

The adrenergic response to intense perioperative stimuli, such as tracheal intubation or surgical incision, can be attenuated with β antagonism. However, it is unclear if this attenuation is sufficient to protect patients from the possible harm associated with the adrenergic response to intense perioperative stimulation. At present, the adrenergic response to surgical stress is probably best managed through a combination of anesthetic agents, opioids, and, when appropriate, β antagonists.

18. How might complications of β blockade be treated intraoperatively?

Bradycardia and heart block will usually respond to atropine or glycopyrrolate; refractory cases may require β_1-agonism with epinephrine, dobutamine, or isoproterenol. Other treatment options include glucagon, calcium, insulin and glucose, and even lipid emulsion therapy.

19. Review α_2 agonists and their role in anesthesia.

α_2-Agonists inhibit adenylate cyclase and decrease cAMP production, thereby decreasing sympathetic outflow from presynaptic nerve terminals in the CNS. The α_2-agonist used most commonly in the perioperative setting is dexmedetomidine. It produces excellent sedation, contributes to analgesia, lowers anesthetic requirement, and reduces heart rate and blood pressure, all without significantly depressing ventilation. Side effects include bradycardia, which can easily be treated with glycopyrrolate. Clonidine, another α_2 agonist, is used as an antihypertensive. It can lead to rebound hypertension if stopped abruptly, leading up to surgery.

20. Discuss the role of muscarinic antagonists in the reversal of pharmacological neuromuscular blockade.

Nondepolarizing muscle relaxants can be reversed with AChE inhibitors, which increases ACh at the neuromuscular junction (nicotinic receptor). However, AChE inhibitors also increase ACh at the parasympathetic innervated organs (muscarinic receptor) causing bradycardia, defecation, secretions, and bronchospasm. To minimize these latter side effects, muscarinic antagonist (e.g., glycopyrrolate) should be coadministered with AChE inhibitors (e.g., neostigmine).

21. Which muscarinic antagonist is most frequently given in the operating room to reverse neuromuscular blockade? Why?

Glycopyrrolate is the muscarinic antagonist that is most frequently administered. It is a quaternary amine (i.e., polar molecule) and therefore does not readily cross the blood-brain barrier, unlike atropine, a tertiary amine (i.e., nonpolar molecule) that readily crosses the blood-brain barrier, causing undesirable CNS anticholinergic effects, such as sedation, confusion, and delayed emergence from anesthesia.

22. What is the significance of autonomic dysfunction?

Patients with ANS dysfunction or dysautonomia are at risk of severe hypotension intraoperatively and aspiration from gastroparesis. Diabetes mellitus and chronic alcohol abuse are risk factors for autonomic dysfunction.

23. How does spinal cord injury affect the autonomic nervous system?

Spinal cord injury can cause various problems of the ANS depending on the site, extent, and timing of the lesion. Autonomic reflexes that are normally inhibited by supraspinal feedback are lost following a high (T6 or above) spinal cord injury. As a result, minor stimuli can produce exaggerated SNS responses.

Initially, for a period of days to weeks, injured patients may experience spinal shock, a condition where the peripheral vascular bed is vasodilated, and compensatory tachycardia predominates. As the injury becomes chronic, hypotension may result in bradycardia, as the vagus nerve is the only component of the baroreceptor reflex that remains intact. In addition, an upregulation of adrenergic receptors may occur, making patients exquisitely sensitive to exogenously administered vasopressors.

Pressure stimuli below the level of the lesion can lead to a dramatic rise in blood pressure and reflexive decline in heart rate, a condition known as *autonomic dysreflexia*, and can be managed by administering vasodilators and/or deepening your anesthetic. Regional anesthesia should strongly be considered in these patients to blunt the exaggerated sympathetic response to painful stimuli.

24. What is a pheochromocytoma, and what are its associated symptoms? How is pheochromocytoma diagnosed?

A pheochromocytoma is a catecholamine-secreting tumor composed of chromaffin tissue, producing either NE or epinephrine. Most are intraadrenal, but some are extraadrenal (within the bladder wall is common), and about 10% are malignant. Computed tomography scan is very accurate in diagnosing and localizing the tumor. Signs and symptoms include paroxysms of hypertension, sudden severe headache, palpitations, flushing, and diaphoresis. Pheochromocytoma is confirmed by detecting elevated levels of catecholamine metabolites (i.e., metanephrine and normetanephrine) in the plasma or from a 24-hour urine.

KEY POINTS: AUTONOMIC NERVOUS SYSTEM

1. Sympathetic nerves originate from the spinal cord at T1–L2.
2. Parasympathetic nerves originate from cranial nerves III, VII, IX, X, and from the spinal cord at S2–S4.
3. The stellate ganglion provides sympathetic innervation to the upper extremity, whereas the celiac plexus (a collection of prevertebral ganglia) provides sympathetic and sensory innervation to the abdominal organs. These are frequent targets for interventional pain procedures, such as complex regional pain syndrome or pancreatic cancer.
4. Patients on β-blockers should take them on the day of surgery and continue them perioperatively. Because the receptors are upregulated, withdrawal may precipitate hypertension, tachycardia, and myocardial ischemia.
5. Patients with high spinal cord injuries (T6 and above) are at risk for autonomic dysreflexia, a condition associated with excessive sympathetic response to painful stimuli below the level of the lesion.
6. Pheochromocytoma is a catecholamine-secreting tumor causing paroxysmal episodes of hypertension, tachycardia, sudden headache, and diaphoresis. It is diagnosed by detecting elevated levels of metanephrine and normetanephrine in the plasma or from a 24-hour urine.

SUGGESTED READINGS

Glick DB. The Autonomic nervous system. In: Miller RD, ed. Miller's Anesthesia. 8th ed. Philadelphia: Elsevier Saunders; 2015: 346–386.

Mustafa HI, Fessel JP, Barwise J, et al. Dysautonomia. Perioperative implications. Anesthesiology. 2012;116:205–215.

Neukirchen M, Kienbaum P. Sympathetic nervous system. Evaluation and importance for clinical general anesthesia. Anesthesiology. 2008;109:1113–1131.

CARDIAC PHYSIOLOGY

John A. Vullo, MD

CHAPTER 5

1. **What is Ohm's law? How does it relate to blood flow in the human body?**

   Ohm's law characterizes the relationship between current and voltage across a resistor:

   $$I = \frac{\Delta V}{R}$$

   I, current; ΔV, voltage gradient; R, resistance

   This law can be applied to calculate the total electrical current through an electrical circuit, or it can be used to calculate the localized current through a specific resistor in a circuit. An analogy of Ohm's law can be made for blood flow in the human body. Where the pressure gradient (ΔP), across the resistance (R), of a vascular bed acts as a driving force for blood flow (Q), through the said vascular bed. The relationship between blood flow, pressure, and systemic vascular resistance (SVR) can be characterized by the following analogous equation:

   $$Q = \frac{\Delta P}{R}$$

   Q, flow; ΔP, pressure gradient; R, resistance

   This equation can be applied to various "resistors" or "circuits" within the human body. Recall, two circuits in series will have the same amount of current or blood flow (i.e., pulmonary and systemic circulation), whereas two resistors in parallel (e.g., mesenteric vs. musculoskeletal circulation) will have varying degrees of blood flow, depending upon their relative resistance. Thus the human body can be described as two circuits in series (i.e., pulmonary and systemic) with multiple resistors in parallel for each circuit. Moreover, the regional blood flow can vary between parallel vascular beds by modulating vascular resistance between sympathetic and parasympathetic tone (i.e., systemic circulation) or by hypoxic pulmonary vasoconstriction (i.e., pulmonary circulation).

   Therefore using Ohm's law, cardiac output can be calculated for the pulmonary and systemic "circuits", respectively:

   $$CO = \frac{mPAP - LAP}{PVR}$$

   Pulmonary circulation

   $$CO = \frac{MAP - CVP}{SVR}$$

   Systemic circulation

   CO, cardiac output; mPAP, mean pulmonary artery pressure; LAP, left atrial pressure; PVR, pulmonary vascular resistance; MAP, mean arterial pressure; CVP, central venous pressure; SVR, systemic vascular resistance

2. **What is the Fick principle?**

   Over 150 years ago, Dr. Fick introduced the principle that the uptake of a substance (e.g., oxygen) is equal to the product of blood flow and the difference between arterial venous concentration of that substance. Most commonly, this equation is solved for cardiac output by calculating the difference between arterial and venous oxygen content and measuring (or approximating) oxygen consumption, $\dot{V}O_2$. The $\dot{V}O_2$ is generally estimated by body weight, or BSA, and not directly measured in a clinical setting. Therefore this is usually the greatest source of error. The Fick principle can be used to calculate cardiac output by the following equation:

   $$CO = \frac{\dot{V}O_2}{CaO_2 - CvO_2}$$

   CO, cardiac output (mL of blood/min); $\dot{V}O_2$, O_2 consumption (mL of O_2/min); $CaO_2 - CvO_2$, difference between arterial and venous O_2 content

3. **What is oxygen content? How do you calculate it?**

   Oxygen content is the amount of O_2 in arterial or venous blood per unit volume. The arterial oxygen content can be calculated from an arterial blood gas, whereas the venous oxygen content is calculated from a mixed venous blood gas using a pulmonary artery catheter to sample blood from the pulmonary artery. Arterial oxygen content, for example, can be calculated by the following equation:

$$O_2 \text{ content} = 1.36 \times [Hg] \times S_aO_2 + 0.003 \times [P_aO_2](mL \text{ of } O_2/dL \text{ of blood})$$

4. What is the most important factor in determining oxygen content?
The most important factor in oxygen content is the hemoglobin concentration and hemoglobin oxygen saturation. Oxygen partial pressure is a minor contributor to oxygen content.

5. What is a typical $\dot{V}O_2$? What are the determinants of myocardial oxygen demand?
Total body oxygen consumption in a healthy adult at rest, a metabolic equivalent equal to one, is 3 to 4 mL O_2/kg/min or about 250 mL O_2/min for a 70-kg person. Metabolic equivalents (MET) are categorized by multiples of the baseline oxygen consumption, $\dot{V}O_2$, at rest. For example, to safely undergo major surgical operations, a patient should have the physiologic reserve to climb greater than one flight of stairs or walk greater than two city blocks (i.e., MET $\geq$4), which yields the following:

$$\dot{V}O_2 \geq \frac{250 \text{ mL } O_2}{min} \times 4 = 1000 \text{ mL } O_2/min$$

Myocardial oxygen demand depends on the amount of work performed by the heart (primarily the ventricles). The primary determinants of myocardial oxygen demand are wall tension (e.g., increases in afterload) and heart rate. Other factors include contractility and ventricular chamber size; however, fundamentally both of these factors are related to wall tension (see question on Laplace's law).

6. What is Laplace's law and how does it apply to myocardial oxygen demand?
The law of Laplace characterizes the relationship between pressure, wall radius, and wall thickness in determining wall tension as depicted subsequently:

$$\sigma = \frac{Pr}{2h}$$

σ, wall tension; P, pressure within the chamber; r, chamber radius; h, chamber wall thickness
This explains the pathophysiological adaptation of the heart to chronic hypertension or aortic stenosis, which cause concentric hypertrophy of the left ventricle. The ventricular wall thickens as an adaptive mechanism to minimize wall tension (i.e., afterload) and hence oxygen demand. It is important to emphasize that afterload can be defined as anything that increases wall tension on the ventricle as depicted by this equation.

7. What is the equation for coronary perfusion pressure?
Coronary perfusion pressure can be explained by the following equation:

$$CPP = P_{aorta} - P_{ventricle}$$

CPP, coronary perfusion pressure; P_{aorta}, aortic pressure; $P_{ventricle}$, ventricular pressure
Although this equation is true for the right heart in both systole and diastole, the left heart is only perfused during diastole, where the equation can be simplified to the following:

$$CPP = dBP - LVEDP$$

CPP, coronary perfusion pressure; dBP, aortic diastolic blood pressure; LVEDP, left ventricular end-diastolic pressure

8. What happens to coronary blood flow during systole and diastole?
The left heart is only perfused during diastole when the aortic pressure (P_{aorta}) is greater than the ventricular pressure ($P_{ventricle}$). Therefore it is important to avoid tachycardia to maintain coronary perfusion to the left heart. The right heart, however, is perfused during systole and diastole, as the aortic pressures are generally higher than the right ventricular pressures in both systole and diastole.

9. Describe the determinants of myocardial oxygen supply and their relationship.
Oxygen delivery to the myocardium is the product of coronary blood flow (CBF) and the oxygen content of arterial blood (CaO_2):

$$Myocardial \text{ } O_2 \text{ } Supply = CBF \times CaO_2$$

Recall, that oxygen content (CaO_2) is determined by the following:

$$CaO_2 = 1.36 \times [Hg] \times S_aO_2 + 0.003 \times [P_aO_2]$$

CBF is governed with the same relationship as $I = \Delta V/R$, where ΔV is the coronary perfusion pressure:

$$CBF = (P_{aorta} - P_{ventricle})/CVR$$

P_{aorta}, aortic root pressure; $P_{ventricle}$, ventricular chamber pressure; CVR, coronary vascular resistance
Therefore myocardial oxygen supply can be rewritten as the following:

$$Myocardial\ O_2\ supply = \frac{P_{aorta} - P_{ventricle}}{CVR}\ CaO_2$$

10. **How can you increase myocardial oxygen supply and delivery?**
From the earlier equation, the myocardial oxygen supply (CaO_2) can be increased by any of the following:
1) Increase [Hg] by transfusing red blood cells.
2) Maintain an S_aO_2 of 100% with supplemental oxygen.
3) Maintain an adequate coronary perfusion pressure ($P_{aorta} - P_{ventricle}$) with vasopressors (i.e., phenylephrine) to increase P_{aorta}.
4) Reduce ventricular pressure ($P_{ventricle}$) with diuretics and/or venodilators (e.g., nitroglycerin).
5) Avoid tachycardia, as ventricular pressure ($P_{ventricle}$) increases during systole, causing coronary blood flow to the left ventricle to approach or equal zero.

11. **How can this be used to understand coronary ischemia? How does this pertain to coronary artery disease, aortic stenosis, and right heart failure because of a pulmonary embolism?**
In referring to the aforementioned equations for coronary blood flow, anything that decreases aortic blood pressure, increases ventricular pressure, increases coronary resistance (e.g., coronary stenosis or thrombosis), or decreases oxygen delivery (e.g., anemia) can cause coronary ischemia.
In patients with coronary artery disease, it is important to avoid tachycardia as the left heart is only perfused during diastole. Further, any medical condition associated with an excessively high ventricular filling pressure (e.g., congestive heart failure, end-stage renal disease, aortic stenosis, pulmonary embolism) can decrease coronary perfusion. Recall, if $P_{ventricle}$ increases, then coronary perfusion pressure decreases, where $CPP = P_{aorta} - P_{ventricle}$. Therefore management of patients with these conditions (e.g., aortic stenosis, right heart failure because of pulmonary embolism) include strategies to optimize coronary perfusion (e.g., diuretics to decrease $P_{ventricle}$ or vasopressors to increase P_{aorta}).

12. **What is Poiseuille's law and how does it relate to blood flow in the human body?**

$$R = (8\eta L)/(\pi r^4)$$

R, resistance; η, viscosity of blood; L, blood vessel length; r, blood vessel radius
Poiseuille's law explains the various factors that affect resistance of flow provided flow is laminar and nonturbulent. For example, low hematocrit blood flowing through a short, wide caliber vessel would have low resistance, whereas high hematocrit blood flowing through a long, narrow caliber vessel would have high resistance to flow. The most important factor affecting resistance to flow is radius, as doubling this parameter will decrease resistance by a factor of 16. The resistance of the arterial vasculature is significantly higher than the venous system, especially at the level of the arterioles.

13. **What is compliance and how does it affect blood flow in the human body?**

$$C = \frac{\Delta V}{\Delta P}$$

C, compliance; ΔV, volume; ΔP, pressure
Compliance reflects the ability of a vessel to distend for a given pressure. Veins are much more compliant than arteries because they lack muscular stiffness. Arteries (and veins) often become stiff with age (i.e., arteriosclerosis) causing decrease compliance. This may contribute or even cause hypertension and will reduce a patient's physiologic reserve in the setting of hemorrhage. Classically, patients with noncompliant, stiff arteries have a larger pulse pressure.
Veins are approximately 20 to 30 times more compliant than arteries and store approximately two-thirds of the entire blood volume. An important concept to appreciate is that this large volume of blood, stored in the venous vasculature, can be recruited in situations associated with hypovolemia or hemorrhagic shock through increased sympathetic tone. In the setting of hypovolemia, increased sympathetic tone stimulates α_1 adrenergic receptors causing venoconstriction, which deceases venous compliance and facilitates venous return to maintain preload.

14. **What is the physiologic response to hemorrhage? How does age affect this response?**
In the setting of hemorrhage, sympathetic tone increases to prevent decreases in blood pressure and cardiac output to ultimately preserve oxygen delivery to tissues. Increased sympathetic tone causes the release of norepinephrine and epinephrine, which stimulate α_1 adrenergic receptors on the arteries (primarily the arterioles) to increase SVR. These same catecholamines also stimulate α_1 adrenergic receptors on the veins to decrease venous

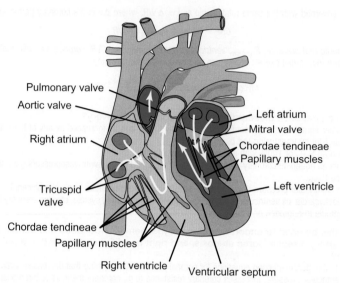

Fig. 5.1 Cardiac anatomy. This figure illustrates the four chambers of the heart, the atrioventricular valves (i.e., mitral and tricuspid), and the semilunar valves (i.e., aortic and pulmonic). (From Feher J. Quantitative Human Physiology: An Introduction. 2nd ed. Cambridge, MA: Elsevier Academic Press; 2017:519.)

compliance, facilitating venous return to maintain preload and cardiac output. Finally, these catecholamines also increase heart rate (i.e., chronotropy) and contractility (i.e., inotropy) to maintain normal cardiac output.

Young, healthy patients tend to have greater physiological reserve and can tolerate relatively large volumes of blood loss before their vitals become abnormal (i.e., tachycardia and hypotension). However, older patients tend to have diminished physiological reserve because of atherosclerosis (decrease venous compliance and ability to recruit blood), decreased cardiac contractility and response to catecholamines, and often are on medications, such as β blockers that blunt their physiological response to hemorrhage.

15. **Describe the basic structure and function of the heart.**
The heart is a muscular organ whose primary purpose is to generate a pressure gradient to drive nutrient and oxygen-rich blood delivery to other organs. The heart consists of four chambers: two atria and two ventricles (Fig. 5.1). The heart is customarily split into two halves: the right side of the heart and the left side. Each successive chamber is separated from the next by a one-way pressure-regulated valve.

All four chambers of the heart contract in a coordinated fashion to generate the movement of blood throughout the entire cardiovascular system. Most of its mass is composed of a continuous band of muscle that is wrapped about the ventricular chambers of the heart to facilitate coordinated contraction.

The left and right sides of the heart are separated by a fibromuscular wall called a *septum*. The septum at the level of the atria is termed the *interatrial septum* and between the ventricles as the *interventricular septum*. The right side of the heart receives deoxygenated blood from the venous system into the right atrium. Blood flows passively and is actively moved across the tricuspid valve (TV) into the right ventricle (RV). This blood is actively pumped across the pulmonic valve (PV) into the pulmonary vascular bed and returns, oxygenated, to the left atrium. Left atrial blood is passively and actively moved across the mitral valve (MV) into the left ventricle (LV). The LV then contracts with enough pressure to pump the oxygenated blood via the aortic valve (AV) throughout the entire cardiovascular system of the body and back to the right atrium.

16. **What are the sequences of the cardiac cycle?**
The cardiac cycle can be separated into two intervals: systole and diastole. Systole is associated with contraction and diastole is associated with relaxation. Technically, each of the four chambers of the heart have their own systolic and diastolic time intervals (e.g., right atrial systole). However, in common practice it is implied that the terms *systole* and *diastole* are with respect to the LV.

Left ventricular systole or "systole" is defined as the time interval between MV closure and AV closure. Similarly, right ventricular systole would refer to the time interval between TV and PV closure. The following events occur during systole:

1) *Isovolumetric contraction*—The ventricle contracts and increases ventricular pressure closing the atrioventricular valve. Both the atrioventricular valves (i.e., mitral and tricuspid) and semilunar valves (i.e., aortic and pulmonic) are closed during this event.

2) *Ejection*—Ventricular pressure is greater than aorta and pulmonary artery pressure causing the semilunar valves (i.e., aortic and pulmonic) to open and blood is ejected from the heart. Ejection and systole terminate when arterial pressure becomes greater than ventricular pressure causing closure of the semilunar valves.

Ventricular diastole is defined as the time interval between semilunar valve closure and atrioventricular valve closure. The following four sequential events occur during ventricular diastole:
1) *Isovolumetric relaxation*—Following ventricular ejection, the ventricle relaxes, while the atrioventricular and semilunar valves remain closed.
2) *Rapid ventricular filling*—The ventricle pressure becomes less than atrial pressure, which opens the atrioventricular valve. The ventricle rapidly fills with atrial blood, moving down an initially steep pressure gradient created by ventricular relaxation.
3) *Diastasis*—Atrial and ventricular pressure equilibrate and flow from atrium to ventricle decreases.
4) *Atrial*—Atria contract forcing any remaining atrial blood to fill the ventricle.

17. Explain the differences between the right and left sides of the heart, specifically between the right and left ventricles.
The RV is significantly thinner and less muscular than the LV. It is one-sixth the mass of the LV and its contractility is significantly less. The RV pumps blood through a low resistance circuit (the pulmonary vascular bed) compared with the LV, which pumps blood through a high resistance circuit. Although both the right and left heart pump approximately the same amount of blood volume (i.e., ~5 L/min), the left heart is thicker, which helps decrease wall tension (see Laplace law) and the RV is more compliant, which helps facilitate venous return. Therefore the anatomic differences between the two correlate with their function. Also they have distinct embryologic origins, which further explain and predict their differences.

18. Describe the determinants of cardiac output in detail.
Cardiac output is the volume of blood delivered per unit time, which can be calculated by the following equation:

$$CO = SV \times HR$$

SV, stroke volume (mL/contraction); HR, heart rate (contractions/min); CO, cardiac output (mL/min)
There are three determinants of stroke volume, which are classically described from the perspective of the LV but apply to the RV as well:
- *Preload*—The amount of stretch placed on the cardiac myocytes, or, clinically, the left ventricular end diastolic volume (LVEDV). All muscles require an appropriate amount of stretch to optimize myosin-actin overlap, which optimizes the force of contraction. However, volume overloaded patients can surpass the stretch reserve of the myocytes leading to decreased contractility.
- *Afterload*—The amount of tension on the cardiac myocytes, or, clinically, the pressure the LV must generate to eject blood through the AV (left ventricular outflow tract) and to the rest of the body. Any cause of increased resistance, such as aortic stenosis, aortic coarctation, elevated systemic vascular resistance (e.g., idiopathic arterial hypertension), will increase the tension on cardiac myocytes requiring them to work harder and consume more energy.
- *Contractility (inotropy)*—The innate ability of the LV to contract. Contractility is influenced by calcium stores, sympathetic tone (endogenous or exogenous beta agonism), thyroid hormone levels, and other medications.

19. What is the Frank-Starling law?
The Frank-Starling law denotes the relationship between stroke volume (SV) and end-diastolic ventricular volume (Fig. 5.2). Fundamentally, it is based on the surface area overlap between actin and myosin, where a certain degree of "stretch" optimizes this overlap, allowing for a greater force of contraction. If the stretch is excessive or inadequate, the force of contractility decreases.
    The basic inference of this relationship is that SV and cardiac output are matched to venous return (end-diastolic volume). Alterations in contractility rotate the curve from the origin. Increased contractility (i.e., β_1 agonism) rotates the curve upwards causing a greater stroke volume for a given end-diastolic volume. The converse is true for decreases in contractility.

20. What is a ventricular pressure-volume loop? Outline the steps in the loop.
A ventricular pressure-volume (P-V) loop describes the complete ventricular cycle with respect to volume on the x-axis and pressure on the y-axis (Fig. 5.3).

21. How do you calculate stroke work? What are its implications?
The area under the P-V loop represents Stroke Work, or the work necessary to produce one SV. The implications are that any increase in preload and/or afterload can increase the amount of "work" the heart performs, which increases cardiac oxygen and energy requirements.

Frank–Starling curves

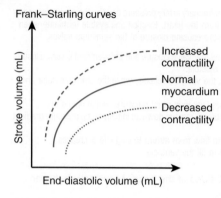

Fig. 5.2 Frank-Starling law. As end-diastolic volume or preload increases so does contractility. Note that excess preload can decrease stroke volume, which is not shown on the figure. (From Hamilton M. Advanced cardiovascular monitoring. Surgery (Oxford). 2013;31(2):90–97.)

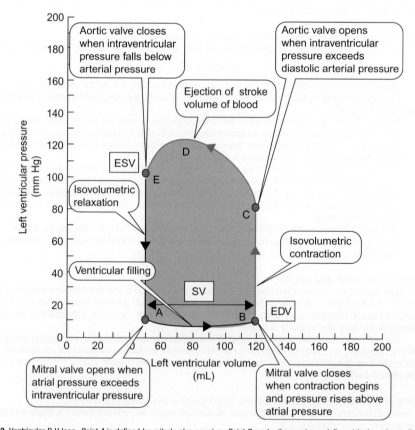

Fig. 5.3 Ventricular P-V loop. *Point A* is defined by mitral valve opening. *Point B* marks the maximum left ventricular volume, the end of diastole and beginning of systole, which occurs at mitral valve closure. *Point C* marks the opening of the aortic valve. *Point D* represents peak left ventricular (LV) pressure and corresponding systolic blood pressure. *Point E* occurs at aortic valve closure, where left ventricular volume is at its smallest, the end of systole, and the start of diastole. *EDV*, end diastolic volume; *ESV*, end systolic volume; *SV*, stroke volume. (From Feher J. Quantitative Human Physiology: An Introduction. 2nd ed. Cambridge, MA: Elsevier Academic Press; 2017:557.)

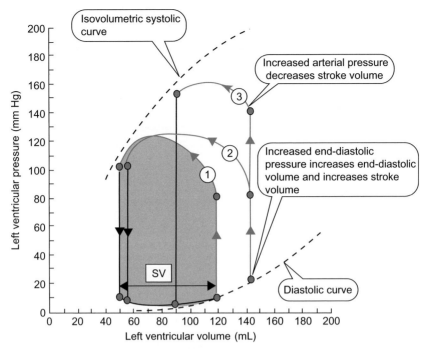

Fig. 5.4 Preload and afterload effects on P-V loop. *Curve #1* illustrates a normal P-V loop. *Curve #2* illustrates increased stroke volume (*SV*) with increased preload (recall Frank-Starling Law). *Curve #3* illustrates decreased stroke volume caused by increased afterload. (From Feher J. Quantitative Human Physiology: An Introduction. 2nd ed. Cambridge, MA: Elsevier Academic Press; 2017:559.)

22. How would changes in preload and afterload affect the pressure-volume loop?
    Please refer to Fig. 5.4.

23. Outline the electrical and physiologic relationship between an electrocardiogram (ECG) tracing and the cardiac cycle.
    An ECG measures electrical signals generated by the heart. Each ECG axis (e.g., lead I) represents a vector projected measurement of electrical activity onto that axis. Please refer to Fig. 5.5.
    - *P wave*—This first wave of the ECG represents atrial depolarization and therefore the impetus for atrial contraction.
    - *PR interval*—Atrial contraction occurs, electrical systole begins with the QRS complex of waves beginning ventricular depolarization, and it represents the AV nodal conduction velocity. This interval represents the time it takes for SA nodal conduction to be relayed through the AV node.
    - *QRS complex*—During this interval, atrial repolarization occurs, which is generally unseen and overshadowed by ventricular depolarization (the onset of electrical systole).
    - *QT interval*—The ventricles completely depolarize and repolarize.
    - *ST segment*—This segment is normally isoelectric and represents the time when ventricles have depolarized.
    - *T wave*—This is ventricular repolarization. The end of the T wave signifies onset of electrical diastole.

KEY POINTS: CARDIAC PHYSIOLOGY

1. Blood flow in the human body can explained by Ohm's law, where the pulmonary circulation and systemic circulation occur in series.
2. The primary determinants of myocardial oxygen demand are increases in afterload (wall tension) and heart rate.
3. The LV is only perfused in diastole and requires a pressure gradient (coronary perfusion pressure) such that aortic diastolic blood pressure is larger than LV end-diastolic pressure.
4. Maximization of myocardial oxygen supply is paramount and can be achieved by: transfusing red blood cells, achieving S_aO_2 of 100% with supplemental oxygen, maintaining an adequate coronary perfusion pressure, and avoiding tachycardia.
5. Especially in the setting of hemorrhage, older patients tend to have a diminished physiological reserve and may have a blunted response to catecholamines (endogenous and exogenous).

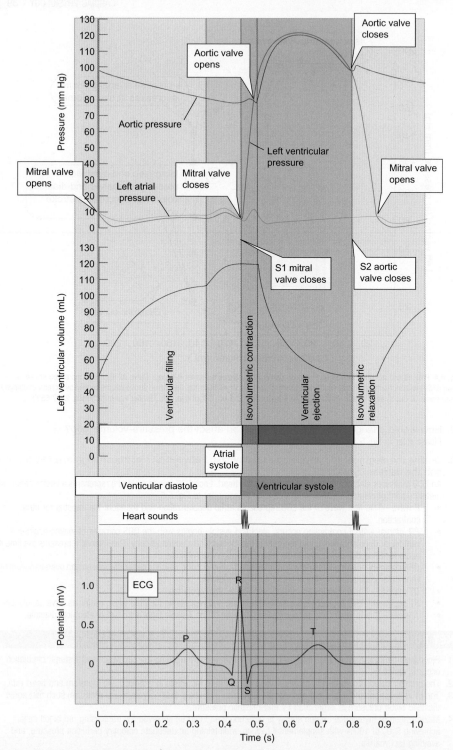

Fig. 5.5 Wiggers diagram. Note how electrical physiology as denoted by the electrocardiogram (*ECG*) proceeds mechanical physiology (e.g., QRS and T waves proceed ventricular systole and diastole, respectively). (From Feher J. Quantitative Human Physiology: An Introduction. 2nd ed. Cambridge, MA: Elsevier Academic Press; 2017:545.)

Suggested Readings

Costanzo LS. Physiology. 6th ed. Philadelphia: Wolters Kluwer Health/Lippincott Williams & Wilkins; 2018.

Feher J. Quantitative Human Physiology: An Introduction. 2nd ed. Cambridge, MA: Elsevier Academic Press; 2017:516–524.

Sun LS, Schwarzenberger J, Dinavahi R. Cardiac physiology. In: Miller RD, ed. Miller's Anesthesia. 8th ed. Philadelphia: Elsevier Saunders; 2015:473–491.

CHAPTER 6

PULMONARY PHYSIOLOGY

Ryan D. Laterza, MD

1. **Define lung volumes and capacities.**
   - Tidal volume (TV) = Volume of gas inspired and passively expired with normal breathing
   - Expiratory reserve volume (ERV) = Volume of gas that can be maximally exhaled from rest
   - Residual volume (RV) = Volume of gas remaining in the lung after maximal exhalation
   - Functional residual capacity (FRC) = ERV + RV
   - Inspiratory reserve volume (IRV) = Volume of gas that can be maximally inhaled above a TV
   - Inspiratory capacity (IC) = IRV + TV
   - Vital capacity (VC) = IRV + TV + ERV
   - Total lung capacity (TLC) = IRV + TV + ERV + RV
   (Fig. 6.1).

2. **Describe the mechanics of respiration.**
   The combination of surface tension of water within the alveoli and the intrinsic elastic properties of the lung create a force (F_{lung}) favoring collapse, whereas the chest wall force (F_{chest}) favors expansion. These two forces directly oppose one another, creating a spring-like physiology, opposing any deviation in lung volume above or below FRC. For example, following a forced inhaled volume above FRC, the recoil force of the lung (F_{lung}) is greater than the expansion force of the chest wall (F_{chest}), facilitating a passive return to FRC. Likewise, following a forced exhaled volume below FRC, F_{chest} is greater in magnitude than F_{lung}, causing a passive return to FRC.

3. **What is FRC? What factors affect it?**
   FRC results when the opposing forces of the expanding chest wall and the recoil forces of the lung are equal. In other words, lung volume is at FRC when $F_{chest} + F_{lung} = 0$. The average FRC for a 70-kg, 5'10", male in the supine position around 2.5 L.
   FRC is increased by:
   - Body size (increases with height)
   - Age (increases slightly with age)
   - Asthma and chronic obstructive pulmonary disease (COPD)
   FRC is decreased by:
   - Female sex (females have a 10% decrease in FRC compared with males)
   - Muscle relaxation (anesthetic agents and neuromuscular blocking agents decrease diaphragmatic muscle tone and other accessory muscles of respiration)
   - Posture (FRC is greatest in standing >sitting >prone >lateral >supine)
   - Decreased chest wall compliance (e.g., obesity, thoracic burns, kyphoscoliosis, abdominal compartment syndrome, ascites, laparoscopy)
   - Decreased lung compliance (e.g., interstitial lung disease, acute respiratory distress syndrome [ARDS])

4. **How long will it take for an apneic patient to develop hypoxemia following induction of anesthesia?**
   In a healthy, 70-kg, 5'10" (body mass index [BMI] 22), male preoxygenated (or denitrogenated) to an end-tidal O_2 = 100%, it will take approximately 10 minutes. At rest (i.e., a metabolic equivalent of 1), the O_2 consumption (3.5 mL/kg/min) for a 70-kg adult male is approximately 250 mL/min. Following induction in the supine position, this patient's lung volume will equal FRC, which is approximately 2.5 L. Assuming this lung volume contains 100% O_2, it will take 2500 mL O_2/(250 mL O_2/min) = 10 minutes.
   However, the earlier is under ideal conditions for a healthy, nonobese patient, assuming an FRC volume equal to 100% oxygen. Realistically, preoxygenation would yield a more commonly obtained end-tidal O_2 of approximately 80% (not 100%), which will decrease the effective volume of O_2 in the FRC by 20%. Also muscle relaxation caused by either anesthetic agents or paralytics will reduce FRC by 20%. Therefore the effective FRC volume containing oxygen is 2500 mL O_2 × 80% × 80% = 1600 mL O_2 yielding 6.4 minutes before the onset of hypoxemia.
   Further, given the high prevalence of obesity and its effects on reducing FRC (decreases outward F_{chest}) and increasing O_2 consumption (increased body mass), the time to hypoxemia can be severely reduced in the general population. Assume the aforementioned patient is 30-kg overweight and now weighs 100 kg (BMI 32). Because obesity decreases FRC by approximately 30 mL/kg for each kg above normal body weight, his effective O_2 volume in FRC, although apneic, will be (2500 mL − 900 mL) × 80% × 80% = 1024 mL O_2 and his O_2 consumption will increase to 350 mL O_2/min. Therefore time to hypoxemia will be 1024 mL O_2 /(350 mL O_2/min) = 2.9 minutes. This is a more realistic time to hypoxemia for a large percentage of patients who are obese (BMI 32) but otherwise healthy.

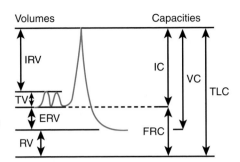

Fig. 6.1 Subdivisions of lung volumes and capacities. *ERV,* Expiratory reserve volume; *FRC,* functional residual capacity; *IC,* inspiratory capacity; *IRV,* inspiratory reserve volume; *RV,* residual volume; *TLC,* total lung capacity; *TV,* tidal volume; *VC,* vital capacity.

5. What is closing capacity and what factors affect it? What is the relationship between closing capacity and FRC?

Closing capacity (CC) is the lung volume at which small, noncartilaginous airways begin to close, resulting in atelectasis and subsequent hypoxemia. It is calculated by the following equation:

$$Closing\ capacity = Closing\ volume + RV$$

In a young, healthy patient, CC is approximately equal to RV. The clinical significance of this is that having a closing volume at RV effectively provides a large physiological oxygen reserve, that is, atelectasis will not occur at FRC. With age, CC increases. At approximately 45 years old, CC equals FRC when supine and at 65 years of age, equals FRC when standing. The end result is a greater likelihood of resting hypoxemia in older patients because of atelectasis.

Although FRC is dependent on position and only slightly correlated with aging, CC is independent of position and increases with aging. CC is thought to be an independent pathological process responsible for decreased pulmonary reserve and hypoxemia in the elderly patient.

6. Discuss the factors that affect resistance to gas flow. How is laminar versus turbulent flow different?

Resistance to gas flow through a tube can be separated into two components: (1) physical properties of the tube (e.g., length and radius), and (2) physical properties of the gas flowing through the tube (e.g., laminar vs. turbulent flow). At low flow rates, flow is laminar and the relationship between flow and pressure is linear as shown by the Hagen-Poiseuille equation:

$$\Delta P = \frac{8l\mu}{\pi r^4} \times \dot{Q}$$

Notice how the pressure gradient (ΔP) increases linearly with increasing flow ($\dot{Q}$) with a slope governed by resistance, $R = 8l\mu/\pi r^4$. Resistance (R) increases with tube length and gas viscosity (μ), while resistance decreases as radius (r) increases by the fourth power. At high flow rates (e.g., bronchospasm, asthma, and COPD), gas velocity significantly increases, resulting in turbulent flow, and the relationship between flow and pressure becomes nonlinear, where $\sqrt{\Delta P} \propto \dot{Q}$ implying a much higher pressure will be necessary for a given flow ($\dot{Q}$) relative to laminar flow, where $\Delta P \propto \dot{Q}$. During turbulent flow, resistance is proportional to the density (ρ) of the gas and inversely proportional to the radius (r) of the tube to the fifth power: $R \propto \rho/r^5$.

7. Give an example of how gas flow resistance applies to clinical practice.

Patients who are intubated must exchange gas through a smaller diameter than their normal airway. Recall, resistance is inversely proportional to radius to the fourth power for laminar flow. Because of the smaller radius of the endotracheal tube, resistance will increase, requiring increased work of breathing if unassisted by the ventilator. This increased work of breathing can be reduced by assisting the patient with a synchronized ventilator mode, such as pressure support. Pressure support allows the patient to trigger the ventilator, which can provide positive pressure to "overcome" the resistance of the endotracheal tube and decrease the work of breathing on inspiration. However, the work of breathing will still be increased on expiration as the ventilator only assists on inspiration. Other examples that pertain to increased airway resistance include bronchospasm, secretions, postextubation stridor, and a kinked endotracheal tube.

8. What determines laminar versus turbulent flow? What are the clinical implications of this?

Laminar flow is more efficient than turbulent flow for gas exchange, as turbulent flow will require a larger pressure gradient to obtain the same amount of flow. Reynolds number (Re) is a dimensionless number that can be used to predict if flow will be turbulent or laminar. A lower Re is associated with laminar flow, and a higher Re is associated with turbulent flow. Re can be calculated by the following equation: Re = $2rv\rho/\eta$, where r is tube radius, v is gas velocity, ρ is gas density, and η is gas viscosity. Notice how increasing gas velocity increases Re, leading to more turbulent flow and decreasing gas density lowers Re, leading to more laminar flow.

9. Discuss clinical interventions that may mitigate turbulent flow.

Increased airway resistance (e.g., bronchospasm) can lead to turbulent flow because of an increased inspiratory flow or gas velocity (see equation for Reynolds number). One method to treat problems related to turbulent flow is to lower the gas density. This can be accomplished with the addition of helium. When helium and oxygen are combined, the result is a gas composition called *heliox*, which has a similar viscosity as air, but importantly, has a much lower density. This accomplishes the following: (1) decreases Reynolds number, allowing for less turbulent and more laminar flow, and (2) decreases turbulent flow resistance. Recall that resistance during turbulent flow is $R \propto \rho/r^5$ (where ρ is gas density). A common mixture is 70% helium and 30% oxygen. Applications where heliox may prove helpful include postextubation stridor and status asthmaticus.

10. What is compliance? How is it calculated?

Compliance is a measurement that reflects the amount of volume the pulmonary system can store for a given pressure. The overall compliance of the pulmonary system is determined by the lung, chest wall, and state of the patient's respiratory cycle (inhalation or exhalation). Pulmonary compliance (C) can be calculated by measuring the change in volume for a given change in pressure:

$$C = \Delta V / \Delta P$$

Two factors that affect the compliance of the lung itself are: (1) water tension, (2) amount of functional lung connective tissue, such as elastin and collagen. A patient may exhibit decreased compliance from the lung itself (e.g., pulmonary fibrosis) or from decreased outward chest wall force (F_{chest}) and/or increased abdominal pressure (e.g., obesity, ascites, pregnancy).

11. Describe how pulmonary compliance changes with inspiration and expiration.

How the state of the respiratory cycle can impact lung compliance can be demonstrated as follows: at the end of exhalation, certain areas of the lung will favor atelectasis (i.e., zone 3 dependent regions) compared with others (i.e., zone 1 nondependent regions). Assume a patient takes a large breath from RV to TLC. At the start of inhalation, pulmonary compliance is low, because the atelectatic regions of the lung contain alveoli that are collapsed and water filled, thereby creating a less energetically favorable state (i.e., requiring more energy to inflate). After these alveoli are recruited, compliance increases until the lung is maximally inflated, at which point lung and chest wall compliance begin to decrease, impairing further inhalation. Here, the elastic recoil forces of the lung itself increase, and the chest wall, which normally favors lung expansion, reaches its maximum limit.

On exhalation, the pulmonary compliance for a given volume or pressure is higher than it is on inhalation. At the beginning of inhalation, atelectatic alveoli are recruited from closed to open, which initially decreases lung compliance (think of blowing up a deflated balloon); however, at the end of inhalation, these formerly atelectatic alveoli are now opened, favoring a higher overall compliance for a given volume or pressure during exhalation (it is easier to keep a balloon inflated once inflated). This concept is known as *hysteresis,* where the current state of a system (i.e., pulmonary compliance) is dependent upon its past state (i.e., inhalation or exhalation).

12. What is surface tension? How does it affect pulmonary mechanics?

Surface tension occurs whenever you have an interface between two mediums (e.g., liquid and gas), where one consists of polar molecules (i.e., water) and the other of nonpolar molecules (i.e., oxygen and nitrogen). To minimize the interface between water (a polar molecule) and air (nonpolar molecules), water will preferentially form the shape of a closed sphere. This shape will yield the largest volume to surface area ratio possible. The large volume of the sphere will facilitate maximum hydrogen bonding between water molecules, while minimizing the exposed surface area (i.e., the interface that is exposed to nonpolar molecules, which cannot undergo hydrogen bonding with oxygen and nitrogen).

In a patent alveolus, water forms a coat on the surface (analogous to a bubble) with a surface tension that wants to collapse this bubble into nature of water (resulting in atelectasis). Surface tension, resulting from hydrogen bonding, is the primary underlying force contributing to lung recoil and the promotion of atelectasis. However other factors, such as alveolar interdependence between walls of shared alveoli, prevent collapse. Further, the structure of alveoli is not spherical but rather more polygonal in shape. Taken together, alveolar interdependence, their polygonal shape, and probably other factors prevent the formation of perfectly spherical, collapsed alveoli, despite the natural tendency of water to do so.

To summarize, alveoli are coated by a layer of water, which creates an alveolar wall surface tension at the liquid-gas interface. This force plays an important role in understanding atelectasis and pulmonary compliance.

13. Discuss Laplace's law. How does it apply to pulmonary physiology?

Laplace's law describes the relationship of pressure across an interface (ΔP), wall-surface tension (T), and the radius (R) of a sphere. It can be used to model the physical properties of an alveolus.

$$\Delta P = 2T / R$$

The Laplace equation states that as the diameter (or radius) of an alveolus decreases, the pressure inside that alveolus will increase, assuming surface tension is constant. This implies that the pressure inside smaller alveoli is greater relative to larger alveoli, causing gas to preferentially flow from small to large alveoli. This would cause small alveoli to get smaller and smaller until atelectasis occurs, although the large alveoli would get larger and larger leading to volutrauma. Note, this phenomenon only occurs if the alveolar surface tension remains constant (i.e., patients who are deficient in pulmonary surfactant). As will be explained, surfactant plays an important role in stabilizing alveoli and preventing this problem from occurring.

14. What is surfactant?

Pulmonary surfactant is a phospholipid substance that contains both polar and nonpolar regions at opposite ends. It is produced in the lung by type II alveolar cells and coats the water already present in the alveoli. This coating forms an interface in the alveoli between the water (polar regions of surfactant) and air (nonpolar regions of surfactant) that reduces surface tension, thereby enabling alveoli to remain open at smaller lung volumes. Because water surface tension is responsible for approximately two-thirds of the recoil force of the lung, pulmonary surfactant plays an important role in preventing atelectasis and increasing pulmonary compliance.

15. What role does surfactant play in pulmonary physiology?

Surfactant plays an important role in stabilizing alveoli. When an alveolus becomes smaller (e.g., during exhalation), the concentration of surfactant increases, thereby decreasing water surface tension. Conversely, when the alveolus becomes larger, the concentration of surfactant decreases, causing water surface tension to increase. Note how surface tension and alveolar radius are intrinsically linked; surface tension increases as radius increases and decreases as radius decreases. Thus this relationship helps minimize any differences in ΔP between smaller and larger alveoli (Laplace's law).

Surfactant also plays a role in elastic recoil. As previously discussed, the concentration of surfactant is a function of alveolar size. Thus surfactant enables the lung to exhibit elastic properties similar to a rubber band, where its recoil force increases as the rubber band is stretched. This property allows the lung to exhibit a higher compliance at low TVs, while also facilitating exhalation at larger TVs. Because surface tension plays such a large role in contributing to the lung's elastic recoil forces, disorders associated with surfactant deficiency are readily apparent.

16. What clinical scenarios might result in an absolute or relative surfactant deficiency?

Patients with surfactant deficiency will exhibit reduced lung compliance and will be more prone to atelectasis and volutrauma (see question on Laplace's law). The classic example of absolute surfactant deficiency is that of the premature newborn, resulting in respiratory distress syndrome. Inflammation and other factors can cause decreased production of surfactant and/or surfactant dysfunction. This may be seen in conditions such as ARDS, asthma, COPD, interstitial lung disease, or following lung transplantation. Although exogenous surfactant is life-saving in the premature newborn, studies to date have not shown benefit in these latter conditions.

17. What are the different zones of the lung?

The physiology of the lung is classically divided into three zones characterized by variations between ventilation ($\dot{V}$) and perfusion ($\dot{Q}$). The three zones of an upright lung begin at the apices (zone 1) and end at the base (zone 3). Note, P_{alv} is alveolar pressure, P_{pa} is pulmonary artery pressure, and P_{pv} is pulmonary vein pressure.

- Zone 1: $P_{alv} > P_{pa} > P_{pv}$, which causes a high ventilation-perfusion mismatch ($\dot{V}/\dot{Q} > 1$) and a propensity for alveolar dead space ($\dot{V}/\dot{Q} = \infty$). Both ventilation and perfusion are at their lowest in this zone; however, ventilation is greater than perfusion
- Zone 2: $P_{pa} > P_{alv} > P_{pv}$, which yields an ideal ventilation-perfusion match ($\dot{V}/\dot{Q} \approx 1$). Both ventilation and perfusion increase whereby ventilation $\approx$ perfusion (oxygen volume for 1 liter of dry air is 210 mL and oxygen capacity for 1 L of blood is 200 mL).
- Zone 3: $P_{pa} > P_{pv} > P_{alv}$, which causes a low ventilation-perfusion mismatch ($\dot{V}/\dot{Q} < 1$) and a propensity for shunt because of atelectasis ($\dot{V}/\dot{Q} = 0$). Both ventilation and perfusion are at their highest in this zone; however, perfusion is greater than ventilation.

Historically, gravity was theorized to explain the variation behind the zones of the lung with the implication that a zero-gravity environment would abolish this variation. However, studies by NASA and on the MIR space station show that ventilation-perfusion matching, as depicted earlier, persist in microgravity. In the upright position, gravity only accounts for about 25% of ventilation-perfusion distribution and 75% of this distribution was retained independent of gravity. The primary mechanism for the different lung zones is resistance to blood and gas flow caused by the geometry of the vasculature and bronchial tree, directing blood and gas to the base of the lungs. Further, these same studies found that perfusion was more evenly distributed throughout the lung in the following order (prone $>>$ supine $>$ upright), thereby, supporting the utility of prone positioning for severe ARDS.

KEY POINTS: PULMONARY PHYSIOLOGY

1. FRC is the volume of the lung at rest.
2. FRC decreases from standing to sitting to supine.
3. Laminar flow is much more efficient than turbulent flow for a given pressure.

Continued

KEY POINTS: PULMONARY PHYSIOLOGY *(Continued)*

4. Two-thirds of the lung's elastic recoil force is caused by surface tension.
5. Surfactant has several benefits: reduces overall lung compliance, stabilizes alveoli by preventing atelectasis and volutrauma, provides the lung with elastic properties facilitating inhalation and exhalation.
6. Disorders associated with surfactant deficiency or dysfunction lead to a loss of these benefits (e.g., premature newborn, ARDS, COPD, and asthma).
7. The lung is heterogeneous and characterized by regional $\dot{V}/\dot{Q}$ mismatch, resulting in dead space (zone one) and shunt (zone three).

18. **What is the alveolar gas equation? What is the normal alveolar oxygen partial pressure at sea level on room air?**
The alveolar gas equation is used to calculate the alveolar oxygen partial pressure P_AO_2:

$$P_AO_2 = F_iO_2\,(P_b - P_{H2O}) - P_aCO_2/R$$

where P_AO_2 is the alveolar oxygen partial pressure, F_iO_2 is the fraction of inspired oxygen, P_b is the barometric pressure, P_{H2O} is the partial pressure of water vapor (47 mm Hg), P_aCO_2 is the partial pressure of carbon dioxide, and R is the respiratory quotient. The respiratory quotient is approximately 0.8 and is dependent on metabolic activity and diet. At sea level, the alveolar partial pressure (P_AO_2) would be the following:

$$P_AO_2 = 0.21\,(760-47) - \frac{40}{0.8} = 99.7\ mm\ Hg$$

19. **How would room air P_AO_2 compare between Denver, CO (elevation 5280 ft) and New York, NY (elevation near sea level)?**
The F_iO_2 at room air (21%) is the same in New York City and Denver. However, because the barometric pressure, P_b, in Denver is lower, the alveolar oxygen partial pressure, P_AO_2, will also be lower.

20. **What are the causes of hypoxemia?**
The five classic pathophysiological causes of hypoxemia are:
- Low inspired oxygen: this can be caused by high altitude, inadvertent swap of nitrous oxide and oxygen gas lines, or simply neglecting to "turn on" the oxygen. Measures to prevent the latter problems include fail-proof safety connectors (i.e., pin indexed safety system and diameter index safety system) and the oxygen analyzer on the inspiratory limb of the anesthesia ventilator
- Alveolar hypoventilation: patients under general anesthesia (breathing spontaneously) and in postanesthesia care unit, following surgery, are often incapable of maintaining an adequate minute ventilation. Reasons for this include the following: residual paralysis from neuromuscular blocking agents, respiratory depressant effects from opioids and other anesthetic agents, shallow breathing from pain (i.e., splinting), or upper airway obstruction (e.g., obstructive sleep apnea). Hypoventilation results in an elevated alveolar CO_2 (P_ACO_2) which, by the alveolar gas equation, decreases alveolar O_2 (P_AO_2), leading to hypoxemia. Of note, hypoventilation affects the arterial partial pressure of CO_2 ($PaCO_2$) to a much greater degree than it does the arterial partial pressure of O_2 (PaO_2). For example, high frequency (jet/oscillatory) ventilation and apneic oxygenation with high-flow nasal cannula are all methods which demonstrate that ventilation, in the traditional sense, is not necessary to oxygenate the blood. Further, pulse oximetry is a poor method to assess for hypoventilation and is often normal despite high levels of CO_2. In addition, it is important to recognize that clinically significant hypoxemia that results from hypoventilation and does not respond to supplemental oxygen is likely because of more than just elevated alveolar CO_2. For example, a patient with multiple bilateral rib fractures may initially hypoventilate because of pain (i.e., splinting), causing a small decrease in PaO2, which is easily treated with supplemental oxygen. However, hypoventilation can lead to atelectasis from small TVs, causing significant hypoxemia.
- Ventilation-perfusion ($\dot{V}/\dot{Q}$) mismatch: alveolar ventilation and perfusion would ideally be close to a one-to-one relationship, promoting efficient oxygen exchange between alveoli and blood. However, when alveolar ventilation and perfusion to the lungs are unequal ($\dot{V}/\dot{Q}$ mismatch), hypoxemia results. Pathological examples of $\dot{V}/\dot{Q}$ mismatch include COPD, asthma, pulmonary embolism, bronchospasm, and mucus plugging. Note, these conditions often contain elements of both elevated and decreased $\dot{V}/\dot{Q}$ mismatching. For example, a patient with a large pulmonary embolism will have increased dead space ($\dot{V}/\dot{Q} = \infty$) in one region of the lung, resulting in high blood flow to another region, potentially causing $\dot{V}/\dot{Q}$ mismatch ($\dot{V}/\dot{Q} < 1$) and subsequent hypoxemia. In general, hypoxemia because of $\dot{V}/\dot{Q}$ mismatch can usually be overcome with supplemental oxygen.
- Right-left shunt: although often listed separately, shunt is really just a subset of $\dot{V}/\dot{Q}$ mismatch, where $\dot{V}/\dot{Q} = 0$. Some of the pathological examples listed later may have an element of $\dot{V}/\dot{Q}$ mismatch in certain regions of the lung where $\dot{V}/\dot{Q} < 1$, but not technically zero. There are two kinds of shunts: (1) physiological shunting, and (2) pathological shunting. Normal physiological shunt (2%–3% of cardiac output) is caused by venous drainage into the left heart by the bronchial and Thebesian veins. Examples of pathological shunt include

arteriovenous malformations, right-to-left cardiac shunt, ARDS, atelectasis, pneumonia, and pulmonary edema. An important distinguishing characteristic of shunt is that hypoxemia cannot easily be overcome with supplemental oxygen alone and, depending upon the pathological condition, often requires alveolar recruitment strategies. Such strategies include: raising the head of bed to greater than 30 degrees, incentive spirometry, ambulation, noninvasive positive pressure ventilation, such as continuous positive airway pressure/bilevel positive airway pressure and, if intubated, increasing positive end expiratory pressure/performing alveolar recruitment maneuvers.
- Impaired diffusion: efficient oxygen exchange depends on a healthy interface between alveoli and the bloodstream. Pulmonary edema, intestinal lung disease, and emphysema are examples of pathological conditions that can impair the diffusion of oxygen into the blood.

21. **What is the most common cause of hypoxemia in the perioperative setting?**
The two most common pathophysiological mechanisms for perioperative hypoxemia is right-left shunt and hypoventilation. Atelectasis (right-left shunt) is likely the most common condition leading to clinically significant hypoxemia, and usually results from factors such as alveolar hypoventilation, obesity, supine positioning, splinting, and "absorption atelectasis" from the use of 100% F_iO_2.

KEY POINTS: CAUSES OF HYPOXEMIA

1. Low inspired oxygen
2. Alveolar hypoventilation
3. $\dot{V}/\dot{Q}$ mismatch
4. Right-left shunt
5. Impaired diffusion

22. **Define anatomic, alveolar, and physiological dead space.**
Physiological dead space (V_D) is the sum of anatomic and alveolar dead space. Anatomic dead space includes the nose, oral cavity, pharynx, trachea, and bronchi. This is about 2 mL/kg in the spontaneously breathing individual and accounts for the majority of physiological dead space. Endotracheal intubation decreases total anatomic dead space because the volume occupied by the endotracheal tube is smaller than the oral cavity, nose, and pharynx. Alveolar dead space is the volume of gas that reaches the alveoli but does not undergo gas exchange because of poor perfusion (i.e., zone 1 of the lung). In healthy patients, alveolar dead space is negligible.

23. **How does dead space affect alveolar ventilation?**
The main goal of ventilation is to facilitate gas exchange at the level of the alveolus. However, as mentioned, there is a significant amount of anatomic dead space between the air we breathe and well perfused alveoli undergoing gas exchange. This can be demonstrated by the following equation: $V_T = V_A + V_D$ where V_T is tidal volume, V_A is alveolar volume, and V_D is physiological dead space volume (anatomic and alveolar). Assuming a (physiological) dead space volume of 2 mL/kg, a 70-kg person would have approximately 140 mL of dead space. Therefore TVs need to be greater than 140 mL to guarantee alveolar ventilation to facilitate gas exchange. Note, this is the classic teaching of this concept and evidence to date shows some alveolar ventilation (and CO_2 gas exchange) can occur with apneic oxygenation using high flow nasal canula (60 LPM) or open-lung ventilation strategies (e.g., high frequency jet/oscillatory ventilation).

24. **How does $PaCO_2$ relate to alveolar ventilation?**
$PaCO_2$ is inversely related to alveolar ventilation and is described by the following equation:

$$PaCO_2 = \dot{V}CO_2 / \dot{V}_{alveolar}$$

$\dot{V}CO_2$, CO_2 production; $\dot{V}_{alveolar}$, alveolar ventilation

Therefore increasing the minute ventilation will decrease the $PaCO_2$, provided TVs are greater than the anatomic dead space.

25. **How can dead space be quantified? How does arterial partial pressure of CO_2 ($PaCO_2$) relate to mixed, expired CO_2 ($PeCO_2$)?**
Dead space can be quantitated using the Bohr equation:

$$V_D/V_T = (PaCO_2 - PeCO_2)/PaCO_2$$

V_D, dead space volume; V_T, tidal volume; $PaCO_2$, arterial CO_2 partial pressure; $PeCO_2$, mixed expired CO_2 partial pressure

The Bohr equation is a method to calculate the physiological dead space (V_D) by measuring the tidal volume (V_T), the mixed expired CO_2, and arterial CO_2 partial pressures. In a healthy 70-kg patient with a $V_D \approx 150$ mL (2 mL/kg) and $V_T \approx 500$ mL (6–8 mL/kg), the dead space is normally 1/3 of the tidal volume (i.e., $V_D/V_T \approx 0.3$). Similarly, in a healthy patent with a $PaCO_2$ of 40 mm Hg, the measured mixed $PeCO_2$ will equal 28 mm Hg. Applying these parameters to the Bohr equation will yield the following: $V_D / V_T = (40 - 28)/40 = 0.3$. The $PeCO_2$ is lower than the $PaCO_2$ (arterial CO_2) because the CO_2 free gas from the physiological dead space dilutes and lowers the P_ACO_2 (alveolar CO_2). Note, that CO_2 is perfusion limited (not diffusion limited like oxygen); therefore in well-perfused alveoli, the $P_ACO_2 \approx PaCO_2$.

26. **What is the difference between end-tidal CO_2 ($ETCO_2$) and mixed, expired CO_2 ($PeCO_2$)? Which one is used clinically?**
The $ETCO_2$ is the CO_2 measured by capnography at the end of exhalation, whereas the $PeCO_2$ is the final CO_2 partial pressure measured in a volume of gas following complete exhalation. Clinically, the $ETCO_2$ is most often used (not $PeCO_2$) and reflects alveolar ventilation (i.e., P_ACO_2). The $ETCO_2$ will decrease in pathological conditions associated with increased alveolar dead space (e.g., pulmonary embolism, cardiac arrest, COPD). Note, because $ETCO_2$ reflects alveolar ventilation, it is less affected by anatomic dead space. Therefore the difference between $PaCO_2$ and $ETCO_2$ is generally minimal (i.e., 4–5 mm Hg), where the $PeCO_2$ will be much lower because it is diluted by both anatomic and alveolar dead space.

27. **How is CO_2 transported in the blood?**
CO_2 exists in three forms in blood: as dissolved CO_2 (7%), as bicarbonate ions (HCO_3^-) (70%), and combined with hemoglobin (23%).

28. **What is hypoxic pulmonary vasoconstriction?**
Hypoxic pulmonary vasoconstriction (HPV) is a localized response of vascular smooth muscle in the pulmonary system that redirects blood flow from hypoventilated regions (i.e., low P_AO_2 and high P_ACO_2) to better ventilated regions. Specifically, low P_AO_2, high P_ACO_2, and low pH cause pulmonary vasoconstriction and high P_AO_2, low P_ACO_2, and high pH cause vasodilation. This serves to improve overall $\dot{V}/\dot{Q}$ matching. It is important to know that this response in the pulmonary system is the opposite of what occurs in the systemic vasculature. Although vasodilating agents and older volatile anesthetic agents (e.g., halothane) may blunt HPV, studies show that the newer volatile agents (i.e., sevoflurane and desflurane) in addition to intravenous agents (i.e., propofol) do not inhibit HPV in commonly used clinical doses.
   Knowledge of HPV plays an important role in managing patients with pulmonary hypertension, as any episode of hypoxemia, hypercarbia, or acidosis will increase pulmonary vascular resistance (PVR). Any increase in PVR will cause the pulmonary artery pressure to increase, potentially leading to right heart failure. Avoiding episodes of hypoxemia and hypercarbia in patients with severe pulmonary hypertension is crucial.

29. **What is arterial oxygen content (CaO_2) and how is it calculated?**
Arterial oxygen content is the amount of oxygen carried in arterial blood (mL of O_2/dL of blood). It is calculated by summing the oxygen bound to hemoglobin (Hgb) and the oxygen dissolved in blood (PaO_2) by the following equation:

$$CaO_2 = (1.34)[Hgb]SaO_2 + (0.003)PaO_2$$

Where 1.34 is the oxygen binding capacity of hemoglobin (mL of O_2/gram of Hgb), SaO_2 is the hemoglobin saturation, Hgb is the hemoglobin concentration (g/dL), 0.003 is the solubility coefficient for oxygen (mL/dL/mm Hg), and PaO_2 is the partial pressure (mm Hg) of arterial oxygen.

30. **What is oxygen delivery?**
One of the primary roles of blood flow is to provide oxygen delivery ($\dot{D}O_2$) to peripheral tissues. This can be represented by the following equation:

$$\dot{D}O_2 = CO \times CaO_2$$

$\dot{D}O_2$, oxygen delivery (mL of O_2/min); CO, cardiac output (liter of blood/min); CaO_2, oxygen content (mL of O_2/dL of blood)
   This equation states that there are two methods to increase oxygen delivery to tissue: (1) increase cardiac output, or (2) increase arterial oxygen content. Because PaO_2 is multiplied by 0.003, dissolved oxygen plays a minor role in determining arterial oxygen content and there is little utility in administering high F_iO_2 to raise the PaO_2 when the SaO_2 is normal. More useful methods to increase oxygen delivery are to maintain normal ($SaO_2 > 90\%$), transfuse packed red cells in the setting of anemia, or administer inotropic agents in the setting of cardiogenic shock. As an example, administering blood to a patient in hemorrhagic shock will increase oxygen delivery by two methods: (1) increasing hemoglobin, which increases CaO_2, and (2) increases stroke volume, thereby increasing cardiac output.

KEY POINTS: USEFUL PULMONARY EQUATIONS

1. Resistance of laminar flow through a tube: $R = 8l\mu/\pi r^4$
2. Compliance: $C = \Delta V/\Delta P$
3. Alveolar gas partial pressure: $P_AO_2 = F_iO_2 (P_b - P_{H2O}) - P_aCO_2/R$
4. Oxygen content of blood: $CaO_2 = (1.34)[Hgb]SaO_2 + (0.003)PaO_2$
5. Oxygen delivery: $\dot{D}O_2 = CO \times CaO_2$
6. $V_D / V_T = (PaCO_2 - PeCO_2)/PaCO_2$

31. Where is the respiratory center located?

The respiratory center is located bilaterally in the medulla and pons. Three major centers contribute to respiratory regulation. The dorsal respiratory center is mainly responsible for inspiration, the ventral respiratory center for both expiration and inspiration, and the pneumotaxic center for controlling breathing rate and pattern. A chemosensitive area also exists in the brainstem just beneath the ventral respiratory center. This area responds to changes in cerebrospinal fluid pH, sending corresponding signals to the respiratory centers. Anesthetics depress the respiratory centers of the brainstem.

32. What role do carbon dioxide and oxygen play in the regulation of breathing?

During hypercapnic and hypoxic states, the brainstem will be stimulated to increase minute ventilation, whereas during periods of hypocapnia and normoxia, minute ventilation will be repressed. Carbon dioxide (indirectly) and hydrogen ions (directly) work on the chemosensitive areas of the brainstem, whereas oxygen interacts with the peripheral chemoreceptors in the carotid and aortic bodies. Of the two, carbon dioxide is, by far, more influential than oxygen in regulating respiration.

33. What are pulmonary function tests, and how are they used?

The term pulmonary function test (PFT) refers to a standardized measurement of a patient's airflow, lung volumes, and diffusing capacity for carbon monoxide. These values are always reported as a percentage of a predicted normal value, which is calculated based on the age and height of the patient. They are used in combination with the history, physical examination, blood gas analysis, and chest radiograph to facilitate the classification of pulmonary disease into an obstructive, restrictive, or mixed disorder.

34. What is the benefit of obtaining PFTs?

The primary goal of obtaining preoperative PFTs, also called *spirometry*, is to recognize patients who are at high risk for developing postoperative pulmonary complications. However, it is important to note that no single test or combination of tests will definitively predict which patients will develop postoperative pulmonary complications.

35. What are the measures of pulmonary function and their significance?

These are effort dependent and require a motivated patient (Fig. 6.2).

- Forced expiratory volume in 1 second (FEV1)
- Forced vital capacity (FVC)
- The ratio of FEV1 and FVC, or FEV1/FVC ratio. The FVC may be normal or decreased as a result of respiratory muscle weakness or dynamic airway obstruction
- Forced expiratory flow at 25% to 75% of FVC (FEF 25–75). A decreased FEF 25–75 reflects collapse of the small airways and is a sensitive indicator of early airway obstruction. It is thought to be the most effort independent measurement

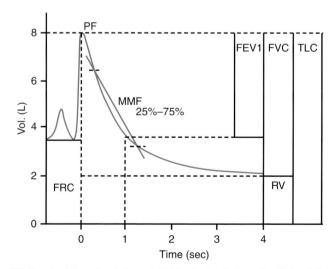

Fig. 6.2 Spirogram. *FEV1*, Forced expiratory volume in 1 second; *FRC*, functional residual capacity; *FVC*, forced vital capacity; *MMF*, mean maximal flow; *PF*, peak flow; *RV*, residual volume; *TLC*, total lung capacity.

KEY POINTS: PULMONARY FUNCTION TESTING

1. Abnormal PFTs identify patients who will benefit from aggressive perioperative pulmonary therapy and in whom general anesthesia should be avoided.
2. FVC, FEV1, the FEV1/FVC ratio, and FEF 25–75 (MMF 25–75) are the most clinically helpful indices obtained from spirometry.
3. No single PFT measurement absolutely contraindicates surgery. Factors, such as physical examination, arterial blood gases, and coexisting medical problems, also must be considered in determining suitability for surgery.

SUGGESTED READINGS

Akella A, Deshpande SB. Pulmonary surfactants and their role in pathophysiology of lung disorders. Indian J Exp Biol. 2013;51(1):5–22.

Feher J. Quantitative Human Physiology: An Introduction. 2nd ed. Cambridge, MA: Elsevier Academic Press; 2017.

Galvin I, Drummond GB, Nirmalan M. Distribution of blood flow and ventilation in the lung: gravity is not the only factor. Br J Anaesth. 2007;98 (4):420–428.

Han S, Mallampalli RK. The role of surfactant in lung disease and host defense against pulmonary infections. Ann Am Thorac Soc. 2015;12 (5):765–774.

Kavanagh BP, Hedenstierna G. Respiratory physiology and pathophysiology. In: Miller RD, ed. Miller's Anesthesia. 8th ed. Philadelphia: Elsevier Saunders; 2015: 444–472.

Lumb AB, Slinger P. Hypoxic pulmonary vasoconstriction: physiology and anesthetic implications. Anesthesiology. 2015;122(4):932–946.

CHAPTER 7

ARTERIAL BLOOD GAS ANALYSIS

Brian M. Keech, MD

1. **What information does an arterial blood gas provide?**
   Arterial blood gas (ABG) machines provide a direct measurement of partial pressure of oxygen in arterial blood (PaO_2), partial pressure of carbon dioxide in arterial blood ($PaCO_2$), pH by using electrodes that measure changes in voltage, current, and resistance. It uses this data to calculate bicarbonate ion (HCO_3^-), base excess, and oxygen saturation. ABG machines may also measure Na, K, iCa, glucose, and lactate.
   - **Oxygenation** (PaO_2). The PaO_2 is the amount of oxygen dissolved in blood and provides information on the efficiency of oxygenation.
   - **Ventilation** ($PaCO_2$). The adequacy of ventilation is inversely proportional to the $PaCO_2$.
   - **Acid-base status** (pH, HCO_3^-, and base excess). A pH greater than 7.45 indicates alkalemia, and a pH less than 7.35 indicates acidemia. The base excess measures the metabolic component of the acid-base disturbance.

2. **What is a CO-oximeter and what information does it provide?**
   A CO-oximeter is a device that measures hemoglobin absorbance of electromagnetic waves of varying wavelength. This can be used to measure total hemoglobin (tHb), oxyhemoglobin (O_2Hb), deoxyhemoglobin (HHb), methemoglobin (MetHb), and carboxyhemoglobin (COHb). A CO-oximeter is similar to a pulse oximeter, except a pulse oximeter only measures two wavelengths, which correspond to deoxyhemoglobin and oxyhemoglobin. However, a CO-oximeter can measure hundreds of wavelengths, which can be used to accurately measure the various molecular configurations of hemoglobin (e.g., COHb). Although some arterial blood gas machines include a CO-oximeter, many ABG machines do not have this functionality.

3. **What are the normal ABG values in a healthy patient breathing room air at sea level?**
   See Table 7.1.

4. **How is the regulation of acid-base balance traditionally described?**
   Acid-base balance is traditionally described using the Henderson-Hasselbalch equation, which states that changes in HCO_3^- and $PaCO_2$ determine pH by the following relationship:

   $$pH = 6.1 + \log\left(HCO_3^- / (0.03 \times PaCO_2)\right)$$

   To prevent a change in pH, any increase or decrease in the $PaCO_2$ should be accompanied by a compensatory increase or decrease in the HCO_3^-, and vice versa. The importance of other physiological noncarbonic acid buffers was later recognized and partly integrated into the base deficit and corrected anion gap (AG), both of which aid in interpreting complex acid-base disorders.

5. **What is meant by pH?**
   pH stands for "Power of the Hydrogen ion" and represents the negative logarithm of the hydrogen ion (H^+) concentration in the extracellular fluid. As with any "p" designation (signifying a negative logarithm), when the entities being measured get larger, the pH, pKa, and so on, get smaller. Normally the $[H^+]$ in extracellular fluid is 40×10^{-9} mol/L, a very small number. By taking the negative log of this value, we obtain a pH of 7.4, a much simpler way to describe $[H^+]$. Note, that because we are using a logarithmic scale, small changes in the pH represent large changes in the $[H^+]$ of the extracellular fluid. For example, a pH of 7.2 corresponds to a $[H^+]$ equal to 60×10^{-9} mol/L, an increase of 50%!

6. **Why is the pH of the extracellular fluid important?**
   The pH of the extracellular fluid is important because hydrogen ions react highly with cellular proteins, altering their function. Avoiding acidemia and alkalemia by tightly regulating hydrogen ions is essential for normal cellular function. Deviations from the normal pH of 7.4 suggest that some physiological processes are in disorder and causes need to be determined and treated.

7. **What are the major consequences of acidemia?**
   Severe acidemia is defined as a blood pH lower than 7.20 and is associated with the following major effects:
   - Impairment of cardiac contractility and cardiac output
   - Impaired responsiveness to catecholamines
   - Increased susceptibility to dysrhythmias
   - Arteriolar vasodilation resulting in hypotension
   - Vasoconstriction of the pulmonary vasculature and subsequent increased pulmonary vascular resistance

Table 7.1 Arterial Blood Gas Values at Sea Level

pH	7.35–7.45
$PaCO_2$	35–45 mm Hg
PaO_2	80–100 mm Hg
HCO_3^-	22–26 mmol/L
BE (base excess)	0 ± 2 mmol/L
Oxygen saturation (SaO_2)	>95%

HCO_3^-, Bicarbonate; $PaCO_2$, partial pressure of carbon dioxide in arterial blood; PaO_2, partial pressure of oxygen in arterial blood.

- Centralization of blood volume, eventually leading to pulmonary edema and dyspnea
- Hyperventilation (a compensatory response)
- Confusion, obtundation, and coma
- Insulin resistance
- Inhibition of glycolysis and adenosine triphosphate synthesis
- Coagulopathy
- Hyperkalemia (occurs primarily with metabolic acidosis but not respiratory acidosis)

8. **What are the major consequences of alkalemia?**
Severe alkalemia is defined as blood pH greater than 7.60 and is associated with the following major effects:
- Increased cardiac contractility until pH greater than 7.7, when a decrease is seen
- Refractory ventricular dysrhythmias
- Coronary artery vasoconstriction
- Hypoventilation (which can lead to hypercapnia and hypoxemia in spontaneously ventilating patients). In patients who are being mechanically ventilated, weaning may be made more difficult as a result of hypoventilation
- Cerebral vasoconstriction
- Neurological manifestations, such as lethargy, delirium, stupor, tetany, and seizures
- Hypokalemia, hypocalcemia, hypomagnesemia, and hypophosphatemia
- Stimulation of anaerobic glycolysis and lactate production

9. **What are the common acid-base disorders and their respective compensations?**
See Table 7.2.

10. **How do you quantify the respiratory and/or renal degree of compensation?**
See Table 7.3.

11. **Can these compensations be represented graphically?**
Yes (Fig. 7.1).

12. **What are the major acid-base buffering systems of the body?**
Bicarbonate, albumin, hemoglobin, and phosphate are the major buffering systems. The major extracellular buffer is HCO_3^-. The major intracellular buffers are the organic phosphates (adenosine monophosphate, adenosine diphosphate, adenosine triphosphate, 2,3-biphosphoglyceric acid), imidazole, and amino groups on proteins and hemoglobin. Phosphate and ammonia are important urinary buffers.

Table 7.2 Major Acid-Base Disorders and Compensatory Mechanisms

PRIMARY DISORDER	PRIMARY DISTURBANCE	PRIMARY COMPENSATION
Respiratory acidosis	↑ $PaCO_2$	↑ HCO_3^-
Respiratory alkalosis	↓ $PaCO_2$	↓ HCO_3^-
Metabolic acidosis	↓ HCO_3^-	↓ $PaCO_2$
Metabolic alkalosis	↑ HCO_3^-	↑ $PaCO_2$

Primary compensation for metabolic disorders is achieved rapidly through respiratory control of CO_2, whereas primary compensation for respiratory disorders is achieved more slowly as the kidneys excrete or absorb acid and bicarbonate. Mixed acid-base disorders are common.
HCO_3^-, Bicarbonate; $PaCO_2$, partial pressure of carbon dioxide in arterial blood.

Table 7.3 Calculating the Degree of Compensation

PRIMARY DISORDER	RULE
Respiratory acidosis (acute)	HCO_3^- increases $0.1 \times (PaCO_2 - 40)$ pH decreases $0.008 \times (PaCO_2 - 40)$
Respiratory acidosis (chronic)	HCO_3^- increases $0.4 \times (PaCO_2 - 40)$
Respiratory alkalosis (acute)	HCO_3^- decreases $0.2 \times (40 - PaCO_2)$ pH increases $0.008 \times (40 - PaCO_2)$
Respiratory alkalosis (chronic)	HCO_3^- decreases $0.4 \times (40 - PaCO_2)$
Metabolic acidosis	$PaCO_2$ decreases 1 to $1.5 \times (24 - HCO_3^-)$
Metabolic alkalosis	$PaCO_2$ increases 0.25 to $1 \times (HCO_3^- - 24)$

Compensatory mechanisms never overcorrect for an acid-base disturbance; when arterial blood gas analysis reveals apparent overcorrection, the presence of a mixed disorder should be suspected.
HCO_3^-, Bicarbonate; $PaCO_2$, partial pressure of carbon dioxide in arterial blood.
Data from Schrier RW. Renal and Electrolyte Disorders. 3rd ed. Boston: Little, Brown; 1986.

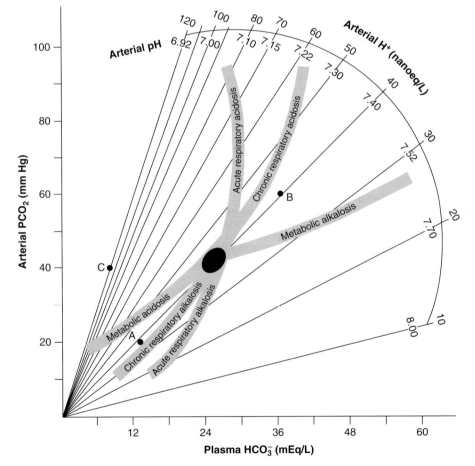

Fig. 7.1 The Davenport Diagram illustrates the relationship between CO_2, HCO_3^-, and pH as governed by the Henderson-Hasselbalch equation.

The extracellular bicarbonate system is the quickest to respond to changes in pH, but has less total capacity than the intracellular systems, which account for 60% to 70% of the chemical buffering of the body. Hydrogen ions are in dynamic equilibrium with all buffering systems through the following relationship:

$$H + HCO_3^- \leftrightarrow H_2CO_3 \leftarrow (Carbonic\ anhydrase) \rightarrow CO_2 + H_2O$$

CO_2 molecules readily cross cell membranes and keep both intracellular and extracellular buffering systems in dynamic equilibrium. In addition, CO_2 has the added advantage of being excreted through ventilation.

13. What are the common causes of respiratory acid-base disorders?

- **Respiratory alkalosis:** sepsis, hypoxemia, anxiety, pain, altitude and central nervous system lesions
- **Respiratory acidosis:** drugs (residual anesthetics, residual neuromuscular blockade, benzodiazepines, opioids), asthma, chronic obstructive pulmonary disease, obesity-hypoventilation syndromes, obstructive sleep apnea, central nervous system lesions (infection, stroke), and neuromuscular disorders

14. What are the common causes of a metabolic alkalosis?

Metabolic alkalosis is commonly caused by vomiting, volume contraction (diuretics, dehydration), alkali administration, and endocrine disorders.

15. What is the anion gap?

The AG is used to further evaluate metabolic acidosis. It is equal to the sum of measured cations minus the sum of measured anions:

$$AG = (Na^+ + K^+) - (Cl^- + HCO_3^-)$$

Note, some sources omit potassium in the earlier equation, in which case the calculated AG would decrease by a commensurate amount (i.e., 2–4 mEq/L).

16. What is the normal anion gap and what accounts for this?

A normal AG is 14 to 18 mEq/L, if potassium is included; otherwise a normal AG is 12 to 14 mEq/L, if only sodium is used. This may lead one to believe that there are more cations than anions in plasma. However, this is not the case. To maintain electroneutrality, the number of Na^+ and K^+ ions, along with all unmeasured cations in plasma, is equal to the number of Cl^-, HCO_3^-, and all unmeasured anions in plasma. What this tells us about the calculated AG is that there are more unmeasured anions than unmeasured cations in plasma under normal circumstances. The primary unmeasured cations include magnesium and calcium, while the primary unmeasured anions include albumin, phosphate, and sulfate.

17. What is the AG used for?

The AG is used to narrow the differential diagnosis of a metabolic acidosis into either normal or high AG metabolic acidosis.

18. What is the effect of albumin on the AG?

Albumin is one of the primary unmeasured anions that need to be considered in interpreting AG calculations. It is often low in critically ill patients, which decreases the unmeasured anions and lowers the AG. This normally is not a problem unless a patient with hypoalbuminemia has a metabolic acidosis causing the AG to appear normal when it would otherwise be elevated. The following equation can be used to correct for hypoalbuminemia:

$$Corrected\ AG = Calculated\ AG + (2.5 \times [normal\ albumin - measured\ albumin])$$

19. What additional laboratory studies are useful in evaluating an elevated anion gap metabolic acidosis?

Additional studies include serum ketones (and beta-hydroxybutyrate), lactate, creatinine, and serum osmolal gap.

KEY POINTS: MAJOR CAUSES OF A HIGH ANION GAP METABOLIC ACIDOSIS

- Lactic acidosis
- Ketoacidosis
- End-stage renal disease
- Toxins (e.g., methanol, salicylates, acetaminophen, ethylene glycol, propylene glycol)

KEY POINTS: MAJOR CAUSES OF A NORMAL ANION GAP METABOLIC ACIDOSIS

- Iatrogenic administration of hyperchloremic solutions (e.g., normal saline)
- Alkaline gastrointestinal losses (e.g., diarrhea)
- Renal tubular acidosis
- Carbonic anhydrase inhibitors
- Ureteric diversion through an ileal conduit

20. **Is the HCO_3^- value on the ABG the same as the CO_2 value on the chemistry panel?**
    No. The ABG HCO_3^- is calculated using the Henderson-Hasselbalch equation and the measured values of pH and $PaCO_2$. In contrast, a chemistry panel reports a measured serum carbon dioxide content (CO_2), which is the sum of the measured bicarbonate (HCO_3^-) and carbonic acid (H_2CO_3). The CO_2 is viewed as an accurate determination of HCO_3^- because the HCO_3^- concentration in blood is about 20 times greater than the H_2CO_3 concentration; thus, H_2CO_3 is only a minor contributor to the total measured CO_2.

21. **What is the base deficit (BD)?**
    The BD or base excess (BE) is a measurement of the metabolic component of the acid-base disturbance. It is defined as the amount of HCO_3^- that needs to be given (or removed) to return the serum pH back to 7.4 under standard conditions ($PaCO_2$ 40 mm Hg and temperature 37°C). BE and BD are often used interchangeably, where BE is the negative of BD.

22. **What is the Δ/Δ? What is its clinical utility?**
    The ratio of the change in AG to the change in HCO_3^- is known as the Δ/Δ and is usually 1:1. If the Δ/Δ is less than 1, a mixed acid-base disorder should be suspected; namely a normal AG metabolic acidosis is occurring with the high AG metabolic acidosis. Conversely, a ratio of greater than 1 suggests a metabolic alkalosis occurring concurrently with the high AG metabolic acidosis. Thus the Δ/Δ is useful for further evaluating the clinical scenario surrounding high AG metabolic acidosis.

23. **Is sodium bicarbonate indicated in the treatment of metabolic acidosis?**
    Sodium bicarbonate is only indicated in the presence of a very low pH (i.e., <7.20). A pH below 7.20 will depress cardiac function, cause severe vasodilation, and increase the heart's susceptibility to a lethal dysrhythmia.
    It is important to note that sodium bicarbonate will produce CO_2, which can readily diffuse across cell membranes. Therefore it is important that the patient has the respiratory reserve to transiently increase their minute ventilation. Otherwise, sodium bicarbonate could worsen the patient's condition as the metabolic acidosis will become respiratory acidosis, and the CO_2 will diffuse across cell membranes causing intracellular acidosis.

24. **How does metabolic acidosis cause hyperkalemia?**
    Various cellular transmembrane proteins act as channels, transporters, and pumps regulating intracellular electrolytes and acid-base balance. The net effect of these transmembrane proteins acting in concert leads to the so-called potassium-hydrogen antiporter, which is a conceptual model describing the net effect where intracellular potassium ions are exchanged for extracellular hydrogen ions depending upon the transmembrane pH gradient.

25. **Does respiratory acidosis cause hyperkalemia?**
    No, only metabolic acidosis causes clinically significant hyperkalemia. Studies show that respiratory acidosis either causes minimal or no change to extracellular potassium. In respiratory acidosis, carbon dioxide readily diffuses across the lipid bilayer causing both intracellular and extracellular acidosis. However, in metabolic acidosis, the acid does not readily diffuse across the lipid bilayer causing primarily extracellular acidosis, which creates a pH gradient facilitating the exchange of intracellular potassium for extracellular hydrogen ions. By this same logic, hyperventilation is not an effective treatment for hyperkalemia.

KEY POINTS:

1. Acid-base balance is traditionally described using the Henderson-Hasselbalch equation, which states that HCO_3^- and $PaCO_2$ determine pH.
2. Bicarbonate, albumin, hemoglobin, and phosphate are the major buffering systems of the body.
3. The AG is used to delineate the causes of metabolic acidosis.
4. The BD (or BE) is the amount of base (i.e., bicarbonate) that would need to be given (or removed) to return the patient's acid-base disturbance back to normal conditions (pH 7.4, $PaCO_2$ 40 mm Hg, and temperature 37° C).
5. Bicarbonate supplementation is only indicated in the presence of a pH less than 7.20, because cardiac function is severely compromised with severe acidosis.
6. Metabolic acidosis can cause hyperkalemia, which is rarely seen with respiratory acidosis.

SUGGESTED READINGS

Berend K. Diagnostic use of base excess in acid-base disorders. N Engl J Med. 2018;378(15):1419–1428.
Kraut JA, Madias NE. Lactic acidosis. N Eng J Med. 2014;371(2):2309–2319.
Morris CG, Low J. Metabolic acidosis in the critically ill. Part 1. Classification and pathophysiology. Anaesthesia. 2008;63:294–301.
Morris CG, Low J. Metabolic acidosis in the critically ill. Part 2. Cause and treatment. Anaesthesia. 2008;63:396–411.
Neligan PJ, Deutschman CS. Perioperative acid-base balance. In: Miller RD, ed. Miller's Anesthesia. 8th ed. Philadelphia: Elsevier Saunders; 2015:1811–1839, e2.
Rastegar A. Use of the $\Delta AG/\Delta HCO_3^-$ ratio in the diagnosis of mixed acid-base disorders. J Am Soc Nephrol. 2007;18:2429–2431.

CHAPTER 8

VOLUME REGULATION AND FLUID REPLACEMENT

David J. Douin, MD, Ryan D. Laterza, MD

1. **Describe the functionally distinct compartments of body water.**
   Total body water comprises approximately 60% of body weight. About two-thirds of body water (40% of body weight) is in the intracellular fluid compartment and one-third (20% of body weight) is in the extracellular compartment. Of the fluid in the extracellular compartment, three-quarters (15% of body weight) is comprised of interstitial fluid and one-quarter (5% of body weight) is plasma volume. An easy way to remember this is to think of body water following the "20-40-60" rule: 20% extracellular, 40% intracellular, 60% total body water. Fig. 8.1 estimates body water compartments in a patient with an ideal body weight of 70 kg. Note, accurate estimations can sometimes be difficult in obese patients.

2. **Describe the dynamics of fluid distribution between plasma and the endothelial glycocalyx.**
   Sterling's principle is the traditional model that describes filtration between the intravascular and interstitial space. Recent evidence suggests this may not capture the entire story of fluid transfer, and a new entity known as the *endothelial glycocalyx* has been proposed. The revised Sterling's principle:

   $$\frac{J_v}{A} = L_p \left[(P_c - P_i) - \sigma(\pi_p - \pi_{sg}) \right]$$

   accounts for the endothelial glycocalyx and supports the theory that filtration continues throughout the length of the capillary bed and that reabsorption from the interstitial space does not occur. Net filtration therefore is governed by endothelial glycocalyx, endothelial basement membrane, and the extracellular matrix.
   Note: J_v/A is volume filtered per area; L_p is hydraulic conductance; P_c is capillary hydrostatic pressure; P_i is interstitial hydrostatic pressure; σ is osmotic reflection; π_p is oncotic pressure on the plasma side of the endothelial layer; π_{sg} is the oncotic pressure in the subglycocalyx space.

3. **What is the normal range for serum osmolarity and how is it calculated?**
   Different sources quote different ranges, but in general, normal serum osmolarity ranges between 285 and 305 mOsm/L. A quick rough estimate is to double the sodium concentration. A more accurate estimate of osmolarity can be obtained using the following equation:

   $$Serum\ Osmolarity \left(\frac{mOsm}{L} \right) = 2 \times [Na] + \frac{Glucose}{18} + \frac{BUN}{2.8}$$

   United States Customary System (imperial system)

   $$Serum\ Osmolarity \left(\frac{mOsm}{L} \right) = 2 \times [Na] + Glucose + BUN$$

   International Systems of Units (metric system)

   Note that the units for the United States Customary System (imperial system) for solutes are sodium (mEq/L), glucose (mg/dL), and BUN (mg/dL), whereas the SI system are all in mmol/L. Some textbooks may use the term osmolality with units mOsm/kg, which is essentially equivalent to osmolarity, because 1 L of water = 1 kg of water. Finally, appreciate the fact that for nation states who have embraced the metric system, the equation is much simpler.

4. **How are body water and tonicity regulated?**
   The response of the kidney to antidiuretic hormone (ADH), also called *vasopressin*, is the primary mechanism by which body water and tonicity are regulated. It is released by the posterior pituitary and circulates unbound in plasma. It has a half-life of approximately 20 minutes and increases the expression of aquaporin channels in the distal convoluted tubule and collecting duct of the nephron. This increases tubular permeability to water, resulting in increased resorption of free water and increased urine concentration. Stimuli for the release of ADH include the following:
   - Hypothalamic osmoreceptors facilitate the release of ADH in response to hyperosmolarity
   - Hypothalamic thirst center neurons regulate conscious desire for water in response to hyperosmolarity
   - Aortic baroreceptors and left atrial stretch receptors respond to hypotension and hypovolemia, respectively, facilitating the release of ADH
   - Increased sympathetic tone from stress, such as in surgery or critical illness

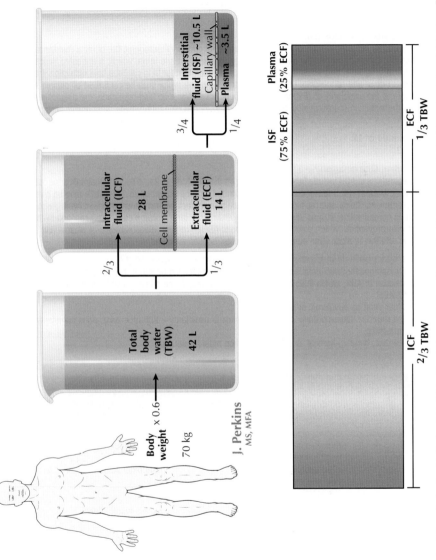

Fig. 8.1 Body water compartments in a patient with an ideal body weight of 70 kg. (From Mulroney, SE., Myers, AK. The cell and fluid homeostasis. In: Netter's Essential Physiology. Philadelphia: Elsevier; 2015:2–11. © 2016. Fig. 1.4.)

Note that hypovolemia and hypotension take precedence over osmolarity; therefore ADH may be secreted to maintain volume at the expense of osmolarity.

5. **Discuss the synthesis of ADH.**
ADH, or vasopressin, is synthesized in the supraoptic and paraventricular nuclei of the hypothalamus. It is transported by carrier proteins down the pituitary stalk in secretory granules to the posterior pituitary gland. There, it is stored and subsequently released into the capillaries of the posterior pituitary in response to stimuli from the hypothalamus. ADH-producing neurons receive efferent innervation from osmoreceptors and baroreceptors.

6. **List the conditions that stimulate and inhibit the release of ADH.**
See Table 8.1.

7. **What is diabetes insipidus (DI)?**
DI can be caused by impaired release of ADH from the posterior pituitary (neurogenic DI), or renal resistance to ADH (nephrogenic DI). The end result is the excretion of large volumes of dilute urine, which, if untreated, leads to dehydration, hypernatremia, and serum hyperosmolarity. The usual test for DI is cautious fluid restriction. Inability to decrease urine output and concentrate urine suggests the diagnosis, which may be confirmed by plasma ADH measurements. If the osmolarity of plasma exceeds that of urine after mild fluid restriction, the diagnosis of DI is suggested. Administration of intravenous desmopressin (DDAVP) can help differentiate nephrogenic versus neurogenic DI.

8. **List the causes of DI.**
See Table 8.2.

9. **How is central DI managed?**
Available preparations of ADH include DDAVP, 2 to 4 mcg intravenously every 2 to 4 hours to maintain urine output less than 300 mL/h. Alternatively, intravenous vasopressin titrated to urine output up to 2.4 units/h may be given. Hypotonic maintenance fluids, such as dextrose 5% may be given to replace the free water deficit. Avoid giving isotonic fluids, such as normal saline (NS) as this can increase serum osmolarity. Incomplete DI may respond to thiazide diuretics or chlorpropamide (which potentiates endogenous ADH). Frequent measurements of plasma and urine osmolarity, in addition to strict urine output measurements, is often indicated.

10. **Define the syndrome of inappropriate ADH. How do you diagnose it?**
Syndrome of inappropriate antidiuretic hormone (SIADH) is characterized by serum hypotonicity caused by the nonosmotic release of ADH, which inhibits renal excretion of water. Three criteria must be met to establish the diagnosis of SIADH:
1. The patient must be euvolemic or hypervolemic
2. The urine must be inappropriately concentrated (plasma osmolarity <280 mOsm/kg, urine osmolarity >100 mOsm/kg)
3. Renal, cardiac, hepatic, adrenal, and thyroid function must be normal

Table 8.1 Conditions that Stimulate and Inhibit Release of Antidiuretic Hormone

	STIMULATES ANTIDIURETIC HORMONE RELEASE	INHIBITS ANTIDIURETIC HORMONE RELEASE
Normal physiological states	Hyperosmolarity Hypovolemia Upright position β-Adrenergic stimulation Pain and emotional stress Cholinergic stimulation	Hypoosmolarity Hypervolemia Supine position α-Adrenergic stimulation
Abnormal physiological states	Hemorrhagic shock Hyperthermia Increased intracranial pressure Positive airway pressure Metabolic and respiratory acidosis	Excess water intake Hypothermia
Medications	Morphine Nicotine Barbiturates Tricyclic antidepressants Chlorpropamide	Ethanol Atropine Phenytoin Glucocorticoids Chlorpromazine
Results	Oliguria, concentrated urine	Polyuria, dilute urine

Table 8.2 Causes of Diabetes Insipidus

VASOPRESSIN DEFICIENCY (NEUROGENIC DIABETES INSIPIDUS)	VASOPRESSIN INSENSITIVITY (NEPHROGENIC DIABETES INSIPIDUS)
Familial (autosomal-dominant)	Familial (X-linked recessive)
Acquired	Acquired
Idiopathic	Pyelonephritis
Craniofacial, basilar skull fractures	Postrenal obstruction
Pituitary tumors, lymphoma, metastasis	Sickle cell disease and trait
Granuloma (sarcoidosis, histiocytosis)	Amyloidosis
Central nervous system infections	Hypokalemia, hypercalcemia
Sheehan syndrome	Sarcoidosis
Hypoxic brain injury, brain herniation, or brain death	Lithium
Pituitary Surgery	

11. How do you manage SIADH? Why can you not just give normal saline to raise the sodium?
The primary therapy for SIADH is water restriction and is usually adequate for asymptomatic hyponatremia. Postoperative SIADH is often stress related and resolves spontaneously. Chronic SIADH may require the addition of demeclocycline, which blocks the ADH-mediated water resorption in the collecting ducts of the kidney, or vaptans, such as tolvaptan, which are ADH receptor antagonists.

Patients with severe symptomatic hyponatremia caused by SIADH should be admitted to the intensive care unit for close monitoring, and treatment with hypertonic saline should be considered. The primary symptom of hyponatremia is altered mental status because of cerebral edema and increased intracranial pressure (ICP) caused by decreased serum osmolarity. Hyponatremia can be fatal if not managed correctly.

Administering isotonic fluid to patients with hyponatremia will not help. In fact, it will worsen the underlying problem of hyponatremia. The kidney can concentrate urine to a maximum of 1200 mOsm/L. Therefore it can concentrate 1 L of NS (308 mOsm/L) into approximately 250 mL of urine. The other 750 mL will be retained as free water, causing a further decrease in serum sodium.

12. What disorders are associated with SIADH?
Central nervous system events are frequent causes, including acute intracranial hypertension, trauma, tumors, meningitis, and subarachnoid hemorrhage. Pulmonary causes are also common, including tuberculosis, pneumonia, asthma, bronchiectasis, hypoxemia, hypercarbia, and positive-pressure ventilation. Malignancies may produce ADH-like compounds. Adrenal insufficiency and hypothyroidism also have been associated with SIADH.

13. Discuss stress-induced hyponatremia. Why is it common intraoperatively and/or in the setting of critical illness and why is urine output a poor indicator of volume status in these situations?
Stressful situations, such as surgery and critical illness, increase sympathetic tone, which facilitates ADH release and activates the renin-angiotensin-aldosterone system. This causes the kidney to reabsorb free water, thereby decreasing urine output despite no change in overall volume status (i.e., the patient is not hypovolemic). This may result in a mild dilutional hyponatremia from the sympathetic-meditated release of ADH, termed *stress-induced* hyponatremia. Therefore urine output in isolation is a poor indicator of intraoperative volume status. Regardless, a low urine output should not be ignored as acute kidney injury is an independent predictor of perioperative mortality.

14. What is aldosterone? What stimulates its release? What are its actions?
Aldosterone is responsible for the control of sodium excretion. The juxtaglomerular cells of the kidney are stimulated to release renin in response to a decrease in renal or systemic arterial blood pressure, hypovolemia, and/or hyponatremia. Circulating angiotensinogen, produced in the liver, is converted by renin to angiotensin I. Angiotensin I is converted to angiotensin II by the angiotensin-converting enzyme, found in the lung. Angiotensin II then stimulates the zona glomerulosa of the adrenal cortex to release aldosterone, a mineralocorticoid. Additional effects of angiotensin II are systemic vasoconstriction and facilitating the release of ADH. Aldosterone acts on the distal renal tubules and cortical collecting ducts, activating sodium/potassium pumps to reabsorb three sodium ions for every two potassium ions excreted. The end result of this is net fluid retention. In addition to hyponatremia and hypovolemia, stimuli for aldosterone release include hyperkalemia, increased levels of adrenocorticotropic hormone, and increased sympathetic tone (e.g., stress from surgery).

15. **What are some of the causes of perioperative fluid status derangements?**
Preoperative hypovolemia may be caused by bowel prep, active blood loss, or inflammatory processes, such as sepsis, pancreatitis, or small bowel obstruction. Of note, fasting for 10 + hours before an elective procedure does not appear to contribute significantly to preoperative hypovolemia. In fact, current evidence does not support the routing replacement of this perceived volume deficit intraoperatively.

Several intraoperative factors can also affect fluid status. Many anesthetic medications or procedures (e.g., spinal anesthesia) cause venous and arterial vasodilation with subsequent hypotension (i.e., decreased preload and vascular resistance, respectively), which may be mistaken as hypovolemia. Decreasing the anesthetic depth or administering a low dose vasopressor (thereby normalizing venous and arterial tone) should be attempted first before replacing perceived fluid losses with significant amounts of volume. Procedure-related blood loss, evaporative losses, and third-spacing are more likely causes of hypovolemia in the perioperative period and should be treated with evidence-based volume resuscitation strategies.

16. **What are the consequences of intraoperative hypovolemia (or hypervolemia)?**
Hypovolemia is common in the perioperative period because of the mechanisms described previously. It can lead to decreased cardiac output and tissue perfusion, which can progress to shock physiology. Hypervolemia can also contribute to perioperative morbidity. It can contribute to pulmonary edema, bowel edema, wound edema, and dilution of coagulation factors, which can exacerbate blood loss. Appropriate volume resuscitation without under- or overresuscitating the patient is of paramount importance.

17. **What is contraction alkalosis and how should it be treated?**
Contraction alkalosis, more accurately termed *chloride depletion alkalosis*, most often occurs in patients who have both hypovolemia and hypochloremia. Common examples include patients who are given diuretics (i.e., hypovolemia) with salt restriction (i.e., hypochloremia), such as in heart failure, or because of upper gastrointestinal losses (e.g., vomiting or nasogastric suction causing loss of volume and chloride,) such as in pyloric stenosis or small bowel obstruction. Without going into the exact detail of the various transporters involved at the level of the nephron, the overall net effect is that bicarbonate is preferentially reabsorbed because of chloride depletion to maintain electroneutrality. Further, aldosterone-mediated renal hydrogen secretion also likely plays an important role in the pathophysiology of contraction alkalosis.

Patients with chloride depletion alkalosis need both chloride and volume resuscitation. If these patients are given chloride supplementation alone without volume resuscitation, the underlying acid-base disturbance will rapidly correct despite remaining hypovolemic. Further, if these patients are given volume without chloride supplementation (i.e., albumin), the metabolic alkalosis will persist despite being euvolemic. Therefore patients with contraction alkalosis really have two problems: hypochloremia and hypovolemia, and both need to be treated as such with high chloride-containing solutions (i.e., NS).

18. **How much fluid is appropriate to administer during a surgical procedure?**
The application of poorly quantifiable methods, such as insensible fluid loss and third-space fluid migration has led to overresuscitation and fluid balances in excess of what is necessary. Arbitrary fluid administration significantly increases the risk of hypervolemia and associated complications.

Recent literature suggests patients undergoing abdominal surgery who received restrictive fluid maintenance intraoperatively (3–5 mL/kg/h) had better outcomes when compared with patients receiving liberal fluid resuscitation (10–12 mL/kg/h). Improved outcomes included quicker return of bowel function, increased hematocrit and serum albumin, improved wound healing, and shorter length of stay. Fluid restriction is particularly important in patients undergoing thoracotomy and lung resections because of concern for postoperative pulmonary edema. Using dynamic measurements of volume status, such as pulse pressure variation and stroke volume variation have recently gained favor as a method to predict fluid responsiveness and decrease inappropriate fluid administration. These are discussed in detail in other chapters. Remember, the goal is optimizing, not maximizing, intravascular volume.

19. **Review the composition of crystalloid solutions and their clinical use.**
Fluid resuscitation in the operating room is usually accomplished with balanced salt solutions, such as Plasma-Lyte or Ringer's lactate (aka lactated Ringer's [LR]). The tonicity and electrolyte composition of balanced salt solutions are more consistent with the extracellular fluid loses that occur during surgery compared with hypotonic solutions or NS.

Patients requiring maintenance fluids are often treated with hypotonic fluids (e.g., 0.45% NS), because their fluid losses are thought to primarily include free water, which is true in healthy patients not suffering from an acute illness. However, patients with an acute illness (i.e., most hospitalized patients) often have elevated circulating levels of sympathetic mediated ADH predisposing these patients to hyponatremia. Evidence to date recommends using isotonic or balanced salt solutions for maintenance fluids instead of hypotonic fluids to minimize this risk. Maintenance fluids often include 5% dextrose to minimize the risk of tissue catabolism and to prevent hypoglycemia. It is important emphasize that the 5% dextrose used in maintenance fluids is inadequate in patients with prolonged malnutrition (e.g., >7 days), or who are already presenting with significant malnourishment. In these situations, total parental nutrition is advised.

Please refer to Table 8.3 to review the composition of NS, LR, and Plasma-Lyte.

Table 8.3 Isotonic Crystalloid Solutions

	OSMOLARITY[A]	pH	Na⁺	Cl⁻	K⁺	Ca²⁺	Mg²⁺	LACTATE	ACETATE	GLUCONATE
NS	308	5.5	154	154	—	—	—	—	—	—
LR	273	6.5	130	109	4	3	0	28	—	—
Plasma-Lyte	294	7.4	140	98	5	—	3	—	27	23

[A]Osmolarity is measured in mOsm/L; other substances are measured in mEq/L.
LR, Ringer's lactate; *NS,* normal saline.

20. Why is the pH of normal saline low and how do balanced salt solutions maintain a normal physiological pH? Why do manufactures not just add bicarbonate to normal saline?
    The pH of NS itself is approximately 5.5; however, when stored in polyvinyl chloride (PVC) packaged bags, which is usually the case, it can be as low as 4.6. This occurs because of the following: (1) atmospheric air contained within the packaged bag of saline contains carbon dioxide, which dissolves in the saline solution and reacts with water to form carbonic acid, yielding a pH of 5.5; and (2) PVC is known to produce small amounts of hydrochloric acid when moist, which further lowers the pH.
    These concerns are attenuated with the use of LR (pH 6.5) or Plasma-Lyte (pH 7.4) because the pH of these solutions more closely mimics that of plasma. LR, also known as *lactated Ringer's solution* or *Hartmann's solution,* contains lactate, which is converted by the liver into bicarbonate. Plasma-Lyte contains gluconate and acetate which, for the most part, are also converted by the liver into bicarbonate.
    Manufactured crystalloid solutions do not use bicarbonate for two reasons. First, bicarbonate will react with water to form carbon dioxide, which after a prolong period of time, will diffuse out of solution and out through the packaging material. Second, bicarbonate may lead to precipitation of calcium and magnesium.

21. How could you make a crystalloid solution using sodium bicarbonate for patients with metabolic acidosis (e.g., end-stage renal disease [ESRD]) which does not contain potassium?
    Sodium bicarbonate may be added to 0.45% NS or 5% dextrose solution to create an alkalotic crystalloid solution for immediate use. One 50 mL ampule of 8.4% sodium bicarbonate (1 mEq/mL) has a pH of 7.0 to 8.5, which can be mixed with 1 L of 5% dextrose solution or 0.45% half-NS to produce solutions that contain a similar or higher pH than balanced salt solutions. Recall from basic chemistry, that an "equivalent" equals the number of moles of an ion multiplied by its valence (positive or negative charge). For example, 1 L of 0.9% NS (308 mOsm/L) has 154 mEq (or 154 mmol) of Na⁺ and 154 mEq (or 154 mmol) of Cl⁻, whereas in comparison, 1 mmol of Ca²⁺ equals 2 mEq of Ca²⁺. Note that equivalence is an antiquated method of measurement that has been replaced by moles in countries outside of the United States, which use the more scientific International System of Units (SI), formerly known as the *metric system.*
    Now back to our example, assuming complete disassociation, 1 mEq/mL (or 1 mmol/mL) of sodium bicarbonate will yield 1 mmol/mL of Na⁺ and 1 mmol/mL of HCO_3^-. Therefore adding sodium bicarbonate (solute) to water (solvent) will increase the solution's osmolarity by 2 mOsm/L for every 1 mL of sodium bicarbonate added. Note, this is neglecting the increase in volume of the solution because of adding the solute. For example, 1.5 ampules of sodium bicarbonate (50 mL/ampule) will contain 75 mmol of Na⁺ and 75 mmol of HCO_3^-. If 1.5 ampules of sodium bicarbonate is added to 1 L of 0.45% (half-normal) saline (77 mmol Na⁺ + 77 mmol Cl⁻) the final solution will have an approximate osmolarity of 304 mOsm/L (77 mmol Na⁺ + 77 mmol Cl⁻ + 75 mmol Na⁺ + 75 mmol HCO_3^- divided by 1 L of H_2O). Note again, this is neglecting the increase in solution volume by adding solute. By this same logic, three ampules of sodium bicarbonate added to 1 L of 5% dextrose solution will yield an isotonic solution with an effective osmolarity of 300 mOsm/L. Patients with ESRD often have metabolic acidosis and may benefit from creating a solution of half-NS with 1.5 ampules of sodium bicarbonate as the solution will have a higher pH than NS but will not contain potassium like other balanced salt solutions.

22. What are the disadvantages of administering large volumes of normal saline versus a balanced salt solution (i.e., Ringer's lactate or Plasma-Lyte)?
    NS contains 154 mEq/L of both sodium and chloride both of which are far greater than normal plasma levels. In addition, the pH of NS is 4.6 to 5.5, well below that of normal plasma pH (7.4). Thus when large volumes of NS are administered, plasma pH decreases and chloride increases, resulting in a hyperchloremic metabolic acidosis. This may exacerbate any acidosis already present (e.g., lactic acidosis because of hemorrhage). Further, balanced salt solutions contain additional electrolytes (i.e., calcium, magnesium, and potassium) and more closely reflects the contents of extracellular fluid.

23. Can Ringer's lactate or Plasma-Lyte safely be used in patients with end-stage renal disease?
    Yes, and evidence to date demonstrates that these solutions result in less hyperkalemia than NS. Although NS is often given in clinical practice because of its lack of potassium, LR and Plasma-Lyte can both be administered safely to patients with ESRD. The amount of potassium in these solutions per liter is 4 mEq and 5 mEq, respectively, which is

very small compared with the total body stores of potassium. Precipitating hyperkalemia from the administration of either LR or Plasma-Lyte is extremely unlikely, as the crystalloid fluid cannot raise the potassium to a higher concentration than that of the fluid itself.

Because ESRD patients often have an associated metabolic acidosis, solutions with increased pH (such as LR or Plasma-Lyte) may be advantageous versus using NS, which has a pH or 5.5 or less. In fact, studies show that potassium levels are lower with balanced salt solutions than NS in patients undergoing kidney transplantation. This is most likely from the metabolic acidosis associated with using NS, which increases serum potassium. Another reasonable option may include using 0.45% half-NS with 1.5 ampules of sodium bicarbonate, which not only increases the pH but is also void of potassium.

24. **What is the concern about administering LR concurrently through the same intravenous line as blood products?**
Calcium is an important cofactor in the coagulation cascade and is removed from blood products by using chelating agents, such as citrate, to prevent clotting during storage. Most crystalloid fluids are void of calcium and therefore will not precipitate clot if mixed with packed red cells. However, LR contains calcium and theoretically could cause packed red blood cells to clot. Note that in common practice, if the blood transfusion is given quickly, this is unlikely to occur. In controlled situations, LR should ideally be avoided when transfusing blood products, unless the situation is emergent.

25. **Are there distinct advantages to using colloids versus crystalloids during resuscitation?**
There is ongoing debate over this issue. Colloid advocates claim that because these solutions have a long intravascular half-life of 3 to 6 hours, they are superior resuscitation fluids. However, when compared with crystalloids in multiple randomized controlled trials, the use of colloids has not been shown to improve outcomes. Further, during situations in which there is increased capillary permeability (e.g., burns, sepsis, trauma), colloids accumulate within the interstitial space, pulling other fluids along, and lead to edema. This is particularly concerning in the setting of traumatic brain injury (TBI), where the use of albumin increases ICP and results in increased mortality.

Although only 250 mL of every 1 L of crystalloid remains intravascular, crystalloids are recommended over albumin for fluid resuscitation. It should be noted that dehydrated patients suffer from fluid deficits both intracellularly and extracellularly, and crystalloids may help to replete both compartments despite being isotonic to the extracellular space. Recall, the kidney can concentrate urine to a maximum of 1200 mOsm/L, therefore it can concentrate 1 L of NS (308 mOsm/L) into 250 mL of urine and retain the other 750 mL as free water if required.

26. **How do the intravascular half-lives of crystalloids and colloids differ?**
Crystalloids have an intravascular half-life around 20 to 40 minutes, whereas albumin has an intravascular half-life around 3 to 6 hours.

27. **Does 1 L of normal saline increase the intravascular volume the same amount as one standard 250 mL solution of 5% albumin?**
Isotonic crystalloids have a short half-life and will primarily increase the extracellular space, whereas colloids will primarily increase the intravascular space. Recall, that the intravascular space is approximately one-quarter of the extracellular space; therefore 1 L of isotonic crystalloid will increase the intravascular space by 250 mL, which is the same volume of one standard unit of isotonic 5% albumin solution.

28. **Review the albumin solutions that are available.**
There are two albumin preparations: 5% albumin and 25% albumin solution. Preparation methods almost completely eliminate the possibility of infection aside from a theoretical risk of prion disease. The 5% solution has a colloid osmotic pressure of about 20 mmHg, which is the approximate colloid osmotic pressure of plasma under normal circumstances. The 25% solution has a colloid osmotic pressure of about 5 times that of normal plasma and its standard volume is 5 times less than the 5% solution (e.g., 50 mL vs. 250 mL). In situations where intravascular volume is depleted but extracellular volume is expanded, this excess colloid osmotic pressure is thought to draw fluid from the interstitial into the intravascular space. However, evidence to date does not support this notion, presumably because of the role of the glycocalyx.

29. **Is albumin suitable for volume replacement?**
In the perioperative environment, there are very few indications for the use of albumin for either volume replacement or for the normalization of serum albumin, and it is far more expensive than crystalloid solutions. Albumin may be considered as a soft recommendation from evidence-based practice guidelines in patients who are hypervolemic but deemed to be volume responsive by dynamic measures, the so-called *hypervolemic intravascular depleted state*.

30. **What situations might be appropriate for the use of hypertonic saline?**
Hypertonic saline (usually 3%) has an osmolarity of 900 mOsm/L and is sometimes used for patients in hypovolemic shock and/or to limit the amount of crystalloid given during large operations. More commonly, hypertonic saline is used to treat symptomatic hyponatremia and elevated ICP. In these situations, it helps decrease the amount of cerebral edema and lower ICP because sodium chloride does not readily cross the blood-brain barrier.

To reduce cerebral edema, hypertonic saline (3%) may be given in 100 to 250 mL boluses over 10 to 30 minutes, titrated to the patient's mental status, ICP, and/or serial sodium levels. Higher concentrations of hypertonic saline (i.e., 23%) may be given when brain herniation is imminent.

31. **What is meant by third-space losses? What are the effects of such losses?**
    In certain clinical conditions, such as major intraabdominal operations, hemorrhagic shock, burns and sepsis, patients develop fluid requirements that are not explained by externally measured losses. These are referred to as *third space* losses. Third-space losses are internal; a temporary sequestration of intravascular fluid into a functionless *third space*. This fluid does not readily participate in the dynamic exchanges seen at the microcirculatory level, and therefore does not contribute functionally to the maintenance of cardiac output and tissue perfusion. The volume of this internal loss is proportional to the degree of injury, and its composition is similar to plasma or interstitial fluid. The creation of the third space (i.e., third-spacing) will necessitate further fluid infusions to maintain adequate intravascular volume. Third-space fluids will generally persist until the patient's primary problem has resolved.

KEY POINTS: VOLUME REGULATION AND FLUID REPLACEMENT

1. Estimating volume status requires gathering as much clinical information as possible because any single variable (e.g., urine output) in isolation may be misleading. Always look for supporting information.
2. Replace intraoperative fluid losses with isotonic fluids.
3. Contraction alkalosis, or chloride deficient alkalosis, is really two separate problems: hypovolemia and hypochloremic metabolic alkalosis. Both volume and chloride need to be replenished, generally with NS.
4. NS, when administered in large quantities, may cause hyperchloremic metabolic acidosis and should not be used as the mainstay fluid for volume resuscitation.
5. Balanced salt solutions, such as LR and Plasma-Lyte are the ideal crystalloid for volume resuscitation. They may also be used for maintenance fluids and in patients with ESRD.
6. Albumin has not been shown to improve outcomes over crystalloids and can increase mortality in patients with traumatic brain injuries.

SUGGESTED READINGS

Boldt J. Use of albumin: an update. Br J Anaesth. 2010;104:276–284.
Chappel D, Jacob M, Hofmann-Kiefer K, et al. A rational approach to perioperative fluid management. Anesthesiology. 2008;109:723–740.
Edwards MR, Grocott MPW. Perioperative fluid and electrolyte therapy. In: Miller RD, editor: Miller's Anesthesia. 8th ed. Philadelphia: Elsevier Saunders; 2015:1767–1810.
Luke RG, Galla JH. It is chloride depletion alkalosis, not contraction alkalosis. J Am Soc Nephrol. 2012;23(2):204–207.
Moritz ML, Ayus JC. Maintenance intravenous fluids in acutely ill patients. N Engl J Med. 2015;373(14):1350–1360.

CHAPTER 9

ELECTROLYTES

Jason C. Brainard, MD, Jessica L. Nelson, MD

QUESTIONS: ELECTROLYTES

SODIUM

1. How is hyponatremia classified?

   Classification is primarily based on the patient's serum osmolality and volume status. Hyponatremia may occur in the presence of low serum osmolality (<285 mOsm/kg), normal osmolality (285–295 mOsm/kg), or high osmolality (>295 mOsm/kg). Elevated total body water is more common than a loss of sodium disproportionate to free water losses. This elevation is typically caused by impaired renal excretion of water, but it can occasionally be caused by excessive intake of water (e.g., primary polydipsia). Additional workup with urine sodium and urine osmolality may be helpful in determining the cause of hyponatremia. Many patients with hyponatremia have a single etiology, although complex or critically-ill patients may have multiple contributing factors. Table 9.1 summarizes causes of hyponatremia and their recommended treatments.

2. List the possible causes of acute hyponatremia in the operating room.

   Administration of hypotonic fluids or absorption of sodium-poor irrigation solutions may result in hyponatremia. Irrigation solutions like glycine and sorbitol can be used to facilitate transurethral resection of the prostate or distend the uterus during hysteroscopies. These solutions are hypotonic to prevent dispersal of the electrical current when monopolar cautery is used.

   The intraoperative use of mannitol, especially in patients with renal dysfunction, may also cause hyponatremia by increasing plasma osmolality. Water moves out of cells, resulting in intravascular volume expansion and a drop in serum sodium. Mannitol is more commonly associated with intracranial surgeries, but can also be used as a flushing solution during transurethral resection of the prostate or bladder, or to promote urine output following renal transplant.

3. What are the symptoms of acute hyponatremia?

   Symptoms often present based on the rate of change, as well as the absolute level of sodium. Typical symptoms include: nausea, vomiting, visual disturbances, muscle cramps, weakness, and bradycardia. Patients may also develop elevated intracranial pressure resulting in mental status changes. These changes can run the spectrum from apprehension and agitation to confusion and obtundation. Patients with severe hyponatremia, usually at levels less than 120 mEq/L, are also at risk for seizures.

4. What degree of hyponatremia is acceptable to continue with a planned elective procedure?

   A normal sodium level is between 135 and 145 mEq/L. Recognizing hyponatremia should prompt an investigation of the cause. In addition to its etiology, the acuity and trajectory of the sodium change will also have an impact on management. Whether the investigation and treatment of hyponatremia should take priority over the surgery depends on the urgency of the procedure and an overall assessment of the patient's condition. In general, mild hyponatremia with a sodium level of at least 130 mEq/L should not result in cancellation of a planned procedure, as long as the patient is not symptomatic, and worsening hyponatremia is not an expected result of the procedure.

5. How should acute hyponatremia be treated?

   The aggressiveness of treatment depends on the extent of symptoms and the rate at which hyponatremia has developed. In the simplest cases, fluid restriction is usually sufficient. Administration of loop diuretics may also be indicated. Correction should occur slowly, with serial sodium concentrations measured. For asymptomatic patients with a sodium concentration of less than 130 mEq/L, serum sodium should be corrected at less than or equal to a rate of 0.5 mEq/L/h.

   Administration of hypertonic saline is reserved for patients with refractory hyponatremia or severe, neurological symptoms, including seizures or coma. For neurological symptoms, the patient can be treated with an initial bolus of 100 mL of 3% saline followed by, if symptoms have not resolved, two additional 100 mL boluses over a total course of 30 minutes. The goal is to rapidly increase the serum sodium by 4 to 6 mEq/L over a few hours, which should be sufficient to decrease intracranial pressure, stop seizure activity, and reduce the risk of herniation.

6. What daily rate of correction for hyponatremia is safe, and what is the risk if this rate is exceeded?

   The rate of sodium increase should not exceed 10 to 12 mEq/L/day. Aggressive correction may result in osmotic demyelination syndrome. As there may be differences between intended and actual correction, it may be safer to

Table 9.1 Causes of Hyponatremia

TOTAL SODIUM CONTENT	CAUSES	TREATMENT (ALWAYS TREAT UNDERLYING DISORDER)
Decreased	Diuretics (including osmotic diuretics); renal tubular acidosis; hypoaldosteronism; salt-wasting nephropathies; vomiting; diarrhea	Restore fluid and sodium deficits with isotonic saline
Normal	SIADH; hypothyroidism; cortisol deficiency	Water restriction
Increased	Congestive heart failure; cirrhosis; nephrotic syndrome	Water restriction, loop diuretics

SIADH, Syndrome of inappropriate antidiuretic hormone.

target lower rates of correction (e.g., 4–6 mEq/L/day), especially in asymptomatic patients. Of note, it is the daily change rather than the hourly change in serum sodium that is associated with osmotic demyelination syndrome. This allows some level of safety for rapid correction in the setting of neurological symptoms, as long as the rapid correction rate does not continue past a period of a few hours. Lastly, osmotic demyelination syndrome is rare in patients who have an initial sodium level higher than 120 mEq/L.

7. **What are the symptoms of osmotic demyelination syndrome? When do they typically develop?**
Clinical manifestations of osmotic demyelination syndrome typically develop 2 to 6 days following rapid sodium changes. Neuromuscular symptoms are the most common and include: confusion, movement disorders, obtundation, seizures, weakness, and myoclonic jerks. Typically, these symptoms are either partially or completely irreversible.

8. **Is there a subset of patients who tend to have residual neurological sequelae from a hyponatremic episode?**
Females of reproductive age, especially during menstruation, have been noted to be at the greatest risk for residual sequelae. There may be an estrogen-related impairment in the ability of the brain to adapt to hyponatremia.
     Brain adaptations that help minimize cerebral edema during hyponatremia also place the brain at risk in the setting of rapid sodium correction. Patients who have had hyponatremia for more than 2 days are especially vulnerable to osmotic demyelination syndrome, because the brain has been given more time to adapt.

9. **What are the common etiologies for hypernatremia?**
Hypernatremia is less common than hyponatremia and is always associated with hypertonicity. Hypernatremia can be present with low, normal, or high total body sodium content. Table 9.2 lists causes and treatment for each category. Frequently, hypernatremia is the result of decreased access to free water, as in elderly or debilitated patients with impaired thirst and decreased oral intake. Other causes include a lack of antidiuretic hormone (central diabetes insipidus) or a lack of response to antidiuretic hormone (nephrogenic diabetes insipidus). In hospitalized patients, hypernatremia is often iatrogenic. Possible etiologies include excess sodium intake from intravenous fluids, usually normal saline, or administration of medications, like sodium bicarbonate or 3% sodium chloride.

10. **What problems does hypernatremia pose for the anesthesiologist?**
Hypernatremia increases minimal alveolar concentration for inhaled anesthetics. More often, though, hypernatremia poses the greater challenge via its association with fluid deficits. Complicating this, hypovolcmia

Table 9.2 Causes of Hypernatremia

TOTAL SODIUM CONTENT	CAUSES	TREATMENT (ALWAYS TREAT UNDERLYING DISORDER)
Decreased	Osmotic diuresis; increased insensible losses	Restore intravascular volume with isotonic fluids first, and then correct sodium with hypotonic fluids
Normal	Diabetes insipidus (neurogenic or nephrogenic); diuretics; renal failure	Correct water loss with hypotonic fluids
Increased	Excessive Na administration ($NaHCO_3$; 3% NaCl); hyperaldosteronism	Slowly correct fluid deficits with D_5W, loop diuretics

D_5W, 5% Dextrose in water.

must be corrected slowly so that cellular edema does not develop. Procedures that involve significant resuscitation and fluid shifts place the patient at increased risk for rapid sodium changes. Elective surgery should generally be delayed if serum sodium levels exceed 150 mEq/L.

POTASSIUM

11. What is a normal serum potassium concentration? What possible etiologies might be considered in a patient with hypokalemia?

A normal serum potassium level is in the approximate range of 3.5 to 5.0 mEq/L. As only about 2% of potassium is extracellular, a low serum potassium concentration represents significant total body potassium depletion. This depletion can occur because of gastrointestinal or renal losses, transcellular shifts, or inadequate intake. Gastrointestinal loss of potassium is often because of diarrhea, although overuse of laxatives and acute, colonic pseudoobstruction can also be triggers. Diuretics, especially loop diuretics, and some forms of renal tubular acidosis (types 1 and 2) are causes of renal losses. β-Adrenergic agonists, insulin, and an elevated serum pH can all shift potassium into the intracellular space. Hypokalemia is not uncommon in pregnant women receiving tocolytic therapy or in patients requiring inotropic support, because β-agonists are used in both instances. Low potassium intake can be seen in patients who are malnourished, but this often just exacerbates hypokalemia from another etiology. If hypokalemia is the primary cause, however, other electrolyte and vitamin derangements will typically be present as well.

12. Describe the dangers of hypokalemia.

Hypokalemia produces electrocardiogram abnormalities (ST segment and T wave depression, prolonged QT, and onset of U waves) and cardiac arrhythmias (often premature ventricular contractions and atrial fibrillation) (Fig. 9.1). It also impairs cardiac contractility. These cardiac abnormalities are usually not seen until serum potassium is below 3 mEq/L. Patients taking digitalis, and those with preexisting arrhythmias or ischemic heart disease, however, may be more sensitive to even mildly decreased levels.

In addition to its cardiac effects, hypokalemia causes muscle weakness, including respiratory muscle weakness, and increases sensitivity to muscle relaxants. In addition, it increases the risk of ileus and, if prolonged, can cause damage to the kidneys. There is no definitive data, however, to suggest that patients having surgery with potassium levels as low as 2.6 mEq/L have adverse outcomes.

13. A patient taking diuretics is found to have a potassium level of 3 mEq/L. Why not rapidly correct it?

The total body deficit of potassium, which is primarily an intracellular cation, is not reflected by serum concentrations. A patient with a serum potassium of 3 mEq/L may have a total body potassium deficit of 100 to 200 mEq. Rapid attempts to correct hypokalemia poorly address the problem and have resulted in cardiac arrest. Hypokalemic patients, without the risk factors previously discussed and who are not undergoing major thoracic, vascular, or cardiac procedures, can tolerate modest hypokalemia to 3 mEq/L and possibly as low as 2.5 mEq/L.

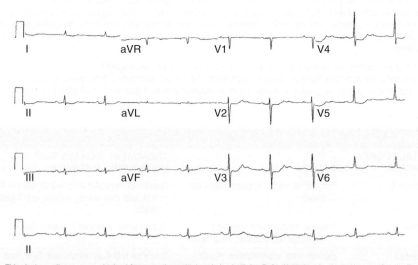

Fig 9.1 This electrocardiogram was obtained from a patient with hypokalemia (3.2 mEq/L). Note the prominent U wave after the T wave in the precordial leads V2–6. There is often TU fusion with hypokalemia, creating a broad T wave and an increase in the measured QT interval. Polymorphic ventricular tachycardia may result from hypokalemia.

14. **If potassium is administered, how much should be given? How fast?**

    For potassium repletion, an often-used heuristic is that every 10 mEq of potassium administered will increase the serum potassium by approximately 0.1 mEq/L. This is less accurate for patients with severe potassium depletion, ongoing losses, or renal insufficiency. Infusion limits are typically 20 mEq/h of potassium via a central line or 10 mEq/h via a peripheral line, as higher concentrations will damage peripheral veins and cause discomfort to the patient during infusion. Injectable potassium chloride should never be given undiluted or as a bolus, and no more than 20 mEq of potassium should ever be connected to a patient's intravenous lines. Patients with mild and asymptomatic hypokalemia are eligible for oral potassium replacement. Oral potassium is often given as 40 to 60 mEq by mouth, 1 to 4 times per day, and usually no more than a total dose of 100 mEq/day.

15. **Discuss the possible symptoms of hyperkalemia?**

    Although hyperkalemia is defined as a serum concentration greater than 5.0 mEq/L, symptoms do not typically develop unless the level is 5.5 mEq/L or higher. Hyperkalemia can produce profound weakness and cardiac conduction abnormalities, including enhanced automaticity and repolarization irregularities. Peaked T waves are usually the earliest finding. Increasing potassium levels are associated with progressive widening of the P wave, lengthening of the PR segment, QRS prolongation, conduction blocks, bradycardia, and ventricular arrhythmias (Fig. 9.2). Development of a sine wave appearance on telemetry or electrocardiogram is usually a precedent to cardiac arrest.

16. **What are some causes of hyperkalemia?**

    Hyperkalemia can be either acute or chronic in etiology. The causes of hyperkalemia are in direct contrast to those previously discussed for hypokalemia and include: increased intake, decreased excretion, and transcellular shifts because of a low serum pH. Hyperkalemia because of increased intake is often iatrogenic (e.g., because of potassium supplementation or potassium-containing medications). Medications that can cause hyperkalemia include angiotensin antagonists and receptor blockers, potassium-sparing diuretics (e.g., spironolactone and triamterene), and succinylcholine. Hyperkalemia can also occur after increased potassium release from cells, such as with severe trauma, rhabdomyolysis, hemolysis, tumor lysis, and massive transfusion. Decreased excretion of potassium is most common because of renal dysfunction, which may be either acute or chronic.

17. **Which patients are at risk of hyperkalemia after the administration of succinylcholine?**

    An increase in serum potassium of approximately 0.5 mEq/L occurs after routine administration of succinylcholine, and it should therefore be avoided in patients who are already hyperkalemic. Other subpopulations of patients, though, may be susceptible to an exaggerated potassium response and subsequent life-threatening hyperkalemia. Examples of such patients include those with spinal cord or denervation injuries, stroke, head injuries, significant burns, rhabdomyolysis, intraabdominal infections, and immobility (e.g., critically-ill patients on bedrest). The timing at which this increased risk develops, however, is debated and often variable. Conservatively, it may be best to avoid the use of succinylcholine in patients with acute burns, stroke, or spinal cord injury after 24 hours.

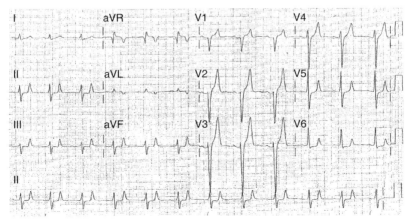

Fig 9.2 This electrocardiogram was obtained from a patient with hyperkalemia (9.2 mEq/L). Note the sharp peaking of T waves, broadening of the QRS complex, and diminished P-wave amplitude.

18. **A patient with chronic renal failure and a potassium of 7 mEq/L requires an arteriovenous fistula for hemodialysis. Discuss the anesthetic concerns?**
Hyperkalemia greater than 6 mEq/L should be corrected before elective procedures. Dialysis is usually the preferred treatment. Intermittent hemodialysis offers faster clearance and may be preferred over continuous renal replacement therapies for patients with significant or symptomatic hyperkalemia.

19. **How is acute hyperkalemia treated?**
Cardiotoxicity, as manifested by changes on electrocardiogram or telemetry, is treated with intravenous calcium chloride or calcium gluconate. Potassium can also be quickly shifted intracellularly by β-adrenergic stimulation (e.g., inhaled albuterol) and intravenous insulin (typically given with intravenous dextrose supplementation). In patients with acidemia, hyperventilation and sodium bicarbonate can be beneficial in shifting potassium intracellularly as well. Bodily excretion of potassium is more time-consuming, but is accomplished using diuretics, sodium polystyrene sulfonate (Kayexalate), and dialysis. Using intravenous fluids (normal saline) may also be helpful in patients who are hypovolemic.

CALCIUM

20. **List some possible causes of hypocalcemia.**
The major causes of hypocalcemia are: hypoparathyroidism, hyperphosphatemia, vitamin D deficiency, malabsorption, rapid blood transfusion (calcium is chelated by citrate), pancreatitis, rhabdomyolysis, and fat embolism (because of free fatty acids binding calcium). Hypocalcemia is a concern after thyroidectomy if no parathyroid tissue is left, and the patient may develop laryngeal spasms and stridor. This must be differentiated from other causes of postoperative stridor, including wound hematoma and injury to the recurrent laryngeal nerves.

21. **Describe the manifestations of hypocalcemia.**
Hypocalcemia impairs cardiac contractility, resulting in hypotension. Serial ionized calcium levels should be checked in patients receiving multiple blood transfusions to ensure that hypocalcemia is not contributing to shock. Hypocalcemia can also cause QT prolongation, although conduction abnormalities are less common than with other electrolyte abnormalities. In addition, patients can develop tetany, perioral paresthesias, seizures, anxiety, and confusion. Trousseau's sign (carpopedal spasm when a blood pressure cuff is inflated above the systolic blood pressure for 3 minutes) and Chvostek's sign (contraction of the ipsilateral facial muscles with tapping of the facial nerve) may be found on examination.

22. **Why would checking an ionized calcium level be helpful in a patient with suspected hypocalcemia?**
Calcium in the serum is bound to proteins, primarily albumin. Consequently, the total serum calcium level may not accurately reflect the ionized (i.e., free) calcium level in the serum, which is the more clinically relevant form of hypocalcemia. Each 1 g/dL reduction in the serum albumin concentration lowers the total calcium concentration by approximately 0.8 mg/dL, although it does not affect the ionized calcium concentration. Of note, the affinity of calcium for albumin is higher in the setting of an alkalosis, so ionized calcium may be decreased in patients with an elevated serum pH.

23. **How is hypocalcemia treated?**
Treatment of acute hypocalcemia is straightforward: administer intravenous calcium chloride or calcium gluconate. Always remember to address the primary disturbance as well. Equivalent calcium chloride dosing provides more active calcium than the gluconate preparation. On the other hand, calcium gluconate may be preferable in patients without central access, as it is less irritating and carries a lower risk of tissue necrosis should extravasation occur.

MAGNESIUM

24. **What is the normal range for serum magnesium? What are the symptoms of hypo- and hypermagnesemia?**
A typical serum magnesium level is 1.3 to 2.2 mEq/L. Hypomagnesemia causes QT prolongation and can lead to torsades de pointes and other arrhythmias. Muscle weakness, tremors, twitches, numbness, and paresthesias are other possible symptoms. Confusion, drowsiness, and seizures can occur with severe hypomagnesemia.

Hypermagnesemia is uncommon and is usually caused by renal dysfunction or excessive intake, which is often iatrogenic (e.g., magnesium is used therapeutically for patients with preeclampsia and eclampsia). Initial symptoms of magnesium toxicity typically occur at levels of 4 to 6 mEq/L and include nausea, headache, drowsiness, and decreased deep tendon reflexes. As the magnesium level continues to increase, patients develop muscle weakness, respiratory insufficiency and failure, absent deep tendon reflexes, hypotension, bradycardia, and possible cardiac arrest.

25. **Does hypomagnesemia pose a problem for the anesthesiologist?**
Hypomagnesemia is increasingly recognized in patients with gastrointestinal losses and patients who are malnourished, addicted to alcohol, or critically ill. Often, hypomagnesemia will be found in association with hypokalemia and hypophosphatemia. Hypokalemia is usually difficult to correct, unless hypomagnesemia is also

treated. The mechanism for this is not fully understood, but it may be because magnesium deficiency exacerbates potassium excretion. Patients with hypomagnesemia have increased susceptibility to muscle relaxants and may be weak after surgery, which can include respiratory insufficiency. They may have impaired cardiac contractility and dysrhythmias (e.g., torsades de pointes) as well. Patients undergoing massive resuscitation are also at risk for hypomagnesemia, and they should be given magnesium chloride (1–2 g), if dysrhythmias or refractory hypotension develop.

CHLORIDE

26. Hyperchloremia has been increasingly recognized after administration of what *standard* resuscitation fluid?

    Hyperchloremia is associated with the use of 0.9% normal saline, which contains 154 mEq/L of chloride. Patients undergoing prolonged surgeries or those who suffer from septic shock or significant trauma are the most likely to be impacted because of their need for large-volume fluid resuscitation. Of note, hyperchloremia also causes a nonanion gap metabolic acidosis.

KEY POINTS: ELECTROLYTES

1. Electrolyte disturbances can be difficult to correct without treating the underlying cause.
2. Emergent treatment of hyponatremic patients with hypertonic saline should be reserved for those with severe, neurological symptoms.
3. Hypernatremia is often associated with fluid deficits, which have to be addressed carefully to prevent cellular edema.
4. Cardiotoxicity because of hyperkalemia should be immediately treated with intravenous calcium chloride or calcium gluconate.
5. Patients who receive high volumes of fluid, especially normal saline, often develop hyperchloremia and a nonanion gap metabolic acidosis.

SUGGESTED READINGS

Asmar A, Mohandas R, Wingo CS. A physiologic-based approach to the treatment of a patient with hypokalemia. Am J Kidney Dis. 2012;60:492–497.

Bagshaw SM, Townsend DR, McDermid RC. Disorders of sodium and water balance in hospitalized patients. Can J Anesth. 2009; 56:151–167.

Elliott MJ, Ronksley PE, Clase CM, et al. Management of patients with acute hyperkalemia. CMAJ. 2010;182:1631–1635.

Gankam Kengne F, Decaux G. Hyponatremia and the brain. Kidney Int Rep. 2017;3:24–35.

Handy JM, Soni N. Physiological effects of hyperchloraemia and acidosis. Br J Anaesth. 2008;101:141–150.

Herroeder S, Schönherr ME, De Hert SG, et al. Magnesium—essentials for anesthesiologists. Anesthesiology. 2011;114:971–993.

Palmer BF. Approach to fluid and electrolyte disorders and acid-base problems. Prim Care Clin Pract. 2008;35:195–213.

1. **How can you identify a patient at risk for perioperative bleeding?**
   Preoperative evaluation for bleeding risk includes a focused history, physical examination, a review of all medications and dietary supplements, appropriate laboratory testing and a consideration of the bleeding risk inherent to the scheduled surgical procedure. Questions should be asked about prior bleeding in nonsurgical settings (e.g., tendency to form large hematomas after minor trauma, severe bleeding while brushing teeth) and significant bleeding with prior surgical procedures not normally associated with significant bleeding (e.g., dental extractions). Prior surgery without the need for transfusion suggests the absence of a clinically significant inherited coagulation disorder. However, it does not rule out the subsequent interim development of an acquired coagulation disorder (liver or renal disease, hematological malignancy, etc.) in a patient who reports "recent easy bleeding/bruising." Preoperative coagulation studies may confirm a clinical suspicion that a patient has a bleeding disorder, but no evidence supports the value of routine preoperative coagulation studies in asymptomatic patients. However, those with a personal history of bleeding will likely bleed again. With regard to von Willebrand disease (vWD), it was demonstrated that a standardized preoperative/antepartum "bleeding questionnaire" was equivalent to laboratory testing for predicting bleeding after dental extractions, and superior to laboratory testing for the prediction of surgical bleeding.

2. **Do dietary supplements and herbal remedies cause bleeding?**
   Many medications unrelated to the coagulation system, herbal remedies, over-the-counter dietary supplements, foods, fruits, vegetables, spices, and vitamins have been demonstrated to have varying degrees of antiplatelet, antithrombotic and/or anticoagulant activity, but most (with a few notable exceptions) have not been unequivocally demonstrated to confer clinically significant bleeding risk in-and-of themselves when taken as directed and/or consumed in normal quantities. Notable exceptions may include certain herbal or dietary supplements (e.g., ginko, ginseng, garlic, omega-3-fatty acids, coenzyme Q_{10}, D vitamins) and some anesthesiologists advise patients to discontinue the use of such supplements for at least 2 weeks preoperatively to decrease the risk of perioperative bleeding and/or complications of planned neuraxial procedures.

3. **What is the difference between hemostasis and coagulation?**
   Hemostasis is the overall process by which bleeding is stopped. Coagulation is the formation of a fibrin clot at the site of blood vessel injury. In nonpathological states, a balance must exist between bleeding and clotting if blood is to remain liquid, and tissue perfusion distal to the site of a vessel injury is to continue, once vessel injuries have been repaired. Thus the overall process of hemostasis must include checks and balances to mitigate the effects of excessive coagulation and dissolution of clots. The hemostatic mechanism therefore includes the following: vasoconstriction of the injured vessel, coagulation at the site of vessel injury, and fibrinolysis.

4. **Describe the process of coagulation.**
   Coagulation (confusingly enough) is subdivided into primary hemostasis and secondary hemostasis.

5. **What is primary hemostasis?**
   Primary hemostasis refers to the formation of a preliminary platelet plug at the site of vessel injury. Exposure of the subendothelial collagen results in the adherence of platelets to the site of injury and their activation. Platelet activation results in degranulation, shape change, aggregation, and exposure of the fibrinogen receptor (glycoprotein IIb/IIIa). A preliminary platelet plug forms as many platelets all bind to the same strands of fibrinogen.

6. **What is secondary hemostasis?**
   Secondary hemostasis refers to the ultimate fibrin crosslinking and reinforcement of the platelet plug developed during primary hemostasis. The additional fibrin needed locally to stabilize the platelet plug and create a true fibrin clot comes from the extrinsic and intrinsic coagulation pathways.

7. **Describe platelet activation.**
   Platelet adherence to exposed subendothelial collagen is via their glycoprotein receptor Gp1b mediated by von Willebrand factor (vWF). Substances like collagen, thrombin, and epinephrine activate phospholipases A and C in the platelet plasma membrane, resulting in the formation of thromboxane A_2 (TXA_2) and the degranulation of platelet alpha- and dense granules. Platelet granules contain a variety of procoagulant factors, including: serotonin, adenosine diphosphate (ADP), TXA_2, vWF, factor V, fibrinogen, and fibronectin, all of which assist in the process by activating platelets, promoting aggregation of platelets, recruiting more platelets to the plug and initiating secondary hemostasis (discussed later). ADP released locally during degranulation initiates shape change (that exposes

electronegatively charged phospholipids on the platelet surface that will activate secondary hemostasis through the "contact activation pathway", as discussed later), as well as a decrease in cyclic adenosine monophosphate (cAMP). Falling cAMP levels in conjunction with other secondary messengers alters the membrane glycoproteins IIb and IIIa to form the activated fibrinogen receptor (GPIIbIIIa). A platelet plug thus forms by many activated platelets binding to fibrinogen through the GPIIbIIIa receptor. Platelet plug formation is referred to as *primary hemostasis*.

8. **What are the extrinsic and intrinsic coagulation pathways?**
   The classic depiction of the extrinsic and intrinsic pathways (Fig. 10.1) as two completely separate processes is no longer accepted because of multiple points of interaction between the two (factors from each can activate factors in the other), although it remains useful conceptually for the interpretation of in vitro tests of coagulation and hemostasis. Both the extrinsic and the intrinsic pathways lead to activation of factor X (which will then cleave prothrombin to thrombin, which will then cleave fibrinogen to fibrin; these latter steps are known as the *common pathway*). Modern terminology for the extrinsic pathway is "the tissue factor pathway," and that for the intrinsic pathway is "the contact activation pathway." The intrinsic pathway is also sometimes known as *the amplification pathway*.

9. **Describe the tissue factor (extrinsic) pathway. What are the laboratory tests for this pathway?**
   The tissue factor (TF) pathway (see Fig. 10.1) is triggered by the exposure of TF at the site of blood vessel damage, which combines with Factor VII to form the activated TF-VIIa complex, which activates Factor X, creating prothrombinase (Xa + Va cofactor). The "extrinsic" or tissue factor pathway thus consists of the activated TF-VIIa complex and the Xa/Va complex (prothrombinase) that cleaves prothrombin to thrombin (thus beginning the "final common pathway" of coagulation resulting in fibrin formation). The prothrombin time (PT) and international normalized ratio (INR) are measurements of clotting via the tissue factor (extrinsic) pathway. The PT uses thromboplastin (mixture of TF + calcium + phospholipid) to activate coagulation in the ex vivo laboratory assay. A normal PT is 10 to 12 seconds. The INR was devised to standardize the results of the PT because different laboratory tests use different formulations of thromboplastin to perform the test. With each batch of

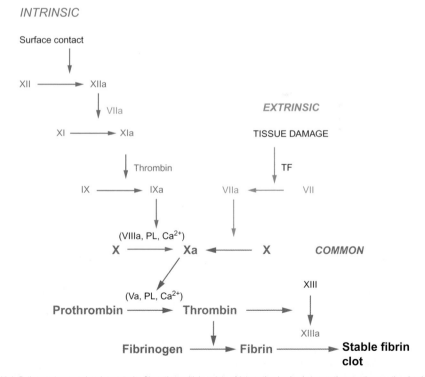

Fig. 10.1 Pathways to secondary hemostasis. Given the multiple points of interaction in vivo between these pathways, the classic and oversimplified depiction of these pathways as truly separate is useful only to aid in the conceptual understanding of laboratory tests of hemostasis and coagulation. Omitted from this diagram, for the purpose of simplification, are the multiple points of interaction, the feedback loops, the counterregulatory factors and inhibitors, and the process of fibrinolysis. *PL*, Phospholipase; *TF*, tissue factor.

thromboplastin, each manufacturer provides an "international sensitivity index rating" (ISI) to which the patient's PT is compared, resulting in the INR. An INR of 0.8 to 1.2 is considered normal. Therapeutic anticoagulation with warfarin generally requires an INR 2 to 3, but an INR of greater than 3 may be desirable for certain anticoagulation indications.

10. Describe the contact activation (intrinsic) pathway. What are the laboratory tests for this pathway?

In vivo, secondary hemostasis can be initiated via the contact activation (intrinsic) pathway in more than one way. When there is vessel injury, the contact activation pathway gets activated by factors from the TF (extrinsic) pathway, as well as by the electronegatively charged phospholipids on the platelet surface and by exposed collagen. Once activated, a series of reactions take place on the activated platelet surface to generate a local burst of thrombin. This contact activation pathway can also be activated by contact with other electronegatively charged surfaces/molecules, such as the electronegatively charged phospholipids in amniotic fluid, or on foreign surfaces, like glass or plastic (e.g., in laboratory tests) or by cardiopulmonary bypass and extracorporeal membrane oxygenation (ECMO) circuits.

The contact pathway is often initiated by contact with collagen (electronegatively charged surface) with three serum proteins: high-molecular-weight kininogen (HMWK), prekallikrein (PK), and factor XII. Although the details are beyond the scope of this text, the result is activation of factor XII, which in turn, causes activation of factor XI, IX, and X, respectively (see Fig. 10.1). However, neither factor XII nor its cofactors (PK and HMWK) are absolutely necessary for clinical hemostasis (because the pathway can be otherwise activated from the TF "extrinsic" pathway), and mild deficiencies of these cofactors do not result in bleeding problems. The partial thromboplastin time (PTT) is a common measure of clotting via the contact activation (intrinsic) pathway. The test is named such because partial thromboplastin is used as the activator (which eliminates the platelet variability had platelet phospholipid been used as the activator). A normal PTT is in the range of 60 to 70 seconds. The activated partial thromboplastin time (aPTT) is a more sensitive version of the PTT and is commonly used to monitor heparin therapy. A normal range for the aPTT is 30 to 40 seconds.

11. Does primary hemostasis happen before secondary hemostasis?

Although the terms primary and secondary hemostasis suggest that one happens after the other, clot initiation, amplification, and propagation all occur concurrently once the process is initiated because of the crossover of multiple factors from and between the various pathways to coagulation.

12. This has gotten confusing. What are the initiation, activation, propagation, and stabilization phases of coagulation? Describe the big picture of how this all happens.

The modern understanding is that the initiation stage of coagulation takes place on TF bearing cells (cells, such as monocytes, that can bind TF and present it to a ligand), which come into play when endothelial injury occurs and TF is exposed. TF is a transmembrane glycoprotein expressed on cells outside the bloodstream and is sometimes referred to as a *cell surface receptor* for the serine protease Factor VIIa. The initiation phase is characterized by presentation of TF to its ligand, factor VII. The activation phase takes place when the TF–VIIa complex activates factors X and IX. Activated factor X (Xa) then binds cofactor V. This TF–Xa/Va complex cleaves prothrombin to thrombin. However, the relatively small amount of thrombin produced thus far by the classic cascades is not sufficient to produce a fibrin clot. A number of other reactions is triggered during all of this, with platelets playing a central role. As previously discussed, platelets are activated during primary hemostasis via receptors for substances, such as collagen and thrombin. The platelets, upon activation, degranulate, releasing procoagulant factors, and change their shape, exposing negatively charged membrane phospholipids. Factors IXa, Xa, and XIa also have negatively charged sites that attach to platelet phospholipid with calcium ions acting as a sandwich-like buffer. Amplification of thrombin production is mediated by enzyme reactions located on the platelet surface. The combination of enzyme, cofactor, calcium, and phospholipid surface increase the speed of these reactions many 1000-fold. This is the propagation phase, in which an explosive increase in thrombin production cleaves large amounts of fibrinogen into fibrin. Finally, the stabilization phase occurs when activated factor XIII (XIIIa) crosslinks fibrin to reinforce the platelet plug to stabilize the clot.

KEY POINTS: BASIC SCIENCE OF COAGULATION

1. Coagulation (the formation of a fibrin-stabilized platelet plug at the site of vascular injury) is only one component of the overall hemostatic mechanism.
2. "Coagulation" is subdivided into "primary" and "secondary" hemostasis.
3. The purpose of "primary hemostasis" is to form a preliminary platelet plug at the site of vessel injury. It is initiated by exposure of subendothelial collagen at the site of vascular injury.
4. The purpose of "secondary hemostasis" is to form fibrin to crosslink the preliminary platelet plug developed during "primary hemostasis." It can be activated by the release of TF from the site of vascular injury and is amplified by positive feedback loops mediated by clotting factors and other events in "primary hemostasis."
5. Checks and balances exist to ensure coagulation does not run wild.

13. **What is the function of Vitamin K in the coagulation pathways?**
Vitamin K facilitates the carboxylation of factors II, VII, IX, X, protein C, and protein S by the enzyme gamma-glutamyl carboxylase.

14. **How does Warfarin work?**
Warfarin (and related coumarins) inhibit "production" of the "vitamin K-dependent" factors II, VII, IX, X, protein C and protein S, by blocking vitamin K epoxide reductase.

15. **Why is the initiation of warfarin therapy associated with hypercoagulability?**
Protein C is an inhibitory counterregulatory factor with a short half-life ($\sim$8 hours) that degrades factors Va and VIIIa, thus limiting the formation of factor Xa (which cleaves prothrombin to thrombin). The initiation of warfarin therapy inhibits the synthesis of anticoagulant protein C, predisposing to hypercoagulability because of the shorter half-life of protein C compared with other procoagulant clotting factors. Warfarin also inhibits the production of anticoagulant protein S but this protein has a much longer half-life ($\sim$30 hours).

16. **How does heparin work?**
Heparin binds to and enhances the activity of antithrombin III, which inhibits the function of activated factors II (thrombin), VII, IX, X, XI, and XII. Heparin is an unfractionated assortment of molecules of varying size all containing a common pentasaccharide sequence. Heparin is also highly electronegatively charged, resulting in nonspecific, pentasaccharide-independent binding to a variety of plasma proteins, (including those secreted by platelets (e.g., platelet factor 4) and endothelial cells (e.g., vWF). Heparin also nonspecifically binds acute phase reactants, macrophages, and endothelial cells. Thus the variable (and sometimes unpredictable) anticoagulant effect of heparin in a given individual is at least in part because of variability in plasma levels of potential binding sites. Chronic heparin therapy is associated with osteoporosis because of heparin binding to osteoclasts.

17. **What is low-molecular-weight heparin?**
Low-molecular-weight heparins (LMWH) are a fractionation of the lower molecular weight heparin molecules. LMWH preparations usually have fragments with a mean molecular weight of 4 to 5 kDa, whereas unfractionated heparin may have molecules on the order of 15 kDa. LMWHs primarily inhibit Factor Xa as their mechanism of action. The LMWHs hold several potential advantages over unfractionated heparin, including less nonspecific binding to plasma proteins (resulting in a more predictable dose-response), less binding to platelets and platelet Factor IV (reducing the incidence of heparin-induced thrombocytopenia), less binding to macrophages and endothelial cells, and less binding to osteoclasts (reducing the risk of osteoporosis). LMWHs are often used clinically for prophylaxis against deep venous thrombosis. LMWH therapy generally does not require specific monitoring (i.e., anti-Xa levels) because its pharmacokinetics and anticoagulant effects are more predictable than heparin. The main limitations of LMWH, in contrast to unfractionated heparin, is that it can only partially be reversed with protamine. Further, it is also dependent upon renal excretion and should be avoided in patients with end-stage renal disease.

18. **What is the ACT?**
The activated clotting time (ACT) measures the time to clot formation ex vivo in fresh whole blood. Either celite or kaolin usually serves as the activator. An ACT of 90 to 120 seconds is considered "normal." The ACT is widely used to monitor heparin therapy in the operating room. Therapeutic prolongation of the ACT depends on the indication. ECMO, for example, requires an ACT of at least 180 to 200 seconds to prevent coagulation in the components of the ECMO circuit, an ACT 300 to 350 seconds is usual during vascular surgery, where vascular clamping is involved, and initiation of full cardiopulmonary bypass classically requires an ACT of more than 480 seconds. Factors that may prolong the ACT include those factors which impair coagulation, including hypothermia, hemodilution, and acquired or inherited coagulopathies.

19. **Why is factor Xa such a key target for many new oral anticoagulants?**
Factor Xa is the central serine protease (in association with cofactor Va) that cleaves prothrombin to thrombin, perhaps the key factor in coagulation (see Fig. 10.1). Thrombin cleaves fibrinogen to fibrin, but thrombin also activates Factor XIII which acts to crosslinks fibrin to stabilize the platelet plug. Thrombin also amplifies its own generation by activating factors XI (in the "intrinsic"/"contact activation"/"amplification" pathway) and VIII (VIIIa also cleaves X to Xa which cleaves prothrombin to thrombin). Importantly, as hemostasis is a balance between bleeding and clotting, thrombin also activates the counterregulatory factor protein C (that inhibits activation of factors V and VIII with the assistance of cofactor protein S).

20. **Explain fibrinolysis.**
The fibrinolytic system is activated simultaneously with coagulation and functions to maintain the overall liquidity of blood during localized coagulation. It also effects clot lysis once tissue repair begins (which is a good thing), but abnormal fibrinolysis is not desirable as it leads to significant coagulopathic bleeding. The ability to lyse a clot is built into every clot (plasminogen is incorporated into every clot formed). When thrombin is present, endothelial cells release tissue plasminogen activator (tPA), which converts plasminogen to plasmin, which degrades fibrin and fibrinogen into small fragments (or "fibrin degradation products [FDPs]"). Plasminogen is also cleaved to plasmin by fragments of factor XII. The FDPs themselves possess relative anticoagulant properties because they compete with fibrinogen for thrombin. FDPs are normally cleared by the monocyte-macrophage system.

21. **What are aminocaproic acid and tranexamic acid used for? How do they work?**
Aminocaproic acid and tranexamic acid are analogues of the amino acid lysine used to prevent fibrinolysis. Binding of these lysine analogues to lysine receptor sites on plasminogen inhibits its activation to plasmin (recall, plasmin

degrades fibrinogen and fibrin). At higher doses, these agents can directly inhibit the activity of plasmin. These agents are frequently used in the setting of severe trauma, postpartum hemorrhage, major orthopedic operations, and in cardiac surgery. Several studies have shown that these agents reduce the risk of bleeding and the need for transfusion, may reduce the risk of complications, such as tamponade, following cardiac surgery, or hysterectomy in postpartum hemorrhage, and may prevent death because of hemorrhage from severe trauma or from postpartum hemorrhage.

22. **Do antifibrinolytics (aminocaproic acid and tranexamic acid) cause clots?**
Despite the perceived theoretical risk of thrombotic complications caused by antifibrinolytics, scientific evidence to date suggests these agents are safe. Several large randomized controlled trials have not shown an increase in thrombotic events associated with antifibrinolytics, including patient populations who are normally considered high risk (patients undergoing liver transplant or large orthopedic operations). Regardless, antifibrinolytics are contraindicated in the setting of secondary fibrinolysis (e.g., disseminated intravascular coagulation [DIC]), as these agents might cause widespread thrombosis.

23. **What is disseminated intravascular coagulation?**
Normally, the liquidity of blood is the result of a balance between clotting and fibrinolysis. In DIC, widespread activation of the clotting mechanism results in an explosive burst of thrombin formation, resulting not only in widespread clotting (which consumes platelets and factors), but in simultaneous widespread fibrinolysis (the enhanced activation of plasmin by thrombin cleaves both fibrinogen and fibrin into FDPs), and thus DIC eventually results in bleeding. The consumption of factors also includes coagulation inhibitory factors, and normal positive feedback loops run wild, with coagulation begetting coagulation, in both the micro- and the macrovasculature.

24. **What causes DIC?**
DIC is not a disease entity, but rather a clinical complication of other problems. It often arises in situations associated with systemic inflammation (i.e., trauma, postcardiac arrest syndrome, sepsis) and/or the release of procoagulant proteins (e.g., TF is abundant in brain and placenta tissue). Common precipitating clinical situations associated with DIC are the following:
- Obstetric conditions (e.g., amniotic fluid embolism, placental abruption, retained fetus, syndrome, eclampsia, saline-induced abortion)
- Septicemia and viremia (e.g., bacterial infections, cytomegalovirus, hepatitis, varicella, human immunodeficiency virus)
- Disseminated malignancy and leukemia
- Traumatic brain injury
- Transfusion reactions, crush injury, tissue necrosis, and burns
- Liver disease (e.g., obstructive jaundice, acute liver failure)
- Whole-body ischemia-reperfusion following cardiac arrest and subsequent return of spontaneous circulation
- Trauma patients requiring massive transfusion

Each clinical condition may have a different mechanism by which DIC is initiated. In sepsis, for example, the release of TF in response to interleukin 1, endotoxin and tumor necrosis factor appears to be the primary trigger. Release of TF may also explain how trauma initiates DIC particularly in the setting of traumatic brain injury. In amniotic fluid, embolism, circulating electronegatively charged phospholipids are apparently to blame. In cancer, malignant cells may express TF on their surface or release TF following cellular lysis.

25. **How is DIC diagnosed? How is it managed?**
DIC is diagnosed when there is an underlying disorder with a known association with DIC, microvascular bleeding, and the presence of the following:
- Prolongation of laboratory tests of secondary hemostasis (e.g., PT/INR and PTT)
- A rapidly falling platelet count and low fibrinogen (reflecting consumption)
- Increased FDPs and D-dimers (reflecting fibrinolysis)

DIC is managed by "treating the cause" and "supportive management" (e.g., by transfusion of needed products, although this "adds fuel to the fire"). In theory, heparin (or another anticoagulant) could stop the excessive coagulation and break the cycle, but few are willing to heparinize an acutely bleeding patient. Heparin is sometimes used to manage chronic DIC.

26. **Why does blood not clot in normal tissue?**
In nonpathological states, blood is normally kept liquid by a variety of endogenous mechanisms, such as the following:
- The monocyte macrophage system scavenges activated clotting factors
- Endothelial cells produce prostacyclin (PGI_2), a potent vasodilator and inhibitor of platelet activation
- Endothelial cells and platelets secrete and express on their cell surface tissue factor pathway inhibitor, which is an anticoagulant protein that inhibits the activation of TF-VIIa and Xa
- Antithrombin III inhibits all coagulation factors except VIIa
- The anticoagulant protein C inactivates Va and VIIIa, where protein S augments the action of protein C

27. **What is an acceptable preoperative platelet count?**
A normal platelet count is 150,000 to 440,000/mm^3. Thrombocytopenia is defined as a count of less than 150,000/mm^3. Intraoperative bleeding can be severe with counts of 70,000 down to 40,000/mm^3, and spontaneous bleeding usually occurs at counts less than 20,000/mm^3. A minimal recommended platelet count before surgery

(or a neuraxial anesthetic technique) is in the range of 70,000/mm^3, but the percentage of platelets in the blood that are actually functioning is important to consider (platelet count alone does not provide the full picture), as is the stability of the platelet count (e.g., preeclampsia is often associated with a rapid falling platelet count). Thrombocytopenic patients with accelerated destruction but active production of platelets have relatively less bleeding than patients with hypoplastic disorders at a given platelet count. A variety of sophisticated point-of-care tests now exist to assess platelet count and function.

28. What are examples of common antiplatelet agents?
Some "antiplatelet" agents prevent platelet activation, while others prevent platelet aggregation. Aspirin, nonsteroidal antiinflammatory drugs (NSAIDs), and P2Y$_{12}$ receptor antagonists (e.g., clopidogrel, ticagrelor, and prasugrel) interfere with platelet activation, whereas GPIIbIIIa inhibitors (e.g., abciximab, eptifibatide, and tirofiban) prevent platelet aggregation. Drugs that prevent platelet aggregation provide a much more potent "antiplatelet" effect than do drugs that interfere with platelet activation because there are a variety of methods/receptors by which platelets can be activated. Aspirin and NSAIDs typically produce only a mild antiplatelet effect, whereas P2Y$_{12}$ receptor antagonists can produce 40% to 60% inhibition of platelet activation.

29. How do aspirin and NSAIDs work as antiplatelet agents?
Aspirin and NSAIDs inhibit the action of platelet membrane cyclooxygenase (COX), which would otherwise convert arachidonic acid into prostaglandin H$_2$, which then gets converted by tissue-specific synthases into the various familiar prostaglandins (e.g., PGE$_2$, PGI$_2$, TXA$_2$) and leukotrienes. As previously stated, TXA$_2$ is a potent activator of platelets. The various prostaglandins exert various effects in different tissues and organ systems. Aspirin appears to inhibit COX for the lifespan of the platelet, whereas other NSAIDs have a more transient effect.

30. How do the antiplatelet agents clopidogrel, ticagrelor, and prasugrel work?
These medications (or their active metabolite) antagonize the platelet P2Y$_{12}$ receptor, preventing the necessary fall in cAMP that facilitates expression of the GPIIbIIIa receptor (fibrinogen receptor). These medications are often used to prevent thrombosis of coronary or other vascular stents, and/or to prevent intracardiac thrombus formation in patients with atrial fibrillation. Clopidogrel is a prodrug that requires hepatic metabolism through a specific P450 isoenzyme to form the active metabolite. Individual variations of that P450 metabolism (and medications that compete for that P450 metabolism) influence if a given patient is a clopidogrel "responder" or not. Ticagrelor does not require hepatic biotransformation to be active and therefore exerts a more predictable antiplatelet effect. Prasugrel (like clopidogrel) is a prodrug, but a combination of intestinal hydrolysis followed by P450 metabolism (via different isoenzymes than clopidogrel) elaborates the active metabolite. Prasugrel has been demonstrated to have less interindividual variation in antiplatelet effect than clopidogrel.

31. My patient in the emergency room needs an urgent exploratory laparotomy. Their medication history includes an oral "antiplatelet agent" but they are not sure which one. Does it matter?
Yes. The active metabolites of both clopidogrel and prasugrel exhibit irreversible binding to the platelet P2Y$_{12}$ receptor, so the effect of the medication can be "reversed" by the transfusion of platelets (the drug does not come off the receptors to which it is already irreversibly bound). In contrast, ticagrelor exhibits reversible binding to the P2Y$_{12}$ receptor, so platelet transfusion would be ineffective to reverse the effects of the medication (transfused platelets would be similarly inhibited by ticagrelor because of its reversible binding).

32. What are abciximab, eptafibitide, and tirofiban?
Abciximab (Reopro$^®$), eptifibitide (Integrilin$^®$), and tirofiban (Aggrastat$^®$) antagonize the platelet fibrinogen receptor, GPIIbIIIa, which prevents platelet binding to fibrinogen and platelet aggregation. Eptafibitide and tirofiban exhibit competitive, reversible binding and "short" durations of action once the infusion is discontinued (elimination half-lives of about 2.5 and 4 hours, respectively), whereas abciximab exhibits noncompetitive, irreversible binding and a very long duration of action (elimination half-life is only about 10–30 minutes from the plasma, but the effect can manifest up to 48 hours, and low levels of GPIIbIIIa blockade are detected for up to 2 weeks after the infusion is discontinued).

33. My patient needs urgent repair of their femoral artery following an attempted catheterization laboratory intervention, where they received an infusion of one of the fibrinogen receptor blockers. Does it matter which one?
Yes. Although the long duration of action of abciximab may be concerning, the binding of the drug to the fibrinogen receptor is irreversible and noncompetitive, and given the very short elimination half-life from the plasma, one can simply transfuse platelets to restore platelet functionality. Thus whereas the drug itself may be "irreversible" in its binding, the effect is "reversible." In contrast, the relatively short duration of action of eptafibitide and tirofiban may be reassuring, but their reversible, competitive binding means that any transfused platelets will be similarly poisoned. Although the drugs themselves are "reversible" in their binding, "reversal" of their effect requires awaiting complete clearance from the plasma.

34. Describe some platelet abnormalities leading to impaired clot formation.

THROMBOCYTOPENIA (QUANTITATIVE PLATELET DISORDERS)

- Absolute or relative thrombocytopenia (e.g., because of dilution after massive blood transfusion)
- Decreased platelet production caused by malignancy (e.g., aplastic anemia, multiple myeloma), drugs (e.g., chemotherapy, cytotoxic drugs, ethanol, hydrochlorothiazide), chronic liver disease (i.e., decreased thrombopoietin), radiation exposure, or bone-marrow depression after viral infection
- Increased platelet consumption caused by HELLP syndrome (hemolysis, elevated liver function tests, and low platelets), hemolytic uremic syndrome, thrombotic thrombocytopenia, DIC, heparin-induced thrombocytopenia (HIT), splenic sequestration (e.g., cirrhosis)

THROMBOCYTOPATHIA (QUALITATIVE PLATELET DISORDERS)

- Inherited disorders, such as von Willebrand disease, Glanzmann thrombasthenia, Bernard-Soulier syndrome
- Acquired disorders, such as uremia, medications (e.g., aspirin, NSAIDs, antiplatelet agents by intention or side effect), vWS, hypothermia

35. When is a platelet transfusion indicated?

As platelets play the central role in primary hemostasis, platelet transfusion might be indicated by either demonstrated thrombocytopenia or thrombocytopathia in the setting of microvascular bleeding (e.g., bleeding because of coagulopathy, as opposed to surgical bleeding). Often, augmentation of fibrinogen can mitigate the number of platelet transfusions required (...*more mortar helps hold the bricks together*...). Such fibrinogen supplementation can be with cryoprecipitate or fibrinogen concentrates. Platelet transfusions may also be part of a "massive transfusion protocol," in which blood and blood products are transfused rapidly in large volumes in the setting of massive hemorrhage (e.g., in the setting of trauma).

36. What is cryoprecipitate and what are the indications for its transfusion in surgical care?

Cryoprecipitate is the cold-insoluble white precipitate formed when fresh frozen plasma (FFP) is thawed. It is removed by centrifugation, refrozen, and thawed immediately before use. Cryoprecipitate contains Factor VIII, vWF, fibrinogen, fibronectin and factor XIII. In the setting of microvascular bleeding, indications for transfusion of cryoprecipitate include the following: low fibrinogen, hemophilia (second-line agent), vWD/vWS (second-line agent), or when fibrinogen concentrates are not available. The "normal" range of plasma fibrinogen is 150 to 400 mg/dL. Fibrinogen supplementation is generally indicated in the setting of microvascular bleeding when fibrinogen levels are less than 150 mg/dL, or when fibrinogen is demonstrated to be insufficient by point-of-care (POC) tests of fibrinogen (e.g., FIBTEM assay of ROTEM). One modern "pool" of cryoprecipitate (5 "units") is estimated to raise plasma fibrinogen levels by 35 to 50 mg/dL. Cryoprecipitate may also be part of a massive transfusion protocol.

37. What is von Willebrand disease?

vWD is an inherited deficiency of vWF (either qualitative or quantitative). It is the most common inherited bleeding disorder (~1% prevalence) with an autosomal inheritance pattern (effects both women and men equally). Symptoms associated with vWD include menorrhagia (up to 20% of cases), epistaxis, and bleeding problems with dental procedures.

Type I vWD is a mild quantitative defect and is the most common cause of vWD (70%–80% of cases). Desmopressin (DDAVP) is commonly used to treat type I vWD to reduce bleeding. It works by increasing vWF plasma levels.

Type II vWD is subclassified into a variety of qualitative defects and is responsible for approximately 20% of cases and also responds to DDAVP. Important, vWD type IIb is a hypercoagulable state, so do not give DDAVP to anyone with vWD type IIb!

Type III vWD is rare (<5% of cases) quantitative defect cause by the complete (or nearly complete) absence of circulating vWF. Type III requires supplementation of vWF (i.e., plasma derived or recombinant vWF [first line] or cryoprecipitate [second line]).

38. What is von Willebrand syndrome?

vWS is an acquired structural or functional defect in vWF. vWS often results from increased destruction (i.e., conformational protein unfolding) of vWF in regions of high shear-stress blood flow (e.g., blood flow through a stenotic aortic valve [i.e., Heyde syndrome] or during mechanical circulatory support with a ventricular assist device), but it can also result from viral, malignant, or pharmacological mechanisms.

39. What is fresh frozen plasma and what are the indications for fresh frozen plasma in surgical care?

Plasma is the liquid portion of blood, once the cells have been separated out by centrifugation. FFP is plasma that has been frozen within 8 hours of collection. It contains all plasma proteins, including both pro- and anticoagulant factors. Transfusion is indicated in the setting of microvascular bleeding when the patient would benefit from the components contained within FFP. FFP may also be indicated in the setting of microvascular bleeding when there is no time to obtain laboratory or POC testing (or it is not available) when the patient would benefit from the components contained within FFP (e.g., as part of a "massive transfusion protocol" in the setting of massive hemorrhage). FFP may also be used to reverse the effects of warfarin (FFP 5–8 mL/kg first dose) and can provide a remedy for acquired heparin resistance (because of the antithrombin III contained within FFP). In the setting of coagulopathic surgical bleeding, it must be remembered that platelets and fibrinogen play the central role in primary hemostasis, and supplementing with FFP will not adequately treat the coagulopathy if the quantity and function of both platelets and fibrinogen is inadequate.

40. What is Thrombate III®?

Thrombate III® (Grifols, USA) is a concentrate of human antithrombin III in lyophilized powder form. It is indicated for the prevention (and treatment) of thromboembolism in patients with a congenital deficiency of antithrombin III. Thrombate III® is frequently used in the cardiac surgical operating room to provide additional antithrombin III in the setting of acquired heparin "resistance."

41. What are PCCs?

Prothrombin complex concentrates (PCCs) are various procoagulant "medications" containing various formulations of vitamin K dependent clotting factors. In the United States, there are two commonly used formulations: three factor PCC (factors II, IX, X) and the more recent US Food and Drug Administration approved four factor PCC (factors II, VII, IX, X, and protein C/S). The main concern with PCC is thrombotic complications, however, most formulations contain heparin to minimize this complication, with recent studies showing no increased risk compared with FFP. The primary indication of PCC is to rapidly reverse the effects of warfarin before emergent surgery or in the case of life-threatening bleeding (e.g., intracranial hemorrhage).

42. What is HIT?

HIT is a result of heparin administration, but it is important to distinguish between HIT type 1 and HIT type 2, as these are different clinical syndromes. HIT type 1 is a nonimmune mediated and self-limited thrombocytopenia that typically develops within the first 48 hours following heparin exposure, as a direct result of heparin-induced activation of platelets. HIT type 2, however, is a hypercoagulable state induced by platelet activation by a complex of antibody, PF4, and heparin. HIT type 2 is also sometimes called *HITT* (heparin-induced thrombocytopenia with thrombosis), as deep venous and arterial thromboses are the hallmark of this syndrome. HIT type 2 generally develops 5 to 10 days after heparin exposure, and the antibodies can persist for months, necessitating immediate discontinuation of and avoidance of all heparin administration (including removal of heparin coated vascular access lines, if present) and prompt initiation of an alternative anticoagulant (e.g., argatroban). Warfarin is not used until the platelet count has recovered. The antibodies mediating HIT type 2 persist for at least 2 to 3 months.

43. How is HIT diagnosed?

The diagnosis of HIT remains largely clinical, as the patient must have exposure to heparin, a decrease in the platelet count by 30% to less than 100,000/mm^3 or a decrease of more than 50% from the patient's baseline platelet count. HIT type 2 is (by definition) also associated with thrombotic events. The demonstration of HIT antibodies are sensitive but not specific for HIT type 2, and the results of the assays can sometimes be inconclusive. Although specific laboratory tests can help confirm the diagnosis when antibody assays are inconclusive, the results of these tests are often not available in a timely manner, and anticoagulation with a heparin alternative should not await the results of such tests. In addition to platelet counts, potentially confirmatory tests for the presence of HIT antibodies include both immunoassays and functional tests (e.g., serotonin release assay, heparin-induced platelet aggregation assay, flow cytometry). The immunoassays have a high sensitivity but low specificity. The serotonin release assay has both high sensitivity and specificity, but is not available in many laboratories, resulting in a prolonged turnaround time. As reexposure to heparin could have devastating consequences for patients with prior HIT type 2, even after the antibodies are demonstrably no longer present, it is generally recommended to use a heparin alternative for future noncardiac surgical procedures where anticoagulation is required. For cardiopulmonary bypass, a one-time heparinization is allowable for patients in whom HIT antibodies can no longer be demonstrated as the significant risk of bleeding with heparin alternatives may outweigh the risk of a heparin reexposure.

44. What are ROTEM and TEG?

ROTEM® (Instrumentation Laboratory, Bedford, MA, USA) and TEG® (Haemonetics Corporation, Braintree, MA, USA) are viscoelastic tests of global hemostasis that measure clot initiation, kinetics, strength, and stability. These tests overcome some of the shortcomings of traditional tests. For example, a cirrhotic patient with thrombocytopenia and an elevated INR is not necessarily coagulopathic (in fact, may even be hypercoagulable because of decreased liver synthesis of anticoagulant proteins), whereas a hypothermic trauma patient with a normal INR and platelet count can be coagulopathic because of hypothermia. Viscoelastic tests can be performed at the POC with results available within 10 to 30 minutes. They are commonly used in the setting of cardiac surgery, liver transplant, and trauma surgery.

ROTEM stands for rotational thromboelastometry, a relatively recent adaptation of TEG (thromboelastography), which has been around since the 1940s. Both provide information about the sufficiency of factors and clottable substrate from small samples of whole blood. Similar measured parameters on both platforms provide information about the quantity and/or quality of coagulation factors and platelets, and the measured values can be used as part of transfusion algorithms and/or blood-product ordering algorithms to guide targeted transfusion of blood products (e.g., platelets, fibrinogen and plasma). Such individualized targeting of appropriate therapies not only helps mitigate the risks and morbidities associated with the transfusion of blood products, but also the cost, by decreasing needless transfusion of products already demonstrated to be adequate to effect hemostasis.

45. What does a normal ROTEM/TEG tracing look like? What are the key measured parameters and what information do they provide?

A prototypical TEG tracing is shown in Fig. 10.2, with examples of abnormal TEG tracings shown in Fig. 10.3. Note, that both TEG and ROTEM yield a similar tracing morphology and provide an assessment of global hemostasis but with different terms. The key measured parameters are compared in Table 10.1.

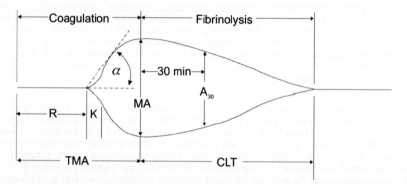

Fig. 10.2 A normal TEG tracing. The tracing morphology and measured parameters with ROTEM are similar. Please see Table 10.1 to correlate measurement terminology between ROTEM and TEG. *A30/LY30*, Amplitude 30 minutes after MA; *CLT*, clot lysis time; *K*, kinetics; *MA*, maximum amplitude; *R*, reaction time; *TMA*, time to maximum amplitude; *α*, alpha angle (From Roshal M, Gil M, Thromboelastography/thromboelastometry. In: Shaz B, Hillyer C, Gil M, ed. Transfusion Medicine and Hemostasis: Clinical and Laboratory Aspects. 3rd ed. Amsterdam: Elsevier Science; 2018:819-826.)

Characteristic Thromboelastograph Tracings

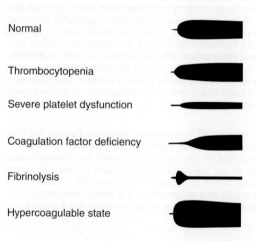

Normal

Thrombocytopenia

Severe platelet dysfunction

Coagulation factor deficiency

Fibrinolysis

Hypercoagulable state

Fig. 10.3 Typical thromboelastography pattern and variables measured as normal values and examples of some abnormal tracings. (From DeCastro M. Evaluation of the coagulation system. In: Faust RJ, ed. Anesthesiology Reviews. 3rd ed. New York: Churchill Livingstone; 2002:352.)

Table 10.1 A Comparison of ROTEM and TEG Nomenclature for the Various Measured Parameters

	ROTEM	TEG	SUGGESTED ACTION IF DEFICIENT
Clot initiation (time to initial thrombin formation)	CT	R	Supplement clotting factors[a]
Clot kinetics (rate of clot stabilization)	CFT, α	K, α	Supplement platelets and/or fibrinogen[b]
Clot strength (maximum strength or firmness)	MCF	MA	Supplement platelets and/or fibrinogen[b]
Clot stability (lysis)	LI30, ML	LY30	Provide an antifibrinolytic

[a]Significant deficiencies of platelets and or fibrinogen can prolong the time to initial thrombin formation, so it is recommended to ensure the adequacy of fibrinogen and platelets before providing factors (unless a factor deficiency is already known or suspected).

[b]The propagation of the clot and the maximum clot formed are dependent on both fibrinogen and platelets, and an effort should be made to understand the contribution of each to the clot before selecting products for transfusion.

CFT, Clot formation time; *CT*, clotting time; *K*, kinetics; *LI*, lysis index 30 minutes after CT; *LY30*, clot lysis at 30 minutes after MA; *MA*, maximum amplitude; *MCF*, maximum clot firmness; *ML*, maximum lysis; *R*, reaction time; α, Alpha angle.

KEY POINTS: CLINICAL ASPECTS OF COAGULATION

1. Warfarin inhibits the synthesis of vitamin K-dependent factors II, VII, IX, X, protein C, and protein S. The anticoagulant protein C has a short half-life and is responsible for the initial hypercoagulability seen when initiating warfarin.
2. Heparin works by enhancing the activity of antithrombin III. A major complication associated with heparin is HIT. A major advantage of heparin is that it can easily be reversed with protamine.
3. LMWH works by inhibiting Factor Xa. Its major advantages over heparin include a more predictable anticoagulation effect which does not necessitate monitoring.
4. Protamine can partially reverse LMWH but not completely. LMWH is renally excreted and contraindicated in patients with end-stage renal disease.
5. Antifibrinolytics (i.e., aminocaproic acid and tranexamic acid) prevent the activation of plasminogen to plasmin. These agents are primarily used to minimize bleeding but may also help reduce surgical complications (cardiac tamponade, hysterectomy, etc.) and the risk of death in certain situations (i.e., trauma, pos-partum hemorrhage).
6. DIC is characterized as systemic activation of coagulation and fibrinolysis, leading to a consumptive coagulopathy (low platelets, low clotting factors). DIC initially presents as a hypercoagulable state followed by a hypocoagulable state.
7. DIC is commonly seen in situations associated with systemic inflammation and/or the release of procoagulant proteins (e.g., TF). It is associated with the following conditions: sepsis, malignancy, pregnancy complications, trauma, traumatic brain injury, etc.
8. The most common type of vWD is type I and can be treated with DDAVP. Type 3 requires vWF supplementation because of the absence of circulating vWF. Do not give DDAVP to patients with type 2B vWD because this subtype causes a hypercoagulable state.
9. vWS is an acquired structural or functional defect in vWF. It is often the result of increased destruction of vWF, such as from high shear-stress blood flow (e.g., through a stenotic aortic valve [i.e., Heyde syndrome] or during mechanical circulatory support with a ventricular assist device).
10. HIT occurs following exposure to heparin. Type 1 is nonimmune and usually self-limited. Type 2 occurs 5 to 10 days following exposure and is associated with thrombotic complications.
11. HIT is often a clinical diagnosis as confirmatory laboratory tests often are not readily available in most hospitals. Treatment includes discontinuing all heparin containing products and to administer anticoagulation (i.e., direct thrombin inhibitors).
12. Viscoelastic tests (i.e., ROTEM/TEG) provide a global assessment of hemostasis that measures clot initiation, kinetics, strength, and stability. These tests are frequently used in the setting of cardiac surgery, liver transplant, and trauma surgery to guide blood product administration.

SUGGESTED READINGS

Gando S, Levi M, Toh CH. Disseminated intravascular coagulation. Nat Rev Dis Primers. 2016;2;(2):16037.
Greinacher A. Clinical practice. Heparin-induced thrombocytopenia. N Engl J Med. 2015;373(3):252–261.
Leebeek FW, Eikenboom JC. Von Willebrand's disease. N Engl J Med. 2016;375(21):2067–2080.
Levy J, Koster A, Quinones Q, et al. Antifibrinolytic therapy and perioperative considerations. Anesthesiology. 2018;128(3):657–670.

CHAPTER 11

TRANSFUSION THERAPY

Ryan A. Lawless, MD, FACS, Ryan D. Laterza, MD

1. **What is the overarching indication for blood transfusion?**
   The overarching indication for transfusing packed red blood cells (RBCs) is to improve oxygen delivery ($\dot{D}O_2$). One of the primary roles of RBCs is to transport oxygen from the lung to tissue to allow aerobic metabolism. $\dot{D}O_2$ is dependent upon the cardiac output (CO) and the arterial oxygen content (CaO_2) by the following equation:

$$\dot{D}O_2 = CO \times CaO_2$$

   Where arterial oxygen content equals the following:

$$CaO_2 = 1.36 \times [Hg] \times S_aO_2 + 0.003 \times [P_aO_2]$$

   Hg, hemoglobin; S_aO_2, arterial oxygen saturation; P_aO_2, arterial oxygen partial pressure
   In other words, oxygen delivery to tissue, $\dot{D}O_2$, is dependent upon the amount of oxygen in the blood, CaO_2, and the rate, CO, that blood is delivered. There are circumstances (e.g., hemorrhage) in which the $\dot{D}O_2$ is inadequate to meet the body's metabolic oxygen demands (VO_2). Transfusing RBCs will increase the Hg level, thereby, increasing CaO_2, which increases $\dot{D}O_2$. Also, transfusing RBCs (and other blood products) will increase the heart's preload and subsequent stroke volume (recall Frank-Starling law), leading to an increase in CO which also increases $\dot{D}O_2$. Recall, CO = stroke volume × heart rate. Therefore transfusing RBCs will increase $\dot{D}O_2$ by increasing both oxygen content and CO.

2. **What happens when there is a mismatch between oxygen delivery and consumption (aka supply-demand mismatch)?**
   $\dot{D}O_2$, usually exceeds oxygen consumption, $\dot{V}O_2$, by a factor of 4 (1000 mL/min vs. 250 mL/min). In other words, oxygen supply to tissue greatly exceeds tissue oxygen demands at rest. However, when $\dot{D}O_2$ is inadequate to meet VO_2 demands, a compensatory increase in "oxygen extraction" occurs to maintain $\dot{V}O_2$. Normally, the oxygen extraction ratio (O_2 ER) is 20% to 30% where O_2 ER = $\dot{V}O_2/\dot{D}O_2$. For example, if $\dot{V}O_2$, is normally 250 mL/min and $\dot{D}O_2$, is 1000 mL/min, then the O_2 ER = 25%. This corresponds to a mixed venous saturation ($S_{mv}O_2$) equal to 70% to 80%. Note, that a $S_{mv}O_2$ requires right heart catheterization with a pulmonary artery catheter to sample blood from the pulmonary artery. Normally, a compensatory increase in CO will occur to maintain adequate $\dot{D}O_2$ in the setting of increased VO_2 (e.g., exercise). If the increase in CO fails to maintain adequate $\dot{D}O_2$, then the oxygen extraction ratio will increase causing the $S_{mv}O_2$ less than 70%. Once these compensatory mechanisms are exhausted, cells switch to anaerobic metabolism (i.e., lactic acidosis). For example, a clinical correlate associated with inadequate $\dot{D}O_2$ is cardiogenic shock caused by inadequate CO or hemorrhagic shock caused by inadequate oxygen content from acute blood loss anemia and inadequate CO from hypovolemia.

3. **What is $\dot{D}O_{2crit}$?**
   $\dot{D}O_{2crit}$ is defined as the critical oxygen delivery needed to satisfy the metabolic demands for oxygen consumption. In a euvolemic patient with normal cardiac function, the $\dot{D}O_{2crit}$ is normally not reached until the Hg concentration decreases to 3.5 g/dL. However, the specific Hg level depends upon the patient's oxygen requirement. For example, in high metabolic states (e.g., sepsis, burns, trauma) there is an increase in VO_2; therefore $\dot{D}O_{2crit}$ is reached at a higher concentration of Hg. Comorbidities, such as coronary artery disease also affects the Hg concentration at which $\dot{D}O_{2crit}$ is reached.

4. **What are some of the surrogate measures for $\dot{D}O_{2crit}$?**
   $\dot{D}O_{2crit}$ cannot be directly measured in the typical clinical setting. Surrogate variables include:
   - Vital signs: hypotension, tachycardia, urine output
   - Labs: lactic acid, base deficit
   - Signs of myocardial ischemia: new ST-segment depression greater than 0.1 mV, new ST-segment elevation greater than 0.2 mV, regional wall motion abnormalities by echocardiography
   - Decreased mixed venous O_2 saturation (<50%)

5. **What are the physiological adaptations to acute normovolemic anemia?**
   Acute normovolemic anemia occurs secondary to the replacement of intraoperative blood loss with crystalloid solution. The compensatory physiological changes include sympathetic stimulation (tachycardia, increased CO), decreased blood viscosity (decreases afterload, increases preload, improves capillary flow), and redistribution of blood flow to tissues that are more oxygen dependent (i.e., heart and brain). Notably, the heart and brain have the highest O_2 ER at baseline and cannot tolerate a decrease in $\dot{D}O_2$ by increasing oxygen extraction compared with other tissues.

6. **What does a low mixed venous saturation suggest in terms of oxygen delivery?**
   A low mixed venous saturation ($S_{mv}O_2$ <60%) implies that the body is increasing its O_2 ER because of decreased $\dot{D}O_2$. This implies that either the CO and/or oxygen content is insufficient to meet the metabolic demands of the body. This is commonly seen in the setting of cardiogenic and hemorrhagic shock.

7. **Can a patient develop lactic acidosis despite a normal mixed venous saturation?**
   Some patients may present with shock physiology (anaerobic metabolism as indicated by lactic acidosis) not because of inadequate $\dot{D}O_2$ but rather because of inability to use oxygen because of impairment of oxidative phosphorylation. This can be seen in septic shock (endotoxin-mediated inhibition of pyruvate dehydrogenase), cyanide toxicity (inhibits electron transport chain), propofol infusion syndrome (inhibits electron transport chain).

8. **Which organ has the highest oxygen extraction ratio?**
   The heart has the highest O_2 ER and consumes more oxygen by mass compare to any other organ. This is evident by the fact that the coronary sinus has the lowest oxygen saturation in the entire body ($SvO_2 \approx 40\%$), which also explains why the mixed venous saturation from the pulmonary artery ($SmvO_2 \approx 70\%$) is lower than the central venous saturation from the superior and inferior vena cava ($ScvO_2 \approx 75\%$). It also explains the rationale in maintaining a higher Hg in patients with coronary artery disease as the heart's oxygen demands can increase up to a factor of five when stressed (e.g., tachycardia caused by shock physiology), but has limited ability to compensate for anemia by increasing its O_2 ER.

9. **What Hg concentration should trigger a blood transfusion?**
   The Transfusion Requirements in Critical Care Trial attempted to answer this question. Within the trial, groups were divided into a restrictive trigger of 7 g/dL (to target a Hg between 7 and 9 g/dL) and a liberal trigger of 10 g/dL (to target a Hg between 10 and 12 g/dL). The 30-day mortality was found to be lower in the restrictive group, with organ dysfunction being comparable between the two groups. Further, the restrictive group received less blood transfusions during the intensive care unit (ICU) stay. It was determined from this trial that the transfusion trigger for most patients in the ICU should be a Hg less than 7 g/dL. However, patients with hemodynamic instability or evidence of cardiac ischemia may need a higher Hg threshold.

   Current American Society of Anesthesiology (2015) guidelines recommend to strongly consider transfusion of RBC when the Hg is less than 6 g/dL, that transfusion is rarely needed when the Hg is greater than 10 g/dL, and that clinical indications (e.g., ongoing blood loss) should guide transfusion triggers when the Hg is between 6 and 10 g/dL.

10. **What is leukoreduction? What are its benefits?**
    Leukoreduction is the process by which white blood cells are removed from donor blood through the use of a filter. It is reported to have the following benefits: (1) reduces the risk of febrile, nonhemolytic transfusion reactions, and (2) reduces the transmission of infectious agents, such as Epstein-Barr virus, cytomegalovirus, human T-cell lymphocytic virus, prion disease (Creutzfeldt-Jakob disease), malaria, leishmaniasis, human granulocytic anaplasmosis, and yersinia enterocolitis. Universal leukoreduction is currently practiced in mostly all developed countries, aside from the United States, where its adherence is not mandated (because of costs/benefit concerns). However, in practice the vast majority (>80%–90%) of hospitals in the United States adhere to universal leukoreduction of all blood products.

11. **What are the risks of blood transfusion?**
    - Infectious transmission
    - Transfusion reactions (see Table 11.1)
    - Immunomodulatory effects

12. **Describe the risk of infection that can occur with blood transfusion.**
    Blood transfusion is extremely safe in this day and age. The risk of transmission of hepatitis C or human immunodeficiency virus (HIV) from a unit of blood is rare in developed nations (one in few million on average) and is highly dependent upon the population. For example, in Canada the risk of hepatitis C and HIV with blood transfusion is reported to be 1 in 13 and 21 million, respectively. However, there will always remain some risk, albeit rare, of infection with blood transfusion. These include pathogens that are routinely tested, including those without a screening test. The pathogens routinely tested include the following: hepatitis, HIV, syphilis, human T-cell lymphotropic virus, West Nile virus, and cytomegalovirus. Other pathogens that may be transmitted include prion-mediated disease (Creutzfeldt-Jakob disease) in the United Kingdom, parasitic diseases, such as Chagas disease, and malaria in underdeveloped regions of the world.

13. **What is the most common adverse reaction to blood transfusion?**
    Febrile, nonhemolytic transfusion reactions are the most common reactions associated with blood product transfusion. The reaction is considered benign, is not associated with hemolysis, and occurs with an incidence ranging between 0.1% and 27% (highest with nonleukoreduced platelets). Symptoms include headache, malaise, and nausea. This reaction is caused by recipient human leukocyte antigen (HLA) antibodies reacting to HLA antigens from donor white blood cells (e.g., neutrophils). It generally occurs in patients with a history of previous blood product transfusion who are thought to develop HLA antibodies. Administering leukoreduced blood can significantly reduce the risk of this complication. Symptoms may be treated with antipyretics for fever and opioids (i.e., meperidine) for shivering.

Table 11.1 Major Transfusion Reactions

DIAGNOSTIC ENTITY	ONSET	MAJOR SIGNS AND SYMPTOMS	DIFFERENTIATING FEATURES
Transfusion-related acute lung injury (TRALI)	Minutes to hours	Dyspnea, respiratory distress, hypoxemia, cyanosis, pulmonary edema, fever, tachycardia	Nonhydrostatic pulmonary edema, frequent fever, transient leukopenia
Transfusion-associated circulatory overload (TACO)	Minutes to hours	Dyspnea, respiratory distress, hypoxemia, cyanosis, pulmonary edema, evidence of hypervolemia (jugular venous distention, peripheral edema, elevated BNP), hypertension	Hydrostatic pulmonary edema, absent fever, hypertension, evidence of hypervolemia, evidence of increased left atrial pressure, elevated BNP, responds to diuretics
Anaphylactic reactions	Minutes to hours	Bronchospasm, respiratory distress, hypotension, cyanosis, generalized erythema and urticaria, mucous membrane edema	Rash, urticaria, and edema present; hypotension and bronchospasm prominent
Bacterial contamination of blood products	Minutes	Fever, rigors, hypotension, and vascular collapse	Fever, rigors, and vascular collapse predominant; most common with platelets
Hemolytic transfusion reaction	Minutes	Fever, rigors, hypotension, hemoglobinuria, disseminated intravascular coagulation	Usually with red blood cell transfusion, hemolysis

Symptoms may be missed while under general anesthesia, and differential diagnosis should be expanded to include common intraoperative problems.
BNP, Brain natriuretic peptide.
Modified from Boshkov LK. Transfusion-related acute lung injury and the ICU. Crit Care Clin. 2005;21:479-495.

14. **What are the risks with administering incompatible blood?**
    Acute hemolytic transfusion reactions are caused by ABO blood group incompatibility. This is usually because of a clerical error at some step in the transfusion process and occurs with a frequency of approximately 1:70,000 units. Symptoms include fevers, chills, nausea, flushing, chest/flank/back pain, hypotension, tachycardia, oliguria, hemoglobinuria, renal failure, and disseminated intravascular coagulation. Symptom onset often occurs shortly after transfusion. Management begins with the cessation of the transfusion and supportive care. Physicians need to maintain a high index of suspicion when a patient is under general anesthesia, as symptoms may not readily be apparent during surgery (patient covered by drapes, general anesthesia causes hypothermia, which may mask fever, etc.).

15. **Can blood products cause anaphylaxis?**
    Allergic reactions (immunoglobulin [Ig]E-mediated histamine release) can occur from blood products and range from urticaria (mild, benign) to anaphylactic shock (severe, life-threatening). Mild allergic reactions are reported to occur at a rate of 1 to 3 per 100 transfusions, whereas severe allergic reactions are on the order of one per 50,000 transfusions. Anaphylactic reactions can present as erythema, urticaria, edema, bronchospasm, tachycardia, and hypotension depending upon severity. Urgent management is necessary and consists of stopping the transfusion, giving epinephrine (e.g., 50 mcg to 1 mg intravenous [IV] depending upon severity), and IV fluid administration. Glucocorticoids and antihistamine medications may also be considered.
    Patients with IgA deficiency have traditionally been considered at high-risk for anaphylactic reactions because of the possibility of circulating IgA antibodies. However, evidence to date suggests most of these patients will not have an anaphylactic reaction to blood transfusion. In elective situations, consider transfusing only IgA deficient donor blood products; however, in emergent situations, blood transfusion in these patients should not be delayed.

16. **Is there convincing evidence that blood transfusions are harmful to immune function?**
    Short answer, no. This has been looked at in multiple studies; however, no difference in long-term mortality because of impaired immune function between liberal and restrictive blood transfusion groups has been found.

17. **What is a blood storage lesion?**
    A blood storage lesion is a change in the blood content or functionality from aging following its collection. Blood storage lesions include a reduction in RBC deformity, depletion of adenosine triphosphate stores, decreased levels of 2,3-diphosphoglycerate (2,3-DPG) causing a shift of the Hg dissociation curve to the left, reducing oxygen offloading

to tissue, and the accumulation of proinflammatory cytokines. To minimize blood storage lesions, the shelf life of packed RBCs is 42 days following collection.

18. **What is TRALI?**

Transfusion-associated acute lung injury (TRALI) is a transfusion reaction that may occur in 1:5000 units transfused. The actual occurrence rate is unknown, as reporting of this complication is voluntary. The majority, 85%, of reported cases are secondary to the infusion of donor HLA antibodies that react with HLA antigens located on recipient neutrophils. The incidence of TRALI was greatly reduced after blood banks updated collection standards to include whole blood, platelets, and plasma from males, never-pregnant females, and females with a history of pregnancy that have tested negative for the HLA antibodies after pregnancy.

Historically, TRALI was responsible for the majority of deaths reported to the US Food and Drug Administration related to blood product administration; however, this trend is now reversing with recent data showing transfusion-associated circulatory overload (TACO) as a slightly higher cause of mortality.

19. **What causes TRALI?**

TRALI can be considered a special form of acute respiratory distress syndrome (ARDS; i.e., nonhydrostatic pulmonary edema) caused by the transfusion of blood products. The pathophysiology of TRALI is explained by the two-hit hypothesis whereby a preexisting condition, making the patient susceptible, causes the first hit. Specifically, the first hit is caused by systemic inflammation (shock, sepsis, alcohol abuse, liver disease, smoking, etc.) leading to pulmonary endothelial activation and cytokine release attracting and priming neutrophils into the lung. The first hit (i.e., systemic inflammation) is also a risk factor for ARDS in general and is not unique to TRALI. The second hit is caused by blood product transfusion and is the distinguishing characteristic of TRALI. Specifically, blood products which contain donor HLA antibodies bind to the activated neutrophils of the recipient within the lung causing a massive inflammatory response, increasing capillary permeability, leading to nonhydrostatic pulmonary edema.

The biggest risk factor for developing TRALI is receiving blood products, especially fresh frozen plasma (FFP) and platelets, from multiparous women, as studies show that up to 50% of this patient population develop anti-HLA antibodies.

20. **What are the diagnostic criteria of TRALI?**
- Acute onset: within 6 hours of transfusion
- Hypoxemia with a PaO_2/FiO_2 of 300 mm Hg or less, regardless of the level of positive end expiratory pressure
- Bilateral infiltrates on chest radiograph
- No circulatory overload signs or symptoms (i.e., no evidence of left atrial hypertension by pulmonary artery catheterization or echocardiography)
- Absence of ARDS before transfusion (if present the diagnosis becomes TRALI Type II)

  *Note, a complete blood count may show a transient leukopenia (or neutropenia), but this is not required for the diagnosis.

21. **What are the therapeutic options for TRALI?**

If TRALI is suspected, the transfusion should immediately be stopped. The remainder of the blood should be sent back to the blood bank for testing. The patient will require respiratory support. This may consist of supplemental oxygen, noninvasive ventilator support (i.e., continuous positive airway pressure/bilevel positive airway pressure), or invasive mechanical ventilation (i.e., endotracheal intubation). Hemodynamic support may be necessary, including IV fluid resuscitation and vasopressors. Diuretic should be avoided, as hypotension is often associated with TRALI and diuresis will worsen the hypotension. Most importantly, TRALI is not associated with hypervolemia, which causes TACO. Finally, steroids are not recommended in the management of TRALI.

22. **Are future transfusions contraindicated in patients with a known TRALI event?**

No. Patients who have suffered from TRALI have the same risk as the rest of the population of a second episode. However, transfusions from the same donor should be avoided.

23. **What is TACO?**

TACO is an acute, hydrostatic pulmonary edema in the setting of transfusion. Patients with TACO often have respiratory distress with marked tachypnea, dyspnea, and hypoxia. TACO is a vascular overload problem, which presents with hypertension, tachycardia, pulmonary edema, and hypervolemia.

24. **Who is susceptible to TACO?**

Patients that are susceptible to TACO include elderly patients ($>$70 years of age), pediatric patients, and patients with heart failure or kidney disease.

25. **What are the differences between TACO and TRALI?**
- The following is seen with TACO but not TRALI:
  - More likely to be associated with a large volume of blood product transfusion
  - Hypertension

- Absence of fever
- Evidence of circulatory overload (pulmonary artery occlusion pressure elevated)
  - Increased vascular congestion on chest radiograph
  - Increased brain natriuretic peptide (BNP) and proBNP
- Responds to diuresis

26. **What are the therapeutic options for TACO?**

If TACO is suspected, all transfusions should be stopped. The transfused unit should be sent to the blood bank for analysis as TACO can be confused with TRALI and other reactions. Careful diuretic administration is necessary to offload the vascular system. Renal function should be monitored carefully to not induce acute kidney injury. The patient may require respiratory support. This consists of supplemental oxygen, noninvasive ventilator support, or invasive mechanical ventilation. The best therapy is prevention. Avoiding unnecessary transfusion by adhering to institutional thresholds and limiting the number of administered units of blood products are important steps in preventing TACO.

27. **What is the 2-hit hypothesis for TRALI and TACO?**

The 2-hit hypothesis consistent of the sequence of events leading to TRALI and TACO. The first hit are the risk factors that predispose a patient to TRALI or TACO. In TRALI, the main risk factor is systemic inflammation, whereas in TACO the main risk factors are kidney disease, heart failure, pediatric patients, and advanced age (>70 years). The second hit is caused by blood product transfusion causing nonhydrostatic (TRALI) and hydrostatic (TACO) pulmonary edema.

28. **Summarize the differences between TACO and TRALI.**

TACO occurs because the circulatory system becomes overloaded from the amount of transfused blood product. TACO causes hydrostatic (aka cardiogenic) pulmonary edema with hypertension and hypoxia being the most common symptoms. The management centers on diuresis as the problem is caused by hypervolemia.

TRALI is a form of nonhydrostatic (aka noncardiogenic) pulmonary edema that may occur with blood transfusion. It is essentially a specific type of ARDS caused by blood transfusion. It is an immune-mediated process that occurs within 6 hours of transfusion. The symptoms include hypoxia, dyspnea, fever, and pulmonary edema. Supportive management of the symptoms is the mainstay of treatment.

29. **Review the ABO and Rh genotypes and the associated antibody patterns (Table 11.2).**

There are three separate alleles involved in blood typing (A, B, and O). Two of the alleles combine to determine a patient's blood type. Patients with type A will have the A antigen present and will form anti-B antibodies over time. Patients with type B will have the B antigen present and will form anti-A antibodies over time. Patients with type AB will have both antigens present and will not form anti-A or anti-B antibodies. This population is considered the universal donor for plasma (i.e., FFP) as there will be no antibodies to blood type alleles in the plasma. Finally, type O patients have neither antigen present on their RBCs, form both anti-A and anti-B antibodies, and are considered the universal donor for RBCs.

The Rhesus (Rh) factor is the (+) or (−) seen when blood is typed. The basis for the Rh factor is the presence or absence of the D antigen. When present, the patient is said to have Rh-positive blood.

An Rh-negative patient can receive Rh-positive blood. However, antibodies can form to the D-antigen in these patients following exposure to Rh-positive blood. This can lead to a delayed, mild, hemolytic transfusion reaction. However, the patient becomes sensitized and can have a significant reaction if reexposed to Rh-positive blood at a later date.

30. **What is the difference between a type & screen and a crossmatch?**

Blood is typed for ABO and Rh group identification. This occurs by mixing the red cells with anti-A and anti-B reagents to reverse type the patient's serum. Blood is then screened for antibodies by mixing the serum with specially selected red cells containing the relevant blood group antigens. A crossmatch is performed to verify in vitro compatibility and detect more unique antibodies (Table 11.3). The latter occurs when the patients' serum is incubated with a small quantity of red cells from the proposed donor unit.

Table 11.2 Blood Types and Constituent Antigens and Antibodies

BLOOD GENOTYPES	BLOOD TYPE	ANTIGENS	ANTIBODIES
OO	O	None[a]	Anti-A and anti-B
OA or AA	A	A	Anti-B
OB or BB	B	B	Anti-A
AB	AB	A and B	None[†]

[a]The absence of antigens makes OO red blood cells (RBCs) the universal RBC donor.
[†]The absence of antibodies makes AB plasma the universal plasma donor.

Table 11.3 Crossmatch and Compatibility

DEGREE OF CROSSMATCH	CHANCE OF COMPATIBLE TRANSFUSION
ABO-Rh type only	99.8%
ABO-Rh type + antibody screen	99.94%
ABO-Rh type + antibody screen crossmatch	99.95%

31. **What blood should be transfused in an emergent situation?**
The quickest choice for emergent situations is type O, Rh-negative packed RBCs and type AB plasma. The next choice is type-specific, uncrossmatched blood, followed by type-specific, partially crossmatched, followed by type-specific, fully crossmatched blood.

32. **What is prothrombin complex concentrate (PCC)?**
Prothrombin complex concentrates (PCCs) are various formulations containing purified vitamin K-dependent clotting factors used for rapid reversal of oral anticoagulants. This classification of drugs includes three-factor (factors II, IX, and X), four-factors (factors II, VII, IX, and X), and activated PCC (activated factors II, VII, IX, and X).

33. **When is PCC used?**
PCCs can be used to reverse warfarin and Factor Xa inhibitors (rivaroxaban, apixaban, or edoxaban). Common indications include urgent reversal of warfarin because of life-threatening bleeding (i.e., intracranial hemorrhage) or to reduce the amount of volume that would normally be needed with plasma in patients who are susceptible to hypervolemia (e.g., heart failure).
Four-factor PCC reverses the anticoagulant effects of the Xa inhibitors better than three-factor PCC. Activated PCC performs even better than the four-factor PCC; however, this formulation is extremely expensive.
PCC has not been universally incorporated into the massive transfusion protocols at this time.

34. **What are the advantages of PCC over plasma transfusion?**
PCC has shown to normalize the international normalized ratio (INR) of patients taking warfarin faster and more reliability than FFP. The volume of PCC required to normalize the INR is significantly less compared with FFP, reducing the risk of TACO. With the smaller volume needed for reversal of INR, the administration time is extremely rapid. Also no blood-typing is necessary with PCC, allowing immediate administration with no risk of ABO incompatibility. Further, there is no known risk of TRALI occurring with PCC.
Further research is needed to determine the pH buffer and oncotic properties of PCC as they compare to plasma. Furthermore, studies are being done investigating the endothelial effects and clot strength effects of PCC.

35. **What are some of the complications of massive blood product transfusion?**
Massive transfusion can lead to multiple complications. These include coagulopathies, such as dilutional thrombocytopenia, decreased coagulation factors secondary to a lack of factors V and VIII in the infused plasma, and disseminated intravascular coagulation. Metabolic disturbances including hyperkalemia, hypocalcemia, and reduced 2,3-DPG occur. Hypothermia can occur with blood transfusion, leading to an increase in blood loss by 16%, for temperatures between 34°C and 36°C. Hypothermia impairs platelet function, as well as the function of coagulation cascade proteins. TACO, TRALI, and the other transfusion reactions can also occur.

36. **What is citrate toxicity?**
Citrate is a calcium chelating agent added to blood products to prevent clotting, as calcium is a necessary cofactor for several clotting factors. Normally, citrate is metabolized by the liver; however, in the setting of massive transfusion or end-stage liver disease citrate toxicity may occur causing hypocalcemia (and hypomagnesemia). This is crucial to recognize and treat as hypocalcemia not only impairs coagulation but also causes vasodilation and impairs cardiac contractility (all detrimental in the setting of hemorrhagic shock). Citrate toxicity can be treated with IV calcium (± magnesium as well). In an emergent situation (e.g., massive transfusion of a trauma patient in hemorrhagic shock), a helpful indicator to guide calcium administration is QT prolongation on electrocardiogram (ECG). FFP and platelets contain the most citrate, but packed RBCs can also cause citrate toxicity to a lesser effect. Hypothermia decreases hepatic clearance and is a risk factor for citrate toxicity.

37. **When suspecting a major transfusion reaction, what management steps should be undertaken?**
    - Immediately stop the transfusion
        - Remove the blood tubing
    - Alert the blood bank
        - Send recipient and donor specimens for compatibility testing
    - Treat hypotension aggressively
        - IV fluid
        - Vasopressors

- Maintain urine output by maintaining a euvolemic state
  - Diuretics and mannitol are used cautiously
- Massive hemolysis can lead to
  - Potential for life-threatening hyperkalemia
    - Follow serum potassium levels
    - Monitor ECG continuously
  - Check urine and plasma Hg levels
  - Direct antiglobulin (Coombs) test
  - Bilirubin level
  - Plasma haptoglobin level
- Disseminated intravascular coagulation may occur
  - Identify the underlying cause if possible
  - Follow the prothrombin time, partial thromboplastin time, fibrinogen, and D-dimer levels

KEY POINTS: TRANSFUSION THERAPY

1. There is no set Hg level at which transfusion is absolutely required. The decision should be individualized to the clinical situation, taking into consideration the patient's age, health status, and risk/benefit ratio of the transfusion.
2. When emergency blood transfusion is necessary, use type O-packed red cells (O-negative is best) and switch to type-specific blood as soon as available.
3. Multiple transfusion-related complications/reactions are possible, and vigilance must be maintained while administering blood, as many of the signs/symptoms can be missed in a prepped and draped patient under general anesthesia.
4. TACO causes hydrostatic pulmonary edema (too much volume), whereas TRALI cause nonhydrostatic pulmonary edema (inflammatory response).
5. The treatment of TACO and TRALI is supportive (supplemental oxygenation, intubation with positive pressure ventilation, etc.). Diuretics are useful for treating TACO but not for TRALI.
6. Recipient HLA antibodies against donor neutrophils causes febrile, nonhemolytic transfusion reactions, whereas donor HLA antibodies against recipient neutrophils causes TRALI.
7. PCC can rapidly reverse warfarin and Factor Xa inhibitors. Indications include urgent reversal of anticoagulation in the setting of life-threatening bleeding (i.e., intracranial hemorrhage) or to reduce the amount of volume in patients at risk for TACO (e.g., heart failure, end-stage renal failure).
8. Citrate toxicity causes hypocalcemia and can occur in the setting of massive transfusion for hemorrhagic shock or in patients with end-stage liver disease. Hypocalcemia is a cofactor for several clotting factors and can worsen coagulopathy, cause vasodilation, and decrease cardiac contractility.
9. Citrate toxicity is treated with calcium ($\pm$ magnesium). Hypocalcemia can be assessed and treated by observing QT prolongation on ECG in an emergent situation.

SUGGESTED READINGS

Chai-Adisaksopha C, Hillis C, Siegal D, et al. Prothrombin complex concentrates versus fresh frozen plasma for warfarin reversal. A systematic review and meta-analysis. Thromb Haemost. 2016;116(5):879–890.

Dunn J, Mythen M, Grocott M. Physiology of oxygen transport. BJA Education. 2016;16(10):341–348.

Semple J, Rebetz J, Kapur R. Transfusion-associated circulatory overload and transfusion-related acute lung injury. Blood. 2019;133 (17):1840–1853.

Vlaar A, Toy P, Fung M, et al. A consensus redefinition of transfusion-related acute lung injury. Transfusion. 2019;59(7):2465–2476.

CHAPTER 12

PERIOPERATIVE PATIENT SAFETY

Colin Coulson, MSNA, CRNA, Thomas B. Moore, MSNA, CRNA,
Ryan D. Laterza, MD

ALLERGIC REACTIONS

1. Review the four types of hypersensitivity reactions and their mechanisms.
   See Table 12.1.

2. What is an anaphylactoid reaction?
   Anaphylactoid reactions clinicaly resemble allergic reactions (e.g., both involve histamine release) but are not immunoglobulin (Ig)E-mediated. Anaphylactoid reactions may present as a severe anaphylactic reaction (i.e., bronchospasm or hypotension), but generally causes more mild reactions (e.g., rash). Red man syndrome caused by vancomycin or pruritis because of morphine are examples of common anaphylactoid reactions.

3. What is the incidence of severe perioperative anaphylactic reactions?
   The overall incidence is approximately one in 10,000.

4. Describe the clinical presentation of anaphylaxis.
   Anaphylaxis can be IgE or non-IgE–mediated with the following signs and symptoms:
   - Hypotension
   - Dysrhythmias
   - Cardiac arrest
   - Bronchospasm
   - Cutaneous symptoms, including flushing, urticaria, and angioedema
   - Gastrointestinal symptoms, including abdominal pain, nausea, vomiting, and diarrhea

5. What is the most common initial presentation for perioperative anaphylaxis? Is rash frequently present with severe reactions?
   The presentation of anaphylaxis is a spectrum ranging from minor cutaneous signs and symptoms (more common) to hemodynamic instability and cardiac arrest (less common). In severe anaphylactic reactions, the most common presentation is hypotension followed by bronchospasm. Cutaneous signs and symptoms are a late finding in severe reactions that often are not present until after the patient is stabilized. Anaphylactic reactions are often a clinical diagnosis and can be IgE-mediated (allergic) or non-IgE–mediated (anaphylactoid), with the former generally presenting as severe reactions and the latter as minor reactions.

6. What are the most common causes of severe perioperative anaphylaxis?
   - Antibiotics
   - Neuromuscular blocking agents
   - Chlorhexidine
   - Latex
   - Blue dyes
     A recent study found antibiotics to be the most common cause of anaphylaxis, with neuromuscular blocking agents a close second. This is contrary to previous studies which found neuromuscular blocking agents to be the most common cause of anaphylaxis. Differences between studies are likely related to medication selection or availability and patient population differences. For example, pholcodine is an over-the-counter cough suppressant available in countries which are associated with a higher incidence of allergy to neuromuscular blocking agents but is rarely prescribed in the United States. Overall, taking various studies in aggregate, the majority of severe anaphylactic reactions seem to be attributed to antibiotics and neuromuscular blocking agents.

7. Which specific antibiotics and neuromuscular agents seem to cause the majority of severe anaphylactic reactions?
   - Glycopeptide (e.g., vancomycin) antibiotics, particularly when given to patients with a history of penicillin allergy and penicillin family antibiotics (e.g., amoxicillin, piperacillin)
   - Succinylcholine and rocuronium cause the majority of severe anaphylactic reactions for neuromuscular blocking agents. Succinylcholine typically presents as bronchospasm, whereas most other agents, including antibiotics, present as hypotension

Table 12.1 Hypersensitivity Classification

TYPE OF REACTION	NAME	MECHANISM	EXAMPLES
Type I	Allergic reaction	Previous exposure to an antigen produces IgE immunoglobulins which binds to mast cells and basophils. Following reexposure, the antigen cross-links two IgE receptors initiating a cascade that ultimately results in release of potent vasodilating mediators (e.g., histamine).	• Anaphylactic shock • Allergic rhinitis • Asthma • Urticaria • Angioedema • Eczema
Type II	Antibody-dependent cellular cytotoxicity	IgG and/or IgM immunoglobulins directed against cellular surface antigens, which activate natural killer cells or activate the complement cascade	• Rheumatic heart disease • Goodpasture disease • ABO incompatible transfusion reactions • Hyperacute transplant rejection
Type III	Antigen-antibody complex reaction	Caused by deposition of this complex into tissue causing inflammatory mediated tissue damage	• Systemic lupus erythematosus • Rheumatoid arthritis • Scleroderma
Type IV	Cell-mediated immunity	Mediated by T lymphocytes	• Contact dermatitis • PPD • Inflammatory bowel disease • Multiple sclerosis • Type 1 diabetes • Chronic transplant rejection

Ig, Immunoglobulin; *PPD*, Purified Protein Derivative.

8. **What are the less common causes of perioperative anaphylactic reactions?**
   - Propofol: A rare allergy. Although propofol includes egg yolk derived lecithin and soybean oil in the emulsion, there is no evidence to suggest that patients with egg or soy allergies have increased risk of an allergic reaction to propofol. Most egg allergies are caused by the egg white proteins ovalbumin and ovomucoid, which are not contained in the propofol emulsion
   - Protamine: An increasingly uncommon allergy with the advent of recombinant protamine. Risk factors include previous exposure to protamine itself or similar medications, such as Neutral Protamine Hagedorn insulin, fish allergies, or vasectomy. Protamine was historically made from salmon sperm and with the increasing use of recombinant protamine, these latter risk factors will likely abate
   - Local anesthetics: Allergies to local anesthetics with amide linkages (e.g., bupivacaine, lidocaine, mepivacaine, ropivacaine) are extremely rare. Allergic reactions to local anesthetics with ester linkages (e.g., procaine, chloroprocaine, tetracaine, benzocaine), while more common than amide local anesthetics, are also rare. Allergic reactions to ester local anesthetics are predominately caused by paraaminobenzoic acid (PABA), a metabolite. Methylparaben, a preservative in amide local anesthetics, may cause allergic reactions because its chemical structure is similar to PABA. Therefore preservative-free amide local anesthetics should be used for patients at risk for local anesthetic allergies.

9. **Review the issues concerning allergic reactions to neuromuscular blockers.**
   IgE immunoglobulins are sensitive to the tertiary or quaternary ammonium groups found in neuromuscular blocking agents. Because these chemical groups are commonly found in foods, cosmetics, and over-the-counter medications, patients may have an anaphylactic reaction to neuromuscular blockers on their initial exposure. When administered rapidly, succinylcholine and some nondepolarizing neuromuscular blocking agents (i.e., atracurium and mivacurium) may cause a mild anaphylactoid reaction resulting in erythema of the chest and face, a mild drop in blood pressure, and a mild increase in heart rate. Steroidal agents (e.g., rocuronium and vecuronium) and cis-atracurium, specifically, are not associated with anaphylactoid reactions even when rapidly administered.

10. **Can a patient with a penicillin allergy receive cephalosporin antibiotics?**
    Current evidence suggests that it is likely safe to administer cephalosporins to penicillin-allergic patients, provided the reaction was not a true "allergic" IgE-mediated anaphylactic reaction and the reaction was greater than

10 years ago. Although penicillin is one of the most commonly reported allergies, fewer than 1% of the general population has a true IgE-mediated allergy to penicillin. Most reported reactions, such as gastrointestinal symptoms or nonspecific rashes, are incorrectly labeled penicillin allergy. An anaphylactic reaction requires at least two symptoms and rash alone is not sufficient. Further, 80% of patients with a known IgE-mediated penicillin allergy will lose their sensitivity after 10 years.

An oft-quoted statistic is that there is a 10% risk of cross-sensitivity between penicillin and cephalosporins, but this is now disputed. Previously, this may have been true, possibly because early generations of cephalosporins may have contained trace amounts of penicillin from contamination during manufacturing. More recent studies show the cross-reactivity between penicillin and cephalosporins is less than 1% to 5% depending upon the generation (higher cross-reactivity with first and second generation and lower cross-reactivity with higher generation cephalosporins).

Therefore patients with a remote history of penicillin allergy causing only a rash and no other signs or symptoms suggesting anaphylaxis may be a candidate for cephalosporin antibiotics, especially if the reported allergic reaction was greater than 10 years ago. Clinical judgement is warranted in these situations with an assessment of the benefit/ risk in administrating cephalosporin antibiotics versus alternative agents, which may be more expensive, less efficacious, and carry their own risk of anaphylaxis as well.

11. **What are the risk factors for a latex allergy?**
- Congenital spinal cord abnormalities (e.g., spina bifida)
- Multiple prior surgical operations
- High occupational exposure to latex (e.g., healthcare workers)
- Atopic individuals (e.g., eczema, asthma, allergic rhinitis)
- Sensitivity to specific foods (e.g., avocado, banana, kiwi, chestnut, papaya, white potato, tomato)

12. **How should an operating room (OR) be prepared for a latex-allergic patient?**
Surgical operations for latex-allergic patients ideally should be scheduled first case of the day, because the quantity of airborne latex particles will be minimized. Use only nonlatex surgical and anesthesia supplies, including nonlatex gloves. Increasingly, latex-free medical supplies are becoming the standard for all patients, but it is important to be familiar with your hospital's equipment.

13. **How should severe anaphylaxis be treated?**
- Epinephrine, either 0.5 mg intramuscular (IM) or 10 to 500 mcg intravenous (IV) depending on severity, patient response, and if the patient is well-monitored (IV) or not well-monitored (IM). IM is more hemodynamically stable and has a longer duration of action but IV has a more rapid onset. Patients frequently require multiple re-doses and some, an epinephrine infusion
- Aggressive volume resuscitation (i.e., bolus 1–2 L of crystalloid repeated as necessary)
- Initiate cardiopulmonary resuscitation if no pulse detected for more than 10 seconds, or systolic blood pressure less than 50 mm Hg
- Administer 100% oxygen to minimize hypoxemia during bronchospasm
- Consider albuterol for bronchospasm. Note, in severe bronchospasm, albuterol may not be adequately delivered to bronchospastic airways and treatment will require IV epinephrine for β-2 mediated bronchodilation
- Consider vasopressin 1 to 2 unit bolus
- Consider intubation for airway edema
- There is no high-quality evidence to support or refute the use of antihistamines (agents with H_1 (e.g., famotidine) or H_2 antagonism (e.g., diphenhydramine) or corticosteroids in the acute management of anaphylaxis)
- Consider admitting the patient for observation of rebound anaphylaxis (4–12 hours after the initial event)

14. **Why is epinephrine the first-line agent for anaphylaxis? How does it work?**
Epinephrine in the most important therapy for anaphylaxis for several reasons. First, it is readily available in most hospitals and has a rapid onset of action. It can be administered in almost every way possible such as IV, endotracheal, subcutaneous, intraosseous, and IM (most common route in the emergency department or outside of the hospital). Second, it stabilizes mast cells preventing further histamine release. Third, it directly treats the pathophysiology of anaphylaxis: (1) β-1 agonism increases cardiac contractility, (2) β-2 agonism causes bronchodilation, and (3) α-1 agonism increases systemic vascular resistance, increases venous return, and may reduce bronchial secretions.

15. **How do you manage anaphylaxis for a patient taking beta-blockers?**
Glucagon. If not readily available, give epinephrine at higher doses.

16. **Should patients with a prior history of allergic reaction be pretreated with histamine blockers or corticosteroids?**
Although premedication with corticosteroids and antihistamines is not uncommon in some settings, such as before IV contrast, chemotherapy, and some immunosuppressant infusions, there is no specific evidence that favors premedication during the perioperative phase as a means of preventing anaphylaxis.

17. **How do you distinguish a perioperative allergic reaction from a nonallergic event? Why is it important to make this distinction?**

Check a serum tryptase level immediately once the patient is stabilized. Serum tryptase levels peak within 15 and 120 minutes after the onset of an IgE-mediated anaphylactic reaction and have a half-life of about 120 minutes.

After a suspected intraoperative allergic reaction, a patient should be referred to an allergist/immunologist for evaluation and prescribed an "epi pen." Detailed reporting of the episode and a serum tryptase level can assist the allergist in distinguishing between an IgE or non-IgE-mediated anaphylactic reaction. However, a positive tryptase does not specify the responsible antigen and only confirms the reaction was IgE-mediated. Often, there are other confounding antigens, such as chlorhexidine and latex, that could also cause anaphylactic reactions in addition to administered medications. If the tryptase is positive, the allergist should perform skin testing for all common antigens exposed to the patient in the perioperative period to confirm the responsible antigen.

OPERATING ROOM FIRES

KEY POINTS: APPROPRIATE PLAN TO MANAGE AN AIRWAY FIRE

1. Without hesitation, remove the endotracheal tube (ETT) or laryngeal mask airway.
2. Stop the flow of all airway gases and flood the surgical field with saline.
3. Mask-ventilate the patient and consider reintubating the patient.
4. Consider performing rigid laryngoscopy and bronchoscopy to assess the damage and remove debris.
5. Assess for inhalation injury and consider admitting the patient.

1. **What are the three essential components necessary to create an OR fire?**

The fire triad consists of:
1. Oxidizers. In the OR this includes oxygen and nitrous oxide.
2. Ignition sources. The three most common are electrosurgical or electrocautery devices, lasers, and argon beam coagulators. Fiberoptic light cables, defibrillator pads, heated probes, and drills and burrs have also been implicated in OR fires.
3. Fuel sources. This includes ETTs (PVC materials are flammable), sponges, drapes, gauze, alcohol-containing preparation solutions, the patient's hair, surgical dressings, gastrointestinal tract gases, and packaging materials. Alcohol containing solutions for skin preparation should be allowed to dry before the patient is draped and ignition sources initiated.

2. **What are high-risk procedures for OR fires?**

Proximity of the procedure to the ETT and an oxidizer source increases fire risk. Common high-risk procedures include head and neck operations, such as tonsillectomies, tracheostomies, removal of laryngeal papillomas, cataract or other eye surgery, burr hole surgery, and removal of lesions about the head, neck, or face.

3. **What strategies can reduce the incidence of airway fires?**
   - Laser-resistant ETTs should be chosen for laser surgery. The cuff should be filled with saline and not air. It is also recommended that the saline contain a small quantity of methylene blue to help identify inadvertent cuff rupture
   - Avoid uncuffed tubes. Verify the cuff is inflated and tightly fit such that no leak is present
   - Avoid nitrous oxide
   - Keep the fraction of inspired oxygen (FiO_2) as low as possible (i.e., FiO_2 <30%)

4. **What are signs that a fire has occurred?**

A flame or flash may be noted, unusual sounds heard (pop or snap), and unusual odors detected. Also smoke, discoloration of the drapes, and/or heat may be noted.

5. **Should an airway fire occur, what are the recommended practices for its management?**
   - Immediately remove the ETT
   - Stop the flow of all airway gases
   - Flood the surgical field with saline and remove all flammable and burning materials
   - Mask-ventilate, avoiding supplemental oxygen and reintubate if necessary
   - Consider performing rigid laryngoscopy or bronchoscopy to assess the damage and remove debris

6. **A patient with chronic obstructive pulmonary disease on 3 L/min of O_2 is scheduled for an operation of the upper lip. Can this be done under monitored anesthesia care (MAC)?**

The FiO_2 from a nasal canula at its source is 100%. Although some head and neck operations can be done under MAC, the clinician should strongly consider intubating all patients undergoing head and neck operations, especially patients with higher oxygen requirements, to minimize the risk of fire during surgery.

PATIENT POSITIONING

KEY POINTS: PATIENT POSITIONING

1. A conscientious attitude toward positioning is required to facilitate the surgical procedure, prevent physiological embarrassment, and prevent injury to the patient.
2. Ulnar neuropathy is the most common positional nerve injury.
3. Keep the extremities less than 90 degrees to prevent brachial plexus injuries.
4. Secure the arms in the supinated position to prevent ulnar nerve injury.
5. In the lithotomy position, ensure adequate padding around fibular head to prevent common peroneal nerve injury.

1. **What is the goal of positioning a patient for surgery?**
   The goal of surgical positioning is to facilitate the surgeon's technical approach, while minimizing any risk to the patient. The anesthetized patient will be unable to inform the clinician of compromised positions; therefore correct patient positioning for surgery is critical for a safe outcome. Proper positioning requires that the patient be securely placed on the operating table; all potential pressure areas padded; the eyes protected; limbs positioned such that no muscles, tendons, or neurovascular bundles are stretched; IV lines and catheters free flowing and accessible; the ETT patent and not kinked or stretched; ventilation and circulation uninterrupted; and that this is maintained for the duration of the surgery. Confer with the patient regarding any impaired mobility at any joint; never attempt to position patients beyond their limitations.

2. **Review the most common positions used in the OR.**
   See Fig. 12.1.

3. **What are the physiological effects caused by a change in body position from standing to supine?**
   - Venous return increases, causing an increase in cardiac output with minimal change in blood pressure secondary to a reflex decrease in heart rate and contractility
   - Intraabdominal pressure increases, which is exacerbated by abdominal tumors, ascites, obesity, pregnancy, or carbon dioxide insufflation for laparoscopy
   - Functional residual capacity (FRC) decreases

4. **How does the supine position decrease functional residual capacity?**
   The supine position decreases FRC by two mechanisms:
   1) It causes the abdominal contents to impinge cephalad on the diaphragm, decreasing FRC. This is exacerbated by obesity, anesthesia, and neuromuscular blocking agents.
   2) The force of gravity is directly perpendicular to anterior chest wall excursion in the supine position, causing decreased chest wall compliance. This is exacerbated by obesity; however, neuromuscular blocking agents may help mitigate this problem by increasing chest wall compliance.

5. **How does supine positioning affect ventilation and perfusion?**
   Supine positioning with positive pressure ventilation increases ventilation/perfusion ($\dot{V}/\dot{Q}$) mismatch. Positive pressure ventilation will preferentially ventilate nondependent regions of the lung because they have a greater compliance compared with the dependent regions of the lung. The opposite is true for perfusion, where the more dependent regions of the lung will preferentially be perfused because of the effects of gravity.

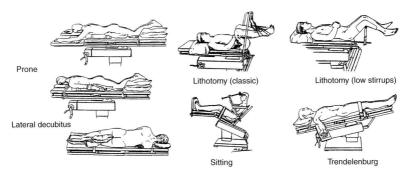

Prone

Lithotomy (classic)

Lithotomy (low stirrups)

Lateral decubitus

Sitting

Trendelenburg

Fig. 12.1 Patient positioning. (From Martin JT. Positioning in Anesthesia and Surgery. 2nd ed. Philadelphia: WB Saunders; 1987.)

6. **Describe the lithotomy position and its risks.**
The patient's hips and knees are flexed, and the patient's feet are placed in stirrups to gain ready access to the genitalia and perineum. The range of flexion may be modest (low lithotomy) or extreme (high lithotomy). The feet may be suspended on vertical structures (known as *candy canes*) or in boots; the knees may also be supported with crutches. With elevation of the legs, pressure is taken off the lower back, and blood is translocated from the lower extremities to the central compartments. The effect on pulmonary physiology is similar to the supine position. The main concern with the lithotomy position is injury to the common peroneal nerve via compression of this nerve against the fibular head.

7. **What are the special concerns for a patient positioned in the lateral decubitus position?**
All patients in the lateral position should have an axillary roll positioned to distribute weight to the patient's rib cage and prevent compression of the neurovascular bundle of the dependent arm. Loss of pulse in the dependent arm may indicate excessive compression; however, the presence of a pulse does not ensure that the brachial plexus is protected. The arms are usually supported and padded in a position perpendicular to the shoulders. The dependent leg is usually flexed at the hip and knee with padding between the legs. The head position should be in line with the vertebral column to prevent stretching the brachial plexus.
    V/Q mismatch is a risk in the lateral position during positive pressure ventilation. The dependent lung is underventilated and relatively overperfused. In contrast, the nondependent lung is overventilated because of the increase in compliance and relatively underperfused. Usually, some physiological compensation (e.g., hypoxic pulmonary vasoconstriction) occurs, and this position is well tolerated, although compromised patients may prove problematic.

8. **What are the physiological effects and risks associated with the Trendelenburg position?**
Head down, or Trendelenburg position, compared with supine position increases translocation of blood to the central compartment, thereby decreasing pulmonary compliance and FRC. Intracranial and intraocular pressure also increase in the Trendelenburg position secondary to decreased cerebral venous drainage, making this position absolutely contraindicated in patients with increased intracranial pressure. Lengthy procedures may result in significant facial and upper airway edema and it may be prudent to check a "cuff leak" to assess if the patient can breathe around the ETT.

9. **What specific concerns are associated with the prone position?**
The prone position results in a cephalad displacement of the diaphragm. Chest rolls are used to decrease abdominal compression, improving diaphragmatic excursion, while limiting compression on the aorta and inferior vena cava. Proper padding of all pressure points, including the face, eyes, ears, arms, knees, hips, ankles, breasts, and genitalia, is necessary in this position. The arms should be placed in a neutral position and abducted less than 90 degrees to avoid traction on the brachial plexus. Electrocardiogram electrodes should not be placed so that the patient is lying on them.

10. **What is the beach chair position?**
This position is often used to improve access and mobility of the upper extremity for shoulder operations. When finally positioned, the anesthesiologist will not have easy access to the head or ETT; thus these structures must be well secured and in a neutral position before initiating surgery. Also perfusion pressure must be closely monitored, because the head is well above the level of the heart. Special care should also be taken to protect the eyes because the surgeon is working very close to the face and instruments could place pressure on the eyes. Protective plastic eye shields are often used for this reason.

11. **What are the indications for the sitting position?**
The sitting position may be used to gain access to the posterior fossa of the cranium and to perform cervical laminectomy. However, these procedures are now usually performed with the patient in the prone position, and the sitting position is rarely used in current practice.

12. **List the dangers of the sitting and beach chair positions.**
    - Anoxic brain injury: This can occur because the circle of Willis is above the brachial artery (where the noninvasive blood pressure [NIBP] is usually measured). Arterial lines should be zeroed or calibrated with the intraarterial transducer at the same height as the external auditory meatus to approximate cerebral perfusion pressure. If a NIBP cuff is used, the difference in blood pressure between the brachial artery and the circle of Willis should be accounted for using the following equation: 1 cm $H_2O = 0.7$ mm Hg
    - Severe neck flexion: This can occur if the patient's head is not properly secured to the table. Complications include spinal cord ischemia and airway obstruction
    - Venous air embolism (VAE): The surgical site is above the level of the right atrium and air may be entrained into the venous circulation

13. What are the concerns for positioning a pregnant patient?

The pregnant patient is susceptible to aortocaval compression secondary to the gravid uterus exerting pressure on these vascular structures, thus potentially decreasing uteroplacental blood flow and venous return to the heart. Left uterine displacement decreases aortocaval compression and is achieved by tilting the patient 15 degrees to the left with the table or supporting the right hip with a pillow or wedge.

14. What peripheral neuropathies are associated with cardiac surgery?

The brachial plexus may be injured because of sternal retraction causing both upward rotation and/or iatrogenic fractures of the first rib (where the brachial plexus is in close proximity).

15. What is the most common perioperative neuropathy?

The ulnar nerve is the most frequently injured peripheral nerve, although its incidence is still relatively infrequent. Ulnar neuropathies tend to be mild and mostly sensory in nature. Of note, patients who suffer positional related ulnar neuropathies tend to have preexisting risk factors (e.g., diabetes) and are often found to have abnormal ulnar nerve conduction studies on the contralateral side.

16. Review the incidence of brachial plexus injuries.

Brachial plexus injuries may be caused by improper patient positioning and/or from regional anesthesia procedures. Risk factors include the use of shoulder braces in head-down positions, abduction of the arm to more than 90 degrees, and excessive rotation of the head. Upper extremity regional anesthetic procedures may result in brachial plexus injuries from direct needle trauma, intraneural injection, or direct neurotoxicity from the local anesthetic.

17. How might upper extremity neuropathies be prevented through proper positioning?

Shoulder abduction should be less than 90 degrees to prevent stretching of the brachial plexus with the arms gently secured to the arm board in the supinated position. Pronation of the arm can cause ulnar nerve compression as it passes between the olecranon process and the medial epicondyle of the humerus. Note that although protective padding is essential to avoid upper extremity neuropathies, it does not necessarily prevent their occurrence.

18. How does the position of the head affect the location of the ETT with respect to the carina?

Flexion of the head may move the ETT toward the carina; extension moves it away from the carina. A general rule is that the tip of the ETT follows the direction of the tip of the patient's nose. The change in tube position is probably more problematic in a child than in an adult, as the distance between the vocal cords and the carina is less. Sudden increases in airway pressure or oxygen desaturation may be caused by inadvertent mainstem bronchial intubation.

OPHTHALMIC COMPLICATIONS

KEY POINTS: OPHTHALMIC COMPLICATIONS

1. Postoperative vision loss (POVL) is a risk in cardiac operations and in spine operations performed in the prone position.
2. Spine operations in the prone position that last longer than 6 hours and are associated with greater than 1 L of blood loss are particularly high risk for POVL.
3. To minimize the risk of POVL, limit the use of crystalloids, use a lower threshold for colloids, such as blood products, and consider using reverse Trendelenburg position to facilitate venous drainage.

1. What perioperative injuries may occur to the eye?

The most common injury is corneal abrasion, but conjunctivitis, chemical injury, direct trauma, blurred vision, and POVL may also occur. Corneal abrasions are usually caused by direct pressure on the eye from facemasks, surgical drapes, chemicals that touch the eye, failure to administer ocular protection, and the patient rubbing their eyes following extubation.

2. What is the treatment for a minor corneal abrasion?

Small uncomplicated corneal abrasions may be treated with artificial tears administered every 30 minutes for 2 to 3 hours. If symptoms do not subside, 0.5% erythromycin ophthalmic ointment may be applied every 6 hours over the following 24 hours. The use of an eye patch has been shown to have no benefit and may even worsen pain and delay recovery.

3. What procedures are associated with postoperative visual loss?

Spine surgery in the prone position and cardiac surgery are the highest risk operations for POVL. The incidence may be as high as 0.2% of all spine and cardiac operations. The majority of cases are caused by ischemic optic neuropathy and retinal ischemia. The mechanism is often caused by decreased oxygen delivery and perfusion caused by hypotension, anemia, venous congestion, increased ocular pressure from direct pressure on the globe, and/or embolism.

4. **What factors may predispose a patient with spine surgery to POVL?**
Patient-specific risk factors for POVL include male gender, history of hypertension, diabetes mellitus, smoking, other vasculopathies, and morbid obesity.
   Surgical risk factors for POVL during spine surgery in the prone position include long duration of operation (i.e., >6 hours) with significant blood loss (i.e., >1 L). Methods to minimize this devastating complication involve reducing venous congestion and optimizing oxygen delivery, including: (1) administer colloids over crystalloids and maintain a higher hematocrit, (2) slight reverse Trendelenburg to minimize venous congestion, (3) avoid hypotension, (4) frequent assessment of the eyes to ensure they are free from mechanical compression, (5) consider staging a single, longer operation into two smaller operations.

VENOUS AIR EMBOLISM

KEY POINTS: VENOUS AIR EMBOLISM

1. Surgical sites above the level of the right atrium are at high risk for venous air embolism (VAE).
2. Methods to decrease this risk involve avoiding positions where the operative site is above the level of the right atrium, avoiding hypovolemia, avoiding nitrous oxide, and avoiding spontaneous negative pressure ventilation.
3. A central venous catheter should be considered for high-risk operations. This can be used both as a diagnostic and therapeutic modality.
4. If a VAE is suspect, flood the surgical site with a saline soaked dressing to prevent continued air entrainment and position the patient such that the surgical site is below the right atrium.
5. Provide supportive measures to optimize right heart coronary perfusion with vasoactive agents. If cardiac arrest ensues, initiate cardiopulmonary resuscitation.

1. **What is a venous air embolism?**
If the surgical site is above the level of the right atrium, venous pressure at this level could become transiently subatmospheric (e.g., during spontaneous negative pressure inspiration) resulting in the venous entrapment of air. Large VAEs may cause an "air-lock," leading to obstruction of the right ventricular outflow tract and/or a pulmonary air embolism; both of which may cause acute right heart failure. If an intracardiac shunt is present, paradoxical air embolism may occur resulting in either a myocardial infarction or an ischemic stroke.

2. **What's the lethal dose for an air embolism? Are small air bubbles in the IV tubing safe for the patient?**
Based on case reports, the volume of air thought to be lethal is 3 to 5 mL/kg or 200 to 300 mL in adults. However, even smaller volumes of air (e.g., 1 mL/kg) may cause hemodynamic instability. If a right to left intracardiac shunt is present, even smaller volumes (e.g., 1–2 mL) could cause stroke or a myocardial infarction. It is important to remember that up to a third of adult patients have a patent foramen ovale (PFO) and that the risks associated with the pediatric population increase with both the incidence of PFO and the lower total lethal dose of air.

3. **Which surgical operations are at risk for VAE?**
Any situation where the surgical site is above the level of the right atrium increases the risk of VAE. Below are examples of operations at particular risk:
   • Sitting craniotomy
   • Caesarian section
   • Central line placement or removal
   • Laparoscopic operations (i.e., CO_2 or gas embolism)

4. **Describe the pathophysiology of VAE.**
VAE creates an "air-lock" that may obstruct the right ventricular outflow tract or cause a pulmonary embolism. In severe cases, this may cause acute right heart failure. The pathophysiology and management has overlap with pulmonary thromboembolism. Both increase right heart afterload and are associated with hypotension and increased right ventricular pressure, leading to decreased right coronary perfusion. Initial treatment should focus on preserving right heart coronary perfusion with supportive measures (i.e., phenylephrine or norepinephrine) to maintain coronary perfusion and judicious use of fluids to minimize right heart overdistention, which may further increase right ventricular pressure and decrease coronary perfusion.

5. Review the sensitivity and limitations of monitors for detecting VAE.

There are numerous monitors for detection of VAE. No single technique is completely reliable; thus the more monitors are used, the greater the likelihood is for detecting VAE. In decreasing order of sensitivity: transesophageal echocardiography >precordial doppler >increases in end-tidal nitrogen fraction >decreases in end-tidal carbon dioxide >increases in right atrial pressure >hypotension, electrocardiogram changes showing right heart strain, or a mill-wheel murmur with an esophageal or precordial stethoscope.

6. How do you treat VAE?

- Avoid hypovolemia, spontaneous negative pressure ventilation, and positions where the surgical site is above the level of the right atrium
- In high-risk operations, consider prophylactic placement of a central venous catheter in the right atrium which can be used to aspirate air
- Avoid or discontinue nitrous oxide as this gas can increase the dimensions of the air-lock bubble
- Flood the surgical site with a saline soaked dressing to prevent continued air entrainment
- Administer vasopressor agents to optimize right heart coronary perfusion
- Chest compressions for cardiac arrest, which may help "break-up" the air bubble
- Trendelenburg and semi left lateral decubitus position may help migrate the air bubble away from the right ventricular outflow tract. Although classically taught, evidence to date suggests this may not be as helpful as previously suggested. The air bubble may migrate away from the right ventricular outflow tract; but the stroke volume remains decreased causing persistent hypotension, increased right ventricular pressures, and decreased right heart coronary perfusion
- Small VAEs will likely reabsorb with supportive measures

KEY POINTS: ALLERGIC REACTIONS

1. To prevent severe allergic reactions, it is important to identify patients at risk and to take a good history.
2. The majority of severe perioperative anaphylactic reactions are caused by neuromuscular blockers and antibiotics.
3. Severe anaphylaxis generally presents as hypotension followed by bronchospasm. Rash and edema are late findings and may not be clinically apparent on presentation.
4. Epinephrine, volume resuscitation, and cardiopulmonary resuscitation are the mainstay treatments for severe anaphylaxis.
5. Although cutaneous signs, such as rash, are helpful in the diagnosis of anaphylaxis, clinicians should not delay treatment in patients with suspected severe anaphylaxis, as there may be a delay before cutaneous signs are evident.

SUGGESTED READINGS

Apfelbaum JL, Caplan RA, Barker SJ, et al. Practice advisory for the prevention and management of operating room fires. Anesthesiology. 2013;118(2):271–290.

Apfelbaum JL, Roth S, Connis RT, et al. Practice advisory for perioperative visual loss associated with spine surgery. Anesthesiology. 2012;116(2):274–285.

Brull SJ, Prielipp RC. Vascular air embolism: a silent hazard to patient safety. J Crit Care. 2017;42:255–263.

Chui J, Murkin JM, Posner KL, Domino KB. Perioperative peripheral nerve injury after general anesthesia. Anesth Analgesia. 2018;127 (1):134–143.

Cook T, Harper N, Farmer L, et al. Anaesthesia, surgery, and life-threatening allergic reactions: protocol and methods of the 6th National Audit Project (NAP6) of the Royal College of Anaesthetists. Br J Anaesth. 2018;121(1):124–133.

Jangra K, Grover V. Perioperative vision loss: a complication to watch out. J Anaesthesiol Clin Pharmacol. 2012;28(1):11.

CHAPTER 13

PERIOPERATIVE MEDICAL ETHICS

Brian M. Keech, MD, Philip Fung, MD

1. **What are the four foundational moral values of medical ethics?**
   - Respect for autonomy: patients have the right to determine what can and cannot be done to their bodies
   - Nonmaleficence: do no harm, or at least, do more good than harm
   - Beneficence: do what is in the best interest of the patient
   - Justice: scarce healthcare resources should be distributed as justly as possible

2. **Why is it important to learn about medical ethics?**
   Ethical questions arise frequently in medicine. Many assume that if they act in good faith and are well intentioned, they do not need to learn about medical ethics; the proper solution will simply present itself. Unfortunately, being a good person and meaning well is not enough. Like other disciplines, medical ethics involves learning to think through ethical dilemmas using reason, knowledge, and problem-solving techniques. Understanding medical ethics provides one with the tools necessary to recognize, analyze, and manage ethical dilemmas as they arise.

3. **What is informed consent?**
   Informed consent is rooted in the ethical principal of respect for patients' autonomy. It is the cornerstone of the patient-physician relationship and no discussion of medical ethics can go far without its consideration. The goal of informed consent is to maximize the ability of patients to make reasonably informed decisions about their care, based on their understanding of the risks and benefits of the proposed intervention.

4. **What are the elements of informed consent?**
   Informed consent generally consists of the following components:
   - Medical decision-making capacity
   - Disclosure: the patient must be given adequate information regarding the nature and purpose of their proposed treatment, as well as risks, benefits, options, and alternatives
   - Voluntariness: their decision must be voluntary and free of coercion or manipulation

5. **How does one determine if a patient has decisional capacity (also known as medical decision-making capacity)?**
   To possess medical decision-making capacity, a patient must:
   - Understand the relevant information about the proposed treatment
   - Appreciate their situation/medical consequences of their situation
   - Use reason to make their decision; applying their life values to their knowledge of the risks and benefits of the proposed treatment or procedure—irrespective if we agree with their conclusion
   - Communicate their choice to their care team

6. **What is the difference between capacity and competence?**
   Competence generally refers to legal decisions, capacity to clinical decisions. In the past, these terms were regarded as separate concepts and their use differed based on locality. However, at present, no distinction between them is usually made.
   When referring to the notion of competence, societies generally determine the level of impairment necessary to render an individual patient incompetent. Societal judgement on this matter reflects the delicate balance between respecting an individual's autonomy and protecting them from harm and/or making bad decisions.

7. **How do we assess for decisional capacity?**
   Unfortunately, an efficacious instrument for the precise assessment of decision-making capacity has not yet been developed. In general, we assume a patient has medical decision-making capacity, until their interactions or behavior suggest otherwise. The Mini Mental Status Evaluation (MMSE), a sensitive instrument to assess cognitive function, has not been demonstrated to correlate highly with decision-making capacity. Although patients who score poorly on the MMSE are less likely to have capacity, and those who score well are more likely to have it, no definitive conclusions regarding a patient's decisional capacity can be drawn from the MMSE. Similarly, other bedside cognitive screening tools, such as the MOCA or SLUMS may be used, but there is no commonly accepted cutoff for determining when a patient lacks decision-making capacity for these either.

8. **What features in a patient's medical history make the assessment of decisional capacity difficult?**
   There are several reversible causes of decisional incapacity that must be ruled out when assessing a patient's decision-making capacity. These include, but are not limited to: intoxication, excessive sedation/analgesia,

polypharmacy, hypoxia, hypercarbia, fever, uremia, and other causes of encephalopathy. Careful inquiry of reversible causes should be pursued before any firm conclusions are drawn. Consultation with our colleagues in psychiatry is often helpful in determining if a patient has decisional capacity.

9. **What process is undertaken once an adult patient is deemed incapable of making medical decisions?**
It is important to note that this process varies according to state and local laws. The following discussion represents, in the authors' opinion, a reasonable approach to this commonly encountered scenario.

Once a patient is determined to lack decisional capacity, the first step is to query if there is some form of substituted judgment, which usually takes the form of an advanced directive. In general, there are three types of advanced directives: the living will, the medical durable power of attorney, and the cardiopulmonary resuscitation (or code status) directive. If an individual has failed to complete any of these documents before becoming decisionally incapacitated, and does not have a legal guardian, many states authorize a separate process for appointing a surrogate decision maker for making medical treatment decisions on their behalf, until they have regained decision-making capacity.

10. **How do you select a surrogate decision maker for a patient that lacks decisional capacity?**
The surrogate decision maker is a person that is either determined by state statute or chosen from a group of "Interested Persons" and may include:
1. The patient's spouse
2. Either parent of the patient
3. Any adult child, sibling, or grandchild of the patient
4. Any close friend (or significant other) of the patient
5. Clergy who are familiar with the person's values
Ideally, the person chosen should have a close relationship with the patient and be most likely to know the patient's values and wishes regarding medical treatment decisions. If there is no proxy decision-maker or disagreement emerges about who should be the proxy, any interested persons may seek legal guardianship through the courts.

The surrogate decision maker has the right, by law, to consent to or refuse care, treatment, and services on behalf of the patient, although some states may have specific exemptions. The care team is authorized to rely, in good faith, on the medical treatment decisions of the surrogate decision maker, until such time as the patient regains decision-making capacity or an individual/party goes to court and is granted guardianship.

11. **What happens if a patient who is decisionally impaired needs to go to the operating room for an urgent case? Or an emergent one? How do we define a surgical emergency?**
Surgical emergencies are defined as injuries or conditions that pose an immediate threat to life or limb if surgery is delayed. Urgent cases must proceed to the operating room within the next 12 to 24 hours to avoid the risk of either becoming emergent or incurring some form of permanent harm to the patient. In the event of a surgical emergency, we can bypass the informed consent process, understanding that if we are to err, we must err on the side of saving life and limb.

12. **How should Do-Not-Resuscitate orders be managed in the perioperative setting?**
The standard practice is to suspend Do-Not-Resuscitate (DNR) orders in the perioperative setting. Because the practice of anesthesiology fundamentally involves resuscitation, such as intubating for respiratory failure or administering inotropic agents for hemodynamic instability, problems may arise in respecting DNR orders during surgery. In general, because these physiological derangements are often temporary and reversible (e.g., because of sedation), DNR orders are often suspended in the perioperative setting and are reinstated following postanesthesia care unit discharge. This practice, however, is not absolute and there are situations where DNR orders may be upheld to varying degrees in the perioperative setting. Such situations generally require a thorough discussion with the patient or their surrogate decision maker, the surgical team, and proper documentation of the discussion in the medical chart, illustrating the patient's wishes.

13. **Is it ethically permissible to withhold or withdraw life-sustaining medical treatment if the clinician disagrees with the patient or surrogate decision maker?**
In general, a clinician should refrain from withdrawing or withholding care he or she believes is likely futile or potentially inappropriate, whenever there is conflict in doing so, with the patient or surrogate decision maker. In these situations, the clinician should seek expert consultation from other specialists, including palliative care and involve the hospital's ethics committee to facilitate dispute-resolution. In time-critical situations, however, clinicians are not obligated to provide medical care they believe is potentially inappropriate (e.g., providing chest compressions to a patient in cardiac arrest who has formally been declared brain dead).

14. **How does our approach to ethical reasoning change for the pediatric population?**
Adolescents and children have limited ability to provide informed consent because of their limited decision-making capacity. In general, as children age, their decision-making capacity, and hence their ability to provide informed consent, increases (Fig. 13.1). In very young children, who possess little to no decision-making capacity, we apply the Best Interest Standard.

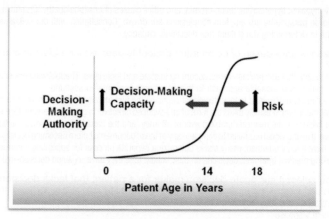

Fig. 13.1 Decision-making authority as a function of age in minors.

15. **What is the Best Interest Standard?**

The ethical principle of the Best Interest Standard simply means doing what is in the best interest of the patient, that is, choosing what we believe is objectively the best care. Unfortunately, there usually is no best care option; there exist several options that lie along a continuum of options. In these instances, parents are usually the appropriate decision makers.

16. **Can physicians and care teams overrule the parents?**

When there is uncertainty regarding which treatments are in the best interests of the child, physicians usually do not overrule the parents. However, physicians and care teams may consider this option if the parents are refusing interventions that are clearly beneficial, or, conversely, wish to pursue treatments that are clearly inadvisable. In such instances, seeking legal assistance is advised.

17. **What does the informed consent process look like for a child?**

It depends on the age of the child. For very young children, who have little to no decision-making capacity, we follow the Best Interest Standard and seek informed permission from the parents. As a child begins to develop decision-making capacity, at around the age of 6 years, we apply the Best Interest Standard, seek informed permission from the parents, and informed assent from the child. As children age and develop more decision-making capacity, they contribute more to the informed consent process. At the age of 18 years, they become adults and are granted complete decision-making authority (Table 13.1).

Note how decision-making authority for a child is affected by the risk associated with the particular situation. In situations where children are deciding between two scenarios that are equally low-risk, they may be granted a high

Table 13.1 Informed Consent in Pediatrics

AGE	MEDICAL DECISION-MAKING CAPACITY	TECHNIQUE USED
<6 years	None	Do what is in the best interest of the child, also known as the Best Interest Standard
6–12 years	Developing	1. Informed Permission of the Parents 2. Informed Assent of the Child
13–18 years	Mostly developed	1. Informed Permission of the Parents 2. Informed Assent of the Child
Mature minor (≥14 years)	Developed, as legally determined by a judge for a specific decision, e.g., Jehovah's Witness and blood administration	Informed Consent
Emancipated minor	Developed, as determined by statutes defining eligible situations, e.g., being married, economically independent	Informed Consent

degree of decision-making authority. However, in situations where the consequences of making a wrong choice are more severe, their decision-making authority should be much more constrained (see Fig. 13.1).

18. **What is informed assent?**
Informed assent is an affirmation of desire from a patient to participate in a planned procedure or treatment.

19. **Are there any instances where patients under the age of 18 years are granted adult status regarding medical decision making?**
Yes, in the instances of mature minors and emancipated minors. Mature minors have been legally determined the ability to make specific decisions regarding their health (e.g., to receive blood products). Emancipated minors, as determined by legal statutes, have the ability to make healthcare decisions once they enter a specific category, for example, being married, economically independent, engaged in military service, and so on (see Table 13.1). The specific criteria are determined by state law and may vary between states. Please refer to your institution's legal counsel for specific questions.

20. **Can adolescent patients under the age of 18 years refuse care if they demonstrate relatively mature decision-making capacity?**
Yes. If their decision is voluntary, and they are substantially informed regarding their decision, they may refuse care. This is referred to as *informed refusal*. To achieve this standard, mature adolescents must be able to imagine and articulate the consequences of their refusal using noncomparative reasoning, articulate opposing views to their decision, thoughtfully engage in discussion, and demonstrate a coherent rationale for their choice. We make adolescents demonstrate this higher standard because the likelihood of a teenager being able to attain this level is less than an adult.

KEY POINTS: PERIOPERATIVE MEDICAL ETHICS

1. Informed consent consists of the following components: (1) medical decision-making capacity, (2) disclosure, and (3) voluntariness.
2. Possessing medical decision-making capacity entails: (1) understanding the proposed treatment, (2) appreciating the severity of the situation, (3) using reason in the decision-making process, and (4) being able to communicate their decision to the care team.
3. There are several reversible causes of decisional incapacity that must be ruled out when assessing a patient's medical decision-making capacity.
4. DNR orders are generally suspended in the perioperative period because of the temporary and reversible nature of anesthesia, leading to respiratory failure and/or hemodynamic instability.
5. Adolescents and children have limited ability to provide informed consent because of their limited decision-making capacity. In these instances, the clinician should apply the Best Interest Standard.

SUGGESTED READINGS

American Society of Anesthesiology Committee on Ethics. Syllabus on Ethics. 2016. Available at: https://www.asahq.org/resources/ethics-and-professionalism. Accessed 10/1/18.
Applebaum PS. Assessment of patients' competence to consent to treat. N Engl J Med. 2007;357:1834–1870.
Cassel EJ. The nature of suffering and the goals of medicine. N Engl J Med. 1982;306:639–646.
Chow G, Czarny M, Hughes M, et al. CURVES: a mnemonic for determining medical decision-making capacity and providing emergency treatment in the acute setting. Chest. 2010;137(2):421–427.
Committee on Bioethics, American Academy of Pediatrics. Informed consent, parental permission, and assent in pediatric practice. Pediatrics. 1995;95:314–317.
Fallat ME, Deshpande JK. Do-not-resuscitate orders for pediatric patients who require anesthesia and surgery. Pediatrics. 2004;114:1686–1692.
Kon A, Shepard E, Sederstrom N, et al. Defining futile and potentially inappropriate interventions: a policy statement from the society of critical care medicine ethics committee. Crit Care Med. 2016;44:1769–1774.
Sessums LL, Zembrzuska H, Jackson JL. Does this patient have medical decision-making capacity? JAMA. 2011;306:420–427.
Van Norman GA, Rosenbam SH. Ethical aspects of anesthesia care. In: Miller RD, ed. Miller's Anesthesia. 8th ed. Philadelphia, 2015:232–250.

CHAPTER 14

INHALED ANESTHETICS

Lee D. Stein, MD, David Abts, MD

1. **What are the most desirable properties of an anesthetic gas?**
   The most desirable properties of an anesthetic gas are predictability in onset and emergence; muscle relaxation, cardiostability, and bronchodilation; nontriggering for malignant hyperthermia or other significant side effects (such as nausea and vomiting); be nonflammable; undergo no transformation within the body; allow easy estimation of concentration at the site of action; and have no environmental impact.

2. **What are the chemical structures of the most common anesthetic gases? Why have some older gases fallen out of favor?**
   Isoflurane, desflurane, and sevoflurane are the most commonly used volatile anesthetics. As the accompanying molecular structures demonstrate, they are substituted halogenated *ethers*. Many older anesthetic agents that are no longer in use had unfortunate properties and/or side effects, such as flammability (cyclopropane and fluroxene), slow induction (methoxyflurane), hepatotoxicity (halothane, chloroform, and fluroxene), nephrotoxicity (methoxyflurane), and the theoretic risk of seizures (enflurane) (Fig. 14.1).

3. **How are the potencies of anesthetic gases compared?**
   The potencies of anesthetic gases are compared using a unitless value known as *MAC*. MAC is the end-tidal concentration of anesthetic gas at 1 atmosphere that abolishes motor response to a painful stimulus (i.e., surgical incision) in 50% of patients, and is analogous to the ED_{50}. Of note, 1.3 MAC is required to abolish this response in 95% of patients. Other definitions of MAC include the MAC-BAR (1.7–2 MAC), which is the concentration required to block autonomic responses to nociceptive stimuli; MAC-Aware (0.4–0.5 MAC), the concentration at which 50% of patients will not form long-term memory, and the MAC-Awake (0.15–0.5 MAC), the concentration at which 50% of patients will open their eyes on command.
   The measurement of MAC assumes that alveolar concentration directly reflects the partial pressure of the anesthetic at its site of action. Also note that MAC is additive, for example, if a patient is receiving 0.5 MAC of sevoflurane and 0.5 MAC of nitrous oxide, they will be receiving 1 MAC total of inhaled anesthetic.

4. **What factors influence MAC?**
   The highest MACs are found in infants aged 1 to 6 months with isoflurane and desflurane. It is highest for sevoflurane during the neonatal period. For all agents, MAC decreases to normal by 1 year of age. With both prematurity and advanced age, MAC decreases. MAC also decreases with body temperature (approximately 2%–5% for every 1° C). Hyponatremia, opioids, barbiturates, α_2 blockers, calcium channel blockers, acute alcohol intoxication, and pregnancy also all decrease MAC. Hyperthermia, chronic alcoholism, and CNS stimulants all increase MAC.
   Factors that do not affect MAC include hypocarbia, hypercarbia, gender, thyroid function, and hyperkalemia.

5. **Define *partition coefficient*. Which partition coefficients are most important?**
   The alveolar concentration of an anesthetic gas ultimately determines its rate of onset. The partition coefficient is used to describe the alveolar concentration by quantifying the distribution of a given anesthetic agent between the phases of blood and gas in the alveolus. A high blood:gas partition coefficient correlates with a greater concentration of anesthetic in the blood (i.e., a higher solubility) than in the alveolus, and thus slower onset of action.
   There are other clinically significant partition coefficients besides blood:gas. Other important partition coefficients include brain:blood, fat:blood, liver:blood, and muscle:blood. Except for fat:blood, all of these coefficients are close to 1 (i.e., equally distributed). Fat has partition coefficients ranging from 30 to 60 for different volatile agents (i.e., the agent continues to enter adipose tissue after equilibration with other tissues has occurred; Table 14.1), allowing fat to serve as a reservoir for more soluble anesthetic agents, and hence, delaying emergence from anesthesia with these agents.

6. **What factors influence speed of induction?**
   Factors that increase the alveolar concentration of an inhalational agent will speed the onset of anesthetic induction. These factors include:
   - Use of low solubility agents (i.e., lower blood:gas partition coefficients). This is because equilibration between alveolus and brain occurs quickly for insoluble volatile anesthetics, and the partial pressure in the alveolus is assumed to match the partial pressure in the brain
   - Increasing the delivered concentration of anesthetic to the alveolus (i.e., high dialed agent concentration, high breathing circuit flows, increased minute ventilation)

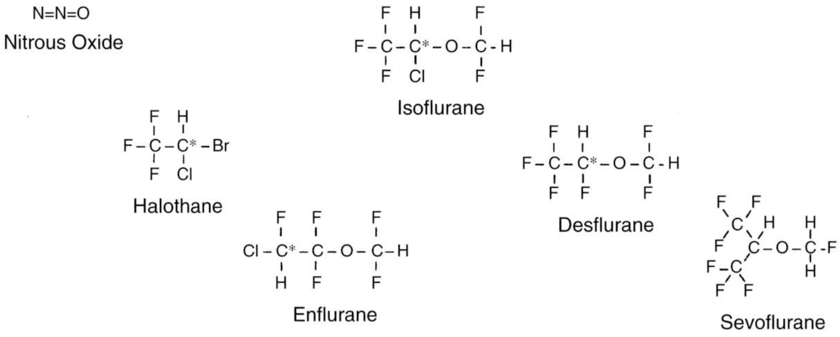

Fig. 14.1 Molecular structures of contemporary gaseous anesthetics.

Table 14.1 Physical Properties of Contemporary Anesthetic Gases					
	ISOFLURANE	**DESFLURANE**	**HALOTHANE**	**NITROUS OXIDE**	**SEVOFLURANE**
Molecular weight (kDa)	184.5	168	197.5	44	200
Boiling point (°C)	48.5	23.5	50.2	−88	58.5
Vapor pressure (mm Hg)	238	664	241	39,000	160
Partition Coefficients at 37°C					
Blood to gas	1.4	0.42	2.3	0.47	0.69
Brain to blood	2.6	1.2	2.9	1.7	1.7
Fat to blood	45	27	60	2.3	48
Oil to gas	90.8	18.7	224	1.4	47.2
MAC (% of 1 atm)	1.15	6	0.77	104	1.7

atm, Atmosphere; *MAC,* minimum alveolar concentration.

- Decreased cardiac output (this effect is more pronounced with insoluble agents)
- Use in pediatric patients (increased minute ventilation relative to functional residual capacity, increased percentage of blood flow to brain)
- Second gas effect (minor)
  Factors that decrease the alveolar concentration of an inhalational agent will slow the onset of anesthetic induction. These factors include:
- Use of high solubility agents. This is because a greater amount of anesthetic will be taken into the blood, therefore acting as a reservoir for the agent, reducing the alveolar concentration and slowing the rate of induction
- Increased cardiac output (this effect is more pronounced with soluble agents)
- Presence of right to left cardiac shunt (as no agent is taken up into shunted blood, thereby diluting arterial concentration)

7. **What is the second gas effect?**
   Classically described for nitrous oxide (N_2O). Because N_2O is insoluble in blood, its rapid absorption from alveoli results in an abrupt rise in the alveolar concentration of the accompanying volatile anesthetic. However, even at high concentrations (70%) of nitrous oxide, this effect accounts for only a small increase in alveolar concentration of the other volatile anesthetic.

8. **Explain diffusion hypoxia.**
   When an insoluble gas (usually N_2O) is discontinued abruptly, its rapid diffusion from the blood to the alveolus decreases the oxygen tension in the lung, leading to a brief period of decreased oxygen concentration known as *diffusion hypoxia.* Administering high flow 100% oxygen at the end of a case can mitigate this.

9. **Describe the ventilatory effects of volatile anesthetics.**
Delivery of anesthetic gases results in dose-dependent depression of ventilation mediated directly through medullary centers and indirectly through effects on intercostal muscle function. Minute volume decreases secondary to reductions in tidal volume, although rate usually appears to increase in a dose-dependent fashion. Respiratory drive in response to hypoxemia can be abolished at 1 MAC and significantly attenuated at lower MACs. Increased delivered anesthetic concentration also attenuates the ventilatory response to hypercarbia.

10. **What effects do volatile anesthetics have on airway caliber, mucociliary function, and hypoxic pulmonary vasoconstriction?**
Volatile anesthetics decrease airway resistance by directly relaxing bronchial smooth muscle. The bronchoconstriction associated with histamine release also appears to decrease when an inhalational anesthetic is administered. Taken altogether, volatile anesthetics are potent vasodilators.
    Mucociliary clearance appears to be diminished by volatile anesthetics as well, principally through interference with ciliary beat frequency. In addition, the effects of dry inhaled gases, positive-pressure ventilation, and high inspired oxygen content will also contribute to ciliary impairment.
    Hypoxic pulmonary vasoconstriction is a locally mediated response of the pulmonary vasculature to reduced alveolar oxygen tension and functions to match lung ventilation to pulmonary perfusion. Inhalational agents attenuate this response, but the clinical significance of this effect is minimal.

11. **Do volatile anesthetics affect intracranial pressure?**
Yes. Volatile anesthetics increase intracranial blood flow and increase intracranial pressure (ICP). Cerebral metabolic rate will be decreased (except in the case of N_2O) and autoregulation of cerebral blood flow impaired. Use of an intravenous anesthetic may be preferred to volatile anesthetics when elevated ICP may impair effective intracranial blood flow.

12. **What effects do volatile anesthetics have on the cardiovascular system?**
See Table 14.2.

13. **Which anesthetic agent is most associated with cardiac dysrhythmias?**
Halothane has been shown to increase the sensitivity of the myocardium to B_1-adrenergic stimulation (i.e., epinephrine), resulting in premature ventricular contractions and tachydysrhythmias. The mechanism of arrythmogenesis may be related to the prolongation of conduction through the His-Purkinje system, thereby facilitating reentry. Compared with adults, children undergoing halothane anesthesia appear to be relatively resistant to this sensitizing effect. However, halothane has been shown to have a cholinergic, vagally induced bradycardic effect in children. Also of note, volatile anesthetics prolong the QT interval.

14. **Do volatile anesthetics affect the renal system?**
Yes. All volatile anesthetics decrease renal blood flow, glomerular filtration rate, and urine output.

15. **Which volatile agents trigger malignant hyperthermia?**
All volatile agents are associated with triggering malignant hyperthermia (MH) except N_2O. MH is not associated with any of the intravenous anesthetics.

Table 14.2 Circulatory Effects of Contemporary Anesthetic Gases

	ISOFLURANE/ DESFLURANE	SEVOFLURANE	HALOTHANE	NITROUS OXIDE
Cardiac output	0	0	− [a]	+
Heart rate	++/0	0	0	+
Blood pressure	− [a]	− [a]	− [a]	0
Stroke volume	− [a]	− [a]	− [a]	−
Contractility	− [a]	− [a]	− [a]	− [a]
Systemic vascular resistance	−	−	0	0
Pulmonary vascular resistance	0	0	0	+
Coronary blood flow	+	+	0	0
Cerebral blood flow	+	+	++	0
Muscle blood flow	+	+	−	0
Catecholamine levels	0	0	0	0

[a], Dose-dependent; +, increase; ++, large increase; 0, no change; −, decrease; —, large decrease.

16. Discus nitrous oxide. Is it harmful to humans?

Nitrous oxide can be harmful to humans because of its ability to prevent cobalamin (vitamin B_{12}) from acting as a coenzyme for methionine synthase. Occasionally, patients may experience signs of toxicity during routine nitrous-based anesthetics, including pernicious anemia and vitamin B_{12} deficiency. There had been concern that using nitrous oxide could increase the risk of cardiac complications; however it is now believed to be safe for noncardiac surgery in patients with known cardiac disease. In general, serious side effects (e.g., myelinopathies, spinal cord degeneration, altered mental status, paresthesias, ataxia, weakness, spasticity) are usually only seen in persons abusing nitrous oxide for long periods of time.

Several surveys have attempted to quantify the relative risk of operating room personal exposure to nonscavenged anesthetic gases. Pregnant women who were exposed frequently to nitrous oxide were reported to have an increased risk of spontaneous abortion and congenital abnormalities. These results, however, could be caused by responder bias and failure to control for other exposure hazards.

Also of note, N_2O, although not flammable, will support combustion, thus increasing the risk of airway fire. It has been associated with an increase in postoperative nausea and vomiting. Lastly, it has been demonstrated to increase pulmonary vascular resistance, especially in patients with preexisting pulmonary hypertension.

17. Are there any conditions in which N_2O administration should be avoided?

N_2O is 20 times more soluble than atmospheric nitrogen (meaning that it diffuses 20 times faster into closed spaces than plain nitrogen gas). This can result in the rapid expansion of air-filled spaces, such as in pneumothorax, bowel gas, venous air embolism, or in the endotracheal tube cuff. It can also increase pressure within noncompliant cavities, such as the cranium (pneumocephalus) or middle ear. Lastly, it can expand intraocular gas bubbles created during ophthalmological surgery.

18. Discuss the biotransformation of volatile anesthetics and relative toxicity of their metabolic by-products.

Desflurane and isoflurane are metabolized less than 1% and sevoflurane is metabolized around 5%. Halothane is metabolized more than 20%, primarily in the liver. Under hypoxic conditions, halothane may undergo reductive (as opposed to oxidative) metabolism, resulting in metabolites that may cause hepatic necrosis. Halothane hepatitis, although rare, occurs secondary to an autoimmune hypersensitivity reaction. This fulminant condition would present postoperatively and substantially contributed to halothane's withdrawal from the market.

Fluoride is another potential by-product of anesthetic metabolism. Fluoride-associated renal dysfunction has been linked to the use of methoxyflurane. Fluoride is also produced by sevoflurane, but this has not been implicated in the development of renal dysfunction.

19. Review the effects of CO_2 absorbents on volatile anesthetic by-products.

Desflurane has been associated with the production of CO. The following conditions must be present for this to occur:

- The volatile compound must contain a difluoromethoxy group (desflurane, enflurane, and isoflurane). This group then interacts with the strongly alkaline and desiccated CO_2 absorbent. A base-catalyzed proton abstraction forms a carbanion that can either be reprotonated by water to regenerate the original anesthetic, or form CO if the absorbent is dry
- The incidence of CO exposure is highest in the first case of the day, when machines have not been used for some time, or when fresh gas flow has been left on for a protracted period of time (i.e., over the weekend). For this reason, absorbents should be changed routinely despite lack of apparent color change, and moisture levels should be monitored
- Potassium hydroxide (KOH)—containing absorbents are the stronger alkalis and result in greater CO production. From greatest to least, KOH-containing absorbents are baralyme (4.6%) > classic soda lime (2.6%) > new soda lime (0%) > calcium hydroxide lime (Amsorb) (0%)
- Choice of volatile anesthetic also determines the amount of CO produced, and at equiMAC concentrations: desflurane >enflurane >isoflurane. Sevoflurane, once thought to be innocent, has been shown to also produce CO when exposed to dry absorbent (especially KOH-containing)

20. What is Compound A? What is its clinical significance?

Older, strong-base containing carbon dioxide absorbers (e.g., soda lime, baralyme) can produce a degradation by-product from sevoflurane known as *Compound A*. Although Compound A has been shown to demonstrate nephrotoxicity in rats, no organ dysfunction in has been noted in humans. It is also important to note that in these animal studies, rats were exposed to Compound A specifically, not to sevoflurane.

Compound A may accumulate during low-flow anesthesia, during longer cases, while using dry CO_2 absorbent and with high sevoflurane concentration. However, multiple randomized controlled trials and metaanalyses have failed to demonstrate any sevoflurane-induced nephrotoxicity under low-flow conditions compared with other volatile anesthetics (e.g., isoflurane). Furthermore, modern CO_2 absorbers contain only small amounts of strong base and are largely nonreactive with respect to Compound A formation.

21. What is the environmental impact of inhaled anesthetics?

All volatile anesthetic agents, as well as nitrous oxide, act as greenhouse gases. For most healthcare systems, the perioperative environment is responsible for the largest share of carbon emissions in the hospital. Within the perioperative environment, volatile anesthetics themselves are responsible for the greatest share of carbon emissions—often over 50% of total emissions. Atmospheric lifetimes of volatile anesthetics have a wide range—1 year for sevoflurane, 3 years for isoflurane, 14 years for desflurane, and 114 years for nitrous oxide. In addition, they vary in their respective carbon emission potentials. Relative to carbon dioxide, sevoflurane is 130 times more potent; however desflurane is 2540 times more potent. When delivered at equivalent flow rates, desflurane is responsible for over 40 times the carbon emissions of sevoflurane. Besides carbon emission, volatile anesthetics and N_2O also contribute to depletion of the ozone layer.

To summarize, the environmental impacts of our anesthetic practice should be considered when making clinical choices, recognizing that there are significant differences with respect to our volatile anesthetics.

22. **Review the historical hypotheses regarding how volatile anesthetics work.**
At the turn of the last century, Meyer and Overton independently observed that an increasing oil-to-gas partition coefficient correlated with anesthetic potency. Their Meyer-Overton lipid solubility theory dominated for nearly 50 years. Next, Franks and Lieb discovered that an amphophilic solvent (octanol) correlated better with potency than lipophilicity and concluded that the anesthetic site must contain both polar and nonpolar sites. Further modifications to Meyer and Overton's membrane expansion theory include the excessive volume theory, stating that anesthesia occurs when polar cell membrane components and amphophilic anesthetics act synergistically to expand cellular volume, and the critical volume hypothesis, stating that anesthesia results when the cell volume at the anesthetic site reaches a critical size. These theories rely on the effects of membrane expansion on ion channels.

These early 19th-century theories oversimplified the mechanism of anesthetic action and were abandoned. Newer theories propose distinct molecular targets and anatomic sites of action rather than nonspecific actions on cell membrane or volume. Volatile anesthetics are presently thought to enhance inhibitory receptors on ion channels, including γ-aminobutyric acid type A and glycine receptors. Blockade of excitatory ion channels are also a feature and are mediated through excitation of NMDA (*N*-methyl-D-aspartate) receptors.

Most likely, the actions of immobilization and amnesia are caused by separate mechanisms at different anatomic sites. At the spinal cord level, anesthetics lead to suppression of nociceptive motor responses and are responsible for immobilization of skeletal muscle. Supraspinal effects on the brain are responsible for amnesia and hypnosis. The thalamus and midbrain reticular formation are more depressed than other regions of the brain during general anesthesia. It is important to remember that amnesia, lack of awareness, and immobility are not guaranteed, especially when the patient has received a neuromuscular blocking drug. At present, the exact mechanism of action of how volatile anesthetics provide anesthesia has yet to be fully understood. Stay tuned!

KEY POINTS: VOLATILE ANESTHETICS

1. Speed of onset of volatile anesthetics is increased by increasing the delivered concentration of anesthetic, increasing the fresh gas flow, increasing alveolar ventilation, and using nonlipid-soluble anesthetics.
2. Volatile anesthetics lead to a decrease in tidal volume and an increase in respiratory rate, resulting in a rapid, shallow breathing pattern.
3. Minimal alveolar concentration (MAC) is decreased by old age or prematurity, hyponatremia, hypothermia, opioids, barbiturates, α_2 blockers, calcium channel blockers, acute alcohol intoxication, and pregnancy.
4. MAC is increased by hyperthermia, chronic alcoholism, hypernatremia, and acute intoxication with central nervous system (CNS) stimulants (e.g., amphetamine).
5. The physiological response to hypoxia and hypercarbia is blunted by volatile anesthetics in a dose-dependent fashion.
6. Because of its rapid egress into air-filled spaces, nitrous oxide should not be used in the setting of pneumothorax, bowel obstruction, or pneumocephalus, or during middle ear or ophthalmological surgery.
7. Degradation of desflurane and sevoflurane by desiccated CO_2 absorbents may lead to carbon monoxide (CO) production and poisoning.

SUGGESTED READINGS

Campagna JA, Miller KE, Forman SA. Mechanisms of actions of inhaled anesthetics. N Engl J Med. 2003;348:2110–2124.
Coppens MJ, Versichelen LFM, Rolly G, et al. The mechanism of carbon monoxide production by inhalational agents. Anaesthesia. 2006;61:462–468.
Leslie K, Myles PS, Kasza J, et al. Nitrous oxide and serious long-term morbidity and mortality in the Evaluation of Nitrous Oxide in the Gas Mixture for Anaesthesia (ENIGMA)-II trial. Anesthesiology. 2015;123:1267–1280.
MacNeill AJ, Lillywhite R, Brown CJ. The impact of surgery on global climate: a carbon footprinting study of operating theatres in three health systems. Lancet Planet Health. 2017;1:e381–e388.
Obata R, Bito H, Ohmura M, et al. The effects of prolonged low-flow sevoflurane on renal and hepatic function. Anesth Analg. 2000;91:1262–1268.
Ong Sio LCL, Dela Cruz RGC, Bautista AF. Sevoflurane and renal function: a meta-analysis of randomized trials. Med Gas Res. 2017;7(3):186–193.
Sherman J, Le C, Lamers V, et al. Life cycle greenhouse gas emissions of anesthetic drugs. Anesth Analg. 2012;114:1086–1090.

CHAPTER 15

INTRAVENOUS ANESTHETICS

Scott Vogel, DO

1. **What qualities would the ideal intravenous anesthetic agent possess?**

   The ideal intravenous induction would produce amnesia, analgesia, hypnosis, and muscle relaxation. Adverse effects and interactions would be rare. Administration would be painless via multiple routes of delivery. Interindividual dose variability would be low and the agent would have a predictably rapid onset and offset. There would be no cardiac, renal, hepatic, immune system, or central nervous system (CNS) toxicity. Hemodynamic and respiratory changes would be minimal. It would be low-cost, shelf-stable, nonhabit forming, and not used outside of medical means. Lastly, it would be manufactured by multiple companies in different geographic areas, precluding a shortage because of local production chain issues.

2. **List the commonly used induction agents and their properties.**

   - Propofol is a γ-aminobutyric acid (GABA)$_A$ receptor agonist that results in a more profound decrease in mean arterial pressure (MAP) compared with etomidate. This is caused by a combination of arterial and venous vasodilation, baroreceptor inhibition (no reflex tachycardia), and a decrease in myocardial contractility. By itself, it has antiemetic properties. It can be associated with significant pain on injection
   - Ketamine inhibits *N*-methyl-D-aspartate (NMDA) receptors, causing dissociative anesthesia with profound analgesia. It is purported to be a direct myocardial depressant, but its sympathomimetic effects usually result in an overall increased cardiac output (CO), MAP, and heart rate (HR)
   - Dexmedetomidine is a selective α_2 adrenergic agonist with sedative, amnestic, and analgesic effects. Its administration results in sedation with very minimal respiratory depression. Adverse effects include bradycardia and dose-dependent hypotension
   - Etomidate is an imidazole derivative with selective GABA$_A$ receptor modulator activity noted for its hemodynamic stability. CO and contractility are preserved with only a mild decrease in MAP. Side effects include pain on injection, nausea, myoclonus, seizures, and adrenal suppression
   - Midazolam is the principal benzodiazepine used perioperatively. Benzodiazepines provide anxiolysis, sedation, amnesia, and in high doses, hypnosis through GABA$_A$ receptor activation and potentiation. Midazolam has minimal myocardial or respiratory depression when used as a sole agent. There is no effect on MAP or CO; HR may increase slightly
   - Opioids are morphine-like drugs used for analgesia and adjunctively during induction. High doses of most opioids have a vagolytic effect, resulting in bradycardia. The exception is meperidine, which has sympathomimetic effects that produce tachycardia. Although they are relatively hemodynamically stable and frequently used in higher doses during cardiac anesthesia, decreased MAP may be noted secondary to bradycardia, vasodilation, and histamine release (especially evident with morphine and meperidine)

   Larger doses of multiple classes of induction agents and sedation medications may result in undesirable hemodynamic effects. Hence a preferred technique requires multiple medications used in smaller doses. This is termed *balanced anesthesia* and takes advantage of the synergism of these agents, while minimizing the adverse effects of each. Muscle relaxants ordinarily are also portions of balanced anesthesia. The effects of intravenous bolus-dosed anesthetics primarily terminate through redistribution as opposed to metabolism (Tables 15.1 and 15.2).

3. **When should one avoid using etomidate?**

   Etomidate causes epileptiform activity on an electroencephalogram and should be used with caution in patients with epilepsy. It has also been associated with adrenal suppression (interfering with hydroxylases during the synthesis of cortisol). Thus it should be used cautiously, if at all, in patients who are critically ill.

4. **Describe the properties of propofol.**

   2,6-Diisopropylphenol, or propofol, has become a highly preferred intravenous anesthetic. It may be administered by bolus or continuous dosing. Hemodynamic effects have been described earlier. It is important to recognize that propofol does not have any analgesic properties and is primarily used for hypnosis. Propofol is water insoluble and must be formulated in a 1% lipid emulsion. This emulsion contains: soybean oil, glycerol, and egg yolk lecithin. These agents are prone to bacterial infection, thus requiring strict sterile management and administration within 12 hours once drawn up in the operating room.

   Of note, most patients with documented egg allergies are allergic to egg white antigens, making propofol an acceptable agent for use in this population. However, it is reasonable to consider avoiding this agent in patients with a history of anaphylaxis to eggs, especially children (see later). Lastly, prolonged infusion with propofol has been associated with a rare, but potentially fatal form of cardiac failure because of arrhythmias, hyperlipidemia, and

Table 15.1 Dosing Guidelines for Anesthetic Induction and Sedation

AGENT	CLASS	DOSE FOR ANESTHETIC INDUCTION	DOSE FOR SEDATION
Ketamine	Phencyclidine derivative	1–2 mg/kg IV 2–4 mg/kg IM	0.2–0.5 mg/kg IV
Etomidate	Imidazole derivative	0.2–0.5 mg/kg IV	Inappropriate use
Propofol	Substituted phenol	1–4 mg/kg IV bolus 50–200 mcg/kg/min infusion	25–100 mcg/kg/min IV
Midazolam	Benzodiazepine	0.1–0.4 mg/kg IV	0.01–0.1 mg/kg IV
Dexmedetomidine	α_2 Adrenergic agonist	N/A	1 mcg/kg loading dose given over 10 minutes, 0.2–0.7 mcg/kg/h

Doses of medications should be adjusted for intravascular volume status, comorbidities, and other medications.
IM, Intramuscular; *IV*, intravenous.

Table 15.2 Cardiovascular Effects of Intravenous Anesthetic Agents

AGENT	MAP	HR	SVR	CO	CONTRACTILITY	VENODILATION
Ketamine	++	++	+	+	+ or −[a]	0
Midazolam	0 to −	0 to +	0 to −	0 to −	0 to −	+
Propofol	−	+	−	0	−	+
Etomidate	0	0	0	0	0	0
Dexmedetomidine	+ or −	+ or −	0	+ or −	0	0

[a]The effect of ketamine depends on patient's catecholamine levels.
CO, Cardiac output; *HR*, heart rate; *MAP*, mean arterial pressure; *SVR*, systemic vascular resistance; *0*, no effect; ++, increases significantly; +, increases; −, decreases.

metabolic acidosis, termed *propofol infusion syndrome* (PRIS). Incidents of PRIS have generally been restricted to patients receiving high doses (≥ 4 mg/kg/h) for 48 hours or more (see later).

5. Discuss the use of propofol in patients who are allergic to eggs and/or soy.
The original accounts of allergic reactions to propofol were not validated with postoperative allergy testing, and therefore resulted in possible misdiagnosis because of the multiple intravenous medications commonly used during an anesthetic. This being said, patients typically have an allergic reaction to the egg protein, ovalbumin, which is present in the egg white but not the egg yolk. Egg lecithin, the egg component in propofol, is produced from the yolk and is processed to remove almost all of that protein. The current body of evidence suggests that propofol is safe for all adult patients with egg allergies, regardless of their reaction type. The remaining caveat, however, is children with anaphylaxis to eggs, where it is still considered prudent to avoid propofol. Soy allergies do not preclude propofol use.

6. Are there other conditions which limit the use of propofol?
Propofol has cardiac depressant effects; thus patients with cardiomyopathies and hypovolemia may not be ideal candidates for its use. Also in patients with disorders of lipid metabolism, such as primary hyperlipoproteinemia, diabetic hyperlipidemia, mitochondrial disease and pancreatitis, it should be used with caution.

7. In general, how do induction agents affect respiratory drive?
All intravenous induction agents, with the exception of ketamine, produce dose-dependent respiratory depression. This manifests as a decreased tidal volume, minute ventilation, and response to hypoxia, as well as a rightward shift in the arterial carbon dioxide dose-response curve, eventually culminating in hypoventilation and/or apnea.

8. Describe the properties of ketamine.
Ketamine is an NMDA receptor antagonist that is chemically related to phencyclidine, resulting in a dose-dependent dissociative state and unconsciousness. It is a potent analgesic but its amnestic ability is weak. Concurrent administration of a benzodiazepine may decrease the incidence of adverse dysphoric effects.

Ketamine causes a centrally mediated increase in sympathetic outflow, resulting in tachycardia, increased CO, and increased MAP. However, it also has direct myocardial depressant effects that tend not to become manifest because of overriding sympathetic stimulation. Therefore in catecholamine-depleted states, the myocardial depressant effects may be unmasked. Ketamine is considered an ideal induction agent in patients with conditions, such as shock, significant hypovolemia, and cardiac tamponade.

Other desirable side effects include bronchodilation and preserved respiratory drive. Undesirable side effects include increased cerebral blood flow and cerebral metabolic rate, increased oral secretions, and potentially unpleasant psychotomimetic reactions.

9. Discuss the use of etomidate in the critically ill patient.

Etomidate inhibits the enzyme 11-β-hydroxylase in the cortisol synthesis pathway. In some studies, a single dose of etomidate resulted in clinically significant adrenal suppression and increased morbidity and mortality in critically ill patients, and those with septic shock. A recent Cochrane review did not find conclusive evidence either way. However, the stable hemodynamic properties of etomidate make it a desirable induction agent for patients in shock. Hydrocortisone supplementation may mitigate the adrenosuppressive effects of etomidate in these patients, but study results are contradictory.

10. Describe propofol infusion syndrome.

First described in 1990, PRIS occurs in critically ill patients receiving high-dose propofol infusions over long periods of time (>4 mg/kg/h for >48 hours). PRIS seemingly results from interference with mitochondrial energy production although the exact mechanism is not fully understood. The syndrome presents with bradycardia in association with one of the following: enlarged liver, lipemic plasma, metabolic acidosis, or rhabdomyolysis. Mortality results from lethal arrhythmias, renal failure, or progressive circulatory failure because of severe lactic acidosis.

11. What would be an appropriate induction agent for a 47-year-old healthy male with a parietal lobe tumor and evidence of increased ICP scheduled for craniotomy?

When used at appropriate doses, propofol is an agent that preserves cerebral blood flow autoregulation, lowers cerebral metabolic rate, and preserves flow-metabolism coupling. Thus it should have a minimal effect on ICP, while maintaining cerebral perfusion pressure.

12. Describe the mechanism of action of benzodiazepines.

GABA is the primary inhibitory neurotransmitter of the CNS and its receptor is found in postsynaptic nerve endings. The GABA receptor is composed of two α subunits and two β subunits. The α subunits are the binding sites for benzodiazepines, the β subunits are the binding sites for GABA, and a chloride ion channel is located in the center.

Benzodiazepines produce their effects by enhancing the binding of GABA to its receptor. GABA activates the chloride ion channel, which hyperpolarizes the neuron and thereby inhibits it.

Benzodiazepines are metabolized in the liver by microsomal oxidation and glucuronidation and should be used with caution in the elderly. The potency, onset, and duration of action of benzodiazepines depend on their lipid solubility. Onset of action is achieved by rapid distribution to the vessel-rich brain. Termination of effect occurs as the drug is redistributed to other parts of the body.

13. What benzodiazepines are commonly administered intravenously?

- Midazolam has the most rapid onset and shortest duration of action. Unlike other benzodiazepines, midazolam is water soluble and therefore can be manufactured without the pain-inducing solvent, propylene glycol. It is by far the most common benzodiazepine used perioperatively for anxiolysis and amnesia. Active metabolites are renally cleared and thus duration of action is prolonged with compromised renal function
- Lorazepam is slightly slower in onset and slightly longer in duration of action versus midazolam. It is most commonly used in the intensive care unit and postanesthesia care unit, where anxiolysis is needed. There are no active metabolites
- Diazepam is the slowest in onset and longest in duration of action. It has the unique property of producing muscle relaxation, which can be beneficial after some surgeries (i.e., hip arthroscopies). Duration of action is prolonged in the elderly and in patients with hepatic impairment because of an active metabolite

14. How should oversedation induced by benzodiazepines be managed?

As a first principle, always provide supportive care. Open the airway and mask-ventilate, if needed. Assess the adequacy of the circulation. Lastly, consider administering the benzodiazepine antagonist flumazenil. Flumazenil works by competitive inhibition, reversing sedation and respiratory depression in a dose-dependent fashion. Onset starts in 45 seconds and peaks within 1 to 3 minutes. It should be titrated to effect by administering doses of 0.2 mg intravenously for a maximum dose of 3 to 5 mg. It should be used with caution, if at all, in patients with a history of epilepsy managed with benzodiazepines. Although only approved for intravenous use, it has been suggested that flumazenil is effective when used intramuscularly, rectally, or sublingually.

15. What are the possible side effects of flumazenil?

The elimination half-life of midazolam is 2 to 3 hours, whereas the elimination half-life of flumazenil is 1 hour, so resedation is a risk. Flumazenil may be repeated at that time or administered as an infusion at 0.5 to 1 mg/h.

KEY POINTS

1. Propofol, ketamine, etomidate, midazolam, opioids (primarily fentanyl), and dexmedetomidine are the intravenous anesthetics used most prevalently in contemporary anesthetic practice.
2. Appropriate dosing of intravenous anesthetics requires consideration of intravascular volume status, comorbidities, age, and chronic medications.
3. Propofol, although used ubiquitously in the practice of anesthesia, is associated with significant myocardial depression and must be used with caution.
4. Propofol is generally regarded as safe for use in adult patients with documented egg allergies, but should be avoided in children with known anaphylaxis to eggs.
5. Ketamine is the best induction agent for hypovolemic trauma patients, as long as there is no risk for increased intracranial pressure (ICP). It is also a good agent for patients with active bronchospastic disease.

SUGGESTED READINGS

Bruder EA, Ball IM, Ridi S, et al. Single induction dose of etomidate versus other induction agents for endotracheal intubation in critically ill patients. Cochrane Database Syst Rev. 2015;CD010225.

Harper NJ. Propofol and food allergy. Br J Anesth. 2016;116:11–13.

Vanlander AV, Okun JG, de Jaeger A, et al. Possible pathological mechanism of propofol infusion syndrome involves coenzyme Q. Anesthesiology. 2015;122:343–352.

OPIOIDS

Christopher L. Ciarallo, MD, FAAP

CHAPTER 16

1. **What is an opiate? An opioid? A narcotic?**
   Opiates are analgesic and sedative drugs that contain opium or an opium derivative from the poppy plant (*Papaver somniferum*). Opiates include opium, morphine, and codeine. An opioid is any substance with morphine-like activity that acts as an agonist or antagonist at an opioid receptor (i.e., δ-, κ-, and μ-receptors). Opioids may be exogenous or endogenous (such as endorphins) and may be natural, derived, or synthetic. The term *narcotic* is not specific for opioids and refers to any substance with addictive potential that induces analgesia and sedation (e.g., cannabis and cocaine).

2. **What are endogenous opioids?**
   Endorphins, enkephalins, and dynorphins are the three classes of endogenous peptides that are derived from prohormones and are functionally active at opioid receptors. Although their physiological roles are not completely understood, they appear to modulate nociception via glutamate inhibition or alteration in potassium channel conductance. Endorphins are not limited to the central nervous system (CNS) and may even be expressed by activated leukocytes.

3. **Differentiate opioid tolerance, dependence, and abuse.**
   Tolerance is a diminution in the physiological effects of a substance, resulting from repeated administration. Dependence may be physical or psychological and refers to the repeated use of a substance to avoid withdrawal symptoms. Tolerance may be necessary to establish the diagnosis of dependence. Abuse refers to the habitual use of a substance, despite adverse consequences, including social and interpersonal problems.

4. **Name the opioids commonly used in the perioperative setting, their trade names, equivalent morphine doses, half-lives, and chemical classes.**
   See Table 16.1.

5. **Describe the various opioid receptors and their effects.**
   See Table 16.2.

6. **What is an opioid agonist-antagonist?**
   Drugs, such as pentazocine, butorphanol, buprenorphine, and nalbuphine, were initially thought to be μ-receptor antagonists and κ-receptor agonists. However, they are now classified as μ- and κ-receptor partial agonists. These drugs provide analgesia, but with less euphoria and risk of dependence as compared with pure agonists. Agonist-antagonists, in general, cause less respiratory depression than do agonists and may reverse the respiratory depression and pruritus caused by pure agonists.

7. **Explain the mechanism of action, duration, and side effects of the opioid antagonist naloxone.**
   Naloxone is a μ-, κ-, and δ-receptor antagonist that will reverse the effects of agonist drugs. The peak effect occurs within 1 to 2 minutes of intravenous administration. The duration of action is between 20 and 60 minutes and may be shorter than the duration of the offending opioid agonist. Incremental doses of 0.2 to 0.5 mcg/kg should initially be used to reverse respiratory depression to minimize side effects, such as acute opioid withdrawal, severe hypertension, ventricular dysrhythmias, or pulmonary edema. Naloxone can also be used intranasally with approximately 47% bioavailability of parenteral dosing.

8. **Describe the various routes of administration of opioids.**
   Typical routes of administration include oral, intravenous, intramuscular, epidural, subarachnoid, and rectal. Intranasal, nebulized, and subcutaneous may also be used. Lipophilic opioids (such as fentanyl) are also available in transdermal, transmucosal, and sublingual formulations.

9. **What are the typical side effects of opioids?**
   Opioid side effects include respiratory depression, nausea and vomiting, pruritus, cough suppression, urinary retention, and biliary tract spasm. Some opioids may induce histamine release and cause hives, bronchospasm, and hypotension. Intravenous opioids may cause abdominal and chest wall rigidity. Most opioids, with the notable exception of meperidine, produce a dose-dependent bradycardia.

10. **Which opioids are associated with histamine release?**
    Parenteral doses of meperidine, morphine, and codeine have been associated with histamine release and resultant cutaneous reactions and hypotension. The incidence and severity, at least with morphine, appear to be dose dependent.

Table 16.1 Comparison of Commonly Used Opioids

GENERIC NAME	TRADE NAME	EQUIPOTENT IV/IM (mg)	EQUIPOTENT PO (mg)	PLASMA HALF-LIFE (h)	CHEMICAL CLASS
Morphine	Roxanol	10	30	2	Phenanthrene
Morphine CR	MS-Contin	—	30	15	Phenanthrene
Diacetylmorphine	Heroin	5	45–60	0.5	Phenanthrene
Alfentanil	Alfenta	1	—	1.5	Phenylpiperidine
Fentanyl	Sublimaze	0.1	—	3–4	Phenylpiperidine
Sufentanil	Sufenta	0.01–0.02	—	2.5–4	Phenylpiperidine
Remifentanil	Ultiva	0.04	—	9 min	Phenylpiperidine
Hydromorphone	Dilaudid	1.3–2	7.5	2–3	Phenanthrene
Oxymorphone	Opana	1	10	7–9	Phenanthrene
Meperidine	Demerol	75	300	3–4	Phenylpiperidine
Methadone (Acute) (Chronic)	Dolophine	10 2–4	20 2–4	15–40	Diphenylheptane
Codeine	Tylenol #3[a]	130 IM	200	2–4	Phenanthrene
Hydrocodone	Vicodin, Lortab[a]	—	30	4	Phenanthrene
Oxycodone	Percocet[a]	—	20	4–5	Phenanthrene
Oxycodone Sr	OxyContin	—	20	5–6.5	Phenanthrene
Tramadol	Ultram	100	120–150	5–7	Cyclohexanol

[a]Opioid compounded with acetaminophen.
CR, Controlled release; *IM*, intramuscular; *IV*, intravenous; *SR*, sustained release.

Table 16.2 Opioid Receptor Subtypes

OPIOID RECEPTOR SUBTYPE	AGONISTS	AGONIST RESPONSE
Mu-1 (μ-1)	Enkephalin Beta-endorphin Phenanthrenes Phenylpiperidines Methadone	Supraspinal analgesia Euphoria Miosis Urinary retention
Mu-2 (μ-2)	Enkephalin Beta-endorphin Phenanthrenes Phenylpiperidines Methadone	Spinal analgesia Respiratory depression Bradycardia Constipation Dependence
Kappa (κ)	Dynorphin Butorphanol Levorphanol Nalbuphine Oxycodone	Spinal analgesia (Kappa-1) Supraspinal analgesia (Kappa-2) Dysphoria Sedation
Delta (δ)	Enkephalin Deltorphin Sufentanil	Spinal analgesia (Delta-1) Supraspinal analgesia (Delta-2) Respiratory depression Urinary retention Dependence
Nociceptin/orphanin FQ (N/OFQ)	Nociceptin/OFQ	Spinal analgesia Supraspinal hyperalgesia

Modified from Stoelting RK, Miller RD. Basics of Anesthesia. 4th ed. New York: Churchill Livingstone; 2000:71; Al-Hashimi M, Scott WM, Thompson JP, et al. Opioids and immune modulation: more questions than answers. Br J Anaesth. 2013;111:80–88.

Table 16.3 Antiemetic Drugs and Their Chemical Receptors

CHEMICAL RECEPTOR	ABBREVIATION	PHARMACOLOGICAL ANTAGONIST
Dopamine	D_2	Haloperidol Droperidol Prochlorperazine Olanzapine Metoclopramide[a]
Histamine	H_1	Promethazine Diphenhydramine
Serotonin	$5\text{-}HT_3$	Ondansetron Dolasetron Palonosetron Granisetron
Acetylcholine	ACh	Scopolamine
Tachykinin	NK-1	Aprepitant
Cannabinoid	CB_1	Dronabinol

[a]Ineffective for prevention of postoperative nausea and vomiting at 10-mg dose.

11. **Describe the mechanism of opioid-induced nausea.**
Opioids bind directly to opioid receptors in the chemotactic trigger zone, in the area postrema of the medulla and stimulate the vomiting center. They exert a secondary effect by sensitizing the vestibular system. The incidence of nausea and vomiting is similar for all opioids and appears irrespective of the route of administration.

12. **What commonly used agents may counteract opioid-induced nausea and vomiting?**
Pharmacological agents, such as glucocorticoids, benzodiazepines, and propofol, are also antiemetic, but their mechanisms of action and functional receptors have not been identified (Table 16.3).

13. **What are the considerations when administering systemic opioids to a breastfeeding mother?**
All opioids are transferred to various degrees into human breast milk. Surprisingly, very few reports of opioid-induced toxicity in breastfeeding infants exist. Clinical toxicology recommendations include the following:
- Avoid opioids or doses that induce maternal sedation, as maternal CNS depression has a high correlation with infant CNS depression
- Infants less than 2-months-old represent the majority of case reports, and newborns in the first few weeks of life appear to be at highest risk for opioid-induced toxicity
- Codeine and tramadol are associated with an increased rate of complications and have an US Food and Drug Administration warning against their use in breastfeeding mothers
- Oxycodone is highly transferred and is associated with a 20% incidence of infant CNS depression
- Methadone is poorly transferred and appears safe to use in breastfeeding mothers
- Breast milk should be discarded (i.e., "pump and dump") in circumstances involving maternal CNS depression or vulnerable infants (e.g., preterm or afflicted by an underlying medical condition)

14. **What are peripheral-acting μ-opioid receptor antagonists?**
Peripheral-acting μ-opioid receptor antagonists (PAMORAs) are a diverse class of medications used to treat opioid-induced constipation by antagonizing peripheral opioid receptors, without significantly compromising central opioid receptor-mediated analgesia. Alvimopan, naloxegol, and naldemedine are oral medications with slightly different mechanisms of action, whereas methylnaltrexone can be administered subcutaneously.

15. **Describe the cardiovascular effects of opioids.**
As a group, opioids have minimal effects on the cardiovascular system. With the exception of meperidine, they cause dose-dependent bradycardia through vagal nucleus stimulation. Other than meperidine, opioids have minimal negative inotropic effect on the myocardium. Some opioids may induce histamine release and significantly reduce systemic vascular resistance (SVR), but most effect only a moderate reduction of SVR, even at anesthetic doses.

16. **Describe the typical respiratory pattern and ventilatory response to carbon dioxide in the presence of opioids.**
Opioids reduce alveolar ventilation in a dose-dependent manner. They slow the respiratory rate and may cause periodic breathing and/or apnea. Represented graphically, opioids shift the alveolar ventilatory response to carbon

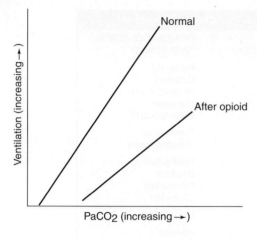

Fig. 16.1 Ventilatory response to arterial partial pressure of carbon dioxide ($PaCO_2$) in the presence of opioids.

dioxide curve down and to the right (Fig. 16.1). Accordingly, for a given arterial carbon dioxide level, the alveolar ventilation will be reduced in the presence of opioids. Furthermore, an increase in arterial carbon dioxide will not stimulate an appropriate increase in ventilation. Opioids also impair hypoxic ventilatory drive.

17. **How do opioids affect intracranial pressure?**
   During controlled ventilation, opioid infusions maintain or reduce intracranial pressure (ICP). Paradoxically, parenteral opioid boluses increase ICP. This effect is likely because of a transient reduction in mean arterial pressure and subsequent cerebral vasodilation to maintain cerebral blood flow. During spontaneous ventilation, opioids reduce minute ventilation, increase arterial carbon dioxide concentrations, and consequently, increase ICP.

18. **Describe the risk factors and management of opioid-induced chest wall rigidity.**
   Chest wall rigidity after opioid administration is described as pronounced skeletal rigidity and increased thoracic and abdominal muscle tone, often with concurrent glottic closure. It is most common with the phenylpiperidines (fentanyl, sufentanil, alfentanil, and remifentanil). Central μ-receptors and dopaminergic pathways appear to be involved at the level of the pons and basal ganglia. Risk factors include: large doses, rapid administration, extremes of age (e.g., newborns, infants, and elderly patients), critical illness, and medications that modify dopamine levels. Management includes assisted ventilation, reversal with naloxone, and/or the administration of neuromuscular blockade.

19. **Describe the analgesic onset, peak effect, and duration of intravenous fentanyl, morphine, and hydromorphone.**
   See Table 16.4.

20. **Explain how fentanyl can have a shorter duration of action but a longer elimination half-life than morphine.**
   Elimination half-lives correspond with duration of action in a single-compartment pharmacokinetic model. Lipophilic opioids, such as fentanyl, are better represented by a multicompartment model, as redistribution plays a much larger role than elimination in determining their duration of action.

21. **Explain the concept of context-sensitive half-time and its relevance to opioids.**
   Context-sensitive half-time is the time required for a 50% reduction in the plasma concentration of a drug after termination of a constant infusion. This time is determined by both elimination and redistribution, and it varies considerably as a function of infusion duration for commonly used opioids (Fig. 16.2).

Table 16.4 Commonly Used Intravenous Opioids			
OPIOID	**ONSET (min)**	**PEAK EFFECT (min)**	**DURATION (h)**
Fentanyl	1–3	3–5	0.5–1
Morphine	5–15	20–30	2–4
Hydromorphone	5–10	15–30	1–3

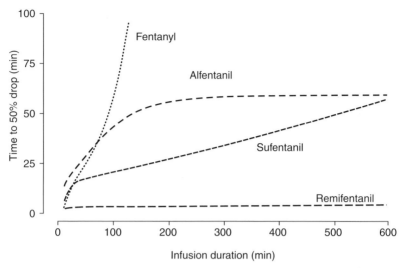

Fig. 16.2 Context-sensitive half-times of commonly used opioids, as a function of infusion duration. (Modified from Egan TD, Lemmens HJM, Fiset P, et al. The pharmacokinetics of the new short-acting opioid remifentanil (GI87084B) in healthy adult male volunteers. Anesthesiology. 1993;79:881.)

22. Explain why morphine may cause prolonged ventilatory depression in patients with renal failure.

    Some 5% to 10% of an administered morphine dose is excreted unchanged in the urine. The remainder is primarily conjugated in the liver as morphine-3-glucuronide (50%–75%) and morphine-6-glucuronide (10%), then renally excreted. Morphine-3-glucuronide is inactive, but morphine-6-glucuronide is approximately 100 times more potent than morphine as a μ-receptor agonist.

23. Which opioids may be associated with seizure activity in patients with renal failure?

    Hydromorphone and meperidine. Rarely, the metabolites hydromorphone-3-glucuronide and normeperidine can accumulate in renal failure and promote myoclonus and seizures.

24. What is remifentanil and how does it differ from other opioids?

    Remifentanil is an ultrashort-acting opioid with a duration of 5 to 10 minutes and a context-sensitive half-time of 3 minutes. It contains an ester moiety and is metabolized by nonspecific plasma esterases. Although remifentanil is most commonly administered as a continuous infusion, it can be used as an intravenous bolus to facilitate intubation. However, when bloused, it may occasionally induce bradycardia, chest-wall rigidity, and involuntary glottic closure. Remifentanil has been shown to induce hyperalgesia and acute opioid tolerance, and its use should be questioned in patients with chronic pain syndromes.

25. What is opioid-induced hyperalgesia?

    Opioid-induced hyperalgesia (OIH) is more than decreased analgesic efficacy. It is nociceptive sensitization resulting in decreased pain thresholds, increased pain intensity over time, and diffuse or spreading pain during or after opioid administration. It is most common following high doses of fentanyl, sufentanil, alfentanil, and remifentanil, and is mediated by N-methyl-D-aspartate (NMDA) and serotoninergic pathways. The use of regional anesthesia, the NMDA antagonist ketamine (>0.33 mg/kg), and gabapentinoids may reduce the incidence of OIH, following high doses of opioids.

26. Describe the metabolism of codeine.

    Codeine is metabolized by cytochrome P-450 2D6 (CYP2D6) and undergoes demethylation to morphine. Genetic polymorphisms in the *CYP2D6* gene lead to patient stratification into poor metabolizers, extensive metabolizers, and ultrafast metabolizers. Poor metabolizers may obtain only marginal analgesia from codeine, whereas ultrafast metabolizers may generate up to 50% higher plasma concentrations of morphine and morphine-6-glucuronide than extensive metabolizers. As a result, ultrafast metabolizers may be at significant risk of opioid intoxication and/or apnea with typical perioperative doses of codeine.

27. What are some particular concerns with methadone dosing?

    Because methadone has a particularly long and variable half-life, repeated dosing may lead to excessive plasma levels, particularly on days 2 through 4 after initiating therapy. It acts both as an agonist at μ-opioid receptors and as an antagonist at the NMDA receptor. The NMDA-receptor antagonism may potentiate the μ-receptor effects and prevent the development of opioid tolerance. Importantly, methadone may prolong the electrocardiographic QT interval and increase the risk of torsades de pointes. Expert panel recommendations include a baseline electrocardiogram (ECG) and follow-up ECG at 30 days and annually, while continuing methadone.

28. What is tramadol?
Tramadol is a codeine analog that acts as a μ-, δ-, and κ-receptor agonist and a reuptake inhibitor of norepinephrine and serotonin. It is a moderately effective analgesic with a lower incidence of respiratory depression, constipation, and dependence compared with other μ-receptor agonists. Rarely, tramadol may induce seizures, and is contraindicated in patients with a preexisting seizure disorder. It is also contraindicated for patients less than 12 years old and for analgesia, following adenotonsillectomy in patients less than 18 years old.

29. What are some of the unique characteristics of meperidine?
Unlike other opioids, meperidine has some weak local anesthetic properties, particularly when administered neuraxially. It does not cause bradycardia and may induce tachycardia, perhaps related to its structural homology to atropine. As a κ-receptor agonist, meperidine may be used to suppress postoperative shivering. Notably, meperidine is contraindicated for use in patients taking monoamine oxidase inhibitors, as the combination may lead to serotonin toxicity, hyperthermia, and even death.

30. Describe the site and mechanism of action of neuraxial opioids.
Neuraxial opioids bind to receptors in the Rexed lamina II (substantia gelatinosa) in the dorsal horn of the spinal cord. Activation of μ-receptors appears to reduce visceral and somatic pain via gamma-aminobutyric acid–mediated descending pain pathways. Activation of κ receptors appears to reduce visceral pain via inhibition of substance P. The effect of δ receptors is not entirely elucidated but appears minimal in some animal models.

31. Discuss the effect of lipid solubility on neuraxial opioid action.
Lipophilic opioids (such as fentanyl) diffuse across spinal membranes more rapidly than do hydrophilic opioids. As a result, lipophilic opioids have a more rapid onset of analgesia. However, they also diffuse across vascular membranes more readily, typically resulting in increased serum concentrations and a shorter duration of action. Hydrophilic opioids (such as morphine and hydromorphone) achieve greater cephalocaudal spread when administered into the epidural or subarachnoid space. They attain broader analgesic coverage than do lipophilic opioids but may result in delayed respiratory depression following cephalad spread to the brainstem.

32. Discuss the incidence and evolution of respiratory depression following neuraxial morphine administration.
The incidence of respiratory depression ranges from 0.01% to 7%, following intrathecal morphine and from 0.08% to 3%, following epidural morphine. The respiratory depression may be biphasic, with an early presentation at 30 to 90 minutes and a delayed presentation between 6 and 18 hours after neuraxial administration. The delayed respiratory depression is likely because of cephalad spread within the cerebrospinal fluid and direct brainstem penetration (specifically, inhibition of the neurokinin-1 receptors in the medullary pre-Bötzinger complex). As a result, the American Society of Anesthesiologists recommends monitoring respiratory rate, depth of respiration, oxygenation, and level of consciousness every hour for 12 hours, and then every 2 hours for the subsequent 12 hours, following a single injection of neuraxial morphine.

33. Describe the advantages of combining local anesthetics and opioids in neuraxial analgesia.
Despite their analgesic benefits, epidural local anesthetics have troublesome side effects, such as motor blockade and systemic hypotension. Epidural opioids can cause pruritus and nausea. When combined, opioids and local anesthetics function in a synergistic manner to optimize analgesia, while attenuating unwanted side effects.

34. Describe the controversial influence of opioids in immunomodulation and cancer recurrence.
Opioids inhibit cell-mediated and humoral immunity and the effects are generally agent specific. For example, morphine inhibits the toll-like receptor on macrophages, whereas fentanyl depresses natural killer cell activity. Codeine, methadone, morphine, remifentanil, and fentanyl are stronger modulators than hydromorphone, oxycodone, hydrocodone, buprenorphine, or tramadol. In cell lines and animal models, this immunomodulation results in increased tumor growth or metastasis and appears to be μ-opioid receptor mediated. Opioids also induce angiogenesis and stimulate vascular endothelial growth factor receptors.

KEY POINTS: OPIOIDS

1. Common opioid side effects include nausea, pruritus, bradycardia, urinary retention, and respiratory depression.
2. Morphine and meperidine should be used with caution in patients with renal failure because of the risk of prolonged ventilatory depression and seizures, respectively.
3. Neuraxial opioids and local anesthetics act synergistically to provide analgesia with reduced side effects.

4. Naloxone should be titrated in incremental doses for opioid-induced respiratory depression and may require repeated dosing for reversal of long-acting opioid agonists.
5. Opioids may be used with caution in breastfeeding mothers if maternal sedation is minimized and the exposure to infants less than 2 months old is limited.
6. Opioid equianalgesic conversions are approximations, and they do not account for incomplete opioid cross-tolerance.
7. Opioids inhibit cell-mediated and humoral immunity and may be implicated in cancer recurrence or metastasis.
8. High doses of lipophilic opioids (e.g., fentanyl, sufentanil, alfentanil, and remifentanil) may lead to opioid-induced hyperalgesia.

SUGGESTED READINGS

American Society of Anesthesiologists Task Force on Neuraxial Opioids. Practice guidelines for the prevention, detection and management of respiratory depression associated with neuraxial opioid administration. Anesthesiology. 2009;110:218–230.

Coda BA. Opioids. In: Barash PG, Cullen BF, Stoelting RK, eds. Clinical Anesthesia. 5th ed. Philadelphia: Lippincott Williams & Wilkins; 2006.

Çoruh B, Tonelli MR, Park DR. Fentanyl-induced chest wall rigidity. Chest. 2013;143:1145–1146.

Crawford MW, Hickey C, Zaarour C, et al. Development of acute opioid tolerance during infusion of remifentanil for pediatric scoliosis surgery. Anesth Analg. 2006;102:1662–1667.

Fukuda K. Intravenous opioid anesthetics. In: Miller RD, ed. Anesthesia. 6th ed. Philadelphia: Elsevier; 2006.

Gillman PK. Monoamine oxidase inhibitors, opioid analgesics and serotonin toxicity. Br J Anaesth. 2005;95:434–441.

Heaney A, Buggy DJ. Can anaesthetic and analgesic techniques affect cancer recurrence or metastasis? Br J Anaesth. 2012;109:i17–i28.

Hendrickson RG, McKeown NJ. Is maternal opioid use hazardous to breast-fed infants? Clin Toxicol. 2012;50:1–14.

Kirchheiner J, Schmidt H, Tzvetkov M, et al. Pharmacokinetics of codeine and its metabolite morphine in ultra-rapid metabolizers because of CYP2D6 duplication. Pharmacogenomics J. 2007;7:257–265.

Krantz MJ, Martin J, Stimmel B, et al. QTc interval screening in methadone treatment: the CSAT consensus guideline. Ann Intern Med. 2009;150(6):387–395.

Moss J, Rosow CE. Development of peripheral opioid antagonists: new insights into opioid effects. Mayo Clin Proc. 2008;83:1116–1130.

Reisine T, Pasternak G. Opioid analgesics and antagonists. In: Hardman JG, Limbird LE, eds. Goodman and Gilman's The Pharmacological Basis of Therapeutics. 9th ed. New York: McGraw-Hill; 1996.

Sachs HC, Committee on Drugs. The transfer of drugs and therapeutics into human breast milk: an update on selected topics. Pediatrics. 2013;132:e796–e809.

Smith HS. Peripherally-acting opioids. Pain Physician. 2008;11:S121–S132.

Veevaete L, Lavand'homme P. Opioid-induced hyperalgesia: new insights into the chronicization of pain. Techniques Reg Anesth Pain Manag. 2015;18:100–104.

Viscusi ER, Martin G, Hartrick CT, et al. Forty-eight hours of postoperative pain relief after total hip arthroplasty with a novel, extended-release epidural morphine formulation. Anesthesiology. 2005;103:1014–1022.

CHAPTER 17

NEUROMUSCULAR BLOCKING AGENTS

Brian M. Keech, MD

1. **Describe the morphology of the neuromuscular junction.**
   The neuromuscular junction (NMJ) consists of three cell types: the motor neuron, muscle fiber, and Schwann cell. The motor neuron originates in the ventral horn of the spinal cord or brainstem (in the case of the cranial nerves) and travels uninterrupted to the neuromuscular junction as a large myelinated axon. Upon approaching the muscle, it forms a spray of terminal branches that contact directly with the muscle fiber. Just proximal to the junction, the motor neuron loses its myelin and becomes covered in Schwann cells. The nerve and muscle are separated by a 20-nm gap called a *junctional* or *synaptic cleft*. The presynaptic nerve terminals contain acetylcholine (ACh) filled vesicles that are clustered along the junctional surface. The muscle fiber surface contains invaginations that are laden with nicotinic acetylcholine receptors (nAChR). The enzyme acetylcholinesterase is located within the synaptic cleft (Fig. 17.1).

2. **What is the structure of the nicotinic ACh receptor?**
   The nicotinic acetylcholine (nAChR) exists in two isoforms: mature and immature. The mature nicotinic nAChR consists of five glycoprotein subunits: two α_1 and one each of β_1, δ, and ε. The subunits are arranged in a cylindrical fashion, the center of the cylinder being a cation channel. The α_1 subunits of both isoforms are the binding sites for ACh. The immature nAChR (aka fetal or extrajunctional) differs slightly in structure (the ε subunit is exchanged for the γ subunit) and is a lower conductance cation channel with longer opening times.

3. **Review the steps involved in normal neuromuscular transmission.**
   Once initiated, an action potential is transmitted along the motor neuron, ultimately depolarizing the presynaptic nerve terminal. Depolarization opens voltage-gated calcium channels, leading to calcium influx, and triggers the migration and fusion of ACh containing vesicles with the active zone of the presynaptic nerve terminal. Upon fusing, ACh is released into the synaptic cleft. The amount of ACh released is large; approximately 200 to 400 vesicles are released, where each vesicle contains 5000 to 10,000 ACh molecules. However, this represents only a small amount relative to what is stored in the presynaptic nerve terminal. ACh molecules then traverse the cleft and bind to the α_1 subunits of the nAChR located on the postjunctional muscle membrane. Binding of one ACh molecule to each α_1 subunit for a given nAChR leads to a conformational change, opening the pore of the nAChR, which creates a channel allowing cations (notably sodium) to flow through, causing a minidepolarization known as an *end plate potential*. Note that an ACh receptor will not open unless both α_1 subunits are simultaneously occupied by an ACh molecule (forming the basis for competitive antagonism with nondepolarizing neuromuscular blocking agents). When several end-plate potentials (each associated with an individual nAChR) are combined, the voltage gradient becomes large enough to activate the perijunctional, voltage-gated, sodium channels. These perijunctional sodium channels are located immediately adjacent to the motor end plate of the postsynaptic nerve terminal and are responsible for propagating the depolarization throughout the muscle fiber. ACh molecules interact with the nAChR for only a short time and are released. Upon release, the receptor closes and the ACh molecule is rapidly hydrolyzed by the enzyme acetylcholinesterase.
   In summary, the nAChRs are chemically controlled, whereas the perijunctional sodium channels are voltage controlled. The nAChR is activated by ACh, which creates a mini voltage change, which activates sodium channels, which propagate the depolarization throughout the muscle fiber, causing muscle contraction.

4. **What are the functional differences between the two receptor isoforms?**
   Mature nAChRs are also known as *innervated* receptors. They are tightly clustered at the NMJ end plates and are responsible for normal neuromuscular activation. Immature receptors differ from their mature counterparts in that they are expressed primarily during fetal development and are suppressed by normal neuromuscular activity. Rather than being localized to the NMJ, these are dispersed throughout the muscular membrane and are prone to releasing larger amounts of potassium because of their longer opening times. Immature receptors are upregulated in the presence of certain pathological states (discussed later).

5. **With regards to neuromuscular transmission, list all locations for nACh receptors.**
   - Prejunctional: located on the presynaptic nerve terminal and is responsible for forming a positive feedback loop, which modulates the release of ACh into the NMJ
   - Postjunctional: located on the muscle fiber at the postsynapse and is responsible for facilitating muscle contraction

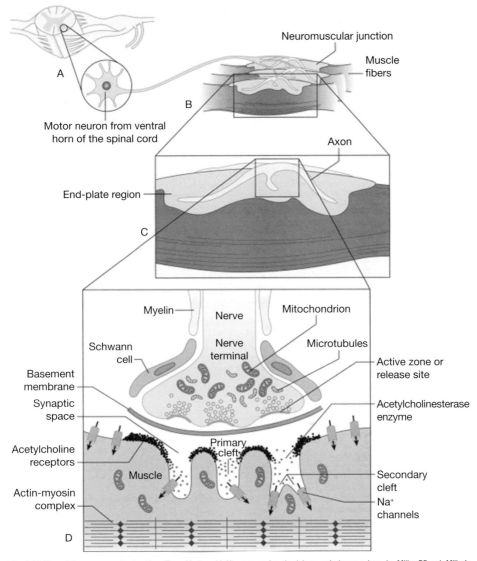

Fig. 17.1 The adult neuromuscular junction. (From Martyn, JJ. Neuromuscular physiology and pharmacology. In: Miller RD, ed: Miller's Anesthesia. 8th ed. Philadelphia: Elsevier Saunders; 2015:426.)

- Extrajunctional: the expression of these receptors is usually low provided the muscle is receiving normal neuromuscular activation. In certain pathological states, their expression will increase

6. How are neuromuscular blocking agents classified, and how do they work?
   - Depolarizing neuromuscular blocking agents (NMBAs) are nAChR agonists that binds to the α_1 subunits of the nAChR. This can be visualized as fasciculations or rapid, small, muscle twitches. Depolarizing NMBAs causes sustained depolarization of the motor end plate potential causing muscle paralysis because of: (1) desensitization of the nAChR, and (2) inactivation of voltage-gated sodium channels because of closure of the time-dependent sodium channel gate. Succinylcholine (SCh) is the only depolarizing NMBA available clinically. It consists of two molecules of ACh bound together
   - Nondepolarizing NMBAs are competitive nAChR antagonists. They need only bind to one of the two α_1 subunits to prevent normal opening of the nAChR cation channel. Nondepolarizing NMBAs can be classified either by

Table 17.1 Neuromuscular Blocking Agent Dosing (mg/kg)

AGENT	ED_{95}[a]	INTUBATING DOSE[b]	MAINTENANCE DOSE
Ultrashort-Acting			
Succinylcholine	0.3	1–1.5	—
Short-Acting			
Mivacurium	0.07	0.2–0.25	0.05–0.1
Intermediate-Acting			
Rocuronium	0.3	0.6–1.2	0.1–0.3
Vecuronium	0.04	0.1–0.2	0.02–0.05
Atracurium	0.2	0.5–0.6	0.1–0.3
Cisatracurium	0.04	0.15–0.2	0.02–0.05
Long-Acting			
Pancuronium	0.07	0.08–0.12	0.02–0.05

[a]Effective dose expected to reduce single-twitch height by 95%.
[b]Intubating dose is generally 2–3 times the ED_{95}.

Table 17.2 Neuromuscular Blocking Agent Onset and Duration (Minutes)

AGENT	ONSET AFTER INTUBATING DOSE	DURATION[a]
Ultrashort-Acting		
Succinylcholine	0.5–1	6–11
Short-Acting		
Mivacurium	2–3	15–20
Intermediate-Acting		
Rocuronium[b]	1–3	40–60
Vecuronium	2–3	40–60
Atracurium	1–3	40–60
Cisatracurium	2–3	40–60
Long-Acting		
Pancuronium	3–5	90

[a]Duration measured as return of twitch to 25% of control.
[b]Rocuronium, when administered in a dose of 1.2 mg/kg, has a similar onset to succinylcholine, although the duration is significantly longer.

duration of action (short-, intermediate-, and long-acting) or by their chemical structure: steroidal (vecuronium and rocuronium) and benzylisoquinolinium (atracurium and cisatracurium)

The dosing, onset, and duration of effect of NMBAs are described in Tables 17.1 and 17.2.

7. What are the indications for using NMBAs?

By interfering with normal neuromuscular transmission, NMBAs (also known as [aka] muscle relaxants) paralyze skeletal muscle, facilitate endotracheal intubation, and optimize surgical operating conditions. Occasionally, they are used to assist with mechanical ventilation in intubated patients (i.e., severe acute respiratory distress syndrome), to prevent elevations in intracranial pressure (ICP) that can be caused by "bucking" or agitation, and to facilitate hypothermia by minimizing shivering with targeted temperature management (formerly called *therapeutic hypothermia*) in comatose patients, following return of spontaneous circulation after cardiac arrest.

8. Should NMBAs always be given to facilitate endotracheal intubation?

The administration of NMBAs help facilitate intubation by paralyzing the vocal cords and muscles of the jaw and neck. Evidence has shown that administration of NMBA, on induction of anesthesia, improves the grade of view on laryngoscopy, reduces the incidence of hypoxemia on induction, and reduces complications associated with endotracheal intubation (i.e., vocal cord lesions, airway trauma, postoperative hoarseness). NMBA administration should strongly be considered in a "can't intubate, can't ventilate" situation if "waking the patient up" is not an option. However, if NMBAs are contraindicated or if the provider wishes to avoid NMBA administration, reasonable alternatives include the use of high-dose opioid on induction (i.e., remifentanil 4–5 mcg/kg, with propofol), which may also yield good to excellent intubating conditions. This combination (high-dose opioid with propofol) can also be useful in situations where rapid sequence induction and intubation are necessary, but NMBAs are contraindicated or need to be avoided. It is important to pretreat with an antimuscarinic (i.e., glycopyrrolate 0.2–0.4 mg intravenous [IV]) because high-dose opioids can cause significant bradycardia.

9. **What are the indications for using succinylcholine?**
   SCh has the fastest onset of all NMBAs (30–60 seconds), with a short duration of action (5–10 minutes). SCh is often used for short operations, patients who will likely desaturate rapidly with apnea (e.g., morbid obesity), and in patients who are at risk for pulmonary aspiration of gastric contents (i.e., rapid sequence induction and intubation). It is important to note, that rocuronium, a nondepolarizing NMBA, given in high doses (1.2 mg/kg aka "double dose"), coupled with sugammadex for reversal, can achieve a similar result to SCh.

10. **Describe risk factors for pulmonary aspiration where administering succinylcholine (or "double dose" rocuronium) would be indicated.**
    Risk factors for pulmonary aspiration of gastric contents include pregnancy, hiatal hernia, diabetes mellitus, opioid abuse or dependence, severe gastroesophageal reflux disease, bowel obstruction, ascites, inadequate fasting, nausea and/or vomiting, and states associated with increased sympathetic tone causing delayed gastric emptying (i.e., trauma, severe pain).

11. **List the side effects of succinylcholine and explain their clinical relevance.**
    - Bradycardia: SCh not only binds to nAChRs within the NMJ, but also binds to cholinergic receptors located elsewhere, namely, the autonomic nervous system. Stimulation of muscarinic cholinergic receptors in the sinus node can result in numerous bradyarrhythmias, including sinus bradycardia, junctional and ventricular escape rhythms, and even asystole. These responses are more common after repeat dosing, particularly when coupled with the intense autonomic stimulation of tracheal intubation or in patients with high vagal tone (i.e., pediatric patients). Prior administration of atropine may help attenuate this response
    - Increases serum potassium: SCh normally increases the potassium level by approximately 0.5 mEq/L, as a result of muscle cell depolarization. However, certain patient populations may have an exaggerated response
    - Increases intraocular pressure (IOP): SCh mildly increases IOP, leading to the theoretical risk of extrusion of intraocular contents in the setting of penetrating eye injury
    - Increases intragastric pressure (IGP): SCh increases IGP presumably from fasciculation of the abdominal skeletal musculature
    - Increases ICP: SCh increases ICP and the mechanism and clinical significance of this is not completely understood
    - Malignant hyperthermia (MH): SCh is a known trigger for MH
    - Myalgia: Skeletal muscle fasciculations caused by SCh have been associated with painful postoperative myalgias. The risks and benefits in administering a nondepolarizing NMBA before administering SCh (aka a defasciculating dose) to prevent myalgia continues to be a matter of debate

12. **Describe the concerns with succinylcholine and hyperkalemia.**
    SCh should carefully be administered, and a recent potassium checked, before administration in pathological conditions associated with hyperkalemia, such as metabolic acidosis (e.g., septic shock) or end-stage renal disease (ESRD). In addition, certain pathological conditions are associated with increased upregulation and expression of immature nAChRs, which can cause an exaggerated hyperkalemic response to SCh, leading to hyperkalemic cardiac arrest. This includes patients with severe burns, various neurological diseases (e.g., stroke, spinal cord injury, multiple sclerosis, Guillan-Barré syndrome) or any other conditions associated with prolonged immobility (e.g., immobile patients in the intensive care unit [ICU]). Upregulation of nAChRs is associated with increased sensitivity to depolarizing NMBAs and resistance to nondepolarizing NMBAs. Of note, patients with ESRD are no more susceptible to an exaggerated hyperkalemic response than those with normal renal function.

13. **Describe the concerns with succinylcholine and masseter muscle spasm.**
    Increased tone in the masseter muscle may be observed in both adults and children after administering SCh. Although this finding may be an early indicator of MH, it is not consistently associated with this syndrome, and no indication exists in changing to a "nontriggering" anesthetic (i.e., avoiding inhaled volatile anesthetic agents) for isolated masseter spasm.

14. **How is succinylcholine metabolized?**
    Unlike ACh, SCh is not hydrolyzed in the synaptic cleft by acetylcholinesterase. For inactivation to occur, SCh must diffuse away from the synaptic cleft to be metabolized in the plasma by pseudocholinesterase (aka butyrylcholinesterase or plasma cholinesterase).

15. **What is pseudocholinesterase deficiency?**
    Pseudocholinesterase is produced in the liver and circulates in the plasma. In patients with normal pseudocholinesterase, 90% recovery of muscle strength, following SCh administration (1 mg/kg), occurs in approximately 9 to 13 minutes. *Quantitative* deficiencies of pseudocholinesterase are observed in severe liver disease,

pregnancy, advanced age, malnutrition, cancer, and in burn patients. In addition, certain medications, such as oral contraceptives, monoamine oxidase inhibitors, cytotoxic drugs, cholinesterase inhibitors, and metoclopramide also interfere with pseudocholinesterase activity. However, from a practical standpoint, the increase in duration of SCh for each of these is probably not clinically significant because of the large enzymatic capacity of normal pseudocholinesterase to metabolize SCh. *Qualitative* deficiencies in pseudocholinesterase occur when a patient possesses an abnormal genetic variant of the enzyme, most commonly known as *dibucaine-resistant cholinesterase deficiency*. Typically, when dibucaine is added to the serum, normal pseudocholinesterase activity will be inhibited by 80%, whereas the genetic variant will be inhibited by only 20%. Therefore a patient with normal pseudocholinesterase is assigned a dibucaine number of 80, and a patient who is homozygous for the genetic variant will have a dibucaine number of 20 to 30. Patients with a dibucaine number of 50 to 60 are heterozygous for the atypical variant. Clinically, the lower the dibucaine number, the longer the SCh blockade will last. Patients with dibucaine number of 50 to 60 will have a moderately prolonged blockade (15–20 minutes), whereas a dibucaine number of 20 to 30 will have a much longer blockade (4–8 hours).

16. **Review the metabolism of nondepolarizing NMBAs.**
    - Steroidal agents (e.g., vecuronium, rocuronium, and pancuronium) undergo both hepatic and renal elimination to various degrees. Vecuronium and rocuronium primarily undergo hepatic elimination ($\sim$75%) and, by a much lesser extent, renal elimination ($\sim$25%). The half-life of these agents may be significantly prolonged in the presence of end-stage liver disease. Pancuronium, however, primarily undergoes renal excretion ($\sim$75%) and, by a much lesser extent, hepatic metabolism and elimination ($\sim$25%). Pancuronium should be avoided in patients with ESRD
    - Benzylisoquinolinium agents (e.g., atracurium, cisatracurium) are unique in that they undergo both ester hydrolysis and spontaneous breakdown at physiological pH and temperature (known as *Hoffmann elimination*). These agents should be strongly considered in patients with compromised hepatic and renal function

17. **Describe the side effects of nondepolarizing NMBAs.**
    Anaphylactoid reactions (i.e., nonimmunoglobulin [Ig]E histamine release) is most significant with atracurium, whereas anaphylactic reactions (i.e., IgE-mediated histamine release) with rocuronium. Cisatracurium is not associated with significant histamine release. Tachycardia is a common side effect of pancuronium because of its vagolytic properties.

18. **Review drug interactions and/or clinical conditions which may potentiate or prolong the duration of NMBAs.**
    - Volatile anesthetics: Mechanism unclear
    - Antibiotics: Specifically, aminoglycosides, tetracyclines, and clindamycin. Note, penicillin and cephalosporins do not affect the duration of NMBA activity
    - Hypocalcemia and hypermagnesemia: Calcium plays an important role in facilitating the release of ACh vesicles from the presynaptic neuron and in muscle contraction itself. Recall that magnesium has a valence of 2^+ and can be considered a physiological calcium channel blocker. Hypermagnesemia may be seen in the obstetric patient population, as magnesium is often used to treat patients with preeclampsia or eclampsia
    - Lithium: Although the mechanism is unclear, it is postulated that it may be caused by its chemical resemblance with other cations (i.e., sodium, magnesium, and calcium)
    - Local anesthetics: Depresses action potential propagation throughout the motor neuron and release of ACh at the NMJ
    - Hypothermia: Decreased metabolism of NMBAs
    - Dantrolene: A medication used for the treatment of malignant hyperthermia, which prevents calcium release from the sarcoplasmic reticulum and depresses skeletal muscle activity.

19. **Which muscles are innervated by the facial and ulnar nerves? Why is this clinically relevant?**
    The orbicularis oculi and the adductor pollicis muscles are innervated by the facial and ulnar nerves, respectively. The facial and ulnar nerves are the most common nerves used clinically for electrical delivery of stimuli with nerve stimulators. Following a delivered impulse by the nerve stimulator, the clinician will assess the response at these muscles to assess the depth of neuromuscular blockade.

20. **Do all muscle groups respond equally to neuromuscular blockade?**
    No. Muscle groups will have different responses to NMBAs, which is likely a function of blood flow. In general, muscles in the central compartments have a shorter onset and offset time compared with peripheral muscles. Muscles characterized with a shorter offset time (i.e., recover from paralysis quicker) are said to be more resistant to neuromuscular blocking agents. The order of most resistant to least is the following: diaphragm > orbicularis oculi (monitored by facial nerve) > adductor pollicis (monitored by ulnar nerve).
    Note that pharyngeal muscles, which are responsible for keeping the airway patent (preventing airway obstruction) and coordinating swallowing (preventing aspiration), correlate best with the adductor pollicis.

21. **Review the clinical signs associated with recovery from neuromuscular blockade.**
    Clinical evaluation for recovery from neuromuscular blockade include the following: 5-second head lift, tongue protrusion, and adequate size of tidal volumes. Clinical evaluation is often performed after the reversal agent is given to

Table 17.3 Clinical Tests for Return of Neuromuscular Function

TEST	RESULTS	% RECEPTORS OCCUPIED
Tidal volume	>5 mL/kg	80
Single twitch	Return to baseline	75–80
Vital capacity	>20 mL/kg	70
Inspiratory force	<−40 cm H_2O	50
Head lift	Sustained 5 seconds	50
Hand grip	Return to baseline	50

ensure the patient is safe for extubation. Patients who have residual neuromuscular blockade may also show signs of generalized weakness resembling a "fish out of water" appearance. Unfortunately, the sensitivity of our clinical assessments in detecting residual neuromuscular blockade is poor (Table 17.3).

22. **How can the depth of neuromuscular blockade be assessed more objectively than by clinical examination?**
    Nerve stimulators are often used to assess the depth of neuromuscular blockade by electrically stimulating nerves using various frequencies and waveform patterns. The most commonly used waveforms are the following: train of four (TOF) at 2 Hz (2 stimulations per second) and tetanic stimulation at 50 or 100 Hz (50 or 100 stimulations per second).

    Although any superficial motor nerve can be used for assessment of neuromuscular blockade, the most common sites are the ulnar and facial nerves. The degree of neuromuscular blockage can be assessed by counting the number of twitches with TOF. For most surgical operations, only one or two twitches is necessary to facilitate surgery. Before emergence of anesthesia, recovery from neuromuscular blockade should be assessed by measuring the degree of fade with TOF.

23. **What are the different modes available with nerve stimulators? Which one is used most often?**
    The modes that are available include the following: single-twitch, TOF, tetanic stimulation, posttetanic count (PTC), double-burst stimulation. The most often used stimulation mode is TOF.

24. **Describe train-of-four stimulation.**
    TOF stimulation delivers four successive electric stimuli at a frequency of 2 Hz (2 stimuli per second). The depth of neuromuscular blockade is assessed by counting the number of twitches observed and, if all four twitches are present, the amplitude ratio of the fourth to the first twitch (T4:T1 ratio). The four twitches of the TOF disappear in reverse order as the degree of blockade deepens (called fade); the fourth disappears when 75% to 80% of receptors are occupied, the third at 85% occupancy, the second at 85% to 90% occupancy, and the first at 90% to 95% occupancy. In general, only one or two twitches are needed to provide adequate surgical operating conditions. Patients are considered recovered from neuromuscular blockade when there is no "fade" by qualitative assessment or when the T4:T1 ratio is greater than 0.9 by quantitative assessment.

    There is accumulating evidence that qualitative assessment of TOF (visual or tactile evaluation of fade) is inferior for evaluating neuromuscular blockade compared with quantitative assessment. Studies show that even with experienced practitioners, qualitative TOF twitch estimations correlate poorly with quantitative TOF fade. Quantitative assessment can be measured using various technologies, such as acceleromyography, strain-gauge monitoring, and electromyography.

25. **Describe tetanic and posttetanic count stimulation.**
    - Tetanic stimulation consists of continuous, high-frequency (50 or 100 Hz), electric stimulation causing sustained muscle contraction. Loss of contraction during sustained tetanic stimulation over 5 seconds is called *tetanic fade* and is a sensitive but not specific indicator of residual neuromuscular blockade. An important drawback in assessing for sustained tetany is that it decreases the validity of any subsequent nerve stimulation at that site, rendering it unhelpful for further assessment of recovery from neuromuscular blockade for approximately 5 minutes
    - PTC consists of tetanic stimulation followed by applying a series of 1 Hz single-twitch stimuli and counting the number of twitches. The number of twitches observed is inversely related to the depth of neuromuscular blockade (similar to a TOF). This mode of stimulation is useful during periods of intense neuromuscular blockade (when there are zero twitches with TOF stimulation) and extends our range of monitoring. It provides an indication as to when recovery of a single twitch is anticipated and thus when reversal of neuromuscular blockade is possible (with a cholinesterase inhibitor), or how much to give (with sugammadex). As with tetanic stimulation, this technique should not be performed more often than every 5 minutes.

26. **What is acceleromyography?**

Acceleromyography is one of the most common methods used for quantitative neuromuscular monitoring. It uses a piezoelectrode accelerometer (small sensor) that is strapped to the thumb and two electrodes (positive and ground) placed over the ulnar nerve. The principle behind acceleromyography is based on Newton's second law of motion, $F = ma$. Because the mass, **m**, of the thumb is constant, the muscular force generated, F, is directly proportional to the measured acceleration, a, of the thumb. The device then calculates the measured acceleration of the fourth twitch to the first twitch to calculate the T4:T1 ratio which quantifies the degree of fade.

27. **What are the problems associated with residual paralysis?**

Studies report that up to 50% of patients arrive to the postanesthesia care unit (PACU) with evidence of residual neuromuscular blockade (T4:T1 < 90%). Residual paralysis is a risk factor for several postoperative complications, including hypercapnia, hypoxemia, upper airway obstruction, aspiration, reintubation, unpleasant symptoms of weakness, prolonged PACU length of stay, and possibly even increased mortality.

28. **Why should quantitative nerve monitoring be used to assess for adequate recovery before extubation?**

Studies show that the sensitivity of clinical evaluation of muscle weakness, such as 5-second head lift, tongue protrusion, and size of tidal volume, is poor in detecting residual paralysis. Qualitative assessment using TOF or sustained tetany, while perhaps better than clinical criteria, is also poor. For example, studies show that subjective assessment of fade either by TOF or sustained tetany cannot be detected when the quantitative T4:T1 ratio is greater than 0.3 to 0.4. Therefore the use of quantitative twitch monitoring, to objectively measure that the T4:T1 is greater than 0.9, is strongly encouraged to assess adequacy of reversal before extubation.

29. **What is a phase I and phase II block?**

- A phase I block is seen with depolarizing NMBAs (SCh). The single-twitch, TOF, and tetanus amplitudes are all uniformly decreased (T4:T1 = 1). There will be no fade in response to TOF or tetanus and there will be no posttetanic facilitation (Fig. 17.2).
- A phase II block is seen with nondepolarizing NMBAs. This twitch pattern is characterized as a "fade" where the amplitude for each successive twitch decreases in amplitude (T4:T1 < 1). A fade will also be present during tetanic stimulation. However, after tetanic stimulation, subsequent responses to TOF will be increased (called *posttetanic facilitation*; Fig. 17.3).

30. **Can a phase II block occur with depolarizing NMBAs?**

Patients who are given large or repeated doses of SCh may develop a phase II block. Note, this may also be seen in patients with pseudocholinesterase deficiency despite appropriate doses of SCh. Although theoretically a phase II block caused by SCh can be reversed, it is recommended to not attempt this, as the response to cholinesterase inhibitors can be unpredictable in this situation.

31. **Review the commonly used acetylcholinesterase inhibitor reversal agents.**

Acetylcholinesterase inhibitors prevent the breakdown of ACh at the NMJ, thereby increasing the amount of ACh available to promote muscle activation. Neostigmine (0.03–0.07 mg/kg) is the most commonly used agent and has a peak effect of 15 to 20 minutes, following administration. It does not cross the blood brain barrier; however, it does cross the placenta. Therefore patients who are pregnant should be given atropine, because glycopyrrolate does not cross the placenta. Physostigmine (0.03–0.04 mg/kg) is another acetylcholinesterase inhibitor that is unique in that does cross the brain barrier, which can be used to treat central anticholinergic syndrome (more common in the ICU).

DEPOLARIZING BLOCKADE

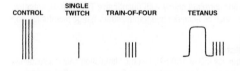

CONTROL SINGLE TWITCH TRAIN-OF-FOUR TETANUS

Fig. 17.2 Response to depolarizing neuromuscular blocking agents. (From Bevan DR, Bevan JC, Donati F. Muscle Relaxants in Clinical Anesthesia. Chicago: Year Book; 1988:49–70.)

NONDEPOLARIZING BLOCKADE

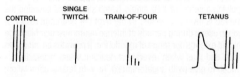

CONTROL SINGLE TWITCH TRAIN-OF-FOUR TETANUS

Fig. 17.3 Response to nondepolarizing neuromuscular blocking agents. (From Bevan DR, Bevan JC, Donati F. Muscle Relaxants in Clinical Anesthesia. Chicago: Year Book; 1988:49–70.)

32. **What are the important side effects of acetylcholinesterase inhibitors?**
Using an acetylcholinesterase inhibitor to increase the amount of ACh at the NMJ (a nicotinic receptor) will also increase the amount of ACh present at muscarinic cholinergic receptors located elsewhere. The main concern is the effect on cardiac conduction. Unopposed muscarinic effects of ACh impair sinus node conduction, resulting in sinus bradycardia, junctional rhythms, and even asystole. To curtail these effects, cholinesterase inhibitors are often administered in concert with an anticholinergic medication. Most often, glycopyrrolate is coadministered with neostigmine, but atropine could also be used if clinically indicated.

33. **Discuss the appropriate time for reversal of neuromuscular blockade with acetylcholinesterase inhibitors, based on nerve stimulation.**
The best method to ensure termination of depolarizing NMBAs are to dose them sparingly and to allow enough time for normal metabolism to occur. Recall that only one α_1 subunit of the postjunctional nAChR needs to be occupied by a depolarizing NMBA to inhibit its function, whereas two molecules of ACh are necessary to stimulate the receptor. Thus receptor dynamics favor NMBAs.
   The most important variable in determining the effectiveness of a reversal agent is the depth of blockade at the time of reversal administration. Reversal agents should only be administered when there are at least two twitches with TOF (ideally performed at the ulnar not facial nerve). Also keep in mind that any recent tetanic stimuli will result in overestimating the TOF. Neostigmine should be administered at least 15 minutes, with at least two twitches present, before anticipated removal of the endotracheal tube to reliably attain a T4:T1 ratio greater than 0.9 at extubation.

34. **Why not just administer cholinesterase inhibitors at a higher dose when the patient exhibits a deep level of blockade (i.e., TOF <2)?**
Cholinesterase inhibitors prevent the breakdown of ACh in the NMJ, which facilitates binding of ACh to the nAChR (recall nondepolarizing NMBAs are competitive nAChR antagonist). However, there is a clinically relevant ceiling effect for ACh that can be achieved at the NMJ with these medications. Once the acetylcholinesterase enzyme is maximally inhibited, a peak concentration of ACh is attained, and any further administration of cholinesterase inhibitors will not increase ACh levels or enhance recovery of neuromuscular blockade. In fact, giving more cholinesterase inhibitor medications at this point may even prolong recovery. For these reasons, reversal of a nondepolarizing NMBA before the TOF contains two twitches is not recommended when using cholinesterase inhibitor medications, such as neostigmine.

35. **What would happen if a patient were to receive succinylcholine after receiving neostigmine?**
Neostigmine inhibits true acetylcholinesterase (located within the NMJ), as well as pseudocholinesterase (located in the plasma). If SCh were administered after reversing a nondepolarizing NMBA with a neostigmine (which may occur as SCh is a treatment for refractory laryngospasm, which can occur after extubation), the effect of the SCh would be significantly prolonged, usually in the range of 10 to 30 minutes.

36. **Review the properties of sugammadex.**
Approved by the US Food and Drug Administration in 2015, sugammadex is a modified cyclodextrin that forms extremely tight water-soluble complexes with steroidal NMBAs (principally rocuronium but also vecuronium). Binding of the NMBA to sugammadex creates a concentration gradient away from the NMJ and subsequent renal excretion of the complex ensues. Note that the efficacy of sugammadex does not depend on renal excretion of the cyclodextrin-relaxant complex. Although cholinesterase inhibitor medications are unable to reverse deeper levels of neuromuscular blockade because of their ceiling effect (discussed previously), sugammadex is effective in reversing moderate and profound levels of blockade. Sugammadex, unlike neostigmine, can therefore be used even if there are zero twitches with TOF stimulation. The recovery to a T4:T1 ratio >0.9 is markedly faster with sugammadex (<1–2 minutes) versus neostigmine (15–20 minutes). Sugammadex has no effect on acetylcholinesterase and does not produce any direct muscarinic side effects. Although sugammadex can bind and sequester steroidal neuromuscular blocking agents, it can also bind to other steroidal agents, such as hormonal birth control medications. Patients taking oral contracepted medications should be advised that sugammadex will make hormonal birth control less effective for several days after its administration.

37. **How is sugammadex dosed?**
Sugammadex is administered at 4 mg/kg as a single dose for reversal of deep blockade (no twitches with TOF and PTC ≥1) and at 2 mg/kg for moderate blockade (TOF ≥2 twitches). Immediate reversal of rocuronium given for rapid sequence induction (i.e., "double dose" rocuronium) can be achieved with 16 mg/kg. Dosing does not need to be adjusted in the presence of renal or hepatic impairment. Sugammadex is not useful for the reversal of benzylisoquinolinium relaxants.

38. **How has sugammadex altered anesthetic practice?**
The role of SCh in facilitating laryngoscopy and intubation has been discussed; unfortunately, this medication has numerous side effects and limitations. Pharmacological innovation in the development of muscle relaxants per se has not yet resulted in a NMBA with a rapid onset, short duration of action, and freedom from worrisome side effects. However, sugammadex provides a useful alternative to SCh, allowing clinicians to administer rocuronium in rapid

sequence intubation (RSI) doses ($\approx$1.2 mg/kg) with an avenue for pharmacological antagonism soon thereafter. In fact, the use of sugammadex after rocuronium provides a fast onset and offset profile similar to SCh (1 mg/kg) for RSI. In addition, it eliminates the need to administer cholinesterase inhibitor medications, thereby reducing unwanted side effects of bradycardia and nausea. Finally, it can be used in patients with residual paralysis who have already received neostigmine.

39. **Should all patients who receive a nondepolarizing NMBA be reversed?**
   Residual neuromuscular blockade, resulting in clinically significant weakness in PACU, occurs frequently (20%–50% of the time). This includes patients who have received only one dose of a nondepolarizing NMBA, generally given on induction of anesthesia, to facilitate laryngoscopy and intubation. Therefore routine reversal of all patients who have received a nondepolarizing NMBA is a prudent practice. Part of the problem of unrecognized residual weakness is likely subjective misinterpretation of the TOF ratio, arguing for more widespread use of quantitative neuromuscular monitoring.

40. **A patient appears weak (i.e., fish out of water) after pharmacological reversal of neuromuscular blockade. What factors should be considered?**
   - Were the proper drugs and dosages administered?
   - Has enough time elapsed to observe peak reversal effect?
   - Was the depth of neuromuscular blockade so intense that reversal was not possible?
   - Did the patient receive SCh before a nondepolarizing NMBA? If so, is it possible they have pseudocholinesterase deficiency?
   - Is your twitch monitor functioning, and are the leads well placed?
   - Are body temperature, acid-base status, and electrolyte status normal?
   - Is the patient receiving any other medications that might potentiate neuromuscular blocking agents?
   - What is the patient's renal and hepatic function?
   - Importantly, if the patient remains weak, do not extubate

---

KEY POINTS: NEUROMUSCULAR BLOCKING AGENTS

1. Depolarizing NMBAs include SCh and nondepolarizing NMBAs include steroidal agents (vecuronium and rocuronium) and benzylisoquinolinium agents (atracurium and cisatracurium).
2. A phase I block is seen with depolarizing NMBAs and a *phase II block* with nondepolarizing NMBAs.
3. Each muscle will have a different onset and offset response to paralytics presumably as a function of blood flow. Onset and offset time (aka resistance) to paralytics is in the following order: diaphragm > orbicularis oculi > adductor pollicis.
4. Rapid sequence induction can be realized with succinylcholine, rocuronium, and high dose opioid (i.e., remifentanil).
5. The best methods to ensure termination of nondepolarizing NMBAs are to dose them sparingly and to allow enough time for normal metabolism to occur.
6. Qualitative nerve monitoring (TOF fade and sustained tetany assessment) is subjective and has been repeatedly demonstrated to underestimate residual neuromuscular blockade.
7. Quantitative nerve monitoring to assess neuromuscular blockade (by measuring the T4:T1 ratio) is strongly encouraged.
8. Neostigmine should be administered at least 15 minutes, with at least 2 twitches present, before anticipated removal of the endotracheal tube to reliably attain a T4:T1 > 0.9 at extubation.
9. It is best practice to administer reversal agents to all patients receiving nondepolarizing NMBAs, unless there is documented evidence that the T4:T1 > 0.9.
10. Leave clinically weak patients intubated and support respirations, until the patient can demonstrate return of strength.

SUGGESTED READINGS

Brull SJ, Kopman AF. Current status of neuromuscular reversal and monitoring: challenges and opportunities. Anesthesiology. 2017; 126(1):173–190.

Hristovska AM, Duch P, Allingstrup M, Afshari A. Efficacy and safety of sugammadex versus neostigmine in reversing neuromuscular blockade in adults. Cochrane Database Syst Rev. 2017;8:CD012763.

Martyn JJ. Neuromuscular physiology and pharmacology. In: Miller RD, ed: Miller's Anesthesia. 8th ed. Philadelphia: Elsevier Saunders; 2015:423–443.

Sørensen MK, Bretlau C, Gätke MR, et al. Rapid sequence induction and intubation with rocuronium-sugammadex compared with succinylcholine: a randomized trial. Br J Anaesth. 2012;108:682.

Szakmany T, Woodhouse T. Use of cisatracurium in critical care: a review of the literature. Minerva Anestesiol. 2015;81:450.

CHAPTER 18

LOCAL ANESTHETICS

David Abts, MD, Brian M. Keech, MD

1. **Discuss the role of local anesthetics in the practice of anesthesiology.**
   Because local anesthetics (LAs) reversibly block nerve conduction, they are used to provide intra- and postoperative regional anesthesia for painful surgical procedures. Beyond regional anesthesia, local anesthetics (most notably lidocaine) can be administered intravenously to attenuate the pressor response to tracheal intubation, decrease coughing during intubation and extubation, and act as systemic analgesics. Lidocaine is also antiarrhythmic.

2. **How are local anesthetics classified?**
   All LAs contain a lipophilic benzene ring linked to an amine group by a hydrocarbon chain of either amide or ester linkage.
   - **Esters:** commonly used ester LAs include procaine, chloroprocaine, benzocaine, tetracaine, and cocaine (Fig. 18.1).
   - **Amides:** commonly used amide LAs include lidocaine, prilocaine, mepivacaine, bupivacaine, levobupivacaine, and ropivacaine. All amide LAs contain the letter "I" in their stem.

3. **Discuss the commonly used local anesthetics. What are their practical applications?**
   - Lidocaine: ubiquitous in its use; short-acting amide LA that is good for topical, subcutaneous, intravenous (IV), regional, and neuraxial anesthesia.
   - Bupivacaine: long-acting amide LA that provides high quality sensory anesthesia with relative motor sparing.
   - Ropivacaine: an amide local anesthetic that is structurally and behaviorally similar to bupivacaine. Like bupivacaine, it is highly protein bound and has a long duration of action. Compared with bupivacaine, it is less cardiotoxic (because of its vasoconstrictive effects) and produces less motor block, thus allowing analgesia with less motor compromise (differential blockade).
   - Chloroprocaine: an ester LA that is useful in obstetrics because of its rapid onset, low risk of systemic toxicity, and/or fetal exposure (rapidly hydrolyzed in blood). Also useful in patients with significant liver disease.
   - Liposomal bupivacaine (Exparel): liposomal suspension promotes extended release (duration up to 72 hours). Used for local infiltration into surgical site rather than for regional anesthesia. Of note, nonbupivacaine LAs can cause immediate release of bupivacaine if coadministered. Avoiding bupivacaine use within 96 hours of infiltration recommended.
   - Cocaine: unique among LAs because of its vasoconstrictive properties. Used as a topical anesthetic, most commonly for sinus surgery and awake fiberoptic intubations. Side effects include hypertension, tachycardia, arrhythmias, coronary ischemia, cardiovascular accident, and pulmonary edema.
   - Mepivacaine: an intermediate duration of action amide LA (longer acting then lidocaine, shorter than ropivacaine or bupivacaine).
   - Benzocaine: use largely limited to orotracheal administration because of its near insolubility in water.
   - EMLA cream (eutectic mixture of local anesthetics): used for topical anesthesia, most commonly for pediatric IV placement. Consists of 2.5% lidocaine and 2.5% prilocaine. Takes 30 to 45 minutes to work. Avoid in glucose-6-phosphate dehydrogenase deficiency.

4. **What is the mechanism of action of local anesthetics?**
   Local anesthetics are hydrophilic tertiary amines with weak basic properties that exist in chemical equilibrium between a charged protonated form and an uncharged neutral basic form. The pK_a of the specific LA determines the relative amounts of each form at a given pH (the lower the pK_a, the more LA molecule exist in uncharged form because they are all weak bases). LAs work by diffusing across nerve cell membranes (while in the uncharged form). Once in the axoplasm, they become protonated (because intracellular pH is <7) and bind to the Na^+ Sodium channel from the inside, thereby blocking subsequent membrane depolarization (Fig. 18.2). Conduction blockade in myelinated nerves will ensue if the sodium channels of three or more consecutive nodes of Ranvier are blocked.

5. **How are they metabolized?**
   Ester LA undergo hydrolysis by pseudocholinesterases, found principally in plasma. Amide LA undergo enzymatic biotransformation primarily in the liver. The lungs may also extract lidocaine, bupivacaine, and prilocaine from the circulation. Chloroprocaine is least likely to result in sustained levels in plasma because of its rapid hydrolysis (most rapid among ester class).
   Risk of toxicity to ester LA is increased in patients with pseudocholinesterase deficiency. Liver disease or decreased liver blood flow, as may occur in patients with congestive heart failure and during general anesthesia, can

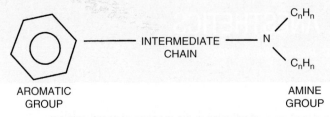

Fig. 18.1 Structure of ester and amide local anesthetics.

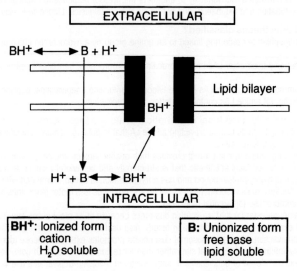

Fig. 18.2 Mechanism of action of local anesthetics.

reduce the metabolism of amide LA as well. Caution should be exercised in all patients at extremes of age, or with low muscle mass, as these conditions can also lead to increases in plasma LA concentration.

6. **What determines their potency?**
   LA potency is determined by lipid solubility. The higher the lipid solubility, the greater the potency (Table 18.1).

7. **What determines local anesthetic onset time?**
   Onset time is largely determined by degree of ionization, which is reflected by an LA pK_a. The lower the pK_a, the greater the number of LA molecules that will be present in the nonionized form, thus facilitating membrane penetration and hastening onset. pK_a is defined as the pH at which the ionized and unionized chemical forms exist in equal concentrations. Because all LAs are weak bases, those with pK_a near physiological pH ($\sim$7.4) will have more molecules in the unionized, lipid-soluble form than in ionized, lipid insoluble form. As mentioned, the unionized form must cross the axonal membrane to initiate neural blockade. Local anesthetic onset time can also be hastened by using a higher concentration, greater total dose, and by adding sodium bicarbonate to the LA solution to increase the number of unionized molecules present. Of note, higher lipid solubility, although increasing LA potency, does slow onset of action, possibly because of compartmentalization of LA within lipid membranes.

8. **What factors influence their duration of action?**
   Local anesthetic duration of action is determined by several factors. The greater the protein binding, the longer the duration of action. Duration is also influenced by peripheral vascular effects of the specific LA. For example, lidocaine, prilocaine, and mepivacaine provide anesthesia of similar duration in an isolated laboratory nerve preparation. However, lidocaine is a more potent vasodilator (all LAs are vasodilators, except ropivacaine and cocaine), thereby increasing absorption and metabolism, resulting in a shorter clinical blockade than that produced by either prilocaine or mepivacaine. Site of LA injection will affect duration; the more vascular the site, the greater the systemic absorption and the shorter the duration. Other factors that prolong duration are increased lipid solubility, presence of liver disease, and presence of pseudocholinesterase deficiency.

Table 18.1 Local Anesthetic Potency

AGENT	LIPID SOLUBILITY	RELATIVE POTENCY	PROTEIN BINDING (%)	DURATION	pK$_a$	ONSET TIME
Procaine	<1	1	5	Short	8.9	Slow
2-Chloroprocaine	>1	3	—	Short	8.7	Very quick
Mepivacaine	1	1.5	75	Medium	7.7	Quick
Lidocaine	3	2	65	Medium	7.9	Quick
Bupivacaine	28	8	95	Long	8.1	Moderate
Tetracaine	80	8	85	Long	8.5	Slow
Ropivacaine	14	8	94	Long	8.1	Moderate

9. **Describe the onset of local anesthetic neural blockade in peripheral nerves. What is the clinical significance of this?**
   Anatomically, conduction blockade proceeds from the outermost (mantle) to the innermost (core) nerve bundles. Generally speaking, mantle fibers innervate proximal structures, and core fibers innervate distal structures. This accounts for the early onset of blockade in more proximal structures, and for the appearance of muscle weakness before sensory blockade if motor fibers are more located more peripherally in the nerve. In terms of individual neurons, small myelinated axons (A gamma motor and A delta sensory fibers) are most susceptible to blockade, followed by large myelinated fibers (A alpha and A beta), and finally nonmyelinated C fibers. This is contrary to the popular belief that C fibers are most sensitive to local anesthetics. Note that some LAs, however, demonstrate the ability to preferentially spare motor neurons. Bupivacaine and ropivacaine are two examples of LAs with this pharmacodynamic profile. Many factors ranging from ion channel subtype to anatomic spread of local anesthetic account for this unexpected characteristic.

10. **Which regional anesthetic blocks are associated with the greatest degree of systemic vascular local anesthetic absorption?**
    Systemic absorption is influenced primarily by the vascularity of the injection site. Degree of systemic absorption for the following sites is as follows:
    Intercostal nerve block > caudal > lumbar epidural > brachial plexus > sciatic-femoral > subcutaneous. The area surrounding the intercostal nerves is highly vascularized, thus facilitating absorption and increasing the likelihood of achieving toxic plasma levels.

11. **What additives are commonly used with local anesthetics?**
    - Epinephrine: causes local tissue vasoconstriction, limiting systemic uptake of LA into the vasculature, thus prolonging their effects and reducing toxic potential. In 1:200,000 concentration (5 mcg/mL), epinephrine is a useful marker for inadvertent intravascular injection. Of note, epinephrine is contraindicated for blocks done in areas with poor collateral circulation (e.g., digits, penis). Also systemic absorption of epinephrine may cause cardiac dysrhythmias and dangerous elevations in blood pressure. Therefore caution is advised regarding its use in patients with ischemic heart disease, hypertension, preeclampsia, etc. Lastly, via alpha-2 adrenergic receptor agonism, epinephrine can activate endogenous analgesic pathways and contribute to block quality.
    - Bicarbonate: used to alkalinize the LA solution. Net effects are to increase the percentage of nonionized form (to aid membrane penetration and decrease onset time) and reduce pain during subcutaneous infiltration.
    - Opiates: increase duration and quality of block.
    - Alpha-2 agonists (such as clonidine and dexmedetomidine): increase duration and quality of block.

12. **What are the maximum safe doses of commonly used local anesthetics?**
    See Table 18.2.

13. **What are the clinical manifestations of local anesthetic systemic toxicity (LAST)?**
    Systemic toxicity results from elevated plasma local anesthetic levels, most often because of inadvertent intravascular injection and, less frequently, from systemic absorption from the injection site. Toxicity involves the cardiovascular and central nervous systems (CNS) primarily. Because the CNS is generally more sensitive to the toxic effects of LAs, it is usually (but not always) affected first. The manifestations of LA toxicity are presented subsequently in chronological order:
    - CNS toxicity:
      - Light-headedness, tinnitus, perioral numbness, confusion
      - Muscle twitching, auditory, and/or visual hallucinations
      - Tonic-clonic seizure, unconsciousness, respiratory arrest

Table 18.2 Maximum Safe Doses of Local Anesthetics

DRUG	MAXIMUM DOSE (mg/kg)	DRUG	MAXIMUM DOSE (mg/kg)
Procaine	7	Mepivacaine	5
Chloroprocaine	8–9	Bupivacaine	2.5
Tetracaine	1.5 (topical)		
Lidocaine	5 or 7 (with epinephrine)		

These doses are based on subcutaneous administration and apply only to single-shot injections. Continuous infusions of local anesthetic, as might occur over several hours during labor epidural anesthesia, allow a greater total dose of anesthetic before toxic plasma levels are reached. Maximum safe dose is also influenced by vascularity of the tissue bed and whether epinephrine is added to the local anesthetic.

- Cardiotoxicity: less common but possibly fatal
  - Hypertension, tachycardia
  - Decreased contractility and cardiac output, hypotension
  - Sinus bradycardia, ventricular dysrhythmias, circulatory arrest

14. **What are some risk factors for LAST?**
    - Patient characteristics
      - Extremes of age: younger than 16 years, or older than 60 years
      - Low muscle mass: neonates, elderly, and debilitated patients
      - Female more common than male
      - Comorbidities: preexisting cardiac disease, liver disease, metabolic disease (including diabetes), low plasma binding states
    - Local anesthetic characteristics
      - Local anesthetic with narrow therapeutic:toxicity window, for example, bupivacaine
      - Administration site
      - Total dose administered
      - Test dosing

15. **Is the risk of cardiotoxicity the same for all local anesthetics?**
    No. The cardiotoxicity of more potent LAs (such as bupivacaine and ropivacaine) differs from that of less soluble LAs (e.g., lidocaine) in the following manner:
    - The ratio of dosage required for irreversible cardiovascular collapse: dosage required to produce CNS toxicity is much lower for bupivacaine than for lidocaine.
    - Conditions, such as pregnancy, acidosis, and hypoxia increase the risk of cardiotoxicity with bupivacaine.
    - Cardiac resuscitation is more difficult following bupivacaine-induced cardiovascular collapse. This may be related to the high lipid solubility of bupivacaine, which results in its slow dissociation from cardiac sodium channels.

    In an effort to minimize the risk of cardiac toxicity, the use of bupivacaine in concentrations greater than 0.5% should be avoided, especially in obstetrics. For postoperative analgesia, bupivacaine concentrations of 0.25% are generally sufficient, providing excellent effect. Note that despite the preceding discussion, there are many reported cases of systemic toxicity with lidocaine. Always be vigilant and use caution when administering any local anesthetic to a patient.

16. **How does one prevent and/or manage LAST?**
    - Patients should be monitored whenever LAs are being used. An oxygen source (tank or wall outlet), as well as emergency airway equipment, should be available to deliver positive pressure ventilation if needed.
    - Most occurrences of LAST can be prevented by careful selection of LA dose and concentration, test dosing with epinephrine, injecting incrementally with frequent pauses for aspiration to confirm needle is not positioned within a vein or artery, constant monitoring for signs and symptoms of toxicity, and the use of ultrasound guidance to minimize the risk of intravascular injection whenever possible. In general, speed of LA injection should not exceed 1 mL/sec, with a 30 second pause every 5 mL to allow for one complete circulation time.
    - Tonic-clonic seizures can quickly lead to hypoxia and acidosis. Recall that acidosis worsens toxicity by trapping local anesthetics in their charged form within the cytoplasm of the cell. Ensuring adequate ventilation with 100% oxygen during these situations is critical.
    - If seizure develops, benzodiazepines, such as IV diazepam or midazolam, may be effective. Small doses of propofol can be considered in hemodynamically stable patients who have failed benzodiazepine therapy.
    - Cardiovascular collapse with refractory ventricular fibrillation or asystole, following local anesthetics, particularly bupivacaine or ropivacaine, can be extremely difficult to treat. Note that bradycardia often precedes these arrhythmias.

- Ensuring adequate ventilation and avoiding hypercapnia should be the first action undertaken in the treatment of LAST, followed promptly by IV lipid emulsion (IVLE).

17. **What is the role of IV lipid emulsion in the treatment of LAST?**
Cardiotoxicity from bupivacaine has historically possessed a high mortality rate, often requiring placement of the patient on cardiopulmonary bypass, while the drug slowly cleared from cardiac muscle tissue. The advent of IVLE has revolutionized the treatment for LAST and dramatically improved survival rates. It works via multiple proposed pathways, namely: shuttling, a cardiotonic effect, and postconditioning. Lipid shuttling acts to transport LA away from high blood flow organs that are particularly sensitive and to redistribute them to organs for storage and detoxification. Evidence also supports the concept that IVLE increases contractility and cardiac performance, increases blood pressure, and protects the heart from ischemic-reperfusion injury.

18. **Describe the step-wise treatment for LAST.**
    - Immediate cessation of LA dosing
    - Prompt, airway management, 100% O_2, consider hyperventilation
    - Seizure control with benzodiazepines (consider low-dose propofol if patient is not in cardiac arrest)
    - Administration of IVLE at the first signs of LAST
        - 20% lipid emulsion bolus
            - 100 mL over 2 to 3 minutes if patient is over 70 kg
            - 1.5 mL/kg lean body weight if patient is less than 70 kg
        - 20% lipid emulsion infusion
            - 200 to 250 mL over 15 to 20 min if patient is over 70 kg
            - 0.25 mL/kg/min if patient is less than 70 kg
            - Consider rebolusing 1 to 2 times, or increasing the infusion rate to 0.5 mL/kg/min if cardiovascular stability is not restored
            - Continue infusion for at least 10 min after cardiovascular stability is restored
            - 12 mL/kg total lipid emulsion is recommended as the upper limit for initial dosing
    - In the event of cardiac arrest:
        - Initiate cardiopulmonary resuscitation
        - Reduced dose of epinephrine (1 mcg/kg/dose)
        - Vasopressin is not recommended
        - Avoid calcium channel blockers and beta-blockers
        - Amiodarone is the preferred treatment for ventricular arrhythmias
        - Failure to respond to lipid emulsion and vasopressor therapy should prompt institution of cardiopulmonary bypass or extracorporeal membrane oxygenation

19. **Apart from cardiovascular and neurological system toxicity, what other risks are associated with local anesthetic usage?**
The following complications associated with LAs have been described:
    - Neural toxicity: prolonged sensory and motor deficits (especially when administered in higher doses) occur. Mechanisms of injury are reported to be mechanical, chemical, and/or ischemic in origin.
    - Transient neurological symptoms can be associated with the use of lidocaine for spinal anesthesia. It may manifest in the form of moderate-to-severe pain in the lower back, buttocks, and posterior thighs. These symptoms appear within 24 hours and generally resolve within 7 days. The delayed onset may reflect an inflammatory etiology.
    - Cauda equina syndrome: prolonged motor weakness and/or paralysis and sensory changes have been reported after spinal anesthesia with local anesthetics. Initially reported in patients receiving continuous spinal anesthesia with 5% lidocaine dosed via microcatheters, the mechanism of neural injury is thought to be the nonhomogeneous distribution of spinally injected local anesthetics, exposing nerve roots to a high concentration of local anesthetic with subsequent neural injury. Rare cases in the absence of microcatheters have also been described.

20. **Which local anesthetics are associated with methemoglobinemia?**
Prilocaine and benzocaine are responsible for most cases of local anesthetic–related methemoglobinemia. Signs/symptoms include shortness of breath, cyanosis, mental status changes, loss of consciousness, and even death. Prilocaine is metabolized in the liver to O-toluidine, which is capable of oxidizing hemoglobin to methemoglobin. Benzocaine, used as a spray for topical anesthesia of mouth and throat, can also result in methemoglobinemia if excessive amounts are used. Methemoglobinemia is treated by the administration of IV methylene blue (1–2 mg/kg), which accelerates the process by which methemoglobin is reduced back to hemoglobin via methemoglobin reductase.

21. **A patient reports allergy to novocaine from a prior dental procedure. Should LA use be avoided in this patient?**
Probably not. Allergic reactions to LA are rare despite their ubiquitous use. Less than 1% of adverse reactions involving LA represent true allergy. Reactions labeled as allergy are much more likely the result of vasovagal response, systemic toxicity, from epinephrine added to the LA solution, or from solution preservatives, than they are from an allergic

reaction. True allergy would be suggested by history of rash, bronchospasm, laryngeal edema, hypotension, elevation of serum tryptase, and positive intradermal testing.

Ester LAs are more likely to produce an allergic reaction than are amides. A significant metabolite of ester LA, p-aminobenzoic acid, is a known allergen. Allergic reactions may also be caused by methylparaben or other preservatives found in commercial amide LA preparations (amide and ester).

KEY POINTS: LOCAL ANESTHETICS

1. Local anesthetic agents are classified as either esters or amides. The two classes differ primarily in their allergic potential and method of biotransformation.
2. Lipid solubility, pK_a, and protein binding determine the potency, onset, and duration of action, respectively, of local anesthetics.
3. Local anesthetic–induced CNS toxicity manifests with excitation, followed by seizures, then loss of consciousness. Hypotension, conduction blockade, and cardiac arrest are signs of local anesthetic cardiovascular toxicity.
4. Bupivacaine has the highest risk of producing severe cardiac dysrhythmias and irreversible cardiovascular collapse. Use of more than 0.5% concentration should be avoided, especially in obstetric epidurals.

Website

Checklist for Local Anesthetic Systemic Toxicity: www.asra.com/advisory-guidelines/article/3/checklist-for-treatment-of-local-anesthetic-systemic-toxicity

---

SUGGESTED READINGS

Heavner JE. Local anesthetics. Curr Opin Anaesthesiol. 2007;20:336–342.

Mulroy ME. Systemic toxicity and cardiotoxicity from local anesthetics: incidence and preventive measures. Reg Anesth Pain Med. 2002;27:556–561.

Neal JM, Barrington MJ, Fettiplace MR. et al. The Third American Society of Regional Anesthesia and Pain Medicine Practice Advisory on Local Anesthetic Systemic Toxicity Executive Summary 2017. Reg Anesth Pain Med. 2018;43:113–123.

Rosenblatt MA, Abel M. Successful use of a 20% lipid emulsion to resuscitate a patient after a presumed bupivacaine-related cardiac arrest. Anesthesiology. 2006;105:217–218.

Strichartz GR, Berde CB. Local anesthetics. In: Miller RD, ed. Anesthesia. 8th ed. Philadelphia: Saunders; 2015:1028–1054:

Weinberg GL. Lipid emulsion infusion: resuscitation for local anesthetic and other drug overdose. Anesthesiology. 2012;117:180–187.

CHAPTER 19

VASOACTIVE AGENTS

Ryan D. Laterza, MD, Michael Kim, DO, Nathaen Weitzel, MD

1. **What are the benefits of vasoactive agents?**
   All major components governing the physiology of cardiac output, such as preload, afterload, inotropy, and chronotropy can be modulated by vasoactive agents. An underlying concept is the Frank-Starling principle, which states that increased myocardial fiber length, or preload, improves contractility up to an optimal state, then decreases with excess preload. Vasoactive agents, such as inotropes, can increase contractility, which can be conceptualized as a shift in the Frank-Starling curve (Fig. 19.1). Other agents, such as vasopressors can increase or decrease arterial resistance (afterload) and venous compliance (preload). Other agents can increase or decrease heart rate (chronotropy), which affects cardiac output and coronary perfusion. Recall, blood pressure is the product of cardiac output and resistance, where cardiac output is the product of stroke volume and heart rate, and where stroke volume is determined by contractility, preload, and afterload. The anesthesiologist can modulate each of these physiologic variables using vasoactive agents to optimize the patient's physiology.

2. **Is epinephrine an inotrope or a vasopressor?**
   Trick question. It is both. Although some medications (e.g., phenylephrine) are pure vasopressors, several of the medications discussed in this chapter have mixed physiologic effects. Medication that have both vasopressor and inotrope characteristics are referred to as an *inopressor* (e.g., epinephrine) and agents that have both vasodilating and inotrope characteristics are referred to as an *inodilator*. See Fig. 19.2 as a general overview illustrating the various characteristics of the medications discussed in this chapter.

3. **What physiological role does calcium play in the setting of managing shock?**
   All inotropic, vasopressor, and vasodilating medications share one common denominator as a final endpoint: calcium. Both vascular smooth muscle and cardiac muscle require calcium as a cofactor to allow myosin and actin filaments to cross-bridge to facilitate muscle contraction. In the resting state, myosin and actin binding sites are blocked by tropomyosin. When intracellular calcium increases, calcium binds to troponin. Troponin, a small protein attached to tropomyosin, when bound to calcium causes tropomyosin to move away from the actin-myosin binding sites, allowing them to cross bridge and muscle contraction ensues.

   Calcium administration can have a profound effect in improving cardiac contractility and increasing systemic vascular resistance in the setting of hypocalcemia. Hypocalcemia frequently occurs in the setting of massive blood transfusion as blood products often contain calcium chelating agents, such as citrate.

4. **What are the physiological goals in managing patients with systolic heart failure?**
   Patients with impaired contractility, such as in systolic heart failure may present with excess preload (i.e., hypervolemia) and afterload (i.e., increased systemic vascular resistance), which can decrease stroke volume and cardiac output. Vasodilators, in addition to diuretics, can help in "unloading the heart" by reducing both preload and afterload to a more optimal physiological state, thereby improving stroke volume or forward flow.

5. **What is the problem with administering vasopressors to a patient with impaired contractility?**
   Because blood pressure is the product of cardiac output and systemic vascular resistance, inappropriate vasopressor administration to normalize the blood pressure can make the vitals "look good" at the expense of elevated systemic vascular resistance, and decreased cardiac output. Ultimately, the most important goal of the cardiovascular system is to deliver oxygen to tissue and a normal blood pressure itself does not guarantee an adequate cardiac output.

   Vasopressors, such as phenylephrine, vasoconstrict both venous vasculature (increase preload) and arterial vasculature (increase afterload) through α_1 mediated vasoconstriction. Healthy patients with normal cardiac contractility generally tolerate the increase in afterload and, depending upon the situation, venoconstriction may improve preload and cardiac output. For most patients undergoing surgery with either general anesthesia or neuraxial anesthesia, phenylephrine is often a good choice to counteract the anesthetic induced vasodilation. However, in patients with decreased contractility, simultaneously increasing preload and afterload with vasopressors can "overload" the heart's physiological reserve, leading to a decrease in cardiac output, therefore careful administration should be used to strike the appropriate balance.

6. **Discuss the mechanisms of action and hemodynamic profile of milrinone.**
   Milrinone is an inotropic agent, classified as a phosphodiesterase (PDE) inhibitor, which decreases the degradation of cyclic adenosine monophosphate, leading to increased contractility and vasodilation. Right ventricular function, in particular, can be favorably impacted, as milrinone can decrease pulmonary vascular resistance to reduce right heart afterload.

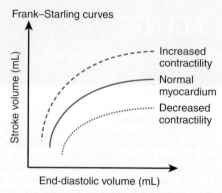

Fig. 19.1 Frank–Starling curves illustrating functional assessment changes in stroke volume secondary to changes in end-diastolic volume, under varying states of cardiac contractility. (Modified from Hamilton M. Advanced cardiovascular monitoring. Surgery (Oxford). 2013;31(2): 90–97.)

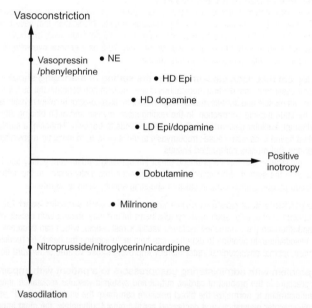

Fig. 19.2 Physiological response to vasoactive agents. *Epi*, Epinephrine; *HD*, high dose; *LD*, low dose; *NE*, norepinephrine.

7. **Describe the hemodynamic profiles of isoproterenol and dobutamine.**
   Isoproterenol is a potent nonselective β agonist with no alpha stimulating properties. Isoproterenol administration will increase heart rate and contractility (β_1), while also decreasing afterload (β_2). Clinically, it is often used for provoking dysrhythmias in electrophysiology procedures and for the treatment of bradycardia in a denervated nonpaced transplanted heart.

   Dobutamine acts principally on β-adrenergic receptors ($\beta_1 > \beta_2$), causing less vasodilation than isoproterenol. Dobutamine is often used as a first-line agent for cardiogenic shock because β_1 receptor agonism improves contractility and partial β_2 receptor agonism causes arterial vasodilation reducing afterload.

8. **How are milrinone and dobutamine similar? What are their differences?**
   Both milrinone and dobutamine increase cardiac contractility (i.e., positive inotrope) and cause vasodilation (i.e., reduces afterload), which together increases cardiac output. Both are considered first-line agents to treat cardiogenic

shock. Although both can cause hypotension and dysrhythmias, hypotension is more evident with milrinone, whereas dysrhythmias tend to occur more often with dobutamine. Dobutamine has a much shorter half-life (2–3 minutes) and is therefore easier to titrate than milrinone, which has a longer half-life (2–3 hours).

9. Describe the hemodynamic profiles of epinephrine, norepinephrine, and dopamine.

The effects of a low-dose epinephrine infusion (e.g., <0.05 mcg/kg/min) are primarily limited to the stimulation of β_1 and β_2 adrenergic receptors in the heart and skeletal muscle, respectively. This results in positive β_1-mediated chronotropy (heart rate), dromotropy (conduction velocity), inotropy (contractility), increased automaticity, and β_2-mediated vasodilation in skeletal muscle. At higher doses (e.g., >0.05 mcg/kg/min), epinephrine stimulates α_1-adrenergic receptors. This increases overall systemic vascular resistance because the α_1-mediated vasoconstriction is greater than the β_2-mediated vasodilation.

Norepinephrine primarily stimulates α_1 adrenergic receptors and partially stimulates β_1 adrenergic receptors. It has very little β_2 receptor selectivity. This results in α_1-mediated increased systemic vascular resistance. The partial β_1-mediated effects help prevent reflex bradycardia that can be seen with pure α_1 agonists (e.g., phenylephrine) and helps preserve cardiac output despite an increase in afterload.

Dopamine, at high doses, is an indirect vasopressor facilitating the release of catecholamines, such as norepinephrine, and at low doses, a direct vasodilator, stimulating specific dopamine receptors in the renal, mesenteric, and coronary arterial beds. These dopaminergic effects occur at low doses (0.5–2.0 mcg/kg/min). At intermediate doses (5–10 mcg/kg/min), β_1-adrenergic stimulation becomes evident. At higher doses (10–20 mcg/kg/min), α_1-adrenergic stimulation predominates, overcoming the vasodilating dopaminergic effects, leading to an overall increased systemic vascular resistance. Dopamine has fallen out of favor as a vasoactive agent, as evidence to date shows increased mortality and a higher incidence of dysrhythmias in patients with septic or cardiogenic shock.

10. How are norepinephrine and epinephrine similar and how are they different? In what situations would you use one or the other?

Both agents are short acting with a half-life of approximately 90 seconds, which often requires an infusion. This short half-life helps facilitate rapid titration in situations where acute changes in hemodynamics are expected. Both agents are α and β receptor agonists, with norepinephrine a more selective α than β receptor agonist and the corollary is true for epinephrine, particularly at low doses.

The differences and clinical utility between these two agents are primarily attributed to their mechanism of action. Inhaled or intravenous (IV) epinephrine can be useful for severe bronchospasm through β_2-mediated bronchodilation. Epinephrine is a mast cell stabilizer, preventing histamine release, and is a first-line agent for anaphylactic shock. In septic or cardiogenic shock, epinephrine is often used as a second-line agent. Norepinephrine, however, is often used as a first-line vasopressor in situations associated with low systemic vascular resistance (e.g., septic shock).

11. What are the adverse effects of epinephrine and norepinephrine?

Epinephrine is generally associated with more side effects than norepinephrine. For example, epinephrine is associated with a much higher incidence of dysrhythmias attributed to its higher β_1 receptor stimulation. Epinephrine is also associated with a much higher incidence of hyperglycemia and lactic acidosis because of β_2 receptor stimulation. This is largely thought to be the result of β_2 receptors on the liver causing gluconeogenesis and β_2-mediated reduced skeletal muscle reuptake of lactate from blood. Norepinephrine has a very low β_2 affinity compared with epinephrine and these latter adverse reactions (i.e., hyperglycemia and lactic acidosis) are less common with this agent.

Both agents can cause mesenteric ischemia and renal failure with prolonged excessively high doses. However, this is often confounded by the fact that the very same patient population receiving these agents often have predisposing conditions that also cause these same problems (e.g., renal failure caused by sepsis or heart failure). Furthermore, hypotension itself can cause mesenteric ischemia or renal failure and studies show that maintaining a normal blood pressure with vasopressors reduces the incidence of these same complications. Therefore vasopressors should be used, in most situations, to restore vascular tone to maintain a normal systemic vascular resistance.

12. How can adverse reactions and limitations of vasoactive agents be minimized?

Adverse reactions and limitations can be minimized by appropriate dosage adjustments and combining complimentary vasoactive agents. For example, some providers favor using epinephrine combined with nitroprusside for cardiogenic shock where epinephrine is used to increase contractility and nitroprusside is used to decrease afterload. Other combinations include using vasopressin and milrinone for right heart failure. Because vasopressin does not increase pulmonary vascular resistance, it can be used as an adjunct to counter problems of hypotension caused by milrinone, without increasing right heart afterload.

13. Describe the mechanism of action of vasopressin.

Arginine vasopressin (AVP) works on three subtypes of receptors (V_1, V_2, V_3). The V_1 receptor stimulates vascular smooth muscle contraction, resulting in the vasopressor response of AVP. The V_2 receptors act primarily in the renal collecting tubule of the kidney to produce water retention (antidiuretic hormone) by regulating osmolarity and blood volume, and the V_3 receptors act in the central nervous system (CNS) and modulate corticotropin secretion. The vasopressin system makes up one of the three vasopressor systems in the body; the sympathetic system and the renin-angiotensin system are the other two vasopressor systems. The half-life of vasopressin is relatively long (approximately 20 minutes) and is often given as a bolus in the operating room or as an infusion in the intensive care unit.

14. **How may vasopressin aid in the management of septic shock? What other scenarios is vasopressin helpful?**
Vasopressin is often used as an adjunct or as a second-line vasopressor for septic shock. In the presence of a systemic inflammatory response, patients with septic shock tend to have low plasma vasopressin concentrations because of low vasopressin secretion. Vasopressin has been shown to improve hemodynamics and reduce requirements of adrenergic agents, such as norepinephrine. Vasopressin may be used as a first-line agent in other situations associated with vasodilation. For example, patients taking angiotensin-converting enzyme (ACE) inhibitors or angiotensin-receptor blockers (ARBs) often have profound hypotension with general anesthesia. These patients often respond poorly to α_1 agonists but respond well to vasopressin.
   Vasopressin is often given as an infusion of 0.01 to 0.04 units/min for septic shock, given as a bolus of 1 to 2 units for patients taking ACE-inhibitors/ARBs, while under general anesthesia, and given as a bolus of 20 to 40 units for patients in cardiac arrest.

15. **What are some of the unique properties of vasopressin? What are its adverse reactions?**
   - Severe acidosis can blunt the α adrenergic receptor response to vasoactive agents, making these agents less efficacious. Vasopressin, however, is unique in that it appears to be equally efficacious despite severe acidosis.
   - Vasopressin can be helpful in patients with severe pulmonary hypertension or right heart failure. Vasopressin has little to no effect on the pulmonary vasculature and can increase systemic vascular resistance without increasing pulmonary vascular resistance.
      Adverse reactions to vasopressin, particularly with excessively high doses, include hyponatremia and splanchnic hypoperfusion.

16. **Should dopamine be used as a first-line agent in managing septic or cardiogenic shock?**
Dopamine should not be used as a first-line agent in these situations because studies have shown a higher mortality with dopamine compared with other vasoactive agents. Studies have also shown that low-dose dopamine is ineffective for the prevention or treatment of acute kidney injury, despite common practice in the past. Dopamine, in comparison to norepinephrine, has been shown to have a higher risk of dysrhythmias in patients with septic shock. Lastly, dopamine blunts the ventilatory drive, increasing the risk of respiratory failure in patients who are being weaned from mechanical ventilation.

17. **Discuss the effects of phenylephrine and review common doses of this medication.**
Phenylephrine is a selective α_1 receptor agonist, which decreases venous compliance facilitating venous return of blood (increasing preload and stroke volume) and increases systemic vascular resistance by arteriole vasoconstriction. It is important to emphasize that patients with decreased cardiac contractility may not have the physiological reserve to overcome this increase in preload and afterload, and giving phenylephrine to this patient population can worsen their cardiac output. A notable side effect of phenylephrine is reflex bradycardia, which may be desirable in patients with coronary artery disease or aortic stenosis to improve coronary perfusion. This drug may be administered for hypotension that is primarily caused by vasodilation to restore normal systemic vascular resistance. Examples of hypotension thought to be primarily vasodilatory include septic shock, following induction of general anesthesia, or hypotension because of a spinal anesthetic.

18. **Discuss the effects of ephedrine and review common doses of this medication. Give some examples of medications that contraindicate the use of ephedrine.**
Ephedrine is a CNS stimulant that is chemically indistinct from methamphetamine, aside from the addition of one hydroxyl group. Clinically, it is often used as an indirect vasoactive agent, which facilitates the release of endogenous norepinephrine and epinephrine. Interestingly, as a CNS stimulant, it can increase the monitored anesthesia care requirements for volatile agents. Repeated dosing may lead to diminished responsiveness, a phenomenon known as *tachyphylaxis*, possibly because of exhaustion of norepinephrine stores. Similarly, an inadequate response to ephedrine may be the result of already depleted norepinephrine stores, as in chronic cocaine or methamphetamine users. Ephedrine should not be used when the patient is taking drugs that prevent the reuptake of norepinephrine because of the risk of severe hypertension. Examples include tricyclic antidepressants, monoamine oxidase inhibitors, and acute cocaine intoxication.
   Please see Table 19.1 for a review of vasopressor and inotropic agents.

Table 19.1 Vasopressor and Inotropic Agents

DRUG	COMMON DOSES	MECHANISM OF ACTION
Dopamine[a,c,†]	0.5–20 mcg/kg/min	D_1/D_2, β_1, α_1
Epinephrine[b,†]	0.02–0.5 mcg/kg/min	$\beta_1 \geq \beta_2 \geq \alpha_1$
Ephedrine[c]	5–10 mg bolus	$\alpha_1 = \beta_1$
Norepinephrine	0.02–0.5 mcg/kg/min	$\alpha_1 > \beta_1$
Phenylephrine	50–200 mcg bolus 0.5–6 mcg/kg/min infusion	α_1
Vasopressin	0.01–0.04 units/min	V_1
Dobutamine	2–20 mcg/kg/min	$\beta_1 > \beta_2$
Isoproterenol	0.02–0.2 mcg/kg/min	$\beta_1 = \beta_2$
Milrinone	0.125–0.75 mcg/kg/min	PDE III Inhibitor

[a]Dopamine stimulates dopamine receptors (D_1/D_2) at low doses (0.5–2.0 mcg/kg/min), β_1 at moderate doses (5–10 mcg/kg/min), and α_1 at higher doses (10–20 mcg/kg/min).
[b]Epinephrine stimulates β_1/β_2 receptors at low doses and α_1 receptors at higher doses.
[c]Dopamine and ephedrine are indirect adrenergic agonists.
[†]High-dose epinephrine and dopamine increases net systemic vascular resistance as α_1 mediated vasoconstriction outweighs vasodilatory effects from β_2 and dopamine receptors.
PDE, Phosphodiesterase E.

KEY POINTS: VASOACTIVE AGENTS

1. Norepinephrine is the first-choice vasopressor in managing septic shock.
2. Epinephrine is a second-line agent in septic and cardiogenic shock and a first-line agent in anaphylactic shock.
3. Milrinone and dobutamine are equally effective and are first-line agents in managing cardiogenic shock by improving contractility and reducing afterload.
4. Vasopressin is unique to other vasoactive agents because of its efficacy with severe acidosis and ability to increase systemic vascular resistance, with no effect on pulmonary vascular resistance.
5. Dopamine is associated with increased mortality in septic and cardiogenic shock patients and evidence does not support its utility in preventing or treating acute kidney injury.
6. Two commonly used vasoactive agents in the operating room are phenylephrine and ephedrine. Phenylephrine IV is dosed at 50 to 200 mcg. Ephedrine IV is dosed at 5 to 10 mg.

19. **What are the most commonly used anticholinergics? How are these agents used in anesthesia practice?**
    The most commonly used anticholinergics in anesthesia practices are atropine and glycopyrrolate.
    Anticholinergics are frequently used as an antisialagogue (i.e., glycopyrrolate) to help minimize secretions, while performing procedures, such as an awake fiberoptic intubation. Other agents, such as diphenhydramine, promethazine, or scopolamine can be used as an adjunct for sedation during surgery and as a treatment for postoperative nausea and vomiting.
    Atropine and glycopyrrolate are primarily used in conjunction with acetylcholinesterase inhibitors (e.g., neostigmine) to minimize the risk of bradycardia caused by these latter agents.

20. **What are some of the differences between glycopyrrolate and atropine?**
    Atropine is a naturally occurring tertiary amine (i.e., nonpolar molecule) that readily crosses the blood-brain barrier. Glycopyrrolate is a synthetic quaternary amine (i.e., polar molecule) that does not cross the blood-brain barrier and therefore causes less sedation compared with atropine. Although both glycopyrrolate and atropine can be used to treat bradycardia and reduce secretions, glycopyrrolate tends to be slightly more efficacious as an antisialagogue and atropine more efficacious in treating bradycardia.

21. **What is the mechanism and site of action for nitrovasodilators?**
    Nitrates, such as nitroglycerin and sodium nitroprusside, are prodrugs that penetrate the vascular endothelium and become reduced to nitric oxide (NO). Nitroglycerin requires intact endothelial enzymatic activity, which is not present in the smallest or damaged vessels, whereas nitroprusside nonenzymatically degrades into NO and cyanide (a compound highly toxic to the mitochondrial respiratory chain). NO then stimulates production of cyclic guanosine monophosphate

(cGMP), reducing intracellular calcium levels, facilitating vascular smooth muscle relaxation. Sodium nitroprusside generally causes more arterial than venous dilation, whereas the converse is true for nitroglycerin (although this is less true with higher doses).

22. **Describe the antianginal effects of nitrates.**
Beneficial effects of nitroglycerin and other nitrates in anginal therapy result from improved coronary perfusion, reduced myocardial oxygen consumption (MVO_2), and antiplatelet effects. Coronary artery spasm is ameliorated, and dilation of epicardial coronary arteries, coronary collaterals, and atherosclerotic stenotic coronary segments occurs. Venodilation reduces venous return, ventricular filling pressures, wall tension, MVO_2 and improves subendocardial and collateral blood flow. Platelet aggregation is inhibited by release of NO and increased formation of cGMP.

23. **What is tachyphylaxis? What are the concerns when a patient develops tachyphylaxis to nitroprusside?**
Tachyphylaxis is defined as a decrease in response to a drug following chronic or repeated administration. It is a form of drug tolerance and can be seen in various medications, such as opioids and other medications, such as nitroglycerin and nitroprusside. Tachyphylaxis to nitroglycerin, commonly termed *nitroglycerin tolerance*, is a common problem because many patients are exposed to this medication for prolong periods (e.g., transdermal nitroglycerin patches).
   Tachyphylaxis to nitroglycerin may limit its clinical utility, but is generally not a problem otherwise. However, tachyphylaxis to nitroprusside can be an early warning sign of cyanide toxicity. Cyanide is a metabolite of nitroprusside and cyanide toxicity can be seen in patients on prolonged high-dose nitroprusside infusions, particularly in the setting of renal failure.

24. **Which beta-blockers are frequently given in the perioperative environment?**
Labetalol is a nonselective beta-adrenergic antagonist and a partial α-adrenergic antagonist. Labetalol blocks β_1 and β_2 equally; however, the ratio of β to α blocking is 7:1 (IV) and 3:1 (by mouth). Labetalol and other beta-blocking agents are frequently given for patients with coronary artery disease and for the long-term management in patients with stable congestive heart failure. However, labetalol and other beta-blocking agents should be avoided in patients with acute decompensated heart failure or cardiogenic shock. It has a long half-life of 5 to 6 hours and is commonly given as a bolus with a dose of 5 to 10 mg.
   Esmolol is a highly selective β_1 adrenergic receptor antagonist. It does not appear to have any β_2 adrenergic receptor antagonism and can safely be administered to patients with chronic obstructive pulmonary disease or asthma. It is metabolized by esterase in the cytosol of red cells and has a short half-life of 9 minutes. Its short half-life makes this agent helpful in situations where frequent changes in hemodynamics are anticipated. It may be given as a bolus (e.g., just before emergence) or by an infusion (e.g., aortic dissection).

25. **Discuss hydralazine. What are the difficulties associated with administering hydralazine? What are the side effects of this medication?**
Hydralazine is a selective arterial vasodilator with an unclear mechanism of action. The onset of hydralazine is variable, often within 5 to 20 minutes, the degree of vasodilation is variable, and its duration of action is long (half-life is 3 hours). Therefore hydralazine administration should be carefully titrated in small doses (e.g., 5 mg), titrated over a long period (e.g., 10–15 minutes). Sinus tachycardia is a common side effect and this medication should be avoided in patients with coronary artery disease or severe aortic stenosis.

26. **What is the mechanism of action of nicardipine? Is it a negative inotrope? What about clevidipine?**
Nicardipine is a calcium channel blocker (CCB) characterized as an arterial selective vasodilator that is not associated with impaired contractility compared with other CCB (e.g., diltiazem). Nicardipine is fast acting (onset 1–2 minutes) and has a half-life of 40 to 60 minutes. Clevidipine is a third-generation CCB that is similar to nicardipine in that it selectively vasodilates the arterial vasculature and has no negative inotropic effects. Clevidipine has a rapid onset of

Table 19.2 Vasodilating Agents

DRUG	DOSE	MECHANISM OF ACTION
Labetalol	5–10 mg	$\beta_1 = \beta_2 > \alpha_1$ antagonist
Esmolol	10–30 mg bolus 50–200 mcg/kg/min infusion	Selective β_1 antagonist
Hydralazine	5–10 mg	Unclear mechanism. Arterial selective
Nitroprusside	0.2–2 mcg/kg/min	Nitric oxide (NO) donation. Arterial >venous
Nitroglycerin	10–200 mcg/min	NO donation. Venous >arterial
Nicardipine	1–15 mg/h	Calcium-channel blocker. Arterial selective

action, an ultra-short half-life (1–2 minutes) and is metabolized by plasma esterases. Although nicardipine is an older CCB and a better validated agent, evidence to date suggests clevidipine has a similar efficacy as nicardipine. Please see Table 19.2 for a review of vasodilating agents.

27. **Which agent would you select to treat hypertension in a patient with cardiogenic shock or severely impaired contractility?**
Nitroprusside, nitroglycerin, and nicardipine can all be used to reduce afterload in patients with cardiogenic shock or in patients with severely impaired contractility (e.g., cardiac surgery patients coming off bypass). Although nitroprusside and nitroglycerin can also be used in this setting, nicardipine is unique because it is highly arterial selective and does not appear to have the problems with tachyphylaxis (nitroglycerin) or cyanide toxicity (nitroprusside).

28. **Which agent would you select to manage hypertension for a patient with intracranial hemorrhage? Which agents should you avoid?**
Both nitroglycerin and nitroprusside can invariably cause venodilation, which increases intracranial pressure. These medications should not be used to control hypertension in the setting of intracranial hemorrhage. Nicardipine is a highly selective, easily titratable, arterial vasodilator and is often the agent of choice in managing hypertension in the setting of intracranial hemorrhage. Labetalol and hydralazine can also be used but because of their longer half-lives are more difficult to titrate. Furthermore, hydralazine's onset and clinical effect is less predictable, whereas labetalol is primarily a β-blocker with weak α_1-mediated vasodilatory effects.

KEY POINTS: VASOACTIVE AGENTS

1. Glycopyrrolate is often preferred over atropine in the perioperative setting. Because glycopyrrolate does not cross the blood brain barrier, it is associated with little to no sedation compared with atropine.
2. Both glycopyrrolate and atropine can be used to treat bradycardia. Atropine, however, is more efficacious and is the first-line treatment in emergencies because of bradycardia.
3. Nitroglycerin vasodilates veins more than arteries and the converse is true for nitroprusside.
4. Beneficial effects of nitroglycerin for anginal therapy result from a reduction in cardiac oxygen demand, improved coronary perfusion, and antiplatelet effects.
5. Labetalol is nonselective β-adrenergic antagonist and a partial α-adrenergic antagonist.
6. Esmolol is a highly selective β_1 adrenergic antagonist with no β_2 antagonism. It is unique in that it has a short half-life (9 minutes) and is metabolized by esterase in the cytosol of red cells.
7. Nicardipine is a selective arterial vasodilator. It is one of the few CCBs that has no negative inotropic effects.

Suggested Readings

Belletti A, Castro ML, Silvetti S, et al. The effect of inotropes and vasopressors on mortality: a meta-analysis of randomized clinical trials. Br J Anaesth. 2015;115(5):656–675.

Gamper G, Havel C, Arrich J, et al. Vasopressors for hypotensive shock. Cochrane Database Syst Rev. 2016;2:CD003709.

Jentzer JC, Coons JC, Link CB, et al. Pharmacotherapy update on the use of vasopressors and inotropes in the intensive care unit. J Cardiovasc Pharmacol Ther. 2015;20(3):249–260.

Lewis TC, Aberle C, Altshuler D, et al. Comparative effectiveness and safety between milrinone or dobutamine as initial inotrope therapy in cardiogenic shock. J Cardiovasc Pharmacol Ther. 2018 Sep 2:1074248418797357.

CHAPTER 20

PULSE OXIMETRY

Benjamin Lippert, DO, FAAP, Brian M. Keech, MD

1. Review pulse oximetry.

   Pulse oximetry is a noninvasive method by which arterial oxygenation can be approximated. It is based on the Beer-Lambert law and spectrophotometric analysis. When applied to pulse oximetry, the Beer-Lambert law essentially states that the intensity of transmitted light passing through a vascular bed decreases exponentially as a function of the concentration of the absorbing substances in that bed, and the distance from the source of the light to the detector.

2. How does a pulse oximeter work?

   A sensor is placed on either side of a pulsatile vascular bed, such as the fingertip or earlobe. The light-emitting diodes (LEDs) located on the opposite side of the sensor send out two wavelengths of light: one red (600–750 nm wavelength) and one infrared (850–1000 nm wavelength). These two wavelengths of light pass through the vascular bed to the sensor located on the other side where a photodetector measures the amount of red and infrared light received. Most pulse oximeters use wavelengths of 660 nm (red) and 940 nm (infrared).

3. How is oxygen saturation determined?

   A certain amount of red and infrared light is absorbed by the tissues (including blood) that are situated between the LEDs and photodetector. Therefore not all the light emitted makes it to the detector. Reduced (deoxygenated) hemoglobin absorbs much more of the red light (660 nm) than does oxygenated hemoglobin. Oxyhemoglobin absorbs more infrared light (940 nm) than does reduced hemoglobin. The photodetector measures the amount of light absorbed at each wavelength, which in turn allows the microprocessor to calculate a specific number (the SpO_2) for the amount of deoxygenated and oxygenated hemoglobin present.

4. How does the pulse oximeter determine the arterial hemoglobin saturation?

   In the vascular bed being monitored, the amount of blood present constantly changes because of the pulsatile nature of blood flow. Thus the light beams pass not only through a relatively stable volume of bone, soft tissue, and venous blood, but also through arterial blood, which is made up of a nonpulsatile portion and a variable, pulsatile portion. By measuring transmitted light several hundred times per second, the pulse oximeter is able to distinguish the changing, pulsatile component (AC) of the arterial blood from the unchanging, static component of the signal (DC) comprised of the soft tissue, venous blood, and nonpulsatile arterial blood. The pulsatile component (AC), generally comprising 1% to 5% of the total signal, can then be isolated by canceling out the static components (DC) at each wavelength (Fig. 20.1).

   The photodetector relays this information to the microprocessor, which knows how much red and infrared light was emitted, how much has been detected, how much signal is static, and how much varies with pulsation. The microprocessor then sets up the red/infrared (R/IR) ratio for the pulsatile (AC) portion of the blood. The R and IR of this ratio is the total amount of absorbed light at each wavelength, respectively, for the pulsatile component of the arterial blood.

5. What is the normalization procedure?

   Normalization involves dividing the pulsatile (AC) component of the red and infrared plethysmogram by the corresponding nonpulsatile (DC) component. This scaling process results in a normalized R/IR ratio, which is virtually independent of the incident light intensity.

   $$R/IR \ ratio = (AC_{red}/DC_{red})/(AC_{ir}/DC_{it})$$

6. How does the R/IR ratio relate to oxygen saturation?

   The normalized R/IR ratio is compared with a preset algorithm that gives the percentage of oxygenated hemoglobin in the arterial blood (the oxygen saturation percentage). This algorithm is derived from volunteers, usually healthy individuals who have been desaturated to a level of 75% to 80%; their arterial blood gas is drawn, and saturation is measured in a standard laboratory format. Manufacturers keep their algorithms secret, but in general an R/IR ratio of 0.4 corresponds to a saturation of 100%, an R/IR ratio of 1.0 corresponds to a saturation of about 87%, and an R/IR ratio of 3.4 corresponds to a saturation of 0% (Fig. 20.2).

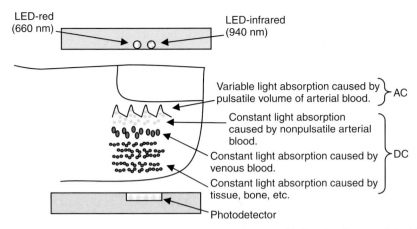

Fig. 20.1 Transmitted light passes through pulsatile arterial blood (AC) and other tissues (DC). The pulse oximeter can distinguish the AC from the DC portion by measuring transmitted light several hundred times per second. *LED*, Light-emitting diode.

7. Review the oxyhemoglobin dissociation curve.

The oxyhemoglobin dissociation curve describes the relationship between oxygen tension, or PaO$_2$, and binding (percent oxygen saturation of hemoglobin) (Fig. 20.3). Efficient oxygen transport relies on the ability of hemoglobin to reversibly load oxygen in the lungs and unload it peripherally, and the sigmoid shape of the oxyhemoglobin dissociation curve is a graphical representation of this capability. In the lungs, where oxygen tension is high, hemoglobin will nearly fully saturate under normal circumstances. As oxygenated blood moves through the peripheral tissues, and oxygen tension begins to lower, oxygen will be released at an accelerating rate from hemoglobin to maintain the necessary oxygen tension needed to facilitate the adequate diffusion gradient for oxygen to move into the cells of the periphery. The curve may be shifted to the left or right by many variables, some pathologic, others to meet the physiological demands of the situation (Table 20.1).

8. Why might a pulse oximeter give a false reading? Part 1 — not R/IR related.
- The algorithm the pulse oximeter uses to determine the saturation loses significant accuracy as hemoglobin saturation drops below 80%.
- Saturation is averaged over a time period of anywhere from 5 to 20 seconds. As a patient is desaturating, the reading on the monitor screen will be higher than the actual saturation. This becomes critical as the patient enters the steep part of the oxyhemoglobin desaturation curve because the degree of desaturation increases

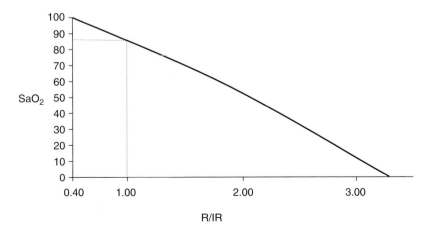

Fig. 20.2 The ratio of absorbed red to infrared light corresponds to the appropriate percentage of oxygenated hemoglobin (SaO$_2$).

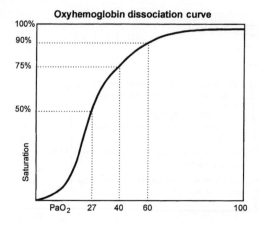

Oxyhemoglobin dissociation curve

Fig. 20.3 Oxyhemoglobin dissociation curve describes the nonlinear relationship between partial pressure of oxygen in arterial blood (PaO_2) and percentage saturation of hemoglobin with oxygen (SaO_2). In the steep part of the curve (50% region), small changes in PaO_2 result in large changes in SaO_2.

Table 20.1 Left and Right Shifts of the Oxyhemoglobin Dissociation Curve

RIGHT SHIFT	LEFT SHIFT
Effects	**Effects**
Decreased affinity of Hb for O_2 (facilitates unloading of O_2 to tissues)	Increased affinity of Hb for O_2 (decreases unloading of O_2 from Hb)
Causes	**Causes**
Increased PCO_2	Decreased PCO_2
Hyperthermia	Hypothermia
Acidosis	Alkalosis
Increased altitude	Fetal hemoglobin
Increased 2,3-DPG	Decreased 2,3-DPG
Sickle cell anemia	Carboxyhemoglobin Methemoglobin

Hb, Hemoglobin; *2,3-DPG,* 2,3-diphosphoglycerate, *PCO_2,* partial pressure of carbon dioxide.

dramatically and may exceed the ability of the monitor to change rapidly enough to show the true level of oxygen saturation. Likewise, as a person's saturation increases, the displayed reading on the screen will be lower than the actual saturation.
- Dark pigmentation of the skin may overestimate oxygen saturation.
- Response time to changes in saturation is related to probe location. Response time is less with ear probes and greater with finger probes.
- Anemia, hypotension; poor perfusion at the site of measurement; and nail polish, especially blue or black, also lead to false readings.

9. Why might the pulse oximeter give a false reading? Part 2—R/IR related: What can affect the R/IR number?
- The R/IR ratio determines the displayed saturation. Any circumstance that erroneously drives the R/IR number toward 1.0 will result in a saturation reading approaching 87%. The majority of times, these circumstances develop in well-oxygenated patients and the displayed saturation is false.
- Motion artifact causes a low signal-to-noise ratio, alters the absorption detection of both the red and infrared light by the photodetector, drives the R/IR ratio toward 1.0, and results in false saturation readings.
- Fluorescent lighting and operating room lights, because of their phased light production (too fast for the human eye to detect), can cause false R/IR readings.
- Dyshemoglobinemias (carboxyhemoglobin [COHb] and methemoglobin [MetHb]) may create inaccurate oxygen saturation measurement. COHb absorbs light at 660 nm, much like oxygenated hemoglobin, causing an

overestimation of true saturation. The influence of methemoglobinemia on SpO_2 readings is more complicated. MetHb looks much like reduced Hb at 660 nm. However, more important, at 940 nm the absorbance of MetHb is markedly greater than that of either reduced or oxygenated Hb. Therefore the monitor reads it as absorption of both species, driving the R/IR number toward 1.0 and the saturation toward 87%. Therefore at a high oxygen saturation (SaO_2) level, the probe underestimates the true value; at a low SaO_2 level, the value is falsely elevated.

10. **What is methemoglobinemia?**
Methemoglobinemia is a blood disorder in which an abnormal amount of MetHb, greater than 1.5%, is found in the blood. MetHb is a form of hemoglobin that contains ferric (Fe_3^+) instead of normal ferrous (Fe_2^+) iron in the hemoglobin molecule. This abnormal hemoglobin species is unable to bind oxygen and causes impaired release of oxygen from other oxygen-binding sites. This prevents supplying oxygen to the body tissues and results in an oxygen-hemoglobin dissociation curve shift to the left.

11. **What are the causes of methemoglobinemia?**
Methemoglobinemia can be either inherited or acquired. The most common form is acquired from exposure to medications or chemicals. These agents include local anesthetics, such as benzocaine, prilocaine, procaine, and lidocaine, vasodilators like nitroglycerin and nitroprusside, antibiotics like sulfonamides and phenytoin, metoclopramide, benzene compounds, and aniline dyes. A common feature of all these is the presence of nitrogen atoms. Nitrogen is capable of extracting electrons from iron, resulting in changes in Fe_2^+ to Fe_3^+.

12. **How does methemoglobinemia affect the pulse oximeter reading?**
With increasing levels of methemoglobin in the blood, the pulse oximetry values decrease until the SpO_2 reads approximately 85%. At that point the SpO_2 reading does not decrease further even though the amount of MetHb may be increasing and the true HbO_2 (Oxyhemoglobin) saturation is much lower. At a pulse oximeter reading of 85%, the amount of MetHb can be 35% or more. Conventional pulse oximetry uses two wavelengths of light and compares absorbance ratios to empirical data. Different hemoglobin species have different absorption coefficients and in MetHb, the ratios of absorbance approximate 1 at an SpO_2 of 85%.

13. **If one suspects methemoglobinemia, what test will establish it?**
If one suspects methemoglobinemia, then a direct measurement of oxyhemoglobin by a cooximeter blood gas analysis is required. A conventional pulse oximeter can neither detect MetHb nor accurately determine SpO_2 when MetHb is present. A cooximeter uses four different wavelengths of light and four species of hemoglobin are quantified; these four are oxygenated Hb, reduced Hb, MetHb, and COHb. The oxyhemoglobin saturation is then the percentage of HbO_2 of all the species determined to be present.

14. **What is the treatment for methemoglobinemia?**
In severe methemoglobinemia, the treatment consists of intravenous methylene blue, increasing the fraction of inspired oxygen to 100%, removing the offending agent, and providing hemodynamic support. Methylene blue acts as a cofactor to speed up the enzymatic reaction that reduces Fe_3^+ to Fe_2^+ (methemoglobin reductase.)
Give 1 to 2 mg/kg over 5 minutes. Dose may be repeated in an hour to a maximum of 7 mg/kg. Methylene blue should not be used in patients with glucose-6-phosphate deficiency (G6PD), hemolytic anemia may result. In patients with G6PD, ascorbic acid can be used to treat methemoglobinemia.

15. **The saturation plummets after injection of methylene blue. Is the patient desaturating?**
No, methylene blue is sufficiently dark and may deceive the pulse oximeter, resulting in a transiently depressed reading.

16. **Does a pulse oximeter reading of 100% indicate complete denitrogenation during preoxygenation?**
Replacing all alveolar nitrogen with oxygen provides a depot (functional reserve capacity) of oxygen that might be needed if mask ventilation or intubation proves difficult. Although hemoglobin may be completely saturated with oxygen during preoxygenation, an SpO_2 reading of 100% in and of itself is not an accurate indication of complete pulmonary denitrogenation.

17. **Is the pulse oximeter a good indicator of ventilation?**
A pulse oximeter gives no indication of ventilation, only oxygenation. For instance, a breathing patient may have an oxygen mask delivering 50% oxygen and an SpO_2 reading in the 90s yet be hypoventilating and hypercapnic. In this situation, the oximeter reading may give a false sense of security. A better approach would be to administer less oxygen, and, as the pulse oximeter values decrease below 90%, arouse the patient from sleep, encourage him or her to breathe deeply, and elevate the head of the patient's bed, rather than just increasing the delivered oxygen concentration more.

18. **Are there complications associated with the use of pulse oximetry probes?**
Pressure necrosis of the skin has been reported in both neonates and adults when the probe has been left on the same digit for prolonged periods of time. Digital burns from the LEDs have been reported in patients undergoing photodynamic therapy.

19. How is the pulse oximeter waveform used to determine fluid responsiveness?

Arterial pulse volume will vary during the inspiratory and expiratory phases of the respiratory cycle. This variation is exaggerated when preload is inadequate, which is usually a result of hypovolemia. Respiratory variations in the pulse oximetry plethysmographic waveform amplitude may predict fluid responsiveness in these patients, when they are mechanically ventilated, and can serve as a useful tool in the assessment of volume status.

KEY POINTS: PULSE OXIMETRY

1. Use of pulse oximetry has allowed anesthesiologists to rapidly detect and treat acute decreases in oxygen saturation.
2. As with all monitors, understanding both the methods of operation and the limitations of pulse oximeters is critical to the delivery of safe care. Pulse oximeters can give falsely high and low numbers; it is important to understand the reasons why this is so.
3. Oxygenation and ventilation are separate processes, and pulse oximetry does not assess the adequacy of ventilation.

SUGGESTED READINGS

Barker S. Motion-resistant pulse oximetry: a comparison of new and old models. Anesth Analg. 2002;95:967–972.

Cannesson M, Attof Y, Rosamel P, et al. Respiratory variations in pulse oximetry plethysmographic waveform amplitude to predict fluid responsiveness in the operating room. Anesthesiology. 2007;106(6):1105–1111.

Jubran A. Pulse oximetry. Crit Care. 2015;19(1):272.

Moyle J. Pulse Oximetry. 2nd ed. London: BMJ Publishing Group; 2002.

Pedersen T, Moller AM, Pedersen BD. Pulse oximetry for perioperative monitoring: systematic review of randomized, controlled trials. Anesth Analg. 2003;96:426–431.

CHAPTER 21

CAPNOGRAPHY

Nick Schiavoni, MD, Martin Krause, MD

1. **What is capnometry?**
   Capnometry is a monitor which detects and measures expired carbon dioxide (CO_2). Capnometry can be qualitative where the device changes color when CO_2 is detected, or quantitative where the device measures the expired CO_2 concentration. The capnogram is a waveform tracing of the quantified CO_2 concentration over time. Interpreting the capnography waveform can be helpful with troubleshooting equipment problems and assessing the patient's physiology.

2. **Describe the most common method of gas sampling/analysis and the associated problems.**
   Sidestream capnography devices aspirate gas (typically 50–250 mL/min), usually from the Y-piece of the circuit, and transport the gas via a small-bore tubing to the analyzer by suction. Sampling can also be performed from a nasal cannula; however, because of room air entrainment causing dilution of the CO_2 concentration, sampling directly from the circuit in an intubated patient provides qualitatively and quantitatively a better sample than nasal cannula. Problems with CO_2 measurement include a finite delay, until the results of the gas sample are displayed and possible clogging of the tubing with condensed water vapor or mucus. Infrared spectrography is the most common method of CO_2 analysis. Because CO_2 absorbs infrared radiation at a specific wavelength (4.25 μm), Beer's law can be used to calculate the CO_2 concentration by measuring the amount of radiation absorbed at this specific wavelength.

3. **Why is measuring end-tidal carbon dioxide important?**
   Measuring end-tidal carbon dioxide ($ETCO_2$) is an important standard of American Society of Anesthetists monitoring. Short of bronchoscopy, CO_2 monitoring is considered the best method to verify correct endotracheal tube (ETT) placement. $ETCO_2$ is dependent upon many important physiological processes, such as metabolic activity, cardiac output, and ventilation. It is often used to assess the following:
   - ETT placement
   - Respiratory ventilation
   - Cardiac output
   - Hypermetabolism (e.g., malignant hyperthermia)

4. **How well does $ETCO_2$ correlate with $PaCO_2$?**
   Because CO_2 can easily diffuse between blood and alveoli approximately 20 times faster than oxygen (O_2), alveolar CO_2 (partial pressure of carbon dioxide [$PACO_2$]) readily reaches equilibrium with blood CO_2 at the level of the alveoli. Recall, O_2 gas exchange at the alveoli is primarily diffusion dependent, whereas CO_2 is perfusion dependent. Therefore the $PACO_2$ in a poorly or nonperfused alveolus (i.e., alveolar dead space) will not reach equilibrium with blood CO_2 in the pulmonary vascular bed. In healthy lungs, this alveolar dead space will dilute expired CO_2, causing a small 3 to 5 mm Hg drop in $ETCO_2$, compared with arterial blood CO_2 ($PaCO_2$). It is important to emphasize that any process which increases alveolar dead space (i.e., asthma, chronic obstructive pulmonary disease [COPD], pulmonary embolism, cardiac arrest) will cause a "drop in $ETCO_2$" and a wider gradient between $PaCO_2$ and $ETCO_2$.

5. **How can $ETCO_2$ be used to assess cardiac output?**
   Because CO_2 is perfusion dependent, anything that decreases perfusion will decrease $ETCO_2$. Stated another way, well-perfused and well-ventilated alveoli have a ventilation/perfusion ($V/\dot{Q} = 1$) and alveolar dead space occurs when ventilation exceeds perfusion ($V/\dot{Q} > 1$), such as in zone 1 of the lung or in diseases processes, such as COPD or asthma. However, decreased perfusion ($\dot{Q}$) can also cause $V/\dot{Q}$ greater than 1, assuming no change in ventilation (V). Therefore any condition associated with decreased cardiac output, such as pulmonary embolism or cardiac arrest, will also cause an increase in alveolar dead space ($V/\dot{Q} > 1$) and a "drop in $ETCO_2$."

6. **How can $ETCO_2$ be helpful in resuscitation for cardiac arrest?**
   As an indirect measurement of cardiac output, $ETCO_2$ levels can be extremely valuable in performing advanced cardiac life support (ACLS). Studies show that high quality chest compressions during cardiopulmonary resuscitation (CPR) can generate a cardiac index of 1.6 to 1.9 L/min/m^2, which correlates to an $ETCO_2$ greater than 20 mm Hg. Other studies have also found that an $ETCO_2$ level of less than 10 mm Hg, after 20 minutes of ACLS, was 100% predictive of failure to resuscitate. As a result, the American Heart Association Guidelines for ACLS recommend quantitative capnometry in all intubated patients undergoing CPR and to target high quality chest compressions to an $ETCO_2$ of at least 10 to 20 mm Hg.

7. **Is it possible to detect exhaled CO_2 after accidental intubation of the esophagus?**
   Yes. Positive pressure ventilation by face mask can result in oropharyngeal air (containing CO_2) to be driven into the esophagus and stomach. In addition, carbonated beverages, certain antacids (i.e., Alka Seltzer, Maalox), and even swallowing exhaled CO_2, while eating or drinking, can result in CO_2 in the stomach. However, the $ETCO_2$ detected upon esophageal intubation is typically less than 10 mm Hg and decreases with each exhaled breath.

8. **What is the most important aspect in using $ETCO_2$ to confirm endotracheal intubation?**
   Because CO_2 can initially be detected on esophageal intubation, it is critical to look for sustained $ETCO_2$ to confirm endotracheal intubation.

9. **Describe the capnography waveform.**
   The important features include baseline level, the extent and rate of rise of CO_2, and the contour of the capnograph. There are four distinct phases to a capnogram (Fig. 21.1). The first phase (A–B) is when the initial stage of exhalation occurs, and the gas sampled is dead space gas and free of CO_2. At point B, there is mixing of alveolar gas with dead space gas, and the CO_2 level abruptly rises. The expiratory or alveolar plateau is represented by phase C–D, and the gas sampled is essentially alveolar. Point D is the maximal CO_2 level, the best reflection of alveolar CO_2, and is known as $ETCO_2$. Fresh gas is entrained as the patient inspires (phase D–E), and the trace returns to the baseline level of CO_2, approximately zero.

10. **What can cause elevation of the baseline capnography waveform?**
    The $ETCO_2$ should return to 0 mm Hg on inspiration. If the baseline CO_2 does not return to zero, the patient is receiving CO_2 during inspiration. This is often termed *rebreathing* (Fig. 21.2). Possible causes of rebreathing include the following:
    - An exhausted CO_2 absorber
    - An incompetent unidirectional inspiratory or expiratory valve

11. **What might result in a sudden complete loss of the capnography waveform?**
    A sudden loss of the capnographic waveform (Fig. 21.3) can be caused by the following:
    - Esophageal intubation
    - Severe bronchospasm

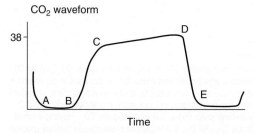

Fig. 21.1 The capnographic waveform. *A–B,* Exhalation of carbon dioxide (*CO_2*) free gas from dead space; *B–C,* combination of dead space and alveolar gas; *C–D,* exhalation of mostly alveolar gas; *D,* end-tidal point (alveolar plateau); *D–E,* inhalation of CO_2 free gas.

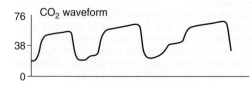

Fig. 21.2 Rebreathing of carbon dioxide (*CO_2*) as demonstrated by failure of the waveform to return to a zero baseline.

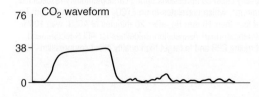

Fig. 21.3 A sudden drop of end-tidal carbon dioxide ($ETCO_2$) to near zero may indicate a loss of ventilation or catastrophic decreases in cardiac output.

- Ventilator disconnection or malfunction
- Capnographic disconnection or malfunction
- Obstructed ETT
- Catastrophic physiological disturbance, such as cardiac arrest or a massive pulmonary embolism

12. **What would cause a decrease in the capnography waveform?**
   A decrease in $ETCO_2$ (Fig. 21.4) can be caused by the following:
   - Hyperventilation
   - Mild or moderate bronchospasm
   - Decreased cardiac output
   - ETT cuff leak

13. **What would cause an increase in the capnography waveform?**
   An increase in $ETCO_2$ (Fig. 21.5) can be caused by the following:
   - Hypoventilation
   - Rebreathing of CO_2
   - Iatrogenic administration of CO_2 (e.g., CO_2 absorption from laparoscopy)
   - Bicarbonate administration
   - Tourniquet release
   - Sepsis and other hypermetabolic conditions (fever, malignant hyperthermia, thyroid storm)

14. **How would obstructive lung disease affect the capnography waveform?**
   Obstructive lung disease, such as asthma and COPD, can cause the $ETCO_2$ waveform to resemble a "shark-fin-like" morphology with a delayed upslope (Fig. 21.6). This is contrast to a normal $ETCO_2$ waveform, which is usually a square wave. Because obstructive lung disease pathology is characterized by an increase in alveolar dead space ($V/\dot{Q} > 1$), the $ETCO_2$ will be low and the gradient between $ETCO_2$ and $PaCO_2$ will be larger than the typical 3 to 5 mm Hg.

15. **What is a "curare-cleft" in the capnography waveform?**
   Spontaneous patient breathing often causes a characteristic "curare-cleft" in the $ETCO_2$ waveform. This occurs when the patient is attempting to inspire during expiration (Fig. 21.7).

Fig. 21.4 A gradual lowering of end-tidal carbon dioxide ($ETCO_2$) indicates hyperventilation, decreased CO_2 production, or decreased cardiac output.

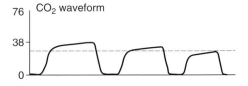

Fig. 21.5 A rising end-tidal carbon dioxide ($ETCO_2$) is associated with hypoventilation, increasing carbon dioxide (CO_2) production, and absorption of CO_2 from an exogenous source, such as CO_2 laparoscopy.

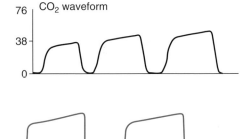

Fig. 21.6 A steep upslope suggests obstructive lung disease.

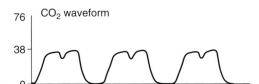

Fig. 21.7 A cleft in the alveolar plateau usually indicates partial recovery from neuromuscular blockade. Surgical manipulation against the inferior surface of the diaphragm or weight on the chest may produce similar, yet irregular, waveforms.

KEY POINTS: CAPNOGRAPHY

1. Sustained $ETCO_2$ detection should be used to confirm proper ETT placement on intubation.
2. In the absence of ventilation-perfusion abnormalities, $ETCO_2$ is approximately 3 to 5 mm Hg less than $PaCO_2$.
3. Abrupt decreases in cardiac output will cause a "drop in $ETCO_2$."
4. Analysis of the capnographic waveform provides supportive evidence for numerous clinical conditions, including decreasing cardiac output; altered metabolic activity; acute and chronic pulmonary disease; and ventilator, circuit, or ETT problems.

SUGGESTED READINGS

American Society of Anesthesiologists. Standards for Basic Anesthetic Monitoring. 2015. Retrieved from https://www.asahq.org/standards-and-guidelines/standards-for-basic-anesthetic-monitoring.

Chitilian H, Kaczka D, Vidal Melo M. Respiratory monitoring. In: Miller RD, ed. Miller's Anesthesia. 8th ed. Philadelphia: Elsevier Saunders; 2015:1541–1579.

Link MS, Berkow LC, Kudenchuk PJ, et al. Part 7: Adult advanced cardiovascular life support. Circulation. 2015;132:S444–S464.

CHAPTER 22

BLOOD PRESSURE MONITORING AND ARTERIAL CATHETERIZATION

Jessica L. Nelson, MD, Tim T. Tran, MD, Ryan D. Laterza, MD

1. **What methods are available to measure blood pressure?**
   Blood pressure (BP) measurements can be divided into direct and indirect methods. Indirect methods include using a cuff or palpation of a pulse, whereas direct methods use an arterial catheter. The most common indirect or noninvasive BP (NIBP) measurement uses a BP cuff, usually on the arm over the brachial artery. An NIBP can be measured using either a stethoscope, listening for Korotkoff sounds (manual method), or by using an oscillometer (automated method). Direct or invasive BP (IBP) monitoring requires the use of a catheter placed into a central or peripheral artery.

2. **How can palpation of a pulse be used to measure blood pressure?**
   Palpation of pulse can also be used in an emergent situation but is not an accurate method. The traditional teaching relies on the 60/70/80 rule, which suggests a minimum systolic BP that is necessary to palpate a pulse based on anatomic location (60 mm Hg for carotid, 70 mm Hg for femoral, and 80 mm Hg for radial). Unsurprisingly, studies show this method does not correlate well with direct measurements. Regardless, these same studies also show that in cardiac arrest, pulses are consistently lost in the following order (radial > femoral > carotid).

3. **How does an oscillometric blood pressure cuff determine blood pressure? Which blood pressure parameters (i.e., systolic, diastolic, mean) are calculated versus measured?**
   The oscillometric (automated) BP measurement is the most common method to measure BP in a hospital setting. It is classified as an indirect or NIBP that works by measuring mean arterial pressure (MAP) and calculating systolic and diastolic BPs. The BP cuff first inflates to a pressure greater than systolic BP. Then it slowly "bleeds" air and, as the cuff pressure approaches MAP, oscillations caused by the pulse are transmitted to the cuff and measured. The oscillations increase in amplitude as the cuff pressure gets closer and closer to MAP. The oscillations are the greatest in amplitude when the cuff pressure equals MAP. As the cuff pressure decreases below MAP, the oscillations become smaller and smaller in amplitude, until they disappear. The cuff pressure corresponding to when oscillations are greatest in amplitude is recorded as MAP.
   Manufacturers have various proprietary methods to calculate systolic and diastolic BP from the MAP measured by the cuff. For example, a common method is to calculate the systolic BP where the ascending slope of the oscillations is maximal or when the ascending oscillations are 50% of the maximum oscillation amplitude. The diastolic pressure is then calculated using the systolic pressure and MAP.

4. **How can an oscillometric NIBP calculate diastolic blood pressure using MAP and systolic blood pressure?**
   Once the MAP and systolic BP are known, the diastolic BP can be calculated using the following equation and solving for diastolic BP:

$$MAP = \frac{sBP + 2 \times dBP}{3}$$

MAP, mean arterial pressure; sBP, systolic blood pressure; dBP, diastolic blood pressure

5. **How do NIBP measurements differ when obtained from auscultation of Korotkoff sounds (manual) versus the oscillometric method (automated)?**
   Auscultation (manual) NIBP measurements rely on Korotkoff sounds caused by turbulent flow that correspond to systolic and diastolic BP. The cuff is inflated above systolic BP and slowly bled. Using a stethoscope, the first Korotkoff sounds correspond to the systolic BP. The cuff is continuously bled more, and the Korotkoff sounds disappear at the diastolic BP. Therefore auscultation NIBP measures systolic and diastolic BP and MAP would need to be calculated. In contrast, oscillometric NIBP measures MAP and calculates systolic and diastolic BPs. Auscultation NIBP measurement is subject to interobserver variability, which is not the case for oscillometric NIBP.

6. **What are the indications for invasive arterial blood pressure monitoring (i.e., arterial line)?**
   - Cardiovascular instability
   - Need for continuous infusions of titratable medications (i.e., vasopressors or antihypertensive agents)

147

- Clinical situations at risk for significant blood loss or fluid shifts, such as intracranial, vascular, or thoracic surgery
- Preexisting cardiovascular disease, such as severe heart failure or valvular heart disease
- Concerns that NIBP monitoring may be inaccurate, as in patients with morbid obesity, atherosclerosis, and essential tremor
- Need for frequent blood samples (e.g., arterial blood gases)

7. **What anatomic locations are available for direct or invasive blood pressure measurement?**
   IBP monitoring can be divided into peripheral and central locations. Peripheral anatomic locations include radial, brachial, and dorsalis pedis arteries, whereas central anatomic locations include axillary and femoral arteries.

8. **What does it mean to level and zero a transducer? Are they the same thing?**
   Leveling and zeroing a transducer are separate processes that are often completed at the same time. Zeroing or calibrating a transducer involves opening the stopcock on the transducer to atmospheric pressure and selecting "zero" on the monitor. This sets the atmospheric pressure as the reference point to 0 mm Hg, which implies that BP measurements will be relative not absolute to atmospheric pressure. Leveling involves setting the vertical position of the transducer with respect to what it is supposed to measure. For example, in the supine position, the transducer is generally leveled at around 5 cm posterior to the sternum (i.e., mid-axillary) to approximate aortic root pressure (arterial line) or right atrial pressure (central venous pressure). While in the sitting position, the arterial line transducer is often leveled to the external auditory meatus to approximate BP within the circle of Willis.

9. **What would happen to the blood pressure if the transducer is inadvertently positioned above or below the patient?**
   If the transducer is vertically positioned above the patient, the patient's measured BP would be falsely decreased. If the transducer is vertically positioned below the patient, the patient's measured BP would be falsely elevated.

10. **If the patient's true MAP is 100 mm Hg and the transducer is lowered 10 cm below the patient, what would the invasive blood pressure now display as the MAP? Why?**
    The relationship between cm H_2O and mm Hg is approximately 10:7. Therefore the displayed MAP is approximately 107 mm Hg. This is because mercury (Hg) is approximately 13.6 times denser than water (H_2O), and the catheter tubing of the arterial line contains normal saline (which is approximately the same density as H_2O). In other words, a 13.6 cm column of H_2O would exert a pressure that is equivalent to a 1 cm column of Hg (or 10 mm Hg), which has an approximate ratio of 10:7.

11. **What are reasons for discrepancies between noninvasive and invasive blood pressure monitoring?**
    Causes of error with NIBP measurements include inappropriate cuff size and positioning, patient obesity, and decreased peripheral blood flow (e.g., septic shock or subclavian artery stenosis). Errors with IBP monitoring can be caused by a problem within the system (e.g., kink in the catheter or tubing, poor calibration, or air in the tubing) or certain patient characteristics (e.g., hypothermia, arterial spasm, subclavian artery stenosis). In practice, the most common cause for BP differences between IBP and NIBP monitoring is an incorrectly leveled transducer.

12. **What is the most common cause for discrepancies between left and right arm blood pressure?**
    Subclavian artery stenosis, arising from peripheral vascular disease (e.g., atherosclerosis), is the most common reason for BP discrepancies. Other causes include aortic dissection, congenital cardiac disease, and unilateral neuromuscular abnormalities. Patients with subclavian artery stenosis often have other cardiovascular diseases, such as coronary artery disease and carotid artery stenosis.

13. **Which is the most accurate blood pressure parameter: systolic, diastolic, or mean arterial pressure? Why?**
    The MAP is the most accurate parameter for both indirect and direct methods of BP measurement.
    The oscillometric NIBP measures MAP and calculates systolic and diastolic BP using proprietary, empirically derived algorithms. Therefore MAP is likely the most accurate NIBP parameter because it reflects a true measurement and is not empirically calculated. Direct, IBP measurements via an arterial line can overshoot or undershoot the systolic and diastolic BP because of overdamping and underdamping, which can lead to inaccurate measurements. MAP, however, is generally unaffected by overdamping and underdamping.

KEY POINTS: BLOOD PRESSURE MONITORING

1. Oscillometric (automated) NIBP measures MAP and calculates systolic and diastolic BP.
2. MAP is the most accurate BP parameter because it is measured with oscillometric NIBP methods and not calculated. MAP is also likely more accurate with direct, IBP monitoring because it is the least likely to be affected by underdamping or overdamping.
3. The relationship between cm H_2O and mm Hg is approximately 10:7.
4. BP discrepancies between left and right arms are most frequently caused by subclavian artery stenosis because of peripheral vascular disease.

14. Describe a typical arterial monitoring system setup.
    An arterial monitoring system consists of the following components: a catheter, tubing, and the transducer. The catheter is placed within the artery and connected to the transducer via noncompliant tubing filled with normal saline. The main role of the transducer is to convert a pressure signal into an electrical signal. The transducer contains a diaphragm that is attached to a circuit called a *Wheatstone bridge*. Pressure waves cause the diaphragm to move inwards and outwards (i.e., oscillate), causing the resistance of the circuit to change. Any changes in resistance will affect the voltage within the circuit, which is used as the electrical signal representing real-time arterial BP.

15. Describe the possible complications of invasive arterial monitoring.
    Complications of arterial catheterization are uncommon. Complications include distal ischemia, arterial thrombosis, hematoma formation, catheter-site infection, systemic infection, necrosis of the overlying skin, pseudoaneurysm, and blood loss caused by disconnection.

16. Explain how the normal blood supply to the hand enables radial artery cannulation.
    The ulnar and radial arteries supply the hand. These arteries anastomose via four arches in the hand and wrist (the superficial and deep palmar arches and the anterior and posterior carpal arches). Because of the dual arterial blood supply, either artery can supply the digits if the other is occluded and thereby avoid ischemic sequelae to the hand.

17. What is the Allen test?
    The Allen test is a physical examination to assess adequacy of collateral circulation to the hand through the ulnar artery, in case of radial artery injury or thrombosis. To perform the test, the clinician applies pressure to both the radial and ulnar artery simultaneously to occlude each artery. The patient then pumps his or her hand to facilitate venous drainage of blood. The clinician then releases pressure from the ulnar artery and looks for color change in the hand to assess perfusion.

18. Is the Allen test an adequate predictor of ischemic complications?
    Evidence does not support the routine use of the Allen test to predict arterial ischemic complications from radial artery cannulation.

19. What sterile precautions are required for arterial line placement?
    For peripheral arterial catheter placement, the Centers for Disease Control and Prevention recommends that an antiseptic, cap, mask, sterile gloves, and small fenestrated drape be used. Maximal sterile barrier precautions should be added for central (femoral and axillary) artery catherization, including a gown and full-body drape.

20. Identify the risks and benefits of each peripheral arterial cannulation site.
    In terms of peripheral sites, cannulation of the radial artery is the most common, given its safety profile and provider familiarity. The ulnar artery may be cannulated if the radial artery provides adequate collateral flow, but it should be avoided if there have been multiple attempts to cannulate the radial artery on the same side. The brachial artery is an end-artery with no collateral flow and has a theoretical risk of ischemic complications with cannulation. However, studies show few complications with brachial artery cannulation and it is a reasonable option if other sites are not available. The dorsalis pedis and posterior tibial sites are also possible cannulation sites but limit patient mobility and are less commonly used. Peripheral arterial sites all carry the benefit of easy compressibility in the event of bleeding or hematoma formation.

21. How does a central arterial waveform differ from a peripheral arterial waveform?
    When the arterial pressure is transmitted from the central arteries to the peripheral arteries, the waveform is distorted (Fig. 22.1). Transmission is delayed, high-frequency components, such as the dicrotic notch, are lost, the systolic peak increases, and the diastolic trough decreases (i.e., increase in pulse pressure). This is known as *distal pulse amplification*. The changes in systolic and diastolic pressures result from a decrease in the arterial wall compliance and from resonance (the addition of reflected waves to the arterial waveform as it travels distally in the arterial tree). Evidence is mixed regarding the consistency between central and peripheral arterial pressure measurements, but some studies have suggested that central cannulation may be preferred for better accuracy in certain subgroups of patients (e.g., those on high-dose vasopressors). Although the systolic and diastolic BP may be different, the MAP is likely to be consistent, regardless of central or peripheral cannulation.

22. What information can be obtained from an arterial waveform?
    - Rhythm: real time waveform analysis can demonstrate dysrhythmias and electromechanical dissociation (e.g., premature ventricular contractions or pulseless electrical activity)
    - Stroke volume: the area under of the curve between systole and diastole is proportionate to stroke volume
    - Hypovolemia: a large variability in pulse pressure or systolic pressure caused by positive pressure ventilation is a reliable indicator of hypovolemia.

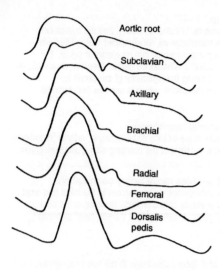

Fig. 22.1 Configuration of the arterial waveform at various sites in the arterial tree. (From Blitt CD, Hines RL. Monitoring in Anesthesia and Critical Care Medicine. 3rd ed. New York: Churchill Livingstone; 1995. With permission.)

23. What are some of the unique problems with invasive blood pressure monitoring equipment that can cause inaccurate measurements?

IBP monitoring is susceptible to inaccurate systolic and diastolic BP measurements because of problems with the damping and natural frequency of the arterial monitoring system (catheter + tubing + fluid + transducer). For example, in an "underdamped" arterial line, the recorded systolic BP will overshoot the true systolic BP and undershoot the true diastolic pressure, causing an elevated pulse pressure because of ringing or oscillations. Conversely, an "overdamped" arterial line may undershoot the systolic BP and overshoot the diastolic BP, causing a narrowed pulse pressure. It is important to emphasize that the MAP is generally unaffected by "overdamped" or "underdamped" arterial waveforms.

24. Define the term *natural frequency*.

The term *natural frequency* (f_n) is the frequency at which a system will naturally oscillate, based upon the physical characteristics of that system. For example, a short guitar string under high tension will naturally oscillate at a higher natural frequency than a long guitar string under low tension. Natural frequency for an arterial monitoring system can be defined by the following equation:

$$f_n = \left(\frac{1}{2\pi}\right)\sqrt{\frac{\pi r^2}{LC}}$$

Natural frequency equation
f_n, natural frequency; L, length; r, radius; C, compliance

The length, radius, and compliance pertain primarily to the catheter and tubing of the arterial monitoring system. Studies show that most arterial monitoring systems have a natural frequency of approximately 15 Hz.

25. Define the term *damping*.

Damping (ζ) is a measurement which reflects the system's resistance to oscillation. In other words, systems that contain high damping will resist oscillating, whereas systems that have no damping will oscillate indefinitely. For example, a guitar string will eventually stop oscillating because of forces that resist oscillation (i.e., damping), such as friction because of air (external resistance), friction between filaments within the string, and other intermolecular forces (internal resistance). Damping for arterial monitoring systems can be defined by the following equation:

$$\zeta = \left(\frac{4\mu}{r^3}\right)\sqrt{\frac{LC}{\pi}}$$

Damping equation
ζ, damping; μ, viscosity; r, radius; L, length; C, compliance

Note that both the damping and natural frequency equations assume density (0.9% normal saline) ≈ 1 (g/mL).

26. What is the fundamental frequency of an arterial waveform?

An arterial waveform can be broken down into the summation of multiple waveforms with various frequencies (i.e., Fourier transform) starting with the fundamental frequency (i.e., first harmonic). The arterial waveform can be reconstructed with reasonable accuracy using only the first eight harmonics. For example, a heart rate of 60 beats per minute can mathematically be described as a sine wave with a frequency of 1 Hz (1 beat or cycle per second). This is the lowest frequency of the arterial waveform and is called the *fundamental frequency* or *first harmonic*. Each following harmonic is a multiple of the fundamental frequency, so the second harmonic would contain the 2 Hz component of the arterial waveform and so on. To reconstruct the arterial waveform with reasonable accuracy, eight harmonics are necessary. This implies that the displayed arterial waveform, assuming a heart rate of 60 beats per minute, will contain a frequency spectrum up to 8 Hz (1 Hz × 8). However, to properly display and measure higher heart rates, most arterial monitors will need to accommodate heart rates up to 180 beats per minute (60 beats per minute × 3). Monitors will therefore need to process and display a waveform that contains a frequency spectrum up to 24 Hz (8 Hz × 3).

27. **What does all this mean?**
The natural frequency of the arterial monitoring system (catheter + tubing + normal saline + transducer) is around 15 Hz, whereas an arterial waveform may contain frequency components up to 24 Hz. As a result, some energy will be transferred from the input signal (pressure in the radial artery) to the arterial monitoring system (tubing and transducer), causing the latter to resonate at its natural frequency of 15 Hz. This occurs when frequencies from the arterial pressure wave contain frequencies that are equal to or near the natural frequency of the arterial monitoring system. Consequently, most arterial pressure monitoring systems at baseline are "underdamped" in that they all have some level of oscillation causing distortion of the systolic and diastolic waveform and pressure readings. Damping, which is the resistance of a system to oscillate, will minimize these oscillations from significantly distorting the arterial waveform and maintain reasonable waveform fidelity. In theory, if the arterial system was designed, such that its fundamental frequency was much higher than the frequency components of the arterial pressure waveform itself, such oscillations would not occur.

28. **Would a kink in the arterial catheter or tubing cause an underdamped or overdamped arterial waveform?**
It will cause an overdamped waveform. One of the most common problems in clinical practice are kinks or blood clots in the arterial catheter that effectively reduce the radius of the catheter. Although a reduced radius will cause the arterial monitoring system to have a lower fundamental frequency promoting oscillations (i.e., underdamped waveform), it has a greater effect on increasing damping as radius is raised to the third power (see dampening and fundamental frequency equations). Therefore small kinks or blot clots in the arterial system can have a large effect in distorting waveform fidelity because of overdamping.

29. **What are the problems with air bubbles in the arterial system tubing? Why is it important that the catheter tubing is well primed with normal saline to minimize air bubbles?**
The first and most obvious problem is air embolism. Because the hand has collateral flow with the ulnar and radial arteries, ischemic complications from an air embolism are uncommon. However, some patients will have inadequate collateral flow and may be at risk.
     The other problem is the complex effects air has on the fundamental frequency and damping of the arterial monitoring system. Because air is compressible (as opposed to liquid, which is not compressible), air will increase compliance of the arterial monitoring system. This will increase the system's damping but will also decrease the system's fundamental frequency (see dampening and fundamental frequency equations). Therefore both "overdamped" and "underdamped" arterial waveforms could occur depending upon the other variables (i.e., radius or resistance, catheter tubing compliance, heart rate). In summary, regardless of whether the arterial waveform is "underdamped" or "overdamped," air in the arterial system tubing could cause either and consequently distort the fidelity of the arterial waveform.

30. **Why is noncompliant (i.e., stiff) tubing used for arterial lines?**
Arterial monitoring systems generally use noncompliant tubing. If compliant tubing is used (e.g., intravenous fluid extension tubing), the compliance of the system will increase causing damping to increase, while also decreasing the natural frequency of the system (see damping and fundamental frequency equations). Increasing the system's damping will cause "overdamped" waveforms, whereas decreasing the systems natural frequency will cause "underdamped" waveforms. Therefore noncompliant tubing prevents these problems from occurring and better maintains arterial waveform fidelity.

31. **How do you determine if the arterial monitoring system is "overdamped" or "underdamped"?**
Pulling back the plunger and releasing it (i.e., fast-flush test) will send an impulse into the arterial system that causes it to resonate at its natural frequency. Most arterial BP systems are slightly "underdamped" and will have some oscillations, which is normal. In general, a system is "underdamped" if there are greater than 2 oscillations, "adequately damped" if there are 1 to 2 oscillations and is "overdamped" if there are no oscillations (Fig. 22.2).

32. **What are possible causes of "overdamped" and "underdamped" arterial monitoring systems?**
Causes of "overdamping" include: air bubbles, loose connections, kinks in the catheter or tubing, blood clots, arterial spasm, tubing that is too long or short.
     Causing of "underdamping" include: air bubbles, catheter whip or artifact, hypothermia, tachycardia, tubing that is too long or short.

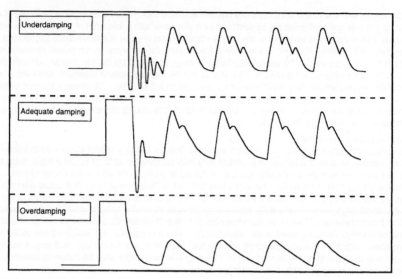

Fig. 22.2 Underdamped, adequately damped, and overdamped arterial pressure tracings after a high pressure or "fast-flush" test.

Note how air bubbles and tubing that is too short or too long can cause either (see damping and fundamental frequency equations). Also note how tachycardia can cause "underdamping." This is attributed to the higher frequency spectrum of arterial waveforms at higher heart rates.

33. **Are there any risks associated with flushing the catheter system?**
    On occasion, arterial catheter systems are flushed to improve the quality of the arterial waveform. Retrograde embolization of air or thrombus into the cerebral vasculature is a theoretical risk. Despite this concern, adverse neurological events associated with arterial cannulation are extremely rare and remain anecdotal.

KEY POINTS: ARTERIAL CATHETERIZATION

1. Evidence does not support the routine use of the Allen test to minimize ischemic complications related to arterial line placement.
2. Peripherally measured arterial waveforms are amplified in comparison to centrally measured arterial waveforms, demonstrating higher systolic pressures and lower diastolic pressures. MAP, however, should be approximately the same.
3. Peripherally measured arterial pressures may be less accurate compared with centrally measured arterial pressures in patients with poor distal perfusion (e.g., severe shock, severe hypothermia, high-dose vasopressors).
4. "Overdamped" waveforms undershoot systolic BP and overshoot diastolic BP, whereas "underdamped" waveforms are the converse.
5. "Underdamped" waveforms are caused by either decreased damping or because the natural frequency of the arterial monitoring system overlaps with the frequency spectrum of the arterial waveform itself.
6. The MAP is the least likely BP parameter to be affected by "overdamped" and "underdamped" waveforms.

Suggested Readings

Brzezinski M, Luisetti T, London MJ. Radial artery cannulation: a comprehensive review of recent anatomic and physiologic investigations. Anesth Analg. 2009;109:1763–1781.

Handlogten KS, Wilson GA, Clifford L, et al. Brachial artery catheterization: an assessment of use patterns and associated complications. Anesth Analg. 2014;118:288–295.

Kim WY, Jun JH, Huh JW, et al. Radial to femoral arterial blood pressure differences in septic shock patients receiving high-dose norepinephrine therapy. Shock. 2013;40:527–531.

Kleinman B. Understanding natural frequency and damping and how they relate to the measurement of blood pressure. J Clin Monit. 1989;5(2):137–147.

Meidert AS, Saugel B. Techniques for non-invasive monitoring of arterial blood pressure. Front Med. 2018;4:231.

CHAPTER 23

CENTRAL VENOUS CATHETERIZATION

Ryan D. Laterza, MD, Thomas Scupp, MD, Samuel Gilliland, MD

1. **Define central venous catheterization.**
   A central venous catheter (CVC) or central line is a catheter that is placed into a large vein such that the catheter's distal orifice is within a central vein. The target central vein for CVCs placed in the internal jugular (IJ) or subclavian is the superior vena cava (SVC), and for the femoral vein, the inferior vena cava (IVC). Please see Fig. 23.1.

2. **What are perioperative indications for placement of a central venous catheter?**
   - Intravenous (IV) access when peripheral access is insufficient or difficult
   - Volume resuscitation (e.g., massive transfusion of blood products)
   - Evaluating cardiac function
   - Drug infusion (e.g., vasopressors)
   - Placement of a pulmonary artery catheter
   - Aspiration of air emboli
   - Frequent blood sampling for laboratory tests

3. **What are additional indications for placement of a central venous catheter?**
   - Placement of a transvenous pacemaker
   - Total parental nutrition
   - Hemodialysis
   - Long-term chemotherapy
   - Plasmapheresis

4. **What are contraindications to central venous cannulation?**
   - Infection or obvious contamination of the site to be cannulated
   - Coagulopathy and choice of a noncompressible venous site (subclavian CVC)
   - Placement of an IJ or subclavian CVC in the setting of raised intracranial pressure (ICP) (Trendelenburg position contraindicated)
   - Thrombus in the vein to be cannulated
   - Patient intolerance

5. **Describe complications associated with placement of the central venous catheter.**
   All CVC placement sites
   - Arterial puncture, dilation, and/or arterial placement of CVC
   - Infection
   - Embolization of a catheter tip or guidewire
   - Air embolism
   - Deep vein thrombus (DVT)
   - Dysrhythmia
   - Extravascular catheter migration

   Internal jugular and subclavian CVC
   - Pneumothorax, particularly with a subclavian CVC, but also possible with an IJ CVC.
   - Hemothorax and bleeding, particularly with subclavian CVC
   - Thoracic duct injury when placing a left IJ CVC
   - Myocardial perforation and cardiac tamponade

   Femoral CVC
   - Retroperitoneal hemorrhage

   It is important to note that some access sites have higher rates of complications than others. For example, femoral CVCs have the highest rate of DVT complications, subclavian CVCs have the highest rate of pneumothorax and bleeding complications (site is noncompressible), and internal jugular CVC has a higher, albeit rare, risk of stroke and death because of cannulation of the carotid.

6. **What types of central venous catheters exist?**
   CVCs can be divided into four categories: nontunneled (e.g., triple lumen catheter or introducer sheath), peripherally inserted central catheters (PICC), tunneled (e.g., Hickman) and totally implantable (e.g., Portacath) (Table 23.1). Nontunneled catheters are by far the most common placed CVC in the perioperative period. Nontunneled catheters allow for quick central access but are more susceptible to infection and are less comfortable for patients

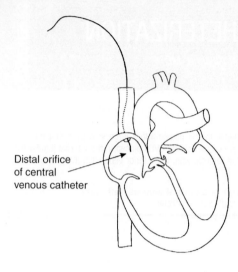

Distal orifice
of central
venous catheter

Fig. 23.1 Placement of a central venous catheter into the superior vena cava.

compared with tunneled, totally implantable catheters (e.g., Portacath®), or PICCs. Although PICCs are associated with less infection in the outpatient setting, PICCs placed in hospitalized patients have the same risk of infection and are associated with increased DVT compared with nontunneled CVCs.

7. Review the different types of nontunneled central venous catheters.
The vast majority of CVC placed in the perioperative domain are nontunneled catheters particularly: (1) multilumen catheters, and (2) introducer sheaths. Multilumen, nontunneled CVCs come in a variety of configurations and sizes. For example, a triple-lumen or quad-lumen catheter has three or four lumens, with orifices at slightly different positions on the distal cannula. This allows separate access to multiple ports on the CVC for simultaneous drug infusion, blood sampling, and central venous pressure (CVP) monitoring. As each port is a separate lumen, the maximum infusion rate will vary based on the diameter and length of that lumen. For example, a typical 7 French (Fr) triple lumen catheter (TLC) has two smaller 18G lumens and one larger 16G lumen. Some catheters are heparin-coated, chlorhexidine, antibiotic-coated lines or silver impregnated to help avoid thrombosis or infection.

Table 23.1 Types of Central Venous Catheters

TYPE OF LINE	INSERTION SITE	DURATION	EXAMPLES
Nontunneled (triple lumen catheter, introducer, hemodialysis catheter)	Internal jugular, subclavian, and femoral vein	Short term (days to weeks)	Difficult intravenous access, vasoactive agents, volume resuscitation, pulmonary artery catheterization, transvenous pacing, hemodialysis
Peripherally inserted central catheter (PICC)	Cephalic, basilic, and brachial veins	Medium term (weeks to months)	Total parenteral nutrition (TPN), chemotherapy, long-term antibiotics, long-term vasoactive agents
Tunneled catheter (e.g., Hickman®, Broviac®)	Internal jugular and subclavian vein	Long term (months to years)	Chemotherapy, hemodialysis
Totally implanted catheter (e.g., Portacath®, Mediport®)	Internal jugular and subclavian vein	Long term (months to years)	Chemotherapy

The other commonly placed nontunneled CVC is an introducer sheath. Introducer sheaths are primarily designed to "introduce" pulmonary artery catheters or transvenous pacing leads into the right heart. However, they are also commonly used for volume resuscitation, particularly in trauma patients and in liver transplant operations. Introducers are typically short- and large-bore (9–12 Fr) with a side-port that allows for infusions or CVP monitoring.

8. **What is the Seldinger technique?**
The Seldinger technique was first described by Dr. Sven-Ivar Seldinger, a radiologist from Sweden, in 1953. His technique allowed for placement of a flexible catheters into the lumen of a blood vessel. The Seldinger technique is often used for arterial and venous catheterization. Before his technique, vascular access for angiography procedures often required large rigid needles or surgical exposure (i.e., cutdown) to facilitate placement of a flexible catheter. His technique involves the following steps:
   1) Puncture the blood vessel with a needle
   2) Thread a guidewire through the needle into the blood vessel
   3) Remove the needle, while keeping the guidewire intravascular
   4) Dilate and thread a CVC over the guidewire into the vessel
   5) Remove the guidewire

9. **What is the modified Seldinger technique?**
Although the Seldinger technique is the traditional approach in placing a CVC, the modified Seldinger is an alternative method that has some unique advantages. The modified Seldinger method uses an angiocatheter as opposed to a straight needle to cannulate the vessel. Once the angiocatheter punctures the lumen of the vessel and blood return into the syringe is visualized, the proceduralist slides the catheter off the needle into the vessel. The proceduralist then uses the Seldinger technique using a guidewire to exchange the smaller catheter to a larger, central venous catheter.
   The modified Seldinger technique may require one extra step compared with the Seldinger technique; however, it is associated with a higher success rate of central venous cannulation. Another advantage of the modified Seldinger technique is that it facilitates manometry before dilating because connecting pressure tubing to a fixed, rigid needle (as opposed to a catheter) can be cumbersome. The modified Seldinger technique may prove difficult with subclavian access and patients with obesity. The clavicle may impede or distort the geometry of the angiocatheter in placing a subclavian CVC and redundant tissue from obesity may create a large distance between the vessel and the skin, preventing one from threading the angiocatheter into the vessel, particularly with the femoral vein.

10. **What are the basic steps in placing a central venous catheter?**
Before cannulation is attempted, various methods should be used to increase venous pressure at the target vessel. The most common method involves using the Trendelenburg position for the IJ and subclavian veins and reverse Trendelenburg position for the femoral veins. Other adjuncts, which may prove helpful, include increasing or doubling positive end expiratory pressure (PEEP) (e.g., PEEP of 10 cm H_2O) for patients intubated on mechanical ventilation. Increasing the target vein pressure with patient positioning and other adjuncts, such as PEEP, will increase the diameter of the vein, facilitating cannulation, and will reduce the risk of air embolism. As the needle is advanced toward the target vessel, gentle, continuous aspiration on the syringe is required. This allows blood to fill the syringe upon entering the blood vessel. Once the needle is within the lumen of the blood vessel, the Seldinger technique can be used to: (1) dilate the tissue creating a tract, and (2) place a CVC into the lumen of the vessel.

11. **Should a CVC be placed using ultrasound guidance or anatomic landmark?**
All CVCs should be placed with ultrasound guidance whenever possible. Ultrasound-guided CVC placement, compared with anatomic landmark technique, has been shown by numerous studies to be associated with significantly less complications, increased first attempt success rate, and reduced time to successful cannulation. Ultrasound-guided CVC placement is endorsed by several evidence-based national guidelines and is the standard for femoral and internal jugular CVC placement.

12. **How do you confirm venous access before dilation? Is blue blood enough?**
Arterial blood may be dark because the patient is hypoxemic, cardiac output is inadequate, or the patient may have methemoglobinemia. Pulsation of arterial blood may prove difficult to appreciate in patients who are hypotensive or in shock. The best way to confirm venous access before dilation and placement of a CVC is by manometry. This can be realized by threading a short, small-gauge catheter (e.g., 20G) into the vein over the guidewire (Seldinger technique) or directly into the vein using an angiocatheter (modified Seldinger technique). A short section of IV tubing is then connected to the catheter and the pressure measured. Although the pressure can be quantitatively measured by connecting the IV tubing to a transducer, most often, a qualitative measurement can easily be performed by allowing the IV tubing to fill with blood and holding the tubing vertically where the height of this column of blood reflects CVP. If the catheter is inadvertently placed in an artery, the height of the column of blood in

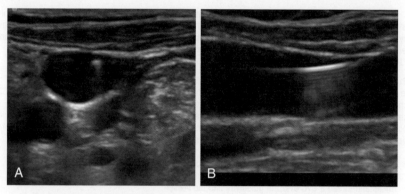

Fig. 23.2 Ultrasound image showing internal jugular guidewire in short (A) and long (B) axis views.

the IV tubing will reflect arterial pressure. Ultrasound can also be used as an adjunct to visualize the guidewire in the vein (Fig. 23.2). Other adjuncts include transesophageal echocardiography, which allows direct visualization of the wire tip in the SVC or right atrium.

13. **What are the shortcomings in only using ultrasound to confirm venous access of the guidewire before dilation?**
    Although ultrasound may be used to visualize the guidewire in the vein before dilation and placement of the CVC, it has limitations. In particular, the guidewire tip is difficult if not impossible to visualize with ultrasound, particularly if the guidewire is placed deep (e.g., 20 cm) into the venous circulation. Recall, the venous vasculature is highly compliant with a thin-walled tunica media. When attempting to puncture the lumen of the vessel with the finder needle, it is not uncommon for the anterior wall to invaginate and "kiss" the posterior wall of the vein. This may result in the needle traveling through and through the vein and possibly puncturing an underlying arterial vessel (i.e., carotid, brachiocephalic, or subclavian artery). If this were to occur and the proceduralists then threads the guidewire, the guidewire would transverse through and through the target vein, and the tip of the guidewire would reside within an arterial vessel. Ultrasound would show a wire located within a vein, but manometry would demonstrate arterial pressure.

14. **Where should the tip of the CVC be placed? What is the problem if the CVC is placed too deep or shallow?**
    The ideal placement for the tip of the CVC is thought to be at the cavoatrial junction, where the SVC meets the right atrium. Using a chest x-ray, this is approximately 3 to 5 cm below the carina. Whereas CVC tips placed in the distal one-third of the SVC or proximal right atrium is acceptable for clinical use, the distal tip may migrate ±2 cm with patient movement and/or respiration. Therefore the ideal placement is likely at the cavoatrial junction to allow safe tip migration with patient movement and/or respiration.
    Complications with shallow CVC tip placement (e.g., brachiocephalic or upper-third of the SVC) are venous thrombus and CVC malfunction. The complications of a distal CVC tip placed in the distal right atrium or right ventricle are dysrhythmias and cardiac tamponade. Although cardiac tamponade remains a rare devastating complication, this was thought to more likely occur in the past because of the more rigid CVCs, whereas most modern CVC are flexible and less likely to cause this complication.

15. **How deep should the CVC be threaded when placing a CVC?**
    When placing right sided CVC (right IJ or right subclavian), the catheter should generally be threaded 14 to 16 cm at the skin and left sided CVC (left IJ and left subclavian), the catheter threaded 16 to 20 cm. This is caused by the longer torturous path through the brachiocephalic vein for left-sided CVCs. In general, it is better to thread the catheter slightly deeper than necessary and confirm tip location with chest x-ray because a CVC can be pulled back, while respecting sterile technique but not advanced deeper.

16. **Is a chest x-ray required before using a CVC that is placed in the operating room?**
    All CVCs, except femoral CVCs, should have a chest x-ray to confirm proper tip location. A chest x-ray can also assess for pneumothorax and help confirm that the tip is not intraarterial, such as the carotid or subclavian artery or migrated up into the IJ vein, which can be seen with subclavian cannulation. Current American Society of Anesthesiology guidelines state a CVC can be used in the operating room following immediate placement, with the chest x-ray delayed until the postoperative period. Therefore in the perioperative setting, it is strongly encouraged that the clinician verifies IV placement with manometry, particularly if the CVC is used before chest x-ray confirmation.

17. You are attempting to cannulate the right internal jugular. In performing the procedure, you inadvertently go through and through the IJ into the carotid with the finder needle. Ultrasound confirmation shows a guidewire that appears to be placed in the IJ and you proceed with dilation and placement of the CVC. Later, you note pulsating, bright red blood in the CVC tubing. Should you immediately pull out the CVC?

NO! Pulling out the CVC can cause significant bleeding and risk causing a carotid dissection and/or stroke. Surgery should be consulted to remove all CVCs that are found to be inadvertently placed in the carotid or subclavian artery. Performing manometry before dilating the blood vessel (in this case the carotid artery) could have prevented this complication. Subclavian arterial cannulation should also be removed by surgery, as the clavicle prevents direct compression. However, inadvertent femoral artery cannulation can safely be removed (although consultation with surgery, cardiology, or interventional radiology should be considered), followed by direct compression over the femoral artery for at least 10 to 15 minutes, while the patient remains flat for several hours.

18. What is the most common first-choice site selection for CVC placement: internal jugular, subclavian, or femoral?

The right IJ vein is generally the first-choice access site for nontunneled CVC placement. This is historically because of several reasons, such as the following: (1) vasculature anatomy facilitating direct placement into the SVC compared with the more torturous vasculature pathway from the left, (2) lower risk of DVT and infection (debatable) compared with femoral, (3) anatomy is more conducive to ultrasound-guided CVC placement compared with subclavian, (4) less risk of bleeding and pneumothorax compared with subclavian, (5) easier access to the CVC ports during surgery compared with a femoral, and (6) familiarity.

19. Why is the femoral vein not used more often as a first-choice site for CVC placement?

Femoral CVC are generally avoided because of concerns of infection and DVT and subclavian CVC because of risk of pneumothorax and bleeding at a noncompressible site. However, historical studies that show a higher risk of femoral CVC infection came from an era before sterile precautions was standardized and enforced. More recent studies show that when a femoral CVC is placed, with strict adherence to sterile technique, its infection risk approaches that of the IJ and subclavian access sites. Furthermore, the risk of devastating neurological complications, either from dilating the carotid artery or infusing vasopressor medications directly into the carotid from a misplaced CVC are virtually impossible with the femoral approach. Therefore, whereas subclavian and IJ infection rates may have a slightly lower risk of infection (although debated), the risks related to performing the femoral CVC placement procedure itself are lower and it may not be unreasonable to place a femoral CVC as first choice, particularly if the CVC is only used for a short period (e.g., 1–2 days). Stated another way, the femoral CVC has reduced short-term risk (i.e., carotid puncture, stroke, pneumothorax, bleeding at a noncompressible site) but higher long-term risk (i.e., infection, DVT) (Fig. 23.3).

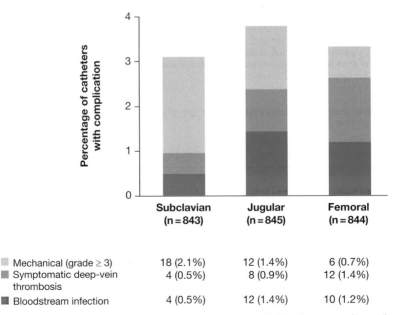

Fig. 23.3 Central line complications by insertion site. Mechanical complications include arterial injury, hematoma, and pneumothorax. (From Parienti J. et al. Intravascular complications of central venous catheterization by insertion site. N Engl J Med. 2015;373:1220–1229.)

20. **What are some clinical situations where a femoral CVC should be considered as the primary access site?**
Clinical situations where a femoral CVC should strongly be considered are the following: (1) emergent quick access (e.g., cardiopulmonary resuscitation), (2) elevated ICP (Trendelenburg positioning with IJ and subclavian sites would raise ICP), (3) unstable cervical spine (cervical collar blocking access to neck), and (4) temporary access for a short period of time where the short-term risks (carotid injury, stroke, pneumothorax, bleeding, etc.) involved with placing the CVC itself are higher than the long-term risks (infection and DVT).

21. **How is CVP measured?**
The CVC tubing is attached to a transducer which converts pressure into an electrical signal that is displayed in mm Hg on a real-time display screen. Please see Chapter 22 Blood Pressure Monitoring and Arterial Catheterization for more details on transducers, including a discussion on leveling and zeroing.

22. **Where on the body should the CVP be measured?**
The CVP should be measured at the right atrium. An external landmark for the right atrium is 5 cm posterior to the sternum or roughly mid-axillary line at the fourth intercostal space. Ongoing adjustment of the transducer is necessary to ensure that the transducer is consistently at this level whenever the patient's position or bed height is changed (Fig. 23.4).

23. **Why is it important that the CVP transducer is correctly leveled?**
It is crucial to place the transducer at the correct level, as a variance of only a few centimeters will result in a significant measurement error, given the low pressures associated with CVP. For example, a 2.7-cm elevation of the transducer will drop the CVP 2 mm Hg (1 cm H_2O = 0.7 mm Hg). For a true CVP of 4 mm Hg, a 2 mm Hg decrease represents an error of 50%!
   Note that this concept also applies when obtaining other low-pressure measurements, such as a wedge or pulmonary artery occlusion pressure (PAOP) using a pulmonary artery catheter.

24. **Should a CVP be measured during inspiration or expiration?**
The CVP is sensitive to respiratory effects and will decrease on inspiration with negative pressure ventilation (i.e., normal spontaneous breathing) and will increase on inhalation with positive pressure ventilation (i.e., intubated on mechanical ventilation). Because the CVP is a small number (0–8 mm Hg), small changes in CVP on inspiration can introduce large percentile errors. Therefore to minimize this problem, the CVP should be measured at the end of expiration.
   Note that this also applies when using a pulmonary artery catheter to measure a wedge or PAOP. Such pressures should also be measured at the end of expiration.

25. **Describe the normal CVP waveform and relate its pattern to the cardiac cycle.**
A normal CVP waveform shows a pattern of three upstrokes (a, c, v) and two descents (x, y) that correspond to events in the cardiac cycle (Fig. 23.5).
* The **a wave** represents an increase in right atrial pressure because of atrial contraction
* Before atrial relaxation is complete, the **c wave** occurs because of bulging of the tricuspid valve into the right atrium during the early phase of right ventricular contraction
* The **x' and x descent** is caused by a decrease in right atrial pressure because of the initial right atrial relaxation (**x'**) and complete right atrial relaxation (**x**)
* The **v wave** is caused by an increase in right atrial pressure that occurs while the atrium fills with blood against a closed tricuspid valve
* The **y descent** occurs when the right ventricle relaxes, allowing the tricuspid valve to open where blood passively fills the right ventricle

26. **What influences CVP?**
CVP is directly related to venous return, venous tone, intrathoracic pressure, and cardiac function. The following perioperative events may change these variables:

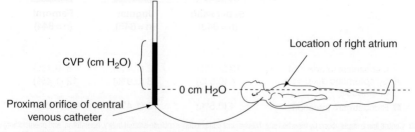

CVP (cm H_2O)

Location of right atrium

0 cm H_2O

Proximal orifice of central venous catheter

Fig. 23.4 Positioning of the patient for central venous catheter measurement. *CVP,* Central venous pressure.

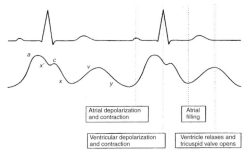

Fig. 23.5 Normal central venous pressure waveform.

- Anesthetic-induced venodilation (decrease CVP) and cardiac depression (increase CVP)
- Severe hypovolemia and hemorrhage (decrease CVP)
- Positive-pressure ventilation and PEEP (increase CVP)
- Increased sympathetic tone from surgical stress or α_1 agonist medications, causing venoconstriction (increase CVP)
- Diastolic dysfunction or systolic heart failure (increase CVP)
- Patient positioning, such as Trendelenburg (increase CVP)

27. **What's the physiologic relevance of a CVP? What is considered a normal CVP?**

The CVP is often interpreted as the right atrial pressure or right ventricular filling pressures and by analogy, the pulmonary artery catheter can be used to measure the PAOP for the left heart. Although a CVP is often used as a surrogate to determine "preload," it is important to understand that there are several other factors that can affect CVP, including ventricular compliance (e.g., diastolic dysfunction may require a higher CVP for adequate preload). Remember, the goal of optimizing a patient's preload is to optimize the frank-starling curve such that the myosin and actin surface area overlap are optimized. Therefore preload is a geometry optimization problem (ventricular end-diastolic volume) not a pressure optimization problem (ventricular end-diastolic pressure). In general, a typical reference range for CVP is 0 to 8 mm Hg. Please see Chapter 25 Volume Assessment for more details.

28. **How can an abnormal CVP waveform be used to diagnose abnormal cardiac events?**

It may be used to assist in diagnosis of pathophysiological events affecting right heart function. For example, atrial fibrillation is characterized by absence of the normal a wave component. Severe tricuspid regurgitation may result in a giant V wave. Contraction of the right atrium against a closed tricuspid valve will cause cannon A waves. This can be seen in conditions, such as atrioventricular dissociation, such as third-degree AV node block or asynchronous atrial contraction during ventricular pacing.

29. **What is a better line to volume resuscitate a patient in hemorrhagic shock: 20G peripherally IV (PIV) or a 7 Fr triple lumen (CVC)?**

A short, 20G PIV will have a higher flow rate than a long, 7 Fr TLC. For example, a typical 7 Fr TLC will be either 16 or 20 cm in length and will have two 18G and one 16G lumens. Because of the long length of a 7 Fr TLC, flow rates, even for the larger 16G lumen, are exceptionally low in comparison with shorter catheters. For example, the flow rate for a 16G lumen in a 7 Fr, 20 cm long TLC is 51 mL/min. In comparison, a short, 16G PIV has a rate flow of 220 mL/min and a 20G PIV has a rate of 65 mL/min! Therefore in the setting of hemorrhagic shock, the ideal line for resuscitation should be "short and fat," such as a 14G PIV, 16G PIV, or an introducer sheath CVC. Please see Table 23.2 for details.

Table 23.2 Flow Rates for Various Catheter Dimensions

GAUGE AND LENGTH	FLOW RATE (CRYSTALLOID) (mL/min)
24G 0.75-inch PIV	20
20G 1-inch PIV	65
18G 1.16-inch PIV	105
16G 1.16-inch PIV	220
16G 20 cm (7 Fr TLC)	51
14G 1.16-inch	450

PIV, Peripheral intravenous catheter; *7 Fr TLC*, 7 French triple lumen catheter.

30. **What is the most important characteristic in determining flow rates through an intravenous catheter: length or radius?**
Although both length and radius can affect flow rate, the most important factor is radius. This is caused by Poiseuille's law, which states flow is proportionate to pressure and radius to the fourth power divided by length for a given fluid viscosity:

$$Q = \frac{\Delta P \pi r^4}{8 \eta l}$$

Poiseuille's law
Q, flow; ΔP, pressure gradient; r, radius of catheter; η, viscosity; l, length

31. **Are any special precautions needed when removing a central venous catheter?**
Before a subclavian or IJ catheter is removed, the patient should be placed in the Trendelenburg position to increase venous pressure at the point of removal to minimize risk of air embolism. Other adjuncts in addition to Trendelenburg position include having the patient "humm" or Valsalva at the same time the CVC is removed. Following removal of the catheter, external pressure should be maintained on the area from which the catheter is withdrawn, until clot formation has sealed the vessel. Removed central lines should have an occlusive dressing placed over the cannulation site to prevent the possibility of a delayed air embolism, until the tract has sufficiently closed, typically within 24 to 48 hours after removal.

KEY POINTS: CENTRAL VENOUS CATHETERIZATION AND PRESSURE MONITORING

1. Complications of CVC include, pneumothorax, arterial injury, bleeding, thoracic duct injury, air embolus, DVT, and infection.
2. The Seldinger technique involves placing a guidewire into a vein, which facilitates the exchange of catheters over the guidewire into the vein.
3. Ultrasound should always be used whenever possible when placing a CVC. Its use is associated with faster CVC placement, fewer complications, and a higher first attempt success rate.
4. The first-choice site for CVC placement is often the right IJ. This is caused by various reasons, including its straight anatomic trajectory to the right atrium, familiarity, ease of access to CVC ports during surgery, anatomy that is amendable to ultrasound-guided CVC placement, and lower rates of infection (debatable) compared with femoral CVC.
5. Manometry should strongly be considered whenever possible to confirm venous placement of the guidewire before dilation, particularly if the CVC is to be used before chest x-ray confirmation and the CVC is placed in the neck near the carotid.
6. CVP is not an accurate method to assess volume status.
7. CVP is prone to errors in measurement, such as from an incorrectly leveled transducer or from taking a CVP measurement during inspiration. The CVP transducer should be carefully leveled to the right atrium and all measurements taken at end-expiration.
8. Triple lumen catheters are slow and are not a good catheter for volume resuscitation. The ideal catheter for volume resuscitation should be "short and fat" (e.g., 14G PIV).

SUGGESTED READINGS

Bodenham Chair A. Association of Anaesthetists of Great Britain and Ireland: Safe vascular access 2016. Anaesthesia. 2016;71(5):573–585.
Higgs ZC, Macafee DA, Braithwaite BD, et al. The Seldinger technique: 50 years on. Lancet. 2005;366(9494):1407–1409.
Parienti J, Mongardon N, Mégarbane B, et al. Intravascular complications of central venous catheterization by insertion site. N Engl J Med. 2015;373:1220–1229.
Rupp SM. Practice guidelines for central venous access: a report by the American Society of Anesthesiologists Task Force on Central Venous Access. Anesthesiology. 2012;116(3):539–573.
Taylor RW, Palagiri AV. Central venous catheterization. Crit Care Med. 2007;35:1390–1396.
Troianos CA, Hartman GS, Glas KE, et al. Guidelines for performing ultrasound guided vascular cannulation. J Am Soc Echocardiogr. 2011;24:1291–1318.

PERIOPERATIVE POINT-OF-CARE ULTRASOUND AND ECHOCARDIOGRAPHY

Bethany Benish, MD, Joseph Morabito, DO

1. **What is the role of point-of-care ultrasound and echocardiography in the perioperative and critical care setting?**
   Ultrasound is a valuable diagnostic tool capable of providing real-time, rapid evaluation of patients. It is mobile, easy to use, safe, and less expensive than other imaging modalities, making its application pertinent to a variety of clinical environments—perioperative, critical care, emergency department, outpatient clinics, or inpatient wards. Ultrasound is progressively decreasing in cost, becoming more available and easier to use. Time-sensitive decisions can be made at the bedside, reducing the burden on sonographers and delay in patient care. Point-of-care ultrasound (POCUS) and echocardiography may prevent unnecessary tests and consults, surgical delay, and placement of invasive monitors, as well as help determine appropriate levels of postoperative monitoring and patient disposition.

   POCUS is a tool that, when combined with history and physical examination, may be used to answer specific clinical questions. These include, but are not limited to, ventricular function, significant structural or valvular cardiac abnormalities, hemodynamic status, and/or severe lung pathology. Formal evaluation of cardiac function/pathology may be further investigated by referral for a diagnostic limited or comprehensive echocardiographic study. POCUS is often performed using transthoracic echocardiography (TTE); however, in the operating room or critical care environment, it may be performed using transesophageal echocardiography (TEE), depending on the physician or provider's level of training.

2. **How are POCUS images obtained?**
   Images result from transmission of ultrasound waves (2–10 mHz) from the TEE/TTE probe through target tissue (heart and great vessels). The time it requires for the wave to be reflected back determines the location of a structure. This can be combined with color flow Doppler to further examine dynamic structures. These high resolution multiplane images and Doppler techniques provide real-time hemodynamic evaluation and assist in the diagnosis of cardiovascular and pulmonary pathology.

3. **Which ultrasound modes can aid in the POCUS examination?**
   The diagnostic utility of two-dimensional ultrasound alone can yield significant information, including global and segmental cardiac function, valve restriction or prolapse, pneumothoraxes, pleural effusions, and hemodynamic status. The availability and understanding of color-flow imaging, spectral Doppler, tissue Doppler, and M-mode will further aid in the clinical examination.

4. **What are some specific pathologies that POCUS can potentially identify?**
   - Left atrial enlargement
   - Left ventricular (LV) hypertrophy, enlargement, and systolic function
   - Right ventricular (RV) enlargement and systolic function
   - Pericardial effusion
   - Intravascular volume status
   - Pneumothorax
   - Pleural effusion
   - Significant aortic and mitral valve pathology

5. **Which TTE views are useful in a POCUS examination?**
   Many protocols exist for perioperative ultrasound evaluation including: FoCUS, FCS, FATE, HEART, HART, FEEL, CLUE, FUSE, RUSH, and so on. Fig. 24.1 is an example of basic transthoracic ultrasound views (FATE) and important pathology that can be identified with these views.

6. **How can POCUS be used to evaluate lung pathology?**
   POCUS pulmonary assessment can be used to rapidly evaluate patients during acute respiratory events. POCUS has been shown to be superior to chest radiography in ruling out pneumothorax and evaluating hemidiaphragmatic paresis. Other pulmonary pathology can be diagnosed with POCUS including lung consolidation, effusion, and pulmonary edema.

161

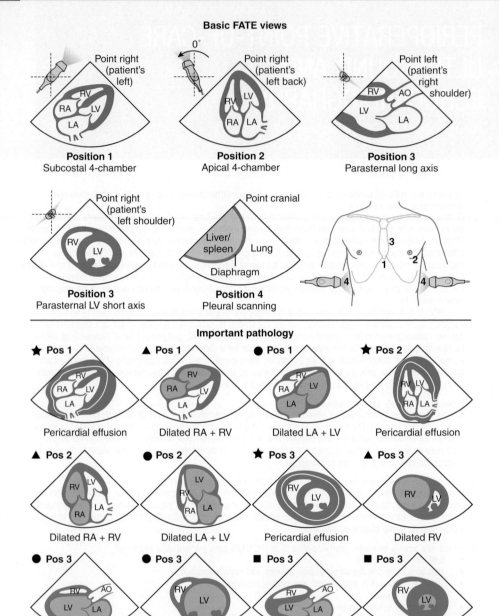

Basic FATE views

Position 1
Subcostal 4-chamber

Position 2
Apical 4-chamber

Position 3
Parasternal long axis

Position 3
Parasternal LV short axis

Position 4
Pleural scanning

Important pathology

★ Pos 1 — Pericardial effusion

▲ Pos 1 — Dilated RA + RV

● Pos 1 — Dilated LA + LV

★ Pos 2 — Pericardial effusion

▲ Pos 2 — Dilated RA + RV

● Pos 2 — Dilated LA + LV

★ Pos 3 — Pericardial effusion

▲ Pos 3 — Dilated RV

● Pos 3 — Dilated LV +LA

● Pos 3 — Dilated LV

■ Pos 3 — Hypertrophy LV + Dilated LA

■ Pos 3 — Hypertrophy LV

Pathology to be considered in particular:

★ Post OP cardiac surgery, following cardiac catheterization, trauma, renal failure, infection

▲ Pulmonary embolus, RV infarction, pulmonary hypertension, volume overload

● Ischemic heart disease, dilated cardiomyopathy, sepsism, volume overload, aorta insufficiency

■ Aorta stenosis, arterial hypertension, LV outflow tract obstruction, hyper trophic cardiomyopathy, myocardial deposit diseases

Fig. 24.1 Basic Focused Assessment of Transthoracic Echocardiography (FATE) views.

7. Describe the evolving role of TEE in the perioperative setting.

Since its introduction in 1976, the use of intraoperative TEE has steadily increased in popularity. Although traditionally used in cardiac surgery, the value of perioperative TEE for noncardiac surgery is becoming widely appreciated.

In 1998 American Society of Echocardiography (ASE) and Society of Cardiovascular Anesthesiologists (SCA) developed a standard comprehensive TEE examination, which includes the 20 views used for full cardiac evaluation and diagnosis of cardiac pathology.

In 2013 ASE/SCA revisited this topic and developed the Basic Perioperative TEE examination for noncardiac surgery, which simplified the examination to 11 views focusing on intraoperative monitoring rather than diagnostics (Fig. 24.2). Various cardiac chambers and vessels are apparent, as well as the TEE probe diagrammed outside the cardiac image.

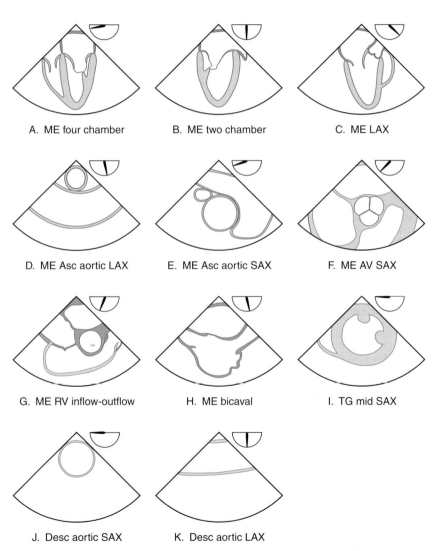

A. ME four chamber B. ME two chamber C. ME LAX

D. ME Asc aortic LAX E. ME Asc aortic SAX F. ME AV SAX

G. ME RV inflow-outflow H. ME bicaval I. TG mid SAX

J. Desc aortic SAX K. Desc aortic LAX

Fig. 24.2 ASE and SCA Basic PTE Examination.

8. **What are the indications for TEE in noncardiac surgery?**

Indications for TEE
- Inadequate transthoracic echo image quality
- Intraoperative assessment of
  - Global and regional LV function
  - RV function
  - Intravascular volume status
  - Basic valvular lesions
  - Thromboembolism or air embolism
  - Pericardial effusion/tamponade
  - Unexplained hypotension or hypoxia
  - Postcardiac arrest
  - Evaluation of preload responsiveness
  - Evaluation of myocardial ischemia

TEE should be considered in cases where the nature of the procedure or the patient's underlying known or suspected cardiovascular pathology might result in hemodynamic, pulmonary, or neurologic instability or compromise. TEE should also be used to assist in diagnosis and management of unexplained life-threatening hemodynamic instability that persists despite initial corrective therapy. This is often referred to as a *rescue TEE*. Of course, proper training is essential before perioperative TEE use to ensure patient safety and diagnostic accuracy.

9. **Are there complications of TEE?**
Although complications of TEE are rare (0.2%), there have been serious and even fatal complications reported. These include:
- Odynophagia/dysphagia
- Dental injury
- Oral/pharyngeal trauma
- Vocal cord injury
- Upper gastrointestinal (GI) bleed
- Esophageal laceration or perforation (0.1%–0.2%)
- Endotracheal tube displacement
- Tracheal compression
- Left atrial compression

10. **What are the contraindications of TEE?**

Relative Contraindications	*Absolute Contraindications*
• Esophageal diverticulum or fistula	• Esophageal obstruction (stricture, tumor)
• Esophageal varices without active bleeding	• Esophageal trauma
• Previous esophageal surgery	• Active upper GI hemorrhage
• Severe coagulopathy or thrombocytopenia	• Recent esophageal/gastric surgery
• Cervical spine disease	• Perforated viscus (known/suspected)
• Mediastinal radiation	• Full stomach with unprotected airway
• Unexplained odynophagia	• Patient refusal

11. **What is the best TEE view to assess volume status?**
The transgastric midpapillary short-axis view (Fig. 24.3) is the most common window to assess volume status using TEE. TEE has been shown to more accurately assess LV preload in patients with normal LV function than pulmonary artery catheters. LV end-diastolic area and diameter can be measured in this view to accurately assess volume status, even in patients with regional wall motion abnormalities. Monitoring the LV in the transgastric midpapillary view provides real-time feedback to fluid resuscitation interventions.

12. **How is TEE/TTE helpful for perioperative ischemia monitoring?**
In the setting of myocardial ischemia, systolic wall motion abnormalities can often be detected before ST segment changes on electrocardiogram (ECG). Complete regional wall motion of the LV is assessed using a 17-segment wall motion score (Fig. 24.4). Rapid assessment of LV function can be done using the transgastric midpapillary short-axis view. In this view, one can visualize areas of the LV perfused by the left anterior descending, circumflex, and right coronary arteries. The midesophageal four-chamber, midesophageal two chamber, and midesophageal long-axis views provide more comprehensive assessment of LV function.

In addition, TEE/TTE can evaluate for complications of myocardial ischemia, including congestive heart failure, new septal defects or ventricular free wall rupture, valvular pathology or new pericardial effusion.

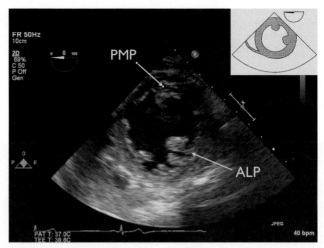

Fig. 24.3 Transgastric mid-papillary short axis view. *ALP*, Anterior lateral papillary muscle; *PMP*, posterior medial papillary muscle. (Reeves ST, Finley AC, Skubas NJ, et al. Basic perioperative transesophageal echocardiography examination: a consensus Statement of the American Society of Echocardiographty and the Society of Cardiovascular Anesthesiologists. Anesth Analg. 2013;117(3):543–558.)

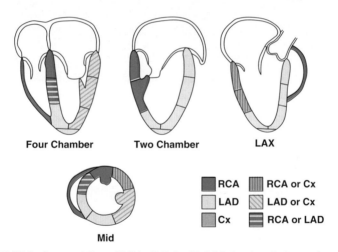

Fig. 24.4 Regional Wall Motion Assessment. (Reeves ST, Finley AC, Skubas NJ, et al. Basic perioperative transesophageal echocardiography examination: a consensus statement of the American Society of Echocardiography and the Society of Cardiovascular Anesthesiologists. J Am Soc Echocardiogr. 2013;26:443–456.)

13. **How can you assess right atrial pressure using TTE or TEE?**
    Elevated right atrial (RA) pressure can be seen in patients with pulmonary hypertension and has been shown to be predictive of mortality in this population. RA pressure can be estimated by measuring inferior vena cava (IVC) diameter and assessing the degree of collapsibility with inspiration. The transthoracic subcostal view images the IVC in long axis, often visualizing the IVC-RA junction. IVC diameter is measured at end-expiration, and again during inspiration or "sniffing." The percent collapse with sniff is used to estimate RA pressure (Table 24.1). One caveat, IVC collapse will not accurately estimate RA pressure in mechanically ventilated patients.

14. **What is TAPSE?**
    • Tricuspid annular plane systolic excursion (TAPSE) is a method of assessing RV function through quantification of the systolic excursion of the tricuspid annulus. The TTE apical four-chamber window or TEE midesophageal four-chamber view are used to visualize the free wall of the RV. M-mode is then used to measure the distance of systolic excursion of the RV annulus along its longitudinal plane (Fig. 24.5). TAPSE under 16 mm is indicative of impaired RV systolic function.

Table 24.1 RA Pressure Estimation

ESTIMATED RA PRESSURE	NORMAL (0–5 mm Hg)	INTERMEDIATE (5–10 mm Hg)	INTERMEDIATE (5–10 mm Hg)	HIGH (15 mm Hg)
IVC diameter	<2.2	<2.2	>2.1	>2.1
Collapse with sniff	>50%	<50%	>50%	<50%

IVC, Inferior vena cava; *RA,* right atrial.

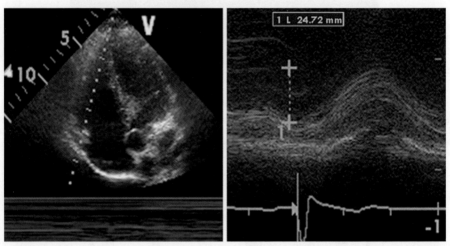

Fig. 24.5 Tricuspid annular plane systolic excursion (TAPSE) to assess RV function. (Rudski LG, Lai WW, Afilalo J, Hua L, et al. Guidelines for the echocardiographic assessment of the right heart in adults: a report from the American Society of Echocardiography endorsed by the European Association of Echocardiography, a registered branch of the European Society of Cardiology, and the Canadian Society of Echocardiography. J Am Soc Echocardiogr. 2010;23(7):685–713; quiz 786–788.)

KEY POINTS

1. POCUS has a variety of roles in the perioperative setting including:
   - Global assessment of LV and RV cardiac function
   - Evaluation of volume status/responsiveness
   - Pulmonary evaluation, including identification of pneumothorax, hemidiaphragm paresis, pleural effusions or consolidations
2. TEE or TTE should be considered in any case in which the nature of the procedure or the patient's underlying known or suspected cardiovascular pathology might result in hemodynamic, pulmonary, or neurologic instability or compromise.

Websites
http://pie.med.utoronto.ca/TEE/
https://echo.anesthesia.med.utah.edu
http://echoboards.org/
http://usabcd.org/FATEcard (free FATE Card app for iPhone and Android)

SUGGESTED READINGS

Reeves ST, Finley AC, Skubas NJ, et al. Basic perioperative transesophageal echocardiography examination: A consensus statement of the American Society of Echocardiography and the Society of Cardiovascular Anesthesiologists. Anesth Analg. 2013;117:543–558.

Reeves ST, Finley AC, Skubas NJ, et al. Basic perioperative transesophageal echocardiography examination: a consensus statement of the American Society of Echocardiography and the Society of Cardiovascular Anesthesiologists. J Am Soc Echocardiogr. 2013;26:443–456.

Rudski LG, Lai WW, Afilalo J, Hua L, et al. Guidelines for the echocardiographic assessment of the right heart in adults: a report from the American Society of Echocardiography endorsed by the European Association of Echocardiography, a registered branch of the European Society of Cardiology, and the Canadian Society of Echocardiography. J Am Soc Echocardiogr. 2010;23:685–713; quiz 786–788.

Spencer KT, Kimura BJ, Korcarz CE, et al. Focused cardiac ultrasound: recommendations from the American Society of Echocardiography. J Am Soc Echocardiogr. 2013;26:567–581.

CHAPTER 25

VOLUME ASSESSMENT

Jeffrey Davis, MD, Ryan D. Laterza, MD

1. **Why do we administer fluids? What is the most important reason perioperatively?**
   Although there are many reasons to administer fluids to patients (correct electrolyte imbalances, administer drugs, nutrients, antibiotics, etc.), the ultimate goal of perioperative fluid administration is to increase cardiac output in an effort to better perfuse end-organs (e.g., heart, brain, kidneys). This goal can be realized when a fluid bolus increases venous return, thereby yielding a more optimal position on the Frank-Starling curve, resulting in increased stroke volume.

   The assessment of volume status (particularly among critically ill patients) and the determination that intravascular volume expansion will ultimately lead to beneficial effects on end-organs is complex. Importantly, inappropriate fluid administration has been shown to cause harm and increased mortality. However, avoiding fluid administration in patients who are hypovolemic also causes harm. Therefore the administration of fluids, like any medication, should be scrutinized for expected benefit and likelihood of potential adverse effects.

2. **What are some complications of fluid imbalance?**
   The risks of fluid imbalance (i.e., hypovolemia and hypervolemia) follow a "U"-shape curve, because both have associated complications, with the least complications occurring at the bottom of the curve when the patient is euvolemic. Complications of hypervolemia include acute renal failure, peripheral edema, delayed ambulation, pulmonary edema, poor wound healing, and ileus. Complications of hypovolemia include acute renal failure, tachycardia, demand cardiac ischemia (i.e., type 2 myocardial infarction), hypotension, end-organ hypoperfusion and mesenteric ischemia.

3. **What is early goal-directed therapy? How does it differ from goal-directed fluid therapy?**
   Early goal-directed therapy (EGDT) is a protocolized resuscitation strategy to specified end-points in the management of sepsis. In particular, titrating crystalloid, blood products, and vasoactive agents to static physiological indices, such as central venous pressure (CVP) of 8 to 12 mm Hg, urine output (UOP) greater than 0.5 mL/kg/h, mean arterial pressure (MAP) greater than 65 mm Hg and mixed venous oxygen saturation ($SmvO_2$) over 65% amongst other end points, including early administration of antibiotics. The original study by Rivers, et al. in 2001 showed significantly improved survival with this approach compared with what was then standard therapy, which did not include the early administration of antibiotics. Following this study, there were major concerns with EGDT, including the rigid, protocol-driven nature of the interventions and the fact that resuscitation goals were not tailored to the unique physiological needs of each patient (e.g., titrating fluid boluses to treat sepsis in a patient with systolic heart failure and chronic kidney disease to a UOP >0.5 mL/kg/h). In particular, this protocolized approach was often associated with problems related to iatrogenic hypervolemia, as many patients required significant amounts of volume to achieve these static physiological endpoints.

   Three large multicenter randomized controlled trials have since reexamined EGDT and found no reduction in all-cause mortality for patients with sepsis compared with current standards of care. Further studies to elucidate the impressive survival benefit realized in the original Rivers study found that the only independent factors in reducing mortality in sepsis were: (1) early recognition of sepsis, and (2) early antibiotic administration. These factors were included in the original Rivers EGDT protocol and were not the standard of care at that time. However, interestingly, early sepsis recognition and antibiotic administration was the standard of care in the latter EGDT trials, which is likely the reason these trials showed no benefit with EGDT. Because volume resuscitation to static physiologicalal endpoints (i.e., CVP) may lead to the aforementioned complications, recent surviving sepsis guidelines now recommend using dynamic measurements to guide volume resuscitation (often referred to as *goal-directed fluid therapy* [*GDFT*]).

4. **Enhanced recovery after surgery protocols frequently recommend GDFT (among other interventions) whenever feasible. What are the clinical benefits of GDFT in the perioperative setting, and how is it instituted?**
   One goal widely proposed in the perioperative setting is "zero fluid balance" at the end of surgery. This implies that the patient's volume status after surgery is the same as it was before surgery, provided the patient was originally euvolemic. Interventions to maintain this perioperative target have been shown to prevent ileus and promote earlier hospital discharge. Judicious fluid administration results in less bowel edema, which, coupled with early oral (PO) intake postoperatively, likely facilitates early return of bowel function.

   To institute GDFT perioperatively, patients should be euvolemic at the beginning of a surgery (i.e., clear liquids should ideally be encouraged up to 2 hours preoperatively), and dynamic indices of preload should be used whenever feasible. Fluid administration with this approach emphasizes the judicious use of maintenance fluids (e.g., <3 mL/kg/h) and to only administered fluid boluses based on clinical assessment of hypovolemia using dynamic physiologicalal measurements. Collectively, this approach is often used using enhanced recovery after surgery (ERAS) protocols, which notably emphasize volume maintenance and resuscitation using dynamic parameters.

5. **What methods are commonly used to assess volume status?**
   There are numerous methods used to assess volume status. In general, these can be categorized as the following:
   - Physical examination: crackles on lung auscultation, orthostatic vital signs, lower extremity edema, jugular venous distention, abnormalities in heart rate, cold-extremities, UOP, dry mucous membranes, delayed capillary refill, etc.
   - Imaging studies: chest radiograph, lung ultrasound, or computed tomography (CT) chest showing evidence of pulmonary edema. Findings on chest radiograph include cephalization, kerley lines, or pleural effusions
   - Static parameters: static physiological measurements: CVP, pulmonary capillary wedge pressure/pulmonary artery occlusion pressure, SmvO$_2$, left ventricular end-diastolic diameter using echocardiography, extravascular lung water (EVLW), or inferior vena cava (IVC) diameter using ultrasound
   - Dynamic parameters: dynamic physiologicalal responses (based on the Frank-Starling law) to provocative tests which affect preload. Measuring dynamic parameters generally requires the use of an arterial-line, esophageal Doppler, pulmonary artery catheter, echocardiography, or pulse contour analysis device to analyze changes in blood pressure (BP), stroke volume, or cardiac output in response to preload alteration. Preload can be altered by producing changes in venous return (generally from positive pressure ventilation, passive leg raises [PLRs], or a small fluid challenges). Dynamic indices are significantly more accurate compared with all other modalities in predicting volume responsiveness

6. **Discuss the Frank-Starling law and its role in using dynamic modalities to assess hypovolemia?**
   The Frank-Starling law correlates stroke volume with preload or end-diastolic volume. As the ventricular volume increases during diastole, the surface area overlap between actin-myosin fibers increases, allowing more cross-bridges to form, which will increase the force of contraction. Patients who are intravascularly hypovolemic are on the "steep" portion of this curve, and any changes in preload will result in a large change in stroke volume. As the end-diastolic volume or preload increases, stroke volume also increases, until optimal actin-myosin overlap occurs and the stroke volume plateaus. Interestingly, if the end-diastolic volume continues to enlarge beyond a certain volume, the actin-myosin overlap may actually spread too far apart and no longer be able to form cross-bridges, leading to decreased contractility and decreased stroke volume (Fig. 25.1).

   Dynamic indices rely on this law to assess volume responsiveness, under the premise that the primary reason to give fluid is to increase stroke volume. The primary goal with using dynamic indices is to optimize the patient's position on the Frank-Starling curve (i.e., so they are on the "flat" rather than the "steep" portion of this curve). Various other approaches may be used to assess the relationship between preload and stroke volume, including PLR, empiric 250 mL fluid challenges, or hemodynamic changes observed from positive pressure ventilation.

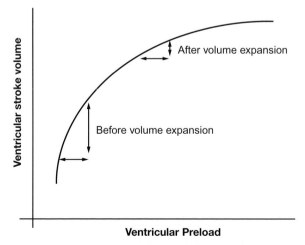

Fig. 25.1 The Frank-Starling curve illustrates the change in stroke volume as cardiac preload is increased. The shape and slope of this curve is dependent on cardiac muscle compliance (lusitropy) and contractility (inotropy). (From Mohsenin V. Assessment of preload and fluid responsiveness in intensive care unit. How good are we? J Crit Care. 2015;30(3):569.)

Table 25.1 Predictive Value of History, Physical, and Chest X-Ray Findings

SYMPTOMS	SENSITIVITY	SPECIFICITY
PND	0.41	0.84
Orthopnea	0.5	0.77
Edema	0.51	0.76
Physical Examination		
Jugular Venous Distention	0.39	0.92
Rales	0.66	0.78
Lower Extremity Edema	0.5	0.78
Chest Radiograph		
Pulmonary Venous Congestion	0.54	0.96
Interstitial Edema	0.34	0.97
Pleural Effusions	0.26	0.92

The specificity of history, physician examination, and chest x-ray findings in predicting hypervolemia is reasonably good, however, its sensitivity is poor.

Data from Wang CS, Fitzgerald JM, Schulzer M before et al. Does this dyspneic patient in the emergency department have congestive heart failure? JAMA. 2005;294(15):1944–1956.

PND, Paroxysmal nocturnal dyspnea.

7. Describe the symptoms, physical examination, and imaging study findings that suggest hypervolemia. How sensitive and specific are these? How do they compare with dynamic modalities in the assessment of volume status?

History, physical examination findings, and imaging studies (Table 25.1) are often used to assess for hypervolemia. Although these modalities in isolation are relatively specific, they are not sensitive and likely have high interobserver reliability because of their qualitative nature. However, using multiple findings together may increase their accuracy, as is often used in clinical practice. For example, a patient with a known history of systolic heart failure, presenting with shortness of breath, and physical examination findings of jugular venous distension, rales, and peripheral edema, is likely hypervolemic.

Whereas history, physical examination, or imaging studies are not as accurate as dynamic modalities, they have a role in clinical practice. Because dynamic tests often require relatively invasive monitoring devices, traditional methods may be helpful in acute situations when rapid assessment and treatment is necessary. Further, it is important to realize that dynamic modalities are meant to predict volume responsiveness and therefore assess hypovolemia, not hypervolemia. However, in a complicated patient presenting with multiple comorbidities, dynamic tests may be helpful to "rule-out" hypovolemia as an etiology for hemodynamic instability.

8. Can a chest radiograph be used to assess volume status?

The chest x-ray (CXR) has moderate positive predictive value for hypervolemia when the following findings are demonstrated: dilated upper lobe vasculature, cardiomegaly, interstitial edema, pleural effusion, and Kerley B-lines. However, these findings have poor sensitivity in detecting hypervolemia, and radiographic findings frequently lag the clinical manifestations of pulmonary edema. Therefore the CXR should be interpreted with caution, as the absence of the earlier findings does not preclude hypervolemia. Further, there are no radiographic findings reliably predictive of intravascular hypovolemia.

9. How accurate are orthostatic vital signs in the assessment of volume status?

Not very. Studies evaluating orthostatic measurements and postural dizziness revealed only a 22% sensitivity in identifying hypovolemia in patients who experienced 500 mL to 1 L of blood loss. Further, other factors, such as deconditioning, autonomic dysfunction, and other logistical barriers (e.g., intubation and sedation) may impair its clinical accuracy or utility. In other words, the very patient population deemed to benefit the most from volume assessment (intensive care unit [ICU] patients) often have pragmatic challenges or contraindications to the widespread use of this modality.

10. What is a base deficit? Can it be used to asses for hypovolemia or as an end point for fluid resuscitation?

Base deficit (or excess) is automatically calculated and reported with an arterial blood gas and quantifies the metabolic component of the acid-base disturbance. It is calculated first by correcting for the pH disturbance because of carbon dioxide and then how much base (i.e., bicarbonate) would need to be added or removed to normalize the pH to 7.40. In other words, base deficit is the amount of bicarbonate that would need to be added or removed to normalize the pH to 7.40 provided the CO_2 is 40 mm Hg at a temperature of 37.0°C.

Base deficit should not be used as the primary end-point in volume resuscitation. In the setting of hemorrhagic shock, often because of trauma, base deficit will also rise because of lactic acidosis. Volume resuscitation with blood products will help normalize the base deficit, assuming the lactic acidosis resolves. However, it is important to recognize that there are other causes for an abnormal base deficit besides a volume deficit. The use of base deficit requires that there are no other underlying conditions that can affect the pH disturbance (e.g., drug toxicity, sepsis), that the liver can receive and metabolize lactate normally, and that there is normal renal function. Patients presenting in shock may have liver dysfunction and acute kidney insufficiency from hypoperfusion, causing the acid base disturbance to persist despite adequate volume resuscitation. Further, other shock states may present with lactic acidosis in patients who are *hypervolemic*, such as in cardiogenic shock or septic shock. Lastly, many critically ill patients have comorbidities at baseline (e.g., end-stage renal disease, heart failure, liver disease) where the base deficit correlates more with hypervolemia than hypovolemia.

11. **Is urine output an accurate measurement to assess for volume status in the perioperative or intensive care setting?**

UOP measured perioperatively and in the ICU is a sensitive but nonspecific indicator of acute kidney injury (AKI) and a poor predictor of volume status. UOP can be affected by several factors aside from hypovolemia, such as MAP, intraabdominal pressure, and abdominal venous pressure, all of which can affect renal perfusion. Further, UOP may be affected by physiological stress, such as from a surgical operation or from a critical illness. Physiological stress and other increased sympathetic tone states (e.g., pain) causes aldosterone and antidiuretic hormone secretion to increase, likely as an adaptive response to anticipated volume loss, resulting in a subsequent decrease in UOP, despite no change in volume status. Therefore a low UOP may be caused by poor renal perfusion, a physiological response to stress, or to intrinsic or postrenal AKI and not necessarily hypovolemia.

In critically ill patients, the assumption that end organ hypoperfusion alone causes AKI is likely inadequate. Among septic patients, for example, renal perfusion is frequently normal or increased, but microcirculatory flow deficits are often present. In conjunction with inflammation and cellular metabolic derangements, oliguria in the setting of septic shock is likely more complex than hypoperfusion alone. Other causes of low UOP, not related to volume status, include AKI from contrast induced nephropathy, acute tubular necrosis, "renal edema" because of congestive heart failure, or other etiologies of chronic kidney disease.

In summary, although a low UOP may be indicative of hypovolemia, in an acutely stressed state (i.e., surgery or critical illness), it may be an appropriate physiological response to stress and/or other factors not related to perfusion (e.g., sepsis). Therefore UOP should not be used in isolation to guide fluid administration. Rather, if abnormal, it should be regarded as a call for further assessment, particularly because acute kidney insufficiency is an independent predictor of perioperative mortality.

12. **What is the formula for mean arterial pressure? Knowing this, can blood pressure be used for volume assessment?**

$$MAP - CVP = CO \times SVR \qquad (25.1)$$
$$MAP = (HR \times SV) \times SVR + CVP \qquad (25.2)$$

BP is a crude marker for assessing volume status, because of a variety of reasons. As can be shown by Equation 25.1 BP is dependent upon systemic vascular resistance (SVR) and cardiac output (CO). Recall, $CO = SV \times HR$ where stroke volume (SV) is dependent upon contractility, preload, afterload, and rhythm. The fundamental reason to give volume is to increase preload; however, preload is only one variable of many that can affect BP as shown by Equation 25.2. BP is poorly correlated to volume status because of the compensatory, sympathetic-mediated mechanisms that maintain BP by increasing heart rate (HR), contractility, and SVR (discussed later).

This is readily apparent in young patients (such as during postpartum hemorrhage) where, because of compensatory mechanisms, hypotension may not occur until a significant amount of blood volume is lost, whereas in older patients with diminished cardiac reserve, hypotension may present with far less blood loss.

13. **How does venous and arterial vasculature differ? Describe the role of each in maintaining a normal blood pressure in the setting of hypovolemia?**

Two of the primary functions of the venous vasculature are to store volume and to minimize variations in venous return in the setting of hypovolemia or hypervolemia. The compliance of veins is approximately 30 times that of arteries, allowing veins to store approximately 70% of the total blood volume (TBV). Conversely, arterial vasculature has low compliance but is responsible for approximately 70% to 80% of SVR (particularly the arterioles). Therefore the physical properties of the venous vasculature include high compliance and low resistance, whereas the arterial vasculature has low compliance and high resistance.

Interestingly, both the arterial and venous vasculature contain alpha-1 receptors that vasoconstrict in response to catecholamines, increasing their resistance and decreasing compliance. However, because of the aforementioned physical properties, alpha-1 agonism of the venous vasculature primarily decreases compliance (facilitating venous return), whereas the primary response of the arterial vasculature is to increase SVR. Because cardiac output must equal venous return, and given the equation: MAP = CO × SVR + CVP, increased sympathetic tone in response to hypovolemia will act synergistically to prevent hypotension by augmenting venous return (cardiac output) and increasing heart rate, contractility, and SVR.

14. **Describe the physiology of the venous system. More specifically, define "unstressed" versus "stressed" volume, and explain why a conceptual understanding of these compartments is necessary to understand venous return.**

   The venous system can be separated into two conceptual volume compartments: unstressed and stressed. The unstressed compartment is that volume necessary to distend the veins from flat to round, and does not increase the transmural pressure across the lumen of a vein (analogous to the first few deciliters of air necessary to initially inflate a deflated balloon before extra pressure is necessary to distend it further). The stressed compartment is that volume that begins to distend and increase transmural pressure across the vein (volume of air blown into a balloon after it is initially inflated). Conceptually, the unstressed volume is the stored blood volume and the stressed volume is the volume contributing to venous return.

   Alpha-1 agonism of the venous vasculature (e.g., phenylephrine) causes venoconstriction, decreasing venous compliance and shifting venous blood from the unstressed to the stressed compartment. This may increase venous return despite no change in TBV. Conversely, decreased alpha-1 agonism (e.g., following a spinal anesthetic) causes venodilation, which increases venous compliance and shifts venous blood from the stressed to the unstressed compartment, thereby decreasing venous return despite, again, no changes in TBV.

15. **How can the ratio of unstressed to stressed volume serve as a marker for physiological reserve?**

   The amounts of stressed and unstressed volume at baseline are determined by the intrinsic compliance of the venous system, which is normally high in younger patients and decreases with age. The sympathetic nervous system can modulate venous system compliance to some degree, shifting blood between the stressed and unstressed compartments to maintain homeostasis, but the impact of this sympathetic stimulation diminishes with age. Patients with a high ratio of unstressed to stressed volume (i.e., young, healthy patients) are thought to have more reserve in the setting of hypovolemia and will therefore exhibit less hemodynamic instability in the face of blood loss, compared with those with a lower ratio (i.e., elderly patients). This difference is likely caused by the reduced venous compliance characteristic of elderly patients, which reduces the amount of blood the venous vasculature can store for a given transmural pressure. This phenomenon has been demonstrated in studies correlating decreased venous compliance with aging and other arteriosclerosis risk factors.

16. **Is CVP an accurate measurement of volume status?**

   CVP is not an accurate measurement of volume status and this has been demonstrated in numerous studies. Recall the Frank-Starling law, which correlates stroke volume with optimal surface area overlap of myocardial actin-myosin filaments. Preload affects the geometry of the ventricle by improving overlap of these filaments to increase contractility, which is better assessed by end-diastolic volume and not end-diastolic pressure (i.e., CVP). Note how elevated extracardiac pressures (e.g., tamponade, positive pressure ventilation) or diastolic dysfunction will confound the relationship between end-diastolic pressure (CVP) and end-diastolic volume (preload), as a higher end-diastolic pressure will be needed to increase end-diastolic volume in these clinical situations.

   Using CVP to assess volume status is analogous to using BP to assess volume status. In dire situations, such as severe hemorrhagic shock, the CVP and BP will be low, but only after exhausting compensatory mechanisms. In less extreme clinical situations, however, there are too many variables that affect these measurements making CVP or BP in isolation inaccurate. For example, in cardiogenic shock, the BP may fall not because the patient is hypovolemic but because of low cardiac output. Similarly, the CVP may rise not because of hypervolemia but because of decreased cardiac output. In the setting of hypovolemia, alpha-1 mediated venoconstriction from increased sympathetic tone facilitates venous return to maintain right heart filling pressure (i.e., CVP) analogous to how arterial vasoconstriction increases SVR to maintain MAP. To maintain homeostasis, the body attempts to compensate to minimize disturbances in CVP and MAP.

17. **List the various factors that can affect CVP**
   - Venous return or right heart filling volume
   - Positive pressure ventilation
   - Extracardiac pressure, such as tamponade
   - Systolic heart failure
   - Ventricular diastolic dysfunction
   - Tricuspid regurgitation
   - Sympathetic mediated venous tone
   - Intrinsic venous compliance
   - Errors, such as improper leveling of the transducer*

   *Note that because the CVP is normally a small number compared with arterial pressure, small errors in leveling the transducer can lead to large errors in diagnosis and management. For example, if the transduce is above or below the right atrium by 10 cm, the CVP will be off by 7 mm Hg.

18. **In a euvolemic patient, how might adding or removing 500 mL of blood affect the CVP?**

   In a healthy, euvolemic patient, administering 500 mL of blood will not necessarily increase the CVP. Because the venous system is highly compliant, it can easily store this added volume by venodilating and shifting the excess from the stressed to the unstressed compartment. Similarly, removing 500 mL of blood from this same patient will not necessarily decrease CVP. In response to hypovolemia, the sympathetic tone will increase, causing venoconstriction and shifting (or recruiting) unstressed volume into the stressed volume compartment and thereby facilitating venous return.

19. How does one define volume responsiveness? How is it measured?

The gold standard for measuring volume responsiveness has traditionally relied on the concept of thermodilution using a pulmonary artery catheter (PAC) to measure the difference in stroke volume after a 250 to 500 mL fluid bolus. Because the measured cardiac output or stroke volume using the PAC has a variability of 5% to 10%, volume responsiveness has been defined as a 10% to 15% increase in cardiac output or stroke volume. Other modalities that measure cardiac output or stroke volume (e.g., pulse contour analyses, esophageal Doppler, bioimpedance) are often validated against the PAC.

20. Describe the dynamic tests used to assess fluid responsiveness. How are they performed?

Dynamic tests for fluid responsiveness rely on the Frank-Starling law to predict if a patient is volume responsive. There are two approaches used to determine a patient's position on the Frank-Starling curve: (1) respirophasic variation, and (2) fluid challenge.

The respirophasic variation approach relies on the physiological interactions with positive pressure breaths and its effect on stroke volume or BP. Respirophasic variation strategies require the following conditions be met: (1) normal heart rhythm, (2) controlled positive pressure ventilation, and (3) tidal volumes 8 mL/kg or more of ideal body weight (IBW). In the ICU, a large percentage of patients do not meet these requirements, as many have atrial fibrillation, are on patient-triggered synchronized ventilator modes, or being ventilated using lung-protection strategies (tidal volumes <8 mL/kg). However, in the operating room (OR), we are often able to use this approach.

The fluid challenge approach involves administering empiric fluid challenges, termed *reversible* or *irreversible*. Reversible fluid challenges entail performing a PLR maneuver, where the patient's legs provide an autologous fluid challenge of 250 to 300 mL of blood to the right heart. This approach has the benefit of preventing the unnecessary administration of fluid boluses and is often used in the ICU more so than in the OR for obvious reasons. Irreversible fluid challenges involve administering 250 to 500 mL of crystalloid, over approximately 10 minutes.

Regardless of which approach is used, each requires a method to measure a change in BP, stroke volume, or cardiac output. The methods most often used in the ICU rely on measuring changes in stroke volume or cardiac output with a continuous monitor. In the OR, monitoring BP variations with an arterial-line and/or stroke volume changes with an esophageal Doppler are more often used. Each approach has different cutoff points used to predict fluid responsiveness. See Table 25.2 for an overview of various dynamic modalities and methods.

Table 25.2 Measures of Volume Responsiveness, Diagnostic Thresholds, and Limitations		
METHODS	**THRESHOLD (%Δ > SV/CO)**	**LIMITATIONS**
Fluid Challenge		
Fluid challenge (250–500 mL)	10%–15%	Giving excess fluid in nonresponders
Passive leg raise (300 mL autologous transfusion)	10%	Requires a continuous measure of cardiac output. Not valid in patients with abdominal compartment syndrome, pregnancy, or lower extremity amputation, Contraindications: Elevated ICP
Respirophasic Variation		
PPV	12%	Spontaneous breathing effort, cardiac dysrhythmias, low tidal volumes, intraabdominal hypertension or open chest
Systolic pressure variation	12%	Same limitations, but slightly less accurate than PPV. Easier to calculate at the bedside
IVC diameter variation	18% (PPV) 40% (NPV)	Poor sensitivity in spontaneously breathing patients and in low tidal volume ventilation
EDM (stroke volume)	14%	Same limitations as PPV. Approximates aortic diameter based on demographic data, makes assumptions to calculate cardiac output as EDM only measures blood flow in descending aorta
Arterial pulse waveform analysis (stroke volume)	9%–15%	Same limitations as PPV Invasive (requires arterial line and ± central line)

CO, Cardiac output; *EDM,* esophageal Doppler monitor; *ICP,* intracranial pressure; *IVC,* inferior vena cava; *NPV,* negative pressure ventilation (or spontaneous breathing); *PPV,* positive pressure ventilation, *SV,* stroke volume.

Data from Monnet X, Marik PE, Teboul J-L. Prediction of fluid responsiveness: an update. Ann Intensive Care. 2016;6:111.

21. Describe the physiology behind stroke volume variation during positive pressure ventilation (i.e., respirophasic changes).

On inhalation, during a positive pressure breath, venous return to the right heart decreases (decreased preload) and pulmonary vascular resistance increases (increased afterload) causing a drop in right heart stroke volume. However, at the same time, venous return to the left heart increases (increased preload) and afterload decreases (positive intrathoracic pressures decreases the transmural pressure across the left ventricle, favoring contraction), each leading to an increase in stroke volume. Conversely, during the expiratory phase, this change is reversed, resulting in an increase in stroke volume for the right heart and a decrease in stroke volume for the left heart.

It is important to note that a sufficient tidal volume (≥ 8 mL/kg IBW) is necessary to produce a measurable effect on stroke volume. The observed difference in stroke volume between inspiration and expiration will be exaggerated in the setting of hypovolemia, as the patient is on the "steep portion" of the Frank-Starling curve (see Fig. 25.1).

Of note, the explanation behind this phenomenon is similar to the commonly taught "Split S2" (temporal difference between pulmonic and aortic valve closure on inhalation) heard during cardiac auscultation. However, the physiological effects are reversed in the setting of positive pressure ventilation, with pulmonic valve closure following aortic valve closure.

22. Respirophasic parameters, such as pulse pressure variation and systolic pressure variation are frequently used in the perioperative setting to determine volume responsiveness. How are these calculated?

Both pulse pressure variation (PPV) and systolic pressure variation (SPV) have been extensively studied to determine volume responsiveness. Although PPV appears to be slightly more accurate for volume responsiveness, both are useful.

To calculate PPV, the inspiratory and expiratory phase pulse pressure (PP) obtained from an arterial line can be calculated as follows:

$$PPV\% = (PP_{max} - PP_{min})/((PP_{max} + PP_{min})/2) \times 100\%$$

To calculate SPV, the inspiratory and expiratory phase systolic blood pressure (SBP) obtained from an arterial line can be calculated as follows:

$$SPV\% = (SBP_{max} - SBP_{min})/((SBP_{max} + SBP_{min})/2) \times 100\%$$

The PPV% and the SPV% can then be used to determine if the patient is volume responsive based on the following: less than 8%, patient is likely not fluid responsive; 8% to 12%, is indeterminate; over 12%, patient is likely fluid responsive. Note that SPV is much easier to calculate by hand and can readily be visualized on the monitor in emergent situations to qualitatively predict volume responsiveness within a reasonable degree of accuracy.

23. How does one perform a passive leg raise maneuver?

The PLR maneuver is performed by transitioning a patient from a 45-degree semirecumbent position to a fully supine position, with bilateral lower-extremity elevation to 45 degrees, flexed at the hip (Fig. 25.2). This maneuver provides a "reversible fluid challenge" of approximately 300 mL of autologous blood when performed correctly. Continuous real time measurements of stroke volume must be made to assess the hemodynamic response to PLR, as the hemodynamic effects of this maneuver reach a maximum at 1 minute and diminish quickly. Of note, a PAC to assess changes in stroke volume will prove challenging, as this modality is too slow, too cumbersome, and too intermittent to reliably measure the transient response with PLR.

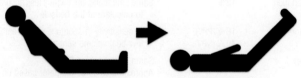

45 degrees Semi-Recumbant   45 degrees Passive Leg Raise

Fig. 25.2 The passive leg raise maneuver consists of the following steps:
1) Measure stroke volume (or cardiac output) in 45-degrees semi-recumbent position.
2) Lay the patient flat and raise the legs to 45 degrees, keeping the knees straight, and keeping the torso flat.
3) Hold this position and repeat the measure of stroke volume (or cardiac output) 30 to 60 seconds after attaining this position. Reposition the patient semi-recumbent when this maneuver is complete.
(From Pitman JT, Thapa GB, Harris NS. Field ultrasound evaluation of central volume status and acute mountain sickness. Wilderness Environ Med. 2015;26(3):320.)

24. What about esophageal Doppler monitoring?

Esophageal Doppler monitoring (EDM) measures the velocity of blood flow in the descending aorta and can be used to predict fluid responsiveness by measuring changes in stroke volume. Fluid responsiveness can be assessed by measuring changes in stroke volume using respirophasic variation, fluid challenges, or PLR. The percentage change in stroke volume variation (SVV%) can be calculated using the following equation:

$$SVV\% = (SV_{max} - SV_{min})/((SV_{max} + SV_{min})/2) \times 100\%$$

Measuring the SVV% has the same requirements as other respirophasic variation measurements, including: (1) tidal volumes greater than 8 mL/kg IBW, (2) sinus rhythm, and (3) controlled positive pressure ventilation. An SVV% over 14% is a predictor of volume responsiveness.

Flow-time corrected (FTc) measures the systolic duration of the left ventricle. This is thought to correlate with stroke volume and is often used as predictor of fluid responsiveness. It is calculated by measuring the flow time of blood moving down the descending aorta, corrected to a heart rate of 60. FTc is considered a static measurement, whereas stroke volume variation is a dynamic measurement. Evidence to date demonstrates that FTc, like other static measurements, is a poor predictor of fluid responsiveness and has an accuracy approximately equal to the flip of a coin (~50%) compared with SVV% (~90%).

25. How do devices using pulse contour analysis (i.e., PiCCO, LiDCO, and FloTrac) calculate stroke volume?

Pulse contour analysis uses arterial BP waveform morphology to calculate stroke volume. It is based on the premise that the stroke volume is proportional to the area under the curve.

PiCCO™ uses thermal transpulmonary dilution, and LiDCO™ uses lithium transpulmonary dilution to measure "true cardiac output." These data are then used to solve for arterial compliance in a process known as *calibration*. Each device requires regular recalibration, as critically ill patients have frequent changes in overall arterial compliance because of fluctuating levels of catecholamines.

FloTrac/Vigeleo™ is a more pragmatic approach, using patient demographic data to estimate arterial compliance, thus forgoing calibration to calculate arterial compliance. It also uses the area under the arterial waveform to calculate stroke volume; however, it makes assumptions for arterial compliance, raising questions about the accuracy of its measurements. Regardless, this modality's ability to predict fluid responsiveness by measuring changes in stroke volume appears reasonably well validated.

26. How can inferior vena cava diameter collapse (or distension) be used to predict fluid responsiveness? How does this technique differ from other dynamic measures?

IVC diameter changes, measured with a standard ultrasound or by echocardiography, occur as a result of respirophasic effects on right atrial pressure. This is the only respirophasic measurement that has been validated in a spontaneously breathing patient. In the inspiratory phase for a spontaneously breathing patient (negative pressure ventilation), the percentage change in IVC diameter because of collapse is measured (% collapse). When patients are on a mechanical ventilator (positive pressure ventilation), the IVC distends and this percentage change can be measured (% distention).

$$\%Collapse = ((D_{max} - D_{min})/D_{max}) \times 100$$

or

$$\%Distention = ((D_{max} - D_{min})/D_{min}) \times 100$$

A patient is likely volume responsive when the % collapse of the IVC is greater than 40% for patient that is spontaneously breathing, or a % distention greater than 18% for patient that is on a mechanical ventilator receiving positive pressure ventilation. IVC collapse is considered less accurate because spontaneously breathing patients will have a variable size and frequency of tidal volumes.

27. What is extravascular lung water?

EVLW is a relatively new static measurement that quantifies the degree of pulmonary edema and can be used to asses for hypervolemia. Specifically, it measures all water in the lungs that is outside the pulmonary vasculature (interstitial, alveolar, intracellular, and lymphatic fluid). An increase in EVLW can be caused by cardiogenic pulmonary edema (i.e., hypervolemia or cardiogenic shock) or noncardiogenic pulmonary edema (i.e., increased vascular permeability).

EVLW increases after a specific hydrostatic pressure threshold is reached. This threshold is primarily affected by capillary permeability. In patients with damage to the endothelial glycocalyx (which occurs in many pathophysiological conditions, including sepsis, surgical stress, and large volume crystalloid administration), permeability increases and the rate of measurable EVLW volume will be higher than in a normal lung for a given hydrostatic pulmonary venous pressure (Fig. 25.3). Increased EVLW is associated with increased hospital mortality among critically ill patients.

28. How does one measure EVLW?

EVLW can be measured in several ways. The gold standard is to simply weigh the lungs of a cadaver. Fortunately, there are other modalities that do not require an autopsy. Devices, such as PiCCO$_2$™ and EV1000™ use transpulmonary thermodilution and arterial pulse contour analysis to approximate EVLW with reasonable accuracy.

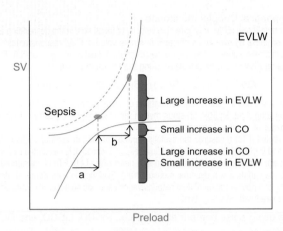

Fig. 25.3 Pulmonary edema (or extravascular lung water [*EVLW*]) can be graphically represented with the Mark-Phillips curve superimposed on the Frank-Starling curve. On the steep portion of the Frank-Starling curve, preload changes effect stroke volume more so than pulmonary capillary pressure. Conversely, on the flat portion of this same curve, preload changes affect pulmonary capillary pressure more so than stroke volume increasing EVLW. Analogous to how systolic or diastolic heart failure can modulate the Frank-Starling curve, patients in sepsis or acute respiratory distress syndrome can shift the Mark-Phillips curve, predisposing patients to pulmonary edema because of increased capillary permeability. *CO*, Cardiac output; *SV*, stroke volume. (From Marik P, Lemson J. Fluid responsiveness: an evolution of our understanding. Br J Anaesth. 2014;112:618.)

Bioreactance (i.e., NICOM™), which measures the phase shift of electric current across the chest, is another technique, which is being used to estimate EVLW. Noninvasive measurements of EVLW include CXR, CT, and ultrasound. However, these measurements are more qualitative in nature and less accurate.

29. "Fluid tolerance" is a term used to describe the margin of safety for fluid administration. Describe a practical approach that may be used to determine fluid tolerance.
    In every patient receiving intravenous fluids, the effects of their administration on stroke volume and EVLW should be considered simultaneously. In patients who are healthy, and who are on the steep portion of the Frank-Starling curve, fluid administration should increase stroke volume, without increasing EVLW, signaling a margin of safety for volume administration. However, patients with impaired myocardial function and damaged, "leaky" pulmonary capillaries may exhibit only limited increases in stroke volume with fluid administration and will more readily incur pulmonary edema.
    A safe approach to volume administration therefore is to sequentially evaluate both volume responsiveness (ideally with a dynamic index of preload), and the observed effect on EVLW (ideally with a direct measure, such as PiCCO™, or at minimum, a measure of pulmonary edema, such as serial lung ultrasound). This approach minimizes harm associated with fluid administration and provides constant feedback about a patient's underlying cardiac and pulmonary physiology.

KEY POINTS: VOLUME ASSESSMENT

1. The fundamental reason to give volume is to increase stroke volume.
2. Dynamic indices use the Frank-Starling law to predict volume responsiveness (i.e., hypovolemia).
3. Dynamic indices are much more accurate than other modalities (static indices, physical exam, imaging studies) in assessing for hypovolemia.
4. Hypervolemia assessment traditionally relies on a combination of physical examination, history, and imaging studies for proper assessment.
5. EVLW is a relatively new static measurement that may be helpful in managing hypervolemia.

Suggested Readings

Funk DJ, Jacobsohn E, Kumar A. The role of venous return in critical illness and shock—part I: physiology. Crit Care Med. 2013;41:255–262.
Gupta R, Gan TJ. Peri-operative fluid management to enhance recovery. Anaesthesia. 2016;71(Suppl 1):40–45.
Marik P, Bellomo R. A rational approach to fluid therapy in sepsis. Br J Anaesth. 2016;116:339–349.
Mohsenin V. Practical approach to detection and management of acute kidney injury in critically ill patient. J Intensive Care Med. 2017;5:57.
Monnet X, Marik P, Teboul J-L. Passive leg raising for predicting fluid responsiveness: a systematic review and meta-analysis. Intensive Care Med. 2016;42:1935–1947.
Monnet X, Marik P, Teboul J-L. Prediction of fluid responsiveness: an update. Ann Intensive Care. 2016;6:111.

CHAPTER 26

THE ANESTHESIA MACHINE

David J. Douin, MD, Ryan D. Laterza, MD

1. What is an anesthesia machine?

    A more modern and correct name for an anesthesia machine is *anesthesia delivery system*. The job of the first anesthesia machines was to supply a mixture of anesthetizing and life-sustaining gases to the patient. Modern anesthesia delivery systems perform these functions, as well as ventilating and monitoring the patient. The most important purpose is to help the anesthesiologist and anesthesia provider keep the patient safe and adequately anesthetized. Currently, there are two major manufacturers available in the United States: Dräger and GE Healthcare (owner of Datex-Ohmeda).

2. Describe the "plumbing" of an anesthesia machine.

    Leaving out the safety features and monitors, the anesthesia machine is divided into three sections:
    - The gas delivery system, which supplies at its outlet a chosen, defined mixture of gases
    - The patient breathing system, which includes the breathing circuit, carbon dioxide absorber, ventilator, and often gas pressure and flow monitors
    - The scavenger system, which collects excess gas and expels it outside of the hospital, thereby reducing exposure of the operating room personnel to anesthetic gases

3. What gases are commonly available on anesthesia machines? What are their sources?

    Oxygen, nitrous oxide, and air are available on almost every anesthesia machine. Usually the gas source for an anesthesia machine is from a centralized wall or pipeline supply. An emergency backup supply for each medical gas is stored in a compressed gas cylinder called an *E-cylinder*, and is attached to the rear of the anesthesia machine. These gas cylinders should be checked daily to ensure they contain an adequate backup supply in case of central pipeline failure.

4. List the uses of oxygen in an anesthesia machine.

    - Contributes to the fresh gas flow
    - Provides gas for the oxygen flush valve
    - Used as a driving gas for bellow ventilators: Ascending bellow ventilators, still used by modern GE machines, use oxygen as a driving gas. Pressure inside the bellows will always be slightly higher than that in the housing chamber (by 1–2 cm H_2O) because of the weight of the bellows itself. This is important because if there was a leak within the bellows, any net gas flow would be out of (not into) the bellows, and would not change the composition of the inspired gas.

5. Because the flow rates of air, nitrous oxide, and oxygen are controlled independently, can the machine ever be set to deliver a hypoxic gas mixture to the patient?

    In a word, no. Both Dräger and GE machines include several safety features, which prevent the provider from delivering a hypoxic gas mixture to the patient. First, software in modern anesthesia machines prevents the provider from digitally prescribing a hypoxic mixture. Further, anesthesia machines have built in "fail-safe devices" to safeguard the patient from the delivery of hypoxic gas mixtures. These "fail-safe devices" are machine specific and include an internal electric gas mixing device (GE) or a sensitive oxygen ratio controller system (Dräger). These devices either proportionally reduce or completely shut off flow from other gases, if the oxygen supply pressure decreases too much. The GE device has a circuit board that relies on pressure sensors and resistors to monitor and control flow, whereas Dräger uses a mechanical device that uses resistors and valves, and controls flow through a mechanical-pneumatic link between the two gas lines. Both devices ensure that the ratio of nitrous oxide to oxygen is such that fraction of inspired oxygen (F_iO_2) remains greater than 25%, provided the anesthesia gas lines have not been swapped and are properly connected (Fig. 26.1).

6. What other mechanisms exist for preventing the administration of a hypoxic gas mixture?

    - In older machines with flowmeters, the oxygen flow knob is larger and distinctively fluted. Knobs for the other gases are smaller and knurled.
    - A color code exists such that the color for each gas knob, flowmeter, tank, and wall attachment are all consistent. In the United States, oxygen is green, air is yellow, and nitrous oxide is blue. International standards may differ.

7. What is a *pressure regulator*? What is a *check valve*? How do these control the flow of gas into the anesthesia machine?

    The medical gases stored in the E-cylinders are under high pressure (i.e., 2000 pressure per square inch gauge [psig] for oxygen, 2000 psig for air, and 750 psig for nitrous oxide), all of which are too high for the anesthesia

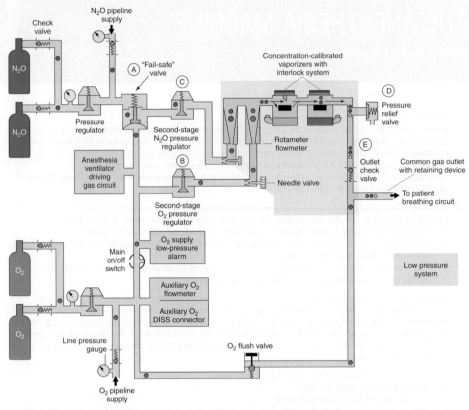

Fig. 26.1 Schematic demonstrating an overview of the gas source, pressure regulators, high- and low-pressure circuits, vaporizers, and flowmeters of a generic anesthesia machine. *N2O*, Nitrous oxide. (From Eisenkraft JB. The anesthesia machine and workstation. In: Ehrenwerth J, Eisenkraft JB, Berry JM, eds. Anesthesia Equipment: Principles and Applications. 2nd ed. Philadelphia: Elsevier Saunders; 2013:28.)

machine, which requires a pressure of approximately 50 ± 5 psig. The function of the pressure regulator is to accept a high-pressure gas from its input, reduce its pressure, and then output that gas at a much lower pressure. Each gas E-cylinder has a separate pressure regulator to ensure its output is 45 psig. The pipeline gas supply has a pressure of approximately 50 to 55 psig and does not need to flow through a pressure regulator.

Each pipeline gas supply and their respective E-cylinder will then converge together before connecting to the anesthesia machine. However, just before their convergence, gas from the pipeline and the E-cylinder, each flow through their own check valve. This valve ensures that gas can only flow in one direction, as determined by the pressure gradient across the valve. The pressure regulator and the two check valves allow gas to flow preferentially from the pipeline gas supply and then from the E-cylinder as a backup. For example, normally the oxygen pipeline supply pressure is 50 to 55 psig and the pressure from the oxygen E-cylinder after the pressure regulator is 45 psig. Because of the check valves, oxygen will not flow from the supply pipeline into the E-cylinder and oxygen will only flow from the supply pipeline to the anesthesia machine. If the supply pipeline were to fail, its pressure would drop and oxygen would then flow from the E-cylinder to the anesthesia machine. Oxygen from the E-cylinder would not be able to flow retrograde because of the check valve on the hospital's oxygen supply pipeline.

8. **How does the hospital pipeline (central) gas supply compare with the use of compressed gas cylinders?**

For practical purposes, wall gases are continuous in volume availability, assuming the central supply is refilled. As mentioned earlier, pipeline gas pressures are typically 50 to 55 psig and the E-cylinder tank pressure is regulated by the "first-stage" pressure regulator to 45 psig. Because of the use of "one-way" check valves, gas will preferentially flow from the source (E-cylinder vs. hospital pipeline) with the highest pressure (45 psig for E-cylinder vs. 50–55 psig for hospital pipeline) to the anesthesia machine. Provided everything is working correctly, the wall supply is used rather than the tank supply. Use of wall supply oxygen is preferable because it is available in greater volume, is cheaper, and preserves the tank supply for emergency situations.

9. Imagine the central supply of oxygen is lost. The gauge on the oxygen tank reads 1000 psi. How long will you be able to deliver oxygen before the tank is empty?

Contemporary anesthesia machines have two supply sources for medical gas: the pipeline supply from the wall and E-cylinders attached to the back of the machine itself. The cylinders are color coded and should be kept off, unless there is a failure of the hospital pipeline supply.

Cylinder Colors (in the United States)

Oxygen—Green
Nitrous Oxide—Blue
Air—Yellow
Carbon Dioxide—Gray
Nitrogen—Black

A full, green E-cylinder of oxygen has a pressure of 2000 psig and contains about 625 L of oxygen. Because the oxygen is a compressed gas, the volume in the E-cylinder correlates linearly with the pressure on the gauge. Therefore a pressure of 1000 psig means that the oxygen E-cylinder has about 312 L of gas remaining.

The oxygen supply to the anesthesia machine may be used for two purposes: (1) to oxygenate the patient, and (2) to pneumatically drive the ventilator bellows. When oxygen is used for both, a large percentage will be lost to drive the bellows (corresponding to the patient's minute ventilation). Thus if a patient is receiving an oxygen fresh gas flow (FGF) of 1 L/min in the breathing circuit, with a minute ventilation of 9 L/min, 10 L of oxygen will be drained from the oxygen E-cylinder every minute. An E-cylinder with 312 L remaining will last for about 30 minutes at this rate. To minimize consumption of oxygen from the E-cylinder, it is recommended to turn off the bellow-driven ventilator and begin hand ventilating the patient.

One of the advantages of a piston-driven ventilator, as opposed to a bellow-driven ventilator, is that the piston is driven by electricity instead of oxygen, greatly reducing the amount that might be otherwise wasted driving the bellows. In this case, given the earlier scenario, only oxygen used by the FGF is consumed and you would have about 300 minutes of oxygen supply, instead of 30 minutes.

10. A new E-cylinder of nitrous oxide is installed, and the pressure gauge reads only 750 psig. Why is the pressure in the nitrous oxide cylinder different than the others?

Air and oxygen are compressed gases. Under normal circumstances, gases can be compressed into their liquid form provided this transformation is conducted below that specific gases' critical temperature (the temperature at which a gas can be compressed into a liquid). Oxygen and air cannot be compressed into liquids at their storage temperature (i.e., room temperature) because at room temperature, the critical temperature is exceeded. Therefore they exist in gas form within their respective E-cylinders.

The relationship between the volume of gas in a cylinder and the pressure displayed on its gauge is linear because of the ideal gas law (P (pressure) × V (volume) = n (no of moles) × R (gas constant) × T (temperature)). As a result, the volume of gas remaining in an oxygen or air cylinder is directly proportional to the gauge pressure. The pressure of a full air or oxygen cylinder is approximately 2000 psig. A pressure reading of 1000 psig would suggest that the tank is half-full.

Nitrous oxide, however, condenses into a liquid at 747 psig. Therefore it exists as a liquid at room temperature. E-cylinders of nitrous oxide contain, in liquid form, the equivalent of about 1600 L of gas when full. The pressure in the cylinder will remain constant, until all of the liquid nitrous oxide has been vaporized into gas form. This point is reached when approximately 25% of the initial volume of nitrous oxide remains in the cylinder. Only then does the pressure displayed on the gauge begin to decrease below 750 psig. An accurate estimation of the volume remaining in the cylinder before this point requires weighing the cylinder and subtracting the empty (tare) weight of the cylinder.

11. Describe the safety systems used to prevent incorrect central and cylinder gas connections to the anesthesia machine.

- All central supply gas connectors are keyed so, for example, only the oxygen supply hose can be plugged into the oxygen connector on the wall, the nitrous oxide hose into the nitrous oxide outlet, and so on. This is known as the *Diameter Index Safety System* (DISS)
- The gas cylinders are keyed using the Pin Index Safety System (PISS—no kidding!) so that only the correct tank can be attached to the corresponding yolk on the anesthesia machine (assuming that the pins have not been sheared off!)
- These safety systems should always include an oxygen analyzer on the inspiratory limb that measures the delivered oxygen concentration to the patient. This is the most important safety feature of the anesthesia machine in preventing a delivery of a hypoxic gas mixture

12. Why are the flowmeters always arranged in a specific order?

In the United States, the oxygen flowmeter must always be on the right, closest to the point of egress into the common gas manifold, just proximal to the anesthesia vaporizers. With the oxygen flowmeter in that position, most leaks tend to selectively lose gases other than oxygen, thereby lessening the likelihood of delivering a hypoxic gas mixture. In addition, requiring the oxygen knob to be in the same relative position on all anesthesia machines helps decrease the risk of accidentally turning the wrong knob. Again, the best way to detect a hypoxic gas mixture is by the oxygen analyzer.

Reasons for this arrangement, other than safety, include National Institute for Occupational Safety and Health government standards, and manufacturer's convention.

13. **Would it be better to have the E-cylinder oxygen tank routinely left open, so as to avoid having to manually open it in the event of pipeline supply failure?**
No. The oxygen supply pipeline pressure, although typically 50 to 55 psig, may occasionally fluctuate below 45 psig. Recall that this is the pressure of the backup tank after the "first-pass" pressure regulator. If left open and a dip in pipeline pressure were to occur, oxygen would then be drawn unnecessarily from the E-cylinder. You may not recognize that this has occurred until the tank is actually needed, only for you to discover that it is empty, while the low oxygen pressure alarm begins to sound. At this point, you would have to quickly scramble to find another oxygen source.

14. **Describe the process of vaporization?**
The saturated vapor pressure of a volatile agent determines the concentration of vapor molecules located just above its surface. As temperature increases, vapor pressure increases. The converse is also true. The energy required to release molecules from the liquid phase to the gas phase is known as the heat of vaporization. Volatile agents, stored in liquid form in the vaporizer, ideally absorb external heat during the process of vaporization; otherwise, the liquid itself would become colder as molecules entered the gas phase. This cooling would cause the vapor pressure to decrease, thereby decreasing volatile agent delivery. To address this issue, vaporizers are constructed of metals possessing high thermal conductivity, thus facilitating the necessary heat transfer required for vaporization from the environment.

15. **What is a variable bypass vaporizer? Why must these remain upright at all times?**
The anesthetic vaporizers are located downstream from the flowmeters. Fresh gas from the flowmeters enters the vaporizer and is then divided into two streams: one stream entering the vaporizing chamber and becoming saturated with volatile agent, and the other entering the bypass chamber. The concentration dial determines what proportion of gas flow enters each chamber. These two streams then reunite near the vaporizer outlet. The fresh gas leaving the vaporizer contains the vapor concentration specified by the concentration dial (Fig. 26.2).

If a variable bypass vaporizer is turned on its side, liquid anesthetic may spill from the vaporizing chamber into the bypass chamber. This would effectively create two vaporizing chambers, increasing vaporizer output, and potentially delivering very high levels of volatile anesthetic to the patient. Most (but not all) modern vaporizers have mechanisms that minimize this problem.

16. **What is temperature compensation?**
During the process of vaporization, liquid anesthetic invariably cools. As this occurs, saturated vapor pressure decreases, thereby decreasing vaporizer output. Vaporizers, with temperature compensation, are better able to maintain a constant output of anesthetic agent, despite the temperature changes caused by vaporization.

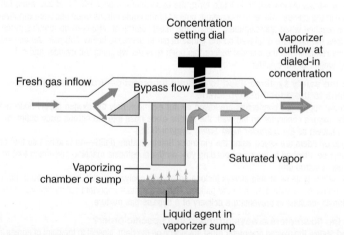

Fig. 26.2 Schematic of concentration calibrated variable bypass vaporizer. (From Eisenkraft JB. Anesthesia vaporizers. In: Ehrenwerth J, Eisenkraft JB, Berry JM, eds. Anesthesia Equipment: Principles and Applications. 2nd ed. Philadelphia: Elsevier Saunders; 2013:68.)

17. **How does altitude affect modern vaporizers?**

The effect of the change in barometric pressure on volume percent output can be calculated as follows: $x' = x\frac{p}{p'}$ where x' is the output in volume percent at the new altitude (p'), and x is the concentration output in volume percent for the altitude (p), when the vaporizer is calibrated.

Consider the following example: a vaporizer calibrated at sea level $(p = 760$ mm Hg) is taken to Denver, Colorado (5280 ft [~1609 m]) $(p' = 630$ mm Hg), and set to deliver 1% isoflurane vapor (x). The actual output (x') is $1\% \times \frac{760}{630} = 1.2\%$. However, recall that it is the partial pressure of the vapor, not the concentration in volume percent, which is the important factor in determining depth of anesthesia. So, 1% at sea level (760 mm Hg) is 7.6 mm Hg; 1.2% in Denver (630 mm Hg) is 7.6 mm Hg. Therefore regardless of altitude, the clinical effect will be unchanged.

18. **What happens if you put the wrong agent in a vaporizer?**

Filling an agent-specific vaporizer with the incorrect agent will typically deliver the wrong dose of agent. The most important factor in determining the direction of error (either under-or overdose) is the vapor pressure of the agent. If an agent with a higher vapor pressure is put into a vaporizer meant for a less volatile agent, output will be excessive. Conversely, if an agent with a lower vapor pressure than the agent intended for the vaporizer is used, the anesthetic output will be lower than anticipated. Vaporizers and volatile anesthetic supply bottles are usually keyed to prevent the incorrect addition of volatile anesthetics to the wrong vaporizers.

19. **Can two vaporizers be operating simultaneously?**

Modern anesthesia machines have an interlocking manifold that allows only one vaporizer to be turned on at a time. However, in anesthesia machines that allow for three vaporizers, the center spot must be occupied for the interlocking manifold to be operational.

20. **What is different about the desflurane vaporizer?**

Desflurane has a vapor pressure of 664 mm Hg at 20°C, which is much higher than the vapor pressures of either isoflurane (238 mm Hg) or sevoflurane (157 mm Hg). Recall that the boiling point of a liquid is the temperature at which its vapor pressure equals atmospheric pressure; 760 mm Hg at sea level. Therefore the boiling point of desflurane is approximately room temperature at sea level and even lower at elevation (i.e., Denver, Colorado).

Vapor pressure increases exponentially with temperature. With desflurane already being on the steep part of the vaporization curve, even at room temperature, passive vaporization would lead to significant variations in vapor pressure. This is because as the liquid agent cools during the process of vaporization, vapor pressure would significantly decrease, changing its position on the curve and, hence its vapor pressure. To overcome this situation, desflurane vaporizers require active compensation to maintain a constant temperature throughout the vaporization process.

The desflurane vaporizer differs from other variable bypass vaporizers by actively heating the liquid to 39°C. At this temperature, the vapor pressure of the agent is approximately 2 atmospheres, or 1550 mm Hg. This pressure allows for a more accurate delivery of agent.

21. **At an altitude of 7000 feet, you have to set the desflurane vaporizer to deliver more gas than usual. Why do you not do this with other anesthetic agents as well?**

Conventional vaporizers (for halothane, isoflurane, and sevoflurane) are altitude compensated. The altitude compensation occurs because the diverting valve is functionally located at the outlet of the vaporizer, a variation in design that minimizes the pumping and pressurizing effects. The output of these vaporizers is a constant partial pressure of agent, not a constant volume percent. The desflurane vaporizer, however, does not divert a portion of the fresh gas flow through a vaporizing chamber, but rather adds vapor to the gas flow to produce a true volume percent output. Because it is the number of molecules of agent (the partial pressure) that anesthetizes the patient, conventional vaporizers provide the same anesthetizing potency at any altitude, whereas the desflurane vaporizer delivers a set volume percent regardless of altitude. However, the delivered partial pressure will decrease with altitude, because a constant percentage of gas represents a decreased partial pressure when the total (barometric) pressure is decreased. This is because of Dalton's law of partial pressures. At 7000 feet (2134 m), the barometric pressure is 586 mm Hg and the delivered partial pressure for one minimum alveolar concentration (MAC) of desflurane (6%) is 35 mm Hg as opposed to 46 mm Hg at sea level. A correspondingly higher percentage of desflurane must be delivered to achieve MAC at 7000 feet.

22. **What is a scavenger?**

Except in a truly closed-circuit situation, gas is always entering and leaving the anesthesia breathing circuit. Exhaust gas is a mixture of exhaled gas from the patient and fresh gas that exceeded the patient's needs, but contains anesthetic agent. To reduce exposure of operating room personnel to trace amounts of anesthetic agents, it is appropriate to capture and expel this anesthetic-laden gas from the operating room environment.

The device used to transfer this gas safely from the breathing circuit to the hospital vacuum system is called a *scavenger.* Because of the periodicity of breathing, gas exits the breathing circuit in bursts. The scavenger provides a reservoir for this exhaust gas until the vacuum system, which works at a constant flow rate, can dispose of it. The scavenger must also prevent both excess suction and any blockage from affecting the patient breathing circuit. It accomplishes this via positive and negative relief valves. Thus if the vacuum is adjusted too high, a negative-pressure relief valve allows room air to mix with the exhaust gas, preventing the buildup of suction on the breathing circuit. If the vacuum system becomes occluded, fails, or its suction flow rate is too low, back pressure exits through a positive-pressure relief valve. (Granted this will contaminate the operating room, but that problem is minimal compared with blowing the patient's lungs up like a balloon.)

KEY POINTS: THE ANESTHESIA MACHINE AND VAPORIZERS

1. Anesthesia machines are integrated systems that not only deliver anesthetic gases but also monitors itself and the patient.
2. When compressed, some gases (nitrous oxide and carbon dioxide) readily condense into a liquid at room temperature, whereas others (oxygen, air, and nitrogen) do not. These properties define the relationship between gas volume supply and tank pressure.
3. Anesthesia machines must have a backup supply of oxygen in case of pipeline oxygen failure.
4. The output of traditional vaporizers depends on the proportion of fresh gas that bypasses the vaporizing chamber compared with the proportion that passes through the vaporizing chamber.
5. The desflurane vaporizer actively injects vapor into the fresh gas stream, whereas all other traditional vaporizers use a passive variable bypass system.

23. What are the different types of anesthesia breathing circuits?

Breathing circuits are usually classified as open, semi-open, semi-closed, or closed. They are configured to allow the patient to breathe spontaneously (negative pressure ventilation) or with manual or mechanical assistance (positive pressure ventilation), using supplemental O_2 and other anesthetic gases, as needed.

An open circuit is the method by which the first true anesthetics were given 160 years ago. A bit of cloth saturated with ether or chloroform was held over the patient's face. The patient inhaled the vapors and became anesthetized. The depth of anesthesia was controlled by the amount of liquid anesthetic on the cloth; thus, it took a great deal of trial and error to become good at the technique.

The various semi-open circuits were described by Mapleson and are commonly known as the *Mapleson A, B, C, D, E, and F circuits* (Fig. 26.3). Common components include a source of fresh gas, corrugated tubing (more resistant to kinking), and a pop-off or adjustable pressure-limiting (APL) valve. The circuits differ based upon the location of the pop-off valve and fresh gas input, and whether or not there is a gas reservoir bag. Advantages of the Mapleson series include simplicity of design, portability, anesthetic titratability, and lack of rebreathing of exhaled gases (provided the fresh gas flow is adequate). Disadvantages include lack of conservation of heat and moisture, limited ability to scavenge waste gases, and the need for high fresh gas flows. Semi-open circuits are rarely used today except during patient transport. Of note, the Mapleson A circuit is the most efficient for a spontaneously breathing patient, and the Mapleson D is the most efficient for controlled ventilation.

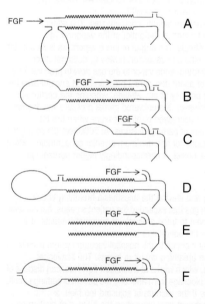

Fig. 26.3 Mapleson A, B, C, D, E, and F circuits. *FGF,* Fresh gas flow. (From Willis BA, Pender JW, Mapleson WW. Rebreathing in a T-piece. Br J Anaesth. 1975;47:1239–1246.)

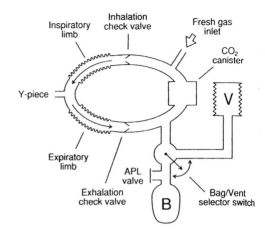

Fig. 26.4 Circle system. *APL*, Adjustable pressure-limiting. (From Andrews JJ. Inhaled anesthetic delivery system. In: Miller RD, ed. Anesthesia. 4th ed. New York: Churchill Livingstone; 1994:185–228.)

An example of a semi-closed circuit is the circle system, which is found in most operating rooms in the United States (Fig. 26.4). Every semi-closed system contains an inspiratory limb, an expiratory limb, unidirectional valves, a carbon dioxide absorber, gas reservoir bag, and an APL or "pop-off" valve, located on the expiratory limb. Advantages of a circle system include conservation of heat and moisture, the ability to use low flows of fresh gas (thereby conserving volatile anesthetic), and the scavenging of waste gases. A notable disadvantage is its complex design; it has approximately 10 connections, each of which has the potential for disconnection and/or leaks.

Like the semi-closed circuit, the closed circuit is a circle system adjusted so the inflow of fresh gas exactly equals the patient's oxygen consumption and anesthetic agent uptake. The exhaled carbon dioxide is eliminated by the CO_2 absorber.

24. Rank the Mapleson circuits in order of efficiency for both controlled and spontaneous ventilation.
    - Controlled: D > B > C > A (mnemonic: *Dog Bites Can Ache*)
    - Spontaneous: A > D > C > B (mnemonic: *All Dogs Can Bite*)

25. How would a breathing circuit disconnection be detected during the delivery of an anesthetic?
    A variety of events would suggest a breathing circuit disconnection during an anesthetic. Breath sounds would no longer be detected with an esophageal or precordial stethoscope, and, if the ventilator parameters are properly set, airway pressure and tidal volume–minute volume monitor alarms would sound. The capnograph would stop detecting carbon dioxide. Eventually, oxygen saturation would decline. However, despite all of this, exhaled carbon dioxide is probably the best monitor to detect disconnections; a decrease or absence of carbon dioxide is sensitive (although not specific) for disconnection.

26. How is carbon dioxide eliminated from a circle system?
    Exhaled gases pass through a canister containing a carbon dioxide absorbent most commonly, soda lime. Soda lime consists primarily of calcium hydroxide ($Ca[OH]_2$), with lesser quantities of sodium hydroxide (NaOH) and potassium hydroxide (KOH). Soda lime reacts with carbon dioxide to form heat, water, and calcium-carbonate. The reaction can be summarized as follows:

$$CO_2 + Ca(OH)_2 = CaCO_2 + H_2O + Heat$$

27. How much carbon dioxide can the absorbent neutralize? What factors affect its efficiency?
    Soda lime can absorb, at most, 23 L of carbon dioxide per 100 g of absorbent. However, the average absorber eliminates 10 to 15 L of carbon dioxide per 100 g absorbent, in a single-chamber system, and slightly more in a dual-chamber system. Factors affecting absorber efficiency include the size of the canister (the patient's tidal volume should be accommodated entirely within the void space of the canister), the size of the absorbent granule (optimal size is 2.5 mm or between 4 and 8 mesh), and the presence or absence of channeling (loose packing allowing exhaled gases to bypass absorber granules in the canister).

28. How do you know when the absorbent has been exhausted? What adverse reactions can occur between volatile anesthetics and carbon dioxide absorbents?
    A pH-sensitive dye added to the granules changes color in the presence of carbonic acid, an intermediary in the carbon dioxide absorption chemical reaction. The most common dye in the United States is ethyl violet, which is white when fresh and turns violet when the absorbent is exhausted.

Inhaled anesthetics passing through an absorbent, particularly soda lime, may produce carbon monoxide. This can increase carboxyhemoglobin levels in the patient and impair tissue oxygen delivery. The magnitude of carbon monoxide production per volatile anesthetic, from greatest to least is: desflurane = enflurane > isoflurane >> halothane = sevoflurane.

Factors which can increase the production of carbon monoxide include the following:

- Dryness of the absorbent
- Type of absorbent (calcium hydroxide > lithium hydroxide)
- Higher anesthetic concentrations
- Low fresh gas flow rates

Other adverse reactions between volatile anesthetics and absorbents are discussed in Chapter 14 *Inhaled Anesthetics.*

29. **What parameters can be adjusted on an anesthesia ventilator?**
Basic adjustable features include:

- Tidal volume
- Respiratory rate
- Inspiratory-to-expiratory (I:E) ratio
- F_iO_2
- Positive end expiratory pressure

30. **What ventilation modes are available on most modern anesthesia ventilators?**

- Volume controlled ventilation
- Pressure controlled ventilation
- Pressure controlled ventilation—volume guaranteed
- Synchronized intermittent mandatory ventilation
- Pressure support ventilation

31. **How and where is tidal volume measured? Why do different sites often yield different measurements?**
Tidal volume is measured via different techniques and at different sites in the breathing circuit. Common measures include the setting on the ventilator control panel, bellows excursion, and flow through the inspiratory (iTV) or expiratory (eTV) limbs of the circuit.

For several reasons, these measures frequently differ. First, circuit tubing is compliant and often absorbs some of the inhaled tidal volume (iTV), thereby reducing the actual tidal volume delivered to the patient. Second, small leaks in the circuit are common and may contribute to a decrease in eTV versus iTV. These include a loose circuit connections, complete disconnections, an under inflated endotracheal tube cuff, or leaks from the lung to the pleural (e.g., pneumothorax). Third, the carbon dioxide sample line removes about 100 to 200 mL/min of fresh gas from the breathing circuit. Lastly, consider the differences between oxygen consumption and carbon dioxide production. For example, a 70-kg patient under general anesthesia will consume about 250 mL of oxygen per minute and produce about 200 mL of carbon dioxide per minute. This creates a discrepancy of 50 mL of gas per minute, further decreasing eTV versus iTV.

32. **When using very low flows of fresh gas, why is there sometimes a discrepancy between inspired oxygen concentration and fresh gas concentration?**
At very low fresh gas flows, concentrations within the breathing circuit are slow to change. Importantly, the patient will consume different gases (removing them from the circuit) at rates different from the rates at which the gases are delivered to the circuit. In the case of oxygen, an average adult patient consumes (permanently removes from the circuit) approximately 250 mL of oxygen per minute. If nitrogen or nitrous oxide is supplied along with the oxygen, the patient will continue to consume oxygen, while the nitrogen or nitrous oxide builds up in the circuit. Therefore it is possible for a hypoxic mixture to develop within the circuit if the volume of oxygen delivered by the fresh gas flow is lower than the patient's metabolic oxygen consumption.

33. **What is included in the checkout of an anesthesia machine?**
Most modern anesthesia machines are able to perform an automated checkout process. Even though minimal manual input is required, it is important to become familiar with what the machine is checking during this process. To start, it ensures the oxygen analyzer is calibrated, typically the reference point is room air (21% F_iO_2). Next, it confirms the oxygen fail safe mechanism is intact, therefore safeguarding against the delivery of a hypoxic gas mixture. After that, both the high- and low-pressure circuits are checked for leaks. The high-pressure circuit includes the oxygen flush valve, inspiratory/expiratory valves, carbon dioxide absorbent, and circle breathing system. The low-pressure system includes the anesthetic vaporizers. Then, the functionality of the ventilator is assessed, as well as the alarm settings. Finally, the gas scavenging system is assessed.

In older machines, a manual checkout is required. This involves closing the pop-off valve, occluding the Y-piece of the circuit, and pressing the oxygen flush valve, until the pressure is greater than 30 cm H_2O. The pressure will not decline if there are no leaks. Next, the pop-off valve should be opened to ensure that it is in working order.

Regardless of the machine you are using, it is important to always perform the nonmachine portion of the anesthesia checkout between each anesthetic. This includes confirming functionality of the suction apparatus, availability of appropriate monitors (pulse oxymeter, end tidal carbon dioxide, noninvasive blood pressure, electrocardiogram, etc.), airway equipment (laryngoscope, endotracheal tube, etc.) and emergency equipment, and having the required pharmacologic agents for the upcoming procedure.

34. **How would you prepare the anesthesia machine for a patient with malignant hyperthermia?**
First, all volatile anesthetic vaporizers should be removed from the anesthesia machine (or, at the very least, made so that they will not be accidentally turned on). Modern GE machines have Aladdin cassette vaporizers, which are easily removed, whereas on Dräger machines, an Allen wrench is required to release them. Next, it is necessary to install a bypass block to the empty vaporizer slot. Note, Dräger recommends that their vaporizers be changed only by authorized service personnel. After that, the anesthesia machine should be flushed using a high fresh gas flow ($\geq$10 L/min) for at least 20 minutes (GE) or 60 minutes (Dräger) to remove all residual volatile anesthetic particles from the machine. Finally, the breathing circuit should be replaced and special charcoal filters, placed near the inspiratory and expiratory valves, should be used.

35. **How do anesthesia ventilators differ from intensive care unit ventilators?**
There are three categories of ventilators: bellow, piston, and turbine. Each refers to the mechanism which drives gas movement during ventilation. GE anesthesia machines use a bellow ventilator (discussed earlier), whereas Dräger machines use a piston. Piston ventilators are powered by electricity, and a driving gas is not required. They deliver more accurate tidal volumes, and a higher inspiratory flow rate compared with bellow ventilators. Most intensive care unit (ICU) ventilators use a turbine design.
ICU ventilators have three distinct advantages when compared with anesthesia machine ventilators. First, turbine ventilators deliver the most accurate tidal volume (turbine is more accurate than piston, which is more accurate than bellows.) This is particularly true when using very low tidal volumes (e.g., in pediatrics.) Second, ICU ventilators come equipped with more ventilation modes than anesthesia machine ventilators. Specialty modes, such as airway pressure release ventilation may be found on ICU ventilators but not on anesthesia machine ventilators. Third, ICU ventilators are able to deliver much higher inspiratory flow rates. This makes spontaneous breathing more comfortable for intubated patients. It also allows for a higher minute ventilation to better compensate for pathologic conditions, such as severe metabolic acidosis. Both instances are more common in the ICU.

KEY POINTS: ANESTHESIA CIRCUITS AND VENTILATORS

1. The semi-closed circuit using a circle system is the most commonly used anesthesia circuit in modern anesthesia machines.
2. Advantages of a circle system include conservation of volatile agents, heat, and moisture. Disadvantages include added complexity in design, multiple sites for leaks, and high compliance.
3. Although the capabilities of anesthesia machine ventilators have improved greatly in recent years, they are still not as sophisticated as a typical ICU ventilator.

SUGGESTED READINGS
Barash PG, Cullen BF, Stoelting RK, et al. Clinical Anesthesiology, 7th ed. Philadelphia: Lippincott Williams & Wilkins; 2013:641–696.
Brockwell RC, Andrews JJ. Inhaled anesthetic delivery systems. In: Miller RD, ed. Miller's Anesthesia. 8th ed. Philadelphia: Elsevier Saunders; 2015:273–316.
Dorsch JA, Dorsch SE. Understanding Anesthesia Equipment. 5th ed. Philadelphia: Lippincott Williams & Wilkins; 2008.

CHAPTER 27

MECHANICAL VENTILATION STRATEGIES

Joanna Olsen, MD, PhD, Ryan D. Laterza, MD

1. **Why might a patient require intubation and mechanical ventilation?**
   There are three main indications:
   1) Hypoxic respiratory failure
   2) Hypercarbic respiratory failure
   3) Airway protection
      These three indications may be caused by primary respiratory pathology (e.g., pneumonia, chronic obstructive pulmonary disease [COPD], acute respiratory distress syndrome [ARDS]), systemic disease or impairment (e.g., Glasgow coma scale <8, Guillain-Barré syndrome, drug intoxication), or airway compromise (e.g., retropharyngeal abscess, head and neck cancer, tracheal stenosis). The decision to intubate and provide mechanical ventilation (is based on both qualitative data (i.e., clinical examination, patient's wishes, and goals) and quantitative data (i.e., oxygen saturation, respiratory rate [RR], arterial blood gas analysis). The decision must be individualized because arbitrary cutoff values for partial pressure of oxygen, partial pressure of carbon dioxide, or pH as indicators of respiratory failure may not be germane to all patients. The principal goal of mechanical ventilation is to support gas exchange and minimize ventilator-induced lung injury until the underlying indication for it is resolved.

2. **Why are patients intubated and placed on MV for general anesthesia?**
   In most surgical operations, patients are intubated and placed on mechanical ventilation for two reasons: (1) airway protection, and (2) hypercarbic respiratory failure because of the neuro and respiratory depressant effects of anesthetic agents and paralytics. Mechanical ventilation may be discontinued and the patient extubated following emergence from general anesthesia, once these two indications are resolved. Specifically, the patient needs to demonstrate that they can protect their airway (e.g., stick out tongue, follow commands, evidence of coughing or gagging from the endotracheal tube [ETT]) and can breathe spontaneously without assistance.

3. **Define tidal volume, respiratory rate, minute ventilation, I:E ratio, PEEP, FiO_2.**
   Tidal volume (TV): The volume of gas delivered to the lungs on inhalation (e.g., 500 mL)
   Respiratory rate (RR): The number of breaths per minute. Sometimes referred to as *frequency* on some ventilators (e.g., 12 breaths per minute)
   Minute ventilation (MV): The amount of gas exchanged with the lung per minute where $MV = RR \times TV$ (e.g., 6 LPM)
   Inspired to expired (I:E) ratio: The ratio of time spent on inhalation versus exhalation (e.g., 1:2). Some ventilators may use inspiratory flow rate or inspiratory time (T_i) as a surrogate for this parameter
   Positive end-expiratory pressure (PEEP): Positive pressure delivered to the lungs to prevent atelectasis during exhalation
   Fraction of inspired oxygen (FiO_2): The percent oxygen delivered to the patient with each TV (e.g., 50%)

4. **Define peak inspiratory pressure, plateau pressure, pulmonary compliance, airway resistance.**
   Peak inspiratory pressure (PIP): The peak pressure during inhalation is measured on the inspiratory limb proximal to the ETT. This measurement is affected by the pulmonary compliance and pulmonary resistance (Fig. 27.1).
   Plateau pressure (P_{plat}): Reflects the pressure within the alveoli and is affected by the pulmonary compliance, but not resistance. Also measured on the inspiratory limb proximal to the ETT, it is done by performing a breath hold immediately following inhalation, when flow = 0 (see Fig. 27.1)
   Pulmonary compliance: This measures the overall compliance of the entire pulmonary system, including both the compliance of the lungs and extrinsic contributions from the abdomen and chest wall
   Airway resistance: This measures the resistance of the pulmonary system and reflects the difference between the PIP and P_{plat}.

5. **How does the plateau pressure (P_{plat}) measure the alveolar pressure (P_{alv})?**
   Recall Ohm's law, $\Delta V = I \times R$, where ΔV is a measure of the voltage drop (or gradient) across a resistor (R) for a given current (I). This equation can be applied to the pulmonary system where $\Delta P = Flow \times R$, with resistors in series between the inspiratory limb of the circuit and alveoli. These resistors are represented by the ETT (R_{ett}) and the distal airways (R_{airway}), each causing a pressure gradient (ΔP) for a given flow. During a breath hold, flow = 0, and the pressure gradient, ΔP across R_{ett} and R_{airway} is also 0. Therefore the inspiratory pressure is the following: $P_{insp} = P_{trach} = P_{alv}$, where P_{insp} is termed P_{plat} when flow = 0.

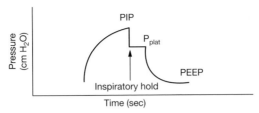

Fig. 27.1 The peak inspiratory pressure (*PIP*) is measured on the inspiratory limb proximal to the endotracheal tube. The plateau pressure (P_{plat}) reflects alveolar pressure and is measured with an inspiratory hold maneuver, immediately following inhalation, and measuring the subsequent pressure when flow = 0. Decreased compliance will increase P_{plat} and increased resistance will increase ($PIP - P_{plat}$). Therefore increases in PIP can be caused by decreased lung compliance or increased airway resistance. *PEEP*, Positive end expiratory pressure. (From Pacheco GS, Mendelson J, Gaspers M. Pediatric ventilator management in the emergency department. Emerg Med Clin North Am. 2018;36(2):409.)

6. List causes for an elevated PIP. How could you differentiate between them with a P_{plat}?
   See Table 27.1.

7. What is the difference between volume control and pressure control ventilation?
   Volume control ventilation provides breaths that are volume constant and pressure variable. This means that the "volume" of the delivered breath is set, or "controlled," by the clinician. The resultant airway pressures with this form of ventilation will depend on the compliance and resistance of the patient's respiratory system, which includes the ETT. Conversely, pressure-control provides breaths that are pressure constant and volume variable. In this mode, the amount of positive "pressure" delivered with each breath is set, or "controlled," by the clinician, and the TV that results from that pressure is again dependent on the resistance and compliance of the patient's respiratory system. Please see Fig. 27.2.
   Remember that in the operating room, events that cause a sudden change in respiratory compliance (e.g., prone positioning, laparoscopy, or paralytics) or airway resistance (e.g., bronchospasm, secretions, mucous plugs, kinked ETT) are common and can cause a dramatic change in the delivered TV, with pressure-control modes of ventilation.

8. How does a volume-controlled breath deliver the prescribed volume?
   Volume-controlled ventilation strategies could arguably be termed *flow-control* based on the mechanism of how the ventilator delivers the TV. The clinician sets the TV, RR, I:E, and the ventilator uses this data to calculate the necessary flow needed to deliver the prescribed TV. For example, assuming a TV of 500 mL, an RR of 10 breaths per minute, and an I:E of 1:2, the ventilator would first calculate the period (time) for one complete breath cycle (inhalation and exhalation) using the RR. In this example, 10 breaths per minute equals 6 seconds per breath. Then it calculates the T_i using the I:E ratio, which equals 2 seconds. The inspiratory flow rate is then calculated, which equals 500 mL/2 sec = 250 mL/sec. Traditionally, this breathe is given at a constant flow (e.g., 250 mL/sec) over the T_i as a "square waveform," but may be given as a "decelerating waveform" to mimic physiological breathing and improve patient comfort.

Table 27.1 Common Causes for an Elevated Peak Inspiratory Pressure	
DECREASED PULMONARY COMPLIANCE (ELEVATED P_{plat})	**INCREASED PULMONARY RESISTANCE (NORMAL P_{plat})**
Obesity	Kinked ETT
Laparoscopy	Small ETT
Trendelenburg position	Bronchospasm (e.g., asthma, COPD)
Abdominal Compartment Syndrome	Secretions
Cardiogenic pulmonary edema	Mucous plug (partially occluding the airway)
Noncardiogenic pulmonary edema (i.e., ARDS)	Bronchial blocker
Pneumonia	Bronchoscopy
Pulmonary fibrosis	
Surfactant deficiency	
Patient-ventilator dyssynchrony	

ARDS, Acute respiratory distress syndrome; *COPD*, chronic obstructive pulmonary disease; *ETT*, endotracheal tube.

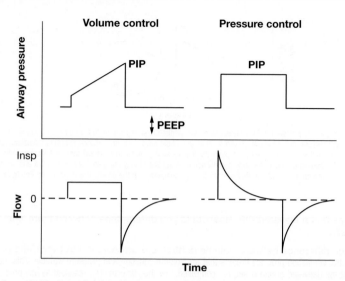

Fig. 27.2 Notice the constant inspiratory flow for volume control and the constant inspiratory pressure for pressure control. The volume control inspiratory flow waveform depicted above is a "square" waveform, which differs from the more natural "exponential decay" waveform of pressure control or spontaneous breathing. Volume control "decelerating flow" waveforms (not shown) attempt to mimic the natural "exponential decay" waveform but are linear and resemble a right-angle triangle with constant deceleration, which is reasonably close, but not as natural as a pressure-control breath. *PEEP,* Positive end expiratory pressure; *PIP,* peak inspiratory pressure.

9. **What are the advantages and disadvantages of a "volume-controlled" breath?**
   The primary advantage is that TVs are constant, minimizing the risk of hypoventilation or hyperventilation. The disadvantage is the nonphysiologic character of the delivered breaths, leading to patient discomfort or patient-ventilator dyssynchrony. This is because of two reasons: (1) flow is constant, and (2) TV is constant (see flow pattern in Fig. 27.2). Normal physiologic breathing is characterized by a high initial flow rate that downslopes toward zero (i.e., exponential decay) with variable TVs. Although most intensive care unit (ICU) ventilators have the ability to also deliver a synthetic "decelerating" flow patterns with volume-controlled breaths to mimic physiological breathing, the TVs are fixed and the decelerating flow pattern is linear (analogous to a right triangle) and not a true exponential decay pattern. In general, volume-controlled breaths are generally used just after induction and during maintenance of anesthesia.

10. **What are the advantages and disadvantages of a "pressure-controlled" breath?**
    The primary advantage is better patient comfort and a higher average inspired airway pressure. Because only the pressure is constant, the patient can determine the delivered inspiratory flow rate and TV which is more comfortable than a volume-controlled breath. Further, the inspiratory flow pattern is not forced but rather governed by the resistance and compliance of the patient's pulmonary system yielding an exponential decay flow pattern (see Fig. 27.2). The "pressure controlled" breath also delivers a higher average airway pressure for a given TV on inspiration compared with a volume-controlled breath. This facilitates alveolar recruitment from atelectasis and marginally increases the arterial partial pressure of oxygen (PaO_2):FiO_2 ratio. The disadvantage is because the TVs are variable, any changes to pulmonary compliance or resistance may lead to problems with hyperventilation or hypoventilation. In general, "pressure-controlled' breaths are most often used just before extubation on awake spontaneously breathing patients.

11. **How does a controlled mandatory ventilation mode, such as strict volume or pressure-controlled ventilation, interact with the patient?**
    Controlled mandatory ventilation modes do not allow the ventilator to interact or synchronize with the patient's respiratory effort. A mandatory mode of ventilation is set to deliver a fixed RR and TV (volume controlled ventilation [VCV]) or inspiratory pressure (pressure controlled ventilation [PCV]), regardless of the patient's efforts. This can be a source of significant distress in an awake patient, as they may attempt to initiate a breath but the ventilator will not allow them to breathe. Therefore these modes of ventilation should be reserved for those who are deeply sedated and not initiating any respiratory effort, such as during general anesthesia.

    Because of historical reasons, VCV and PCV imply controlled mandatory ventilation modes that do not synchronize with patient effort. However, these terms are still used to describe the "control variable" that determines the volume and pressure characteristics for ventilator modes that do synchronize with the patient. This is often a source of confusion. For example, Volume control synchronized intermittent mandatory ventilation (VC-SIMV) delivers a synchronized breath, but the clinician "controls" the delivered "volume."

12. **What are the most commonly used modes of positive-pressure ventilation?**

Modes of ventilation are named based on the control variable set by the clinician: volume or pressure, and the method which the ventilator interacts with the patient: (1) machine triggered, where breaths are fixed and always initiated by the ventilator, and (2) patient triggered, where breaths are initiated by the patient and only by the machine as a backup (Table 27.2).

Ventilator nomenclature can be rather confusing for several reasons. The nomenclature used by various manufactures is not standardized and any attempts to do so have further complicated the subject. For example, "SIMV" or "VC-SIMV" may be termed *SIMV-VC* on some GE Healthcare machines or termed *synchronized volume-controlled ventilation* on some Dräger machines. Historically, "controlled mandatory ventilation" (CMV) was the standard nomenclature for ventilator modes that were strictly machine triggered; however, now CMV stands for "continuous mandatory ventilation" and includes ventilator modes that are patient triggered. For these reasons, the authors of this chapter have endeavored to focus on keeping the terminology as simple as possible with a focus on the concepts behind the ventilator modes.

13. **What are common ventilator settings when initiating MV? Give an example.**

The first setting is usually the mode of ventilation (e.g., PCV, VCV, volume control–assist control [VC-AC]). After that, the other settings are chosen including the RR (or frequency), the I:E ratio, PEEP, FiO$_2$, and, depending upon the mode of ventilation, either a TV or an inspiratory pressure (P$_{insp}$). For example, a common mode in the operating room would be the following: Mode: VCV; TV: 500 mL; RR: 12 breaths per minute; I:E 1:2; PEEP: 5 cm H$_2$O; FiO$_2$: 50%.

14. **How does volume control–assist control mode work?**

The VC-AC mode delivers a set number of breaths at a preset TV. If the patient is initiating breaths, the preset TV will be delivered on these spontaneously initiated breaths. If the patient's RR drops below the preset RR, these breaths will be ventilator initiated. This insures that the patient will receive a mandatory RR or minute ventilation. VC-AC mode thus provides full support for a patient, while also allowing for spontaneous ventilation. In a spontaneously breathing patient, VC-AC may result in respiratory alkalosis or promote autopositive PEEP because the patient is receiving a full preset TV with every breath, even when tachypneic.

15. **How do VC-AC and VC-SIMV differ?**

Both modes guarantee a minimum mandatory RR at a controlled TV that can be machine or patient triggered. This allows both modes to deliver a mandatory minimum minute ventilation regardless of patient effort. The difference between the two is that VC-AC will always provide the same TV, even for patient triggered breaths above the minimum preset RR. VC-SIMV, however, will not provide the same TV for patient triggered breaths above the minimum preset RR. In VC-SIMV, all breaths above this preset rate may either be completely unassisted (uncommon) or assisted with pressure support (common), and the delivered TV will be determined by patient effort. In a patient breathing below the preset RR, VC-AC is indistinguishable from VC-SIMV.

16. **When initiating MV, how do you decide between VC-AC and VC-SIMV?**

VC-AC is considered a "full support" mode, where the work of respiration is completely supported by the ventilator. This is the most common ventilator mode used in the ICU. In addition, it is comfortable for spontaneously breathing patients. VC-SIMV is typically used as a weaning mode, because the breaths taken by the patient above the set rate are either not assisted or only partially assisted by pressure support. This increases the patient's respiratory work and is relatively less comfortable than VC-AC. However, it is still much more comfortable than the machine-triggered breaths of VCV or PCV.

17. **What is pressure support ventilation?**

Pressure support ventilation (PSV) augments spontaneous breathing using patient triggered, positive pressure breaths prescribed or controlled by the clinician. PSV allows patients to establish their own RR, vary their own flow rate, and, consequently, control their own TV and minute ventilation breath-to-breath. Because of this, PSV is reported to be the most comfortable mode of ventilation for a spontaneously breathing patient.

Table 27.2 Standard Mechanical Ventilation Modes		
	MACHINE TRIGGERED	**PATIENT TRIGGERED**[a]
Volume	Volume controlled ventilation (VCV)	Volume controlled-synchronized intermittent mandatory ventilation (VC-SIMV) Volume controlled-assist control (VC-AC)
Pressure	Pressure controlled ventilation (PCV)	Pressure controlled-synchronized intermittent mandatory ventilation (PC-SIMV) Pressure controlled-assist control (PC-AC) Pressure support ventilation (PSV)

[a]Patient triggered ventilator modes generally have a default backup rate that will provide mandatory machine-triggered breaths.

18. **How does pressure-controlled ventilation differ from PSV?**
PCV, unlike PSV, is a machine triggered breath. The exact TV delivered with PCV depends on the prescribed inspiratory time (i.e., I:E ratio) and inspiratory pressure. In general, the longer the inspiratory time or the higher inspiratory pressure, the larger the TV. Furthermore, the delivered TV is also affected by respiratory system compliance and resistance. PCV provides full ventilator support, whereas PSV is optimal for providing partial ventilatory support just before extubation or during a spontaneous breathing trial.

19. **What is a dual-control ventilator mode and how does it work?**
Dual-control mode ventilators combine the benefits of pressure control and volume control into one ventilator mode. The term for this ventilator mode is manufacture specific and is called *pressure control ventilation–volume guaranteed* on GE Healthcare, AutoFlow on Dräger, and *pressure-regulated volume control* on Maquet machines, and so on. These ventilator modes provide a pressure-control breath, while continuously monitoring the delivered TV. Each subsequent breath will be adjusted (e.g., ± 3 cm H_2O) to deliver a consistent TV that is set on the ventilator by the clinician. Although the specific implementation is manufacture specific, the overall concept is the same between manufactures.

KEY POINTS: MECHANICAL VENTILATION

1. The indications for mechanical ventilation and intubation are hypoxic respiratory failure, hypercarbic respiratory failure, or inability to protect the airway.
2. Volume control allows better control of minute ventilation at the expense of ventilator dyssynchrony in a spontaneous breathing patient.
3. Pressure control allows better patient comfort and may slightly improve the PaO_2:FiO_2 ratio because of higher mean airway pressures facilitating alveolar recruitment at the expense of less control of minute ventilation.
4. Dual control ventilation modes combine the advantages of both pressure control and volume control, while minimizing the disadvantages of each.

20. **Describe the four types of ventilator-induced lung injury?**
There are several ways in which mechanical ventilation can create or exacerbate existing lung injury. These are typically broken down into the following:
1) Volutrauma: damage to the alveoli from overdistension because of large TVs
2) Barotrauma: damage to the alveoli from increased transpulmonary pressures
3) Atelectotrauma: damage to patent alveoli that share a wall with collapsed alveoli, or damage to the alveolus itself from repeated collapse and recruitment
4) Oxygen toxicity: damage to the alveoli caused by high FiO_2 (e.g., >60%) over prolonged periods (e.g., >12 hours) because of free-radical induced injury

21. **What is lung-protective ventilation?**
Lung-protective ventilation, also known as *harm reduction ventilation*, refers to mechanical ventilation strategies aimed at protecting the lung from ventilator-induced lung injury. This includes the following:
1) Low TV ventilation: typically, 6 mL/kg (but includes a range from 4–8 mL/kg) of ideal body weight (IBW) with a plateau pressure less than 30 cm H_2O. This protects from volutrauma and barotrauma. Note, TVs should always be calculated based on IBW because lung size correlates with height more than weight
2) PEEP: typically starts at 5 cm H_2O but can go much higher (e.g., 15 cm H_2O)
3) FiO_2: titrate oxygen to the lowest levels necessary to maintain a pulse oximetry (SpO_2) of 88% to 92%. In the operating room, high FiO_2 is permissible as needed, especially surrounding intubation and extubation

22. **Should lung-protective ventilation be used in the operating room, or is it just for ARDS?**
The concept of lung-protective ventilation was born out of the literature on ARDS. However, subsequent studies have demonstrated benefits with lung-protective ventilation strategies, even for healthy patients undergoing elective surgery. Intraoperative lung-protective strategies have been associated with decreased postoperative respiratory complications, as well as shorter hospital length of stay. The parameters for lung protective ventilation in the operating room are generally less stringent than for patients with ARDS. Typically, TVs of less than 8 mL/kg IBW are targeted, along with PEEP of 5 cm H_2O or higher, with regular recruitment maneuvers.

23. **What is the difference between alveolar and dead space ventilation? How does this pertain to lung protection strategies?**
Dead space ventilation refers to the anatomic regions (i.e., mouth, trachea, bronchi, bronchioles) and the physiologic dead space (i.e., alveoli in zone 1 of the lung) that do not participate in gas exchange. Physiological or alveolar dead space is normally negligible in healthy patients. However, anatomic dead space is fixed and measures approximately 150 mL in adult patients. Alveolar ventilation is the region where gas exchange occurs. This can be represented by the following equation:

$$V_T = V_D + V_A$$

V_T, tidal volume, V_D, dead space, V_A, alveolar ventilation

The ultimate goal of a delivered TV is to ventilate the alveoli and facilitate gas exchange. However, lung protection strategies deliver lower TVs and less alveolar ventilation, because a greater proportion of each breath is wasted on dead space ventilation. Decreased alveolar ventilation can contribute to atelectasis and hypercapnia, so it is important to combine lung protective TVs with PEEP and a relatively higher RR.

24. **What is the role of PEEP?**
PEEP refers to the pressure applied to the expiratory circuit of the mechanical ventilator, and, as the name implies, is the pressure on the respiratory system at the end of exhalation. The main goals of PEEP are the following:
- Increase functional residual capacity by preventing alveolar collapse or atelectasis
- Decrease atelectasis and subsequent intrapulmonary shunt
- Minimize atelectotrauma
- Optimize pulmonary compliance

25. **In what situations would you increase PEEP? What maneuver should be done in conjunction with this?**
PEEP increases should be considered in response to periods of desaturation, especially after other etiologies have been ruled out (e.g., bronchospasm, mucous plugging). Increases in PEEP should always be made in combination with recruitment maneuvers. Increasing PEEP, without a preceding recruitment maneuver, may cause overdistension of the already open alveoli, while failing to recruit atelectatic regions. Similarly, a recruitment maneuver performed without increasing PEEP is likely to cause only a temporary increase in the $PaO_2:FiO_2$ ratio, as atelectasis will reoccur.
Recruitment maneuvers are performed either by applying a steady positive pressure of 25 to 40 cm H_2O for 30 seconds, using the breathing bag (i.e., anesthesia machine method), or by increasing the PEEP to 25 to 40 cm H_2O for 1 to 2 minutes (i.e., ICU ventilator method). The patient should be continuously monitored for adverse effects, as high levels of PEEP can impair venous return and increase right ventricular afterload, leading to decreased cardiac output.

26. **How is optimal PEEP identified?**
There are multiple methods to determine the optimal PEEP for a given patient. These include:
- Increasing PEEP empirically (e.g., 3–5 cm H_2O) for hypoxemia (in combination with a recruitment maneuver)
- Follow the ARDSNet PEEP/FiO_2 escalation tables (available at www.ardsnet.org), which adjust PEEP based on the severity of hypoxia
- Titrating PEEP to minimize driving pressure ($P_{plat} - PEEP$). This is a new and promising technique that is strongly correlated with decreased mortality in patients with ARDS and may become a new primary goal for lung protection ventilation
- Less common methods include titrating PEEP to optimize lung compliance (adjust to the lowest inspiratory inflection point using spirometry), or by using esophageal manometry to estimate pleural pressure

27. **What is intrinsic PEEP or auto-PEEP?**
Auto- or intrinsic PEEP is residual positive alveolar pressure that occurs in response to incomplete exhalation. Patients with a high minute ventilation and/or COPD/asthma are at risk for developing auto-PEEP. If the RR is too rapid, or the expiratory time too short, there may be insufficient time for full exhalation to occur. This could result in breath stacking and the subsequent generation of residual positive airway pressure at end exhalation. Small-diameter ETTs may also contribute to auto-PEEP by increasing the resistance to exhalation.
COPD increases the risk of auto-PEEP because of the decreased pulmonary compliance from emphysema and the high airway resistance from bronchitis. Such patients have difficulty exhaling gas because their lung recoil force is low (i.e., emphysema) and airway resistance is high (i.e., bronchitis), even at standard RRs.

28. **How can auto-PEEP be recognized and treated?**
One method to detect and measure auto-PEEP is to occlude the expiratory port at end expiration and monitor airway pressure. Another method is to monitor expiratory flow, ensuring that it returns to zero before the next inhalation. If auto-PEEP occurs, decrease the rate or increase the expiratory time (e.g., I:E ratio to 1:4) to allow time for full exhalation. Administering a bronchodilator may also be helpful to reduce airway resistance and facilitate exhalation. Unrecognized severe auto-PEEP may present as high airway pressures (because of the inspiratory pressure being added to the already high auto-PEEP) and hypotension, from impairment of venous return. The treatment in this scenario is to temporarily disconnect the circuit from the ETT and allow for full exhalation.

29. **What is controlled hypoventilation with permissive hypercapnia?**
Controlled hypoventilation (or permissive hypercapnia) is a pressure- or volume-limiting, lung-protective strategy whereby arterial partial pressure of carbon dioxide ($PaCO_2$) is allowed to rise, placing more importance on protecting the lung than on maintaining eucapnia. The prescribed TV is lowered to a range of approximately 4 to 6 mL/kg/IBW, in an attempt to keep the PIP below 35 to 40 cm H_2O and the static plateau pressure below 30 cm H_2O. The $PaCO_2$ is allowed to rise slowly to a level of 80 to 100 mm Hg.
Permissive hypercapnia is usually well tolerated. A potential adverse effect is cerebral vasodilation, leading to increased ICP. Intracranial hypertension is the only absolute contraindication to using permissive hypercapnia.

30. **How does prone positioning improve ventilation/perfusion matching?**
    The mechanism is slightly complex, but it relates to our understanding of Zone's law of the lung. Studies completed by NASA and Russian space missions have shown that the primary mechanism explaining Zone's law of the lung is anatomic, with gravity providing a secondary mechanism. Specifically, 75% of the normal ventilation/perfusion ($\dot{V}/\dot{Q}$) as depicted by Zone's law persists in a microgravity environment and is therefore independent of gravity. Further studies in space showed that the anatomy of the bronchial tree preferentially ventilates the ventral and superior regions of the lung and the anatomy of the pulmonary vasculature preferentially perfuses the dorsal and inferior regions.
    In the supine position with positive pressure ventilation, the ventral lung regions are more compliant and are preferentially ventilated; however, because of the anatomy of the pulmonary vasculature, in addition to gravity, the dorsal lung regions are preferentially perfused, resulting in $\dot{V}/\dot{Q}$ mismatch. In the prone position, because of the weight of the body (including the mediastinal contents) compressing the ventral lung regions and chest wall, the compliance of the pulmonary system is more homogeneous, facilitating a better distribution of ventilation throughout the lung. The distribution of blood flow is also improved because the anatomic preference to perfuse the dorsal lung regions is balanced by the effects of gravity to perfuse the ventral regions, resulting in the overall improvement of $\dot{V}/\dot{Q}$ matching.

31. **What are some available rescue strategies for patients with ARDS who are difficult to oxygenate?**
    The most commonly used rescue strategies for refractory hypoxemia in ARDS are prone positioning, neuromuscular blockade and venovenous extracorporeal membrane oxygenation (ECMO). Studies have shown that the PaO_2 improves significantly in approximately two-thirds of patients with ARDS, when they are positioned prone. The use of neuromuscular blockade (paralytics) can also facilitate gas exchange by improving chest wall compliance and to reduce metabolic energy consumption when sedation alone is inadequate. Refractory ARDS, unresponsive to prone positioning and paralytic therapy, is an indication for venovenous ECMO, which uses venous inflow and outflow cannulas to pass blood through an extracorporeal oxygenation circuit to provide oxygenation.

32. **Should neuromuscular blockade be used to facilitate MV in the ICU?**
    Neuromuscular blocking agents (NMBAs) in general should not be routinely administered to facilitate MV. However, there are unique situations where their use is warranted and may improve outcomes. Muscle paralysis may be helpful in managing intracranial hypertension, severe ARDS, and unconventional modes of ventilation (e.g., inverse ratio ventilation or extracorporeal techniques) to decrease ventilator dyssynchrony.
    Drawbacks to the use of these drugs include loss of the ability to perform neurological examination, abolished cough, potential for an awake paralyzed patient, numerous medication and electrolyte interactions, potential for prolonged paralysis, critical illness myopathy, and death associated with inadvertent ventilator disconnects. NMBAs are also associated with prolonged mechanical ventilation, ventilator dependence, and delays in weaning. If deemed necessary, the use of NMBAs should be limited to 24 to 48 hours to prevent potential complications.

KEY POINTS: MECHANICAL VENTILATION STRATEGIES

1. Lung protection ventilation strategies should be viewed as harm reduction ventilation strategies and applied to all mechanically ventilated patients not just ARDS.
2. Risk factors for auto-PEEP are high minute ventilation, small ETT, COPD, and asthma.
3. To minimize the risk of auto-PEEP, monitor the expiratory flow to ensure it returns to zero before the ventilator gives the next breath and titrate the I:E ratio accordingly.
4. Prone positioning may increase a patient's PaO_2:FiO_2 ratio and is helpful in managing patients with severe ARDS.
5. Other strategies for managing severe ARDS include neuromuscular blocking agents and venovenous ECMO.

SUGGESTED READINGS

Mechanical Ventilation in the Operating Room

Futier E, Constantin JM, Paugam-Burtz C, et al. A trial of intraoperative low-tidal-volume ventilation in abdominal surgery. New Engl J Med. 2013;369:428–437.

Futier E, Marret E, Jaber S. Perioperative positive pressure ventilation: an integrated approach to improve pulmonary care. Anesthesiology. 2014;121:400–408.

Ventilation Modes

MacIntyre NR. Patient-ventilator interactions: optimizing conventional ventilation modes. Respir Care. 2011;56:73–84.

Neto AS, Cardoso SO, Manetta JA, et al. Association between use of lung-protective ventilation with lower TVs and clinical outcomes among patients without acute respiratory distress syndrome, JAMA. 2012;308:1651–1659.

ARDS

Guérin CG, Reignier J, Richard JC, et al. Prone positioning in severe acute respiratory distress syndrome. N Engl J Med. 2013;368:2159–2168.

Papazian L, Forel JM, Gacouin A, et al. Neuromuscular blockers in early acute respiratory distress syndrome. N Engl J Med. 2010;363:1107–1116.

ELECTROCARDIOGRAM

John A. Vullo, MD, Ryan D. Laterza, MD

CHAPTER 28

1. **Describe the electrical conduction system of the heart.**
   The electrical conduction system of the heart is a network of specialized myocardial cells that generate, regulate, and propagate a series of electrical impulses. These impulses are generated by subtle changes in the resting membrane potential because of the movement of ions through cellular membrane channels.

   The basic structure of this system consists of specialized cells that make up the sinoatrial (SA) node, the atrioventricular (AV) node, the His bundle, the left and right bundles, and the Purkinje fibers (PF).

   The SA node is located within the wall of the RA. It has an unstable resting potential (discussed later), allowing it to spontaneously generate electrical activity that is propagated via specialized atrial cells known as the *internodal tract to the AV node*. The AV node acts as a "gate-keeper" by regulating a small delay before the electrical signal can propagate to the very efficient His-bundle-PF system.

   The purpose of the electrical conduction system is to coordinate contraction between all four chambers of the heart to efficiently generate a stroke volume. Disorders that impair the electrical conduction system, such as AV node block, left bundle branch block (LBBB), or atrial fibrillation, cause mechanical dyssynchrony between the chambers of the heart and impair cardiac output.

2. **What is unique about the action potential at the SA node (and other pacemaker cells)?**
   The SA node is unique in that it can spontaneously depolarize because of inward sodium "funny" current (Fig. 28.1). This "funny" current allows the SA node to have automaticity where it can spontaneously depolarize at an intrinsic rate. Although the SA node is the primary pacemaker for the heart, cells in the AV node and PF also have "funny" current giving them automaticity as well although at a slower rate. The following are the phases for an SA node action potential:
   - *Phase 4*: Slowly depolarizes automatically because of an inward Na^+ current called *funny* current. It is called funny current because this ion channel is activated by negative membrane potentials (hyperpolarization), which contrasts other ion channels, which are activated by positive membrane potentials (depolarization). Pacemaker cells, such as the SA node, contain the property described in this phase because it allows for spontaneous depolarization.
   - *Phase 0*: After a certain membrane potential is reached, the upstroke of the action potential is generated by voltage-gated Ca^{2+} channel opening causing an increase of inward Ca^{2+} current.
   - *Phase 3*: The repolarization phase is caused by inactivation of Ca^{2+} channels and K^+ current out of the cell.

3. **How is the action potential of the atrial and ventricular myocytes different than the SA node?**
   In addition to the funny current giving the SA node automaticity, the SA node only has three phases, whereas the atrial and ventricular myocyte actional potential has five phases (see Fig. 28.1) as depicted later:
   - *Phase 0*: This is the upstroke of the action potential, but here, it is caused by opening of voltage-gated Na^+ channels, which depolarize the membrane.
   - *Phase 1*: The rapid depolarization from phase 0, causes a small overshoot in depolarization, which is corrected by a small repolarization because of a decrease in inward Na^+ current and an increase in K^+ current out of the cell.
   - *Phase 2*: The plateau of the action potential is maintained by an increase in Ca^{2+} current into the cell and by an outward K^+ current. The plateau marks a period of dynamic equilibrium of inward and outward cation currents.
   - *Phase 3*: Repolarization is caused by a predominance of outward K^+ current and inactivation of calcium channels. This hyperpolarizes the membrane.
   - *Phase 4*: The cell is hyperpolarized and is at its resting membrane potential. This reflects a state where a dynamic equilibrium exists between all permeable ions.

4. **So, if the SA node fails, what keeps the heart beating then?**
   Phase 4 depolarization automaticity (just like the SA node) also occurs within the AV node and the PF, albeit at a slower (usually much slower) rate of depolarization. Therefore if there is suppression of the SA node or its signal propagation, these specialized cells can act as the de facto pacemaker of the heart. Therefore patients who lack a functioning SA or AV node (sick sinus syndrome, complete heart block, etc.) will continue to have a heartbeat and can survive until a permanent pacemaker is placed. The automaticity of the AV node is about 40 to 60 beats per minute and for the PF, 30 to 40 beats per minute.

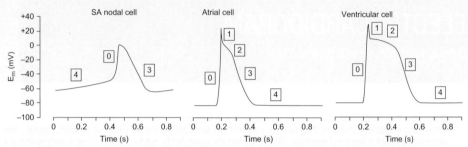

Fig. 28.1 Action potentials. Action potential in the sinoatrial (*SA*) node versus the atrial and ventricular myocyte. Note the steeper slope of phase 4 for the SA node facilitating spontaneous depolarization.

KEY POINTS: ACTION POTENTIALS

1. The SA node is unique in that it can spontaneously depolarize because of inward sodium "funny" current.
2. The AV node and PF also possess automaticity if the SA node is dysfunctional, albeit at slower rates.
3. Note the differences in ion channels necessary for the respective action potentials. These can be exploited as targets of pharmacological therapies.

5. **Explain how an electrocardiogram is obtained from a patient.**
The electrical conduction system of the heart produces small voltage changes that can be measured by attaching electrodes to the body. The electrodes transmit this electrical signal to an electrocardiogram (ECG) machine that filters noise and amplifies the small voltage to a larger voltage, so we can visualize the electrical activity of the heart. Furthermore, when electrodes are placed in standardized locations across the body, we can understand the electrical potential differences of the heart that is conducive to systematic study and clinical interpretation. In other words, we use the electrodes to monitor the direction of electrical signals emitted by the heart to diagnose and treat problems.

6. **What are the customary lead placements sites for a 12-lead ECG?**
A standard 12-lead ECG contains 10 electrodes. The four limb electrodes correspond to each limb (right arm, left arm, right leg, left leg) and measure the ECG voltage changes in the frontal axis. The six precordial leads are placed across the chest from the sternum to the left axilla and measure ECG changes in the transverse axis. Please see Fig. 28.2.

7. **Why are there are only 10 electrodes, but 12 leads?**
There are four limb electrodes (right arm, left arm, right leg, and left leg) and six precordial electrodes (V1–V6). These 10 electrodes create nine axes (three limb axes and six precordial axes) and the last electrode (right leg) serves as a ground. Each axis measures the projected electric field force generated by the atria (P wave) and ventricles (QRS and T waves). The remaining three leads are "virtual" axes created by combining two electrodes to create a new virtual ground that can be used to create an "augmented" axis (i.e., aVR, aVF, aVL).

8. **Describe the limb leads.**
The limb leads measure ECG voltage differences across the frontal plane of the heart:
- Lead I measures the voltage difference between the left arm (LA) and the right arm (RA) electrode: Lead I = LA − RA.
- Lead II measures the voltage difference between the left leg (LL) and the right arm (RA) electrode: Lead II = LL − RA.
- Lead III measures the voltage difference between the left leg (LL) and the left arm (LA) electrode: Lead III = LL − LA.

9. **What is the Wilson central terminal?**
The Wilson central terminal (WCT) is a virtual electrode that is used as a reference point for the augmented limb and precordial leads. It is determined by summing the three limb electrodes and averaging their voltage: $WCT = \frac{LA + RA + LL}{3}$. The WCT mathematically represents a central "virtual" electrode at the center of Einthoven's triangle.

10. **Describe the precordial leads.**
The precordial leads measure ECG voltage differences across the transverse plane of the heart. It consists of six "virtual" axes created by six "positive" electrodes that surround the chest where each electrode uses the virtual WCT as its "negative" reference electrode. Each of the six precordial leads, just like the limb leads, measure the heart's

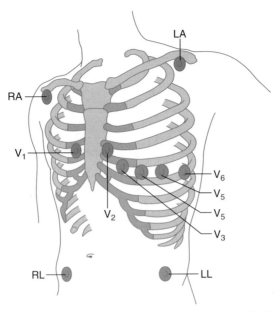

Fig. 28.2 Electrocardiogram electrode placement. The four limb leads: *RA*, right arm; *LA*, left arm; *RL*, right leg; *LL*, left leg. The six precordial leads: V_1, fourth intercostal space, right sternal margin; V_2, fourth intercostal space, left sternal margin; V_3, midway between V_2 and V_4; V_4, fifth intercostal space, left mid-clavicular line; V_5, fifth intercostal space, left anterior axillary line; V_6, fifth intercostal space, left mid-axillary line. (From Landesberg G, Hillel Z. Electrocardiography, perioperative ischemia, and myocardial infarction. In: Miller RD, ed. Miller's Anesthesia. 8th ed. Philadelphia: Elsevier Saunders; 2015:1437.)

electric field force (a vector) projected onto an axis. Each precordial axis is referred to as V_i, where "i" represents the six precordial electrodes. Each precordial lead or axis can be calculated as follows:

$$V_i = \varphi_i - WCT$$

V_i, *precordial voltage lead; φ_i, precordial electrode; WCT, Wilson central terminal; i, corresponding lead/electrode 1 to 6*

Note that some texts refer to the precordial leads as *unipolar,* implying these leads do not require a negative electrode. However, that is false; all ECG leads represent the difference between a positive and negative electrode, whether created virtually by combing multiple electrodes together or by using one single electrode. Lastly, "V" is abbreviated notation for both precordial and augmented leads and may refer to virtual, vector, or voltage.

11. **Describe the augmented leads.**
    The three remaining leads are the *augmented voltage (aV)* left, right, and foot leads:
    - aVL is the voltage difference between the LA electrode and the average voltage of the RA and LL electrodes: $aVL = LA - \frac{RA + LL}{2}$
    - aVR is the voltage difference between the RA electrode and the average voltage of the LL and LA electrodes: $aVR = RA - \frac{LL + LA}{2}$
    - aVF is the voltage difference between the LL electrode and the average voltage of the RA and LA electrodes: $aVF = LL - \frac{RA + LA}{2}$

12. **Why are "augmented leads" augmented? Is this necessary?**
    Originally, these leads were simply referred to as VL, VR, and VF with the same negative virtual electrode, WCT, as the precordial leads. For example, $VL = LA - \frac{RA + LL + LA}{3}$. Unfortunately, the amplitude of the ECG voltage measured on these leads was found to be too small with a low signal-to-noise ratio. To increase the voltage and improve the signal-to-noise ratio, it was found that the voltage of these leads could be "augmented" by using a different virtual negative electrode. Instead of using WCT, all ECG machines today use the average of the two opposite electrodes (i.e., Goldberger's central terminal) and not all three electrodes as in WCT. It is important to emphasize that this was first proposed and implemented in the 1940s, way before digital amplifiers even existed. With current high-fidelity digital amplifiers and filters, a strong argument can be made that voltage augmentation of limb leads using mathematical "trickery" (i.e., Goldberg's central terminal) is no longer necessary and that we should return back to WCT as the reference virtual electrode, so these leads can share the same virtual electrode as the precordial leads. Regardless, the

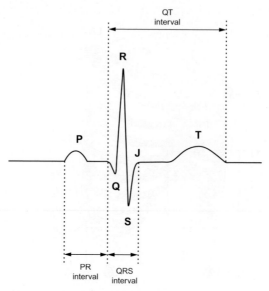

Fig. 28.3 Electrocardiogram waveform and intervals. The normal intervals are the following: PR interval 120 to 200 ms, QRS interval 70 to 100 ms, QTc interval under 440 ms (men) or under 460 ms (women).

effects on Einthoven's triangle in determining axis projection and angles between vectors is unaffected, regardless of which virtual electrode implementation is used.

13. **What are the waveforms of a normal ECG?**
Please refer to Figure 28.3. It is important to understand that electrical activity on ECG does not imply simultaneous mechanical contraction. There is a small latency between the electrical activity detected on ECG and mechanical contraction of the heart.
   The *P wave* is the first upward (positive) deflection during the cardiac cycle, demonstrating atrial depolarization. It is a combination of, first, right atrial, then, left atrial depolarization. Any downward deflection following the *P wave* that precedes the *R wave* is considered a *Q wave*. The *Q wave* represents depolarization of the interventricular septum, which occurs from left to right. Presumably, this is because the electrical conduction velocity of the left heart is slightly faster than the right heart, allowing the larger left heart to contract in synchrony with the smaller right heart. The *R wave* is the first upward (positive) deflection of the QRS complex or the first upward deflection after a *P wave*. It signals early ventricular depolarization. The *S wave* is the first downward (negative) deflection of the QRS complex, which occurs after the *R wave*. It is caused by late ventricular depolarization from the PF. The *ST segment* is normally not elevated and isoelectric starting at the *J point* to the beginning of the *T wave*. The *T wave* is the upward (positive) deflection after a *QRS complex*. It is caused by ventricular repolarization and is normally upright (positive) in all leads except aVR.

14. **What is the "J point"?**
The J point is the junction between the end of the QRS complex and the beginning of the ST segment. This transition point usually occurs at the isoelectric point on the ECG, but deviations above or below the isoelectric point may reflect pathology. Elevated J point is thought to reflect early depolarization. Most often, it is seen in young, healthy, athletic males and is traditionally thought to be benign in the acute setting. However, there is some evidence to suggest a higher incidence of sudden cardiac death and Brugada syndrome in patients with elevated J point.

15. **Describe the normal intervals found on ECG.**
The *PR interval* is the time from the start of a P wave to the start of a QRS complex. It is primarily determined by the conductive delay through the AV node. Its interval is normally 120 to 200 ms (i.e., < 5 small squares). A PR interval over 200 ms indicates first-degree heart block because of delayed conduction through the AV node. This may be caused by high vagal tone (e.g., healthy patients) but is also associated with cardiac disease and is a risk factor for atrial fibrillation. A *PR interval* under 120 ms may occur if there is an accessory pathway between the atria and ventricles, which bypasses the AV node (i.e., Wolff-Parkinson-White [WPW] syndrome).
   The *QRS interval* indicates the time necessary for complete depolarization of the ventricles following conduction through the AV node. A normal *QRS interval* is between 70 and 100 ms (less than three small boxes). A wide *QRS*

interval may be caused by a left or right bundle branch block (RBBB), ventricular tachycardia (VT), supraventricular tachycardia (SVT) with an aberrancy, hyperkalemia, WPW syndrome, or from ventricular pacing.

The *QT interval* is the time from the onset of the Q wave to the completion of the T wave. It reflects the total time of ventricular depolarization and repolarization. The *QT interval* is inversely related to the heart rate in that it decreases as the heart rate increases, which makes *QT interval* assessment problematic. The corrected QT (QTc) interval is a method that allows for more objective assessment of the *QT interval*, independent of heart rate, by determining what the *QT interval* would be at a heart rate of 60 beats per minute. Although there are several different equations that can be used to do this, one of the most common is the Bazett formula: $QTc = QT / \sqrt{RR}$ interval, where the RR interval $= 60/HR$. The QTc is considered prolonged in men if the QTc is greater than 440 ms and in women if the QTc is greater than 460 ms. Long QTc syndrome is associated with lethal dysrhythmias, such as torsade de pointes.

16. **What is Einthoven's triangle?**
Einthoven's triangle is an equilateral triangle that can be realized using three electrodes (RA, LA, and LL), where the electrodes are used to create an axis called a *lead* (e.g., lead I, aVF). Einthoven's triangle is an important concept to understand because it is the fundamental basis for deriving the cardiac axis with the frontal plane leads (Fig. 28.4).

17. **How do you determine the axis of the QRS complex?**
The best method is to first understand the concept of vector projection and how it pertains to the axis created by the various ECG leads, as discussed with Einthoven's triangle. Recall, the measured QRS on ECG represents the gross electric field vector, E_{heart}, for the entire heart during ventricular systole. Each lead corresponds to an axis that measures E_{heart} onto that axis. Recall a vector contains both magnitude and direction and each lead will measure a different voltage, depending on the magnitude and direction of the heart's electric field force.

When E_{heart} is perfectly parallel to the axes measured by a lead, the area under the curve (AUC) of the measured QRS will be maximal. However, if E_{heart} is perpendicular to the axis for a given lead, the projected E_{heart} will be exactly 0 (in theory). In reality, because of motion from the heart contracting and breathing, the projected vector onto the axis will create a "wobble" effect causing positive and negative deflections of equal magnitude. Therefore the best method to assess the projected E_{heart} is to visually measure the AUC of the QRS complex. If the AUC of the QRS complex is positive or negative, then E_{heart} is not perpendicular to that lead; if the AUC of the QRS complex is approximately 0, then E_{heart} is perpendicular to that lead (also termed *isoelectric*). The lead demonstrating the largest positive AUC of the QRS complex is the most parallel axis to E_{heart}. Please see Figure 28.5.

The "take away point" is that the QRS axis can be determined by knowing the axis angles created by the various leads using Einthoven's triangle and answering two questions: (1) where is the AUC of the QRS "most" positive? and (2) where is the AUC of the QRS equal to 0?

18. **What is normal QRS axis? How do you determine a left or right axis deviation?**
A normal QRS axis is between −30 and 90 degrees and is most parallel to lead II (generally). This implies that the AUC for the QRS complex should be positive in both lead I and lead II with the AUC of lead II > lead I (generally). If E_{heart} is between −30 and −90 degrees (left axis deviation), then the AUC of the measured QRS complex in lead II will be

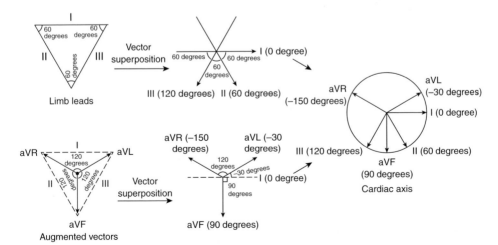

Fig. 28.4 Frontal plane axis determination. Einthoven's triangle can be used to derive the cardiac axis in the frontal plane. Wilson's central terminal is depicted in the center of the triangle for the "augmented vectors." The lead axes created are the following: lead I (0 degrees), lead II (60 degrees), lead III (120 degrees), aVL (−30 degrees), aVF (90 degrees), aVR (−150 degrees).

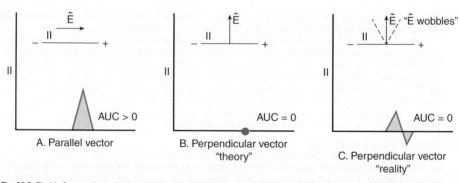

Fig. 28.5 Electric force vector projection onto lead axis. (A) When the heart's gross electric field force (E_{heart}) is parallel, the projected measurement onto that lead will record a large (or negative) deflection, where the total area under the curve (*AUC*) depicts the direction of E_{heart}. (B) In theory, if E_{heart} is perpendicular to the axis, the recorded measurement will not have a deflection and the AUC is 0. (C) In reality, because of cardiac and respiratory motion, the deflection will contain equally positive and negative deflections because of the "wobble effect," as depicted where the AUC will equal 0.

Table 28.1 Limb Lead (Frontal Plane) Axis Deviation	
LEFT AXIS DEVIATION (LAD)	**RIGHT AXIS DEVIATION (RAD)**
Left anterior fascicular block	Left posterior fascicular block
Inferior myocardial infarction	Lateral myocardial infarction
Wolff-Parkinson-White (WPW) syndrome	WPW syndrome
Left ventricular hypertrophy (debated)	Right ventricular hypertrophy
	Right heart strain (e.g., pulmonary embolism)

negative and positive in lead I. If **E_{heart}** is between 90 and 180 degrees (right axis deviation), then the AUC of the measured QRS complex will be positive in lead III and negative in lead I. Please refer to Figure 28.4 for the axes of various leads.

19. What are the criteria for left axis and right axis deviation? What is the differential diagnosis for axis deviation? Why does this occur?
    A left axis deviation (LAD) occurs when the QRS axis is between −30 and −90 degrees and a right axis deviation (RAD) occurs when the QRS axis is between 90 and 180 degrees. See Table 28.1 for causes of axis deviation.
        Axis deviation occurs because the lead measures the gross electric field force generated by the heart, projected onto its axis. In other words, although the individual electrical forces of the right heart may point in the opposite direction to that of the left heart, what is measured by ECG is the heart's overall electric force. For example, an inferior myocardial infarction will decrease the downward electric field forces causing the heart's mean electric field force to point up and to the left (i.e., left axis deviation). Similarly, larger electric field forces because of right ventricular hypertrophy can shift the mean electric field force toward the right (i.e., right axis deviation).

20. Is there a method to assess axis deviation in the transverse plane (i.e., precordial leads)?
    R wave progression in the precordial leads is a method to assess axis deviation in the transverse plane. In this plane, the heart's gross electric field force, **E_{heart}**, will be isoelectric (perpendicular) to V3 or V4 and most parallel to V6. Again, this is because **E_{heart}** represents the gross electric field force for the entire heart. Although the right heart's electric forces will point anteriorly in the transverse plane, the left heart generates a larger electrical force posteriorly causing the AUC of the QRS complex to be most positive at V6, most negative in V1, and isoelectric at V3 or V4. Please refer to Figure 28.6.
        Conditions that cause the right heart to have a weaker electric force (e.g., anterior myocardial infarction) will cause E_{heart} to point more toward the left heart and vice versa. Conditions associated with right heart electric field forces being greater than the left heart electric forces will cause an "early" R wave progression. This will cause the isoelectric point to occur before V3/V4. Conversely, conditions associated with left heart electric forces being greater than right heart electric forces will cause "delayed" R wave progression, causing the isoelectric point to occur after V3/V4. The key in assessing R wave progression is to look for the isoelectric point and determine if it occurs before or after the normal isoelectric point (normally V3/V4).
        Please see Table 28.2 for causes of abnormal R wave progression.

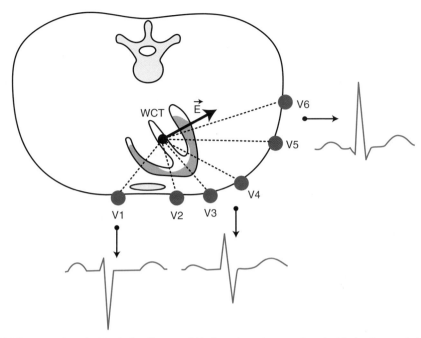

Fig. 28.6 Transverse plane axis determination. The precordial leads can be used to assess the axis of the heart's gross electric field force (E_{heart}) in the transverse plane. The key is to determine the QRS isoelectric point (E_{heart} is perpendicular) and where the area under the curve (AUC) of the QRS is positive and the largest (E_{heart} is parallel). Note, this is the same approach in determining QRS axis for the frontal plane. Normally, the AUC of the QRS is most negative in V1, most positive in V6, and isoelectric in V3/V4. WCT, Wilson central terminal. (Modified From: Jekova I, Krasteva V, Leber R, et al. Inter-lead correlation analysis for automated detection of cable reversals in 12/16-lead ECG. Comput Methods Programs Biomed. 2016 Oct;134:31–41.)

Table 28.2 Causes for Abnormal R Wave Progression in Precordial Leads

REVERSED OR "EARLY" R WAVE PROGRESSION	SLOW OR "DELAYED" R WAVE PROGRESSION
Posterior myocardial infarction	Anterior myocardial infarction
Right ventricular hypertrophy	Left ventricular hypertrophy
Right bundle branch block	Left Bundle Branch Block
Wolff-Parkinson-White (WPW) syndrome	WPW syndrome

KEY POINTS: ECG BASICS

1. ECG electrode positioning is used to monitor the direction of electrical signals emitted by the heart to diagnose and treat problems.
2. Accurate lead placement is paramount to proper ECG interpretation.
3. Einthoven's triangle is the fundamental basis for deriving the cardiac axis with the frontal plane leads.

21. What's the main concern with a prolonged QT interval?

The main concern with prolonged QT is an "R-on-T," such as from a premature ventricular contraction (PVC) or asynchronous pacing causes the ventricle to depolarize during the T wave when the ventricle is in a partially depolarized and repolarized state. This may cause the heart to develop a lethal rhythm, such as torsade de pointes or ventricular fibrillation (VF). Preventing R-on-T is the rationale behind synchronized cardioversion, as opposed to unsynchronized cardioversion (also known as defibrillation), which synchronizes the electrical "shock" to the R wave.

22. **What can cause QT prolongation in the perioperative setting?**
Several causes have been implicated in QT prolongation, such as electrolyte abnormalities, medications, or even the stress of surgery itself. Frequent causes of QT prolongation in the perioperative setting include hypocalcemia, hypomagnesemia, antiemetic medications (i.e., ondansetron, haloperidol, droperidol), opioids (i.e., methadone), antibiotics, amiodarone, and ketorolac. It is important to note that this list is not exhaustive, as many other medications are associated with prolonged QT.
    Patient's with prolonged QT should have their electrolytes checked and replenished namely potassium, calcium, and magnesium. Other considerations include avoiding medications associated with QT prolongation, such as methadone and haloperidol.

23. **What are pathological Q waves? What do they signify?**
Pathological Q waves generally occur from a previous myocardial infarction causing myocardial scar tissue. Q waves are considered pathological if they are greater than 2 mm, over 25% of the amplitude of the R wave, or if they are ever visible in V1–V3.

24. **Can a supraventricular tachycardia present with a wide QRS complex?**
Yes. This is called an *SVT with an aberrancy* and is often caused by an induced RBBB because of tachycardia. This occurs because of the longer refractory period of the right bundle compared with the left bundle. Differentiating an SVT with an aberrancy from monomorphic VT can be very difficult. However, if the patient is unstable but has a pulse, immediate synchronized cardioversion should be delivered regardless.

25. **What are the effects of hyperkalemia on the ECG?**
In general, ECG changes are associated with the degree of hyperkalemia starting and ending in the following order:
    1) Peaked T waves
    2) Prolongation of PR interval
    3) Loss of P wave (third-degree heart block, accelerated junctional rhythm, etc.)
    4) Widening of QRS interval
    5) Sinewave QRS pattern
    6) VF

26. **What are the effects of hypocalcemia on the ECG? What clinical situations is this most likely to occur?**
Hypocalcemia prolongs the QT interval. This most often occurs in the setting of massive transfusion causing acute citrate toxicity. Normally, this does not occur when blood products are given slowly (e.g., 1 unit of packed red blood cells over 1 hour) because the liver has time to metabolize the citrate. However, if large amounts of blood products are being transfused quickly, hypocalcemia can quickly be detected (and treated) in emergent situations by noticing prolongation of the QT interval. This is important as hypocalcemia can impair coagulation, impair cardiac contractility, and decrease systemic vascular resistance.

27. **What is the significance of ST depression on ECG?**
ST depression is most often a sign of myocardial ischemia and can be the result of myocardial oxygen demand exceeding myocardial oxygen delivery. The most common cause of ST depression is subendocardial ischemia; however, it may also reflect reciprocal changes in corresponding leads because of ST elevation in other leads. There are many nonischemic causes of ST depression as well: digoxin side effect, normal variant during sinus tachycardia, hypokalemia, hypothermia, and others.

28. **What is the ECG diagnostic criteria for an ST elevation myocardial infarction?**
ECG diagnostic criteria for an ST elevation myocardial infarction (STEMI) per recent American College of Cardiology Foundation/American Heart Association guidelines requires the following (in addition to clinical signs and symptoms):
    New ST elevation ($\geq$1 mm) at the J point in at least two contiguous leads, except leads V2–V3 where the J point elevation needs to be 2 mm or more in men or 1.5 mm or more in women.
    ST elevation can have a variety of morphologies, which can include anything from a flat ST segment to a more "tombstone" appearance (Fig. 28.7). The following are a few caveats to be aware of in diagnosing a STEMI on ECG:
    1) Acute posterior myocardial infarction will cause reciprocal ST depression (not elevation) in the anterior precordial leads
    2) Diagnosing a STEMI in the setting of a LBBB is challenging. An LBBB is not an automatic STEMI equivalent and requires using specific criteria (i.e., Sgarbossa criteria), along with clinical signs and symptoms for diagnosis. Expert consultation is advised.

29. **What situations may cause ST elevation that is not considered acute coronary syndrome?**
Left ventricular hypertrophy, pericarditis (frequently seen after cardiac surgery), and early repolarization (common finding in young, healthy patients).

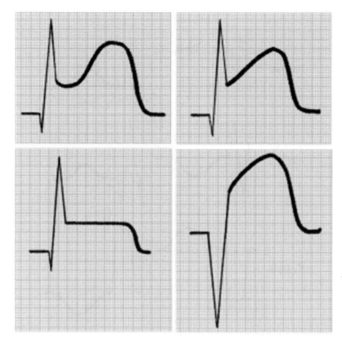

Fig. 28.7 ST elevation morphology. Acute myocardial infarction demonstrating various ST elevation morphologies. Not all acute myocardial infarctions will look the same. (From Goldberger A, Goldberger Z, Shvilkin A. Myocardial ischemia and infarction, part I: ST segment elevation and Q wave syndromes. In: Goldberger A, Goldberger Z, Shvilkin A, eds. Goldberger's Clinical Electrocardiography: A Simplified Approach. 9th ed. Philadelphia: Elsevier; 2018:77.)

30. Describe right and left bundle branch blocks. How are they diagnosed on ECG?

RBBB

All electrical current propagates through the left bundle causing the left ventricle to depolarize normally and the QRS complex will demonstrate a normal appearing positive "r" wave deflection. However, electrical propagation to the right ventricle is delayed, causing a second R wave to occur after the first "r" wave. The ECG will demonstrate the typical bunny ear pattern called rSR'. This rSR' complex is widened (>12 ms) and appears in the V1–V3 precordial leads. Associated ST depression and T wave inversion are also common. The etiology of an RBBB can range from an isolated finding, with no evidence of cardiac disease to coronary artery disease, or right heart strain (e.g., pulmonary hypertension, pulmonary embolism). Please see Figure 28.8.

LBBB

Normal septal depolarization occurs from left to right. In an LBBB, depolarization occurs in the reverse direction from the right bundle branch first then to the left ventricle via the septum. This inefficient sequence results in a prolonged QRS complex greater than 120 ms and the physiological normal small Q waves disappear. The precordial lead V1 will show an almost entirely negative QRS complex and lead V6 will demonstrate a large positive QRS complex with morphology resembling an "M" with T wave inversion. An LBBB is almost always abnormal and a new LBBB requires further workup. Please see Figure 28.8.

Both left and right BBB may be incomplete if the characteristic appearance exists, but the QRS interval is less than 120 ms.

31. How does a BBB impair cardiac contractility? What is the role of cardiac resynchronization therapy?

An LBBB causes the right ventricle to contract before the left ventricle and the converse is true with an RBBB. Normally, the septum is relatively fixed and bows slightly into the right ventricle; however, in the setting of a bundle branch block, the septum bows further (or flattens) into the contralateral ventricle causing a decrease in stroke volume. This is called *interventricular dependence*, where one side of the heart can impair the function of the contralateral side. Cardiac resynchronization therapy or biventricular pacing involves placing two leads: one in the right ventricle and the other at

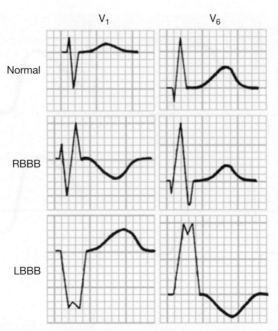

Fig. 28.8 Right and left bundle branch block (*RBBB* and *LBBB*). Note how the RBBB has the rSR' morphology, is widened, and has associated T wave inversion in V1 but not V6. The LBBB has a negative, widened QRS in V1 and in V6 demonstrates a positive, widened QRS with "M" morphology, T wave inversion, and loss of normal physiological Q waves. Both RBBB and LBBB will have a QRS interval over 120 ms. (From Goldberger A, Goldberger Z, Shvilkin A. Ventricular conduction disturbances: bundle branch blocks and related abnormalities. In: Goldberger A, Goldberger Z, Shvilkin A, eds. Goldberger's Clinical Electrocardiography: A Simplified Approach. 9th ed. Philadelphia: Elsevier; 2018:66.)

the left ventricle via the coronary sinus. This allows the left and right ventricle to contract in synchrony and is often indicated in patients with heart failure in the setting of an LBBB.

32. Please see **Figure 28.9**. What is the QRS axis in the frontal plane? Is the QRS complex normal in the precordial leads? Does this rhythm concern you?

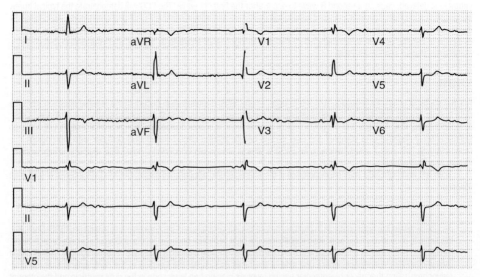

Fig. 28.9 Electrocardiogram in a patient that needs a pacemaker. (From Habash F, Siraj A, Phomakay V, Paydak, H. Pace before it's too late! Second degree AV block with RBBB and LAFB. JACC. 2018;71(11):A2619–A2619. © 2018.)

Frontal Plane

The AUC of the QRS complex is positive in lead I and negative in lead II, therefore a left axis deviation is present. The QRS complex is not isoelectric in any lead, but the AUC of lead II is the closest lead to 0 and is negative, therefore the QRS axis must be less than −30 degrees (see figure on Einthoven's triangle). Further, the AUC of the QRS is the most positive in leads I and aVL; therefore the QRS axis is likely closer to −30 degrees than −90 degrees.

QRS Morphology in Precordial Leads

The QRS complex in the precordial leads V1–V3 is wide (QRS > 120 ms), with the characteristic rSR' morphology, and T wave inversion consistent with an RBBB.

Rhythm

Note that a P wave follows each T wave but there is no corresponding QRS complex and the heart rate is bradycardic. This is consistent with a 2:1 AV block in the setting of a LAD and RBBB. One of the most common causes of an LAD is a left anterior fascicular block. Therefore this patient likely has a bifascicular block, with all electrical conduction occurring through the left posterior fascicle. This patient is at high risk for a third degree AV and should be immediately evaluated for a pacemaker!

33. What are the main categorizations of dysrhythmias? How are they defined?
    Dysrhythmias can be broadly classified into bradydysrhythmias (Table 28.3) and tachydysrhythmias (Table 28.4).

34. What is the differential diagnosis for a wide versus narrow QRS tachycardia? What if the rhythm is regular versus irregular?
    When assessing tachycardia on ECG, there are three questions you need to address:
    1) Does the patient have a pulse? If not, then initiate advanced cardiac life support (ACLS).
    2) Is the QRS complex wide or narrow?
    3) Is the QRS complex irregular or regular?
       Assuming the patient has a pulse, assessing both the QRS interval and its regularity will help you form an initial differential diagnosis. Please see Table 28.5.

Table 28.3 Bradydysrhythmias		
BRADYDYSRHYTHMIA	**DESCRIPTION**	**TREATMENT**
Sinus bradycardia	HR < 60 beats per minute and P wave before each QRS complex	Atropine, Beta-1 agonists (dobutamine, isoproterenol, etc.), or no treatment if asymptomatic
Sick sinus syndrome	Degenerative disease of the electrical conduction system causing symptomatic bradycardia, junctional escape rhythms, and frequent sinus pauses	Permanent pacemaker
First-degree AV block	Prolonged PR interval (>200 ms)	No treatment needed
Second-degree AV block type I (Mobitz I)	Incomplete AV nodal blockade, resulting in progressive PR interval increase until a QRS complex is "dropped"	Atropine or temporary pacemaker if symptomatic, otherwise no treatment
Second-degree AV block type II (Mobitz II)	Incomplete AV nodal blockade, resulting in *randomly* dropped QRS complexes without any change in the PR interval	Permanent pacemaker
Third-degree AV block	Complete AV nodal blockade, resulting in complete dissociation of atrial and ventricular impulses	Permanent pacemaker
Pulseless electrical activity	A form of cardiac arrest: electrical activity, but no mechanical activity	CPR, ACLS protocol
Asystole	A form of cardiac arrest: no electrical activity and no mechanical activity	CPR, ACLS protocol, pacemaker placement

ACPS, Advanced cardiac life support; *AV*, atrioventricular; *CPR*, cardiopulmonary resuscitation; *HR*, heart rate.

Table 28.4 Tachydysrhythmias

TACHYDYSRHYTHMIA	DESCRIPTION	TREATMENT
Sinus tachycardia (ST)	HR >100 bpm and sinus rhythm, that is 1:1 AV conduction - each QRS is preceded by only 1 P wave	Treat underlying cause (pain, hypovolemia, etc.), vagal stimulation, β1 antagonist, etc.
Atrial flutter (A. Flutter)	The atrial rate is near its maximum at roughly 300 beats per minute. Usually there is variable conduction such that not all P wave impulses continue through the AV node and cause a QRS complex. A 2:1 conduction is most common. Characterized by "sawtooth" pattern in Lead II	Cardioversion, antiarrhythmic Rx (amiodarone, etc.), Ablation
Atrial fibrillation (A. Fib)	Irregularly, irregular rhythm insofar as the atrial rate is often near its maximum at roughly 300 beats per minute with variable conduction. The ventricular response rate may be as high as 180 beats per minute. This is called *rapid ventricular response* and is characterized by insufficient cardiac output causing fatigue, heart failure, and rapid decompensation	Cardioversion, antiarrhythmic Rx (amiodarone, etc.), Ablation
Premature atrial contractions (PACs)	If there are ectopic areas of electrical activity within the atrium, they can generate P waves separate from the SA node. These P wave and QRS complexes will occur without the usual pause between regular beats	Decrease caffeine intake, pain control, β1 antagonism
Premature ventricular contractions (PVCs)	Ectopic foci beyond the AV node create a stray ventricular impulse. Defined by a long compensatory pause and by a compensatory increase in the stroke volume of the subsequent heartbeat	Beta-1 antagonism, amiodarone, procainamide, lidocaine, ablation
Monomorphic ventricular tachycardia (VT)	May be sustained or nonsustained, with a pulse or without. Monomorphic VT has a wide complex and regular rhythm. Patients may be asymptomatic, in cardiogenic shock, or cardiac arrest	Synchronized (unstable with pulse) or unsynchronized (no pulse) cardioversion, amiodarone, procainamide, lidocaine, etc.
Polymorphic ventricular tachycardia (PVT)	May be sustained or nonsustained, with a pulse or without. Defined as having an irregular QRS morphology and is more often an irregular rhythm. Patients will be *unstable* and in overt heart failure. It can quickly deteriorate into ventricular fibrillation. PVT is often referred to as *torsade de pointes* when associated with QT prolongation.	Synchronized (unstable with pulse) or unsynchronized (no pulse) cardioversion, Magnesium
Ventricular fibrillation (VF)	No pulse, no coordinated contractions, no cardiac output	Unsynchronized cardioversion

AV, Atrioventricular; *HR*, heart rate; *SA*, sinoatrial.

35. What is the difference between a Mobitz type I and Mobitz type II second-degree AV block? Which one is more concerning?

A Mobitz type I (aka Wenckebach) is often associated with elevated parasympathetic tone states (e.g., sleeping) and is characterized on ECG as increasing prolongation of the PR interval with eventual loss of the QRS complex. It is generally considered benign. A Mobitz type II is characterized as randomly dropped QRS complexes following a P wave. A Mobitz

Table 28.5 Tachycardia Classification

Regular Rhythm and Narrow QRS	Irregular Rhythm and Narrow QRS
• Sinus Tachycardia • Atrial Flutter • AVRT (e.g., WPW) • AVNRT	• Atrial Fibrillation • Multifocal Atrial Tachycardia
Regular Rhythm and Wide QRS	**Irregular Rhythm and Wide QRS**
• VT • SVT with an Aberrancy • Paced Rhythm • AVRT	• Atrial Fibrillation with a Bundle Branch Block • Atrial Fibrillation with an Accessory Pathway (e.g., WPW) • Atrial Fibrillation with an Aberrancy • Polymorphic VT (i.e., Torsade de Pointes)

AVRT, Atrioventricular reentrant tachycardia; *AVNRT*, atrioventricular nodal reentry tachycardia; *SVT*, supraventricular tachycardia (AVRT, AVNRT); *VT*, ventricular tachycardia; *WPW*, Wolff-Parkinson-White.

type II is a much more concern for developing a third-degree complete heart block. These latter patients should strongly be considered for placement of a pacemaker.

36. What is tachy-brady syndrome?

Tachy-brady syndrome occurs in elderly patients who are found to have age-dependent fibrosis of the sinus node tissue and surrounding atrium, causing both sinus node dysfunction (aka sick sinus syndrome), with episodes of paroxysmal atrial fibrillation. These patients may intermittently switch between episodes of sinus bradycardia and atrial fibrillation. Treatment includes placement of a permanent pacemaker and/or catheter ablation of atrial fibrillation.

37. A patient develops symptomatic bradycardia and you need to temporarily pace the patient with transcutaneous pacing. How do you do this? What about transvenous pacing?

Patients that develop symptomatic bradycardia and are unresponsive to atropine will likely need temporary pacing. There are two approaches for temporary pacing: (1) transcutaneous, and (2) transvenous pacing. Transcutaneous pacing involves placing pads (most defibrillators have this ability) to the patient and increasing the amperage, until capture is apparent. The amperage applied should be set to two settings higher than when capture is lost. Transvenous pacing applies a similar approach, however, the temporary pacing leads are placed through an introducer (preferably through the right internal jugular) and increasing the amperage, until capture is apparent. In truly emergent situations, it may be advantageous to initially start with the highest amperage and down titrate, until capture is lost. Temporary transvenous pacing is more comfortable for the patient compared with transcutaneous pacing and less current is needed; however, transcutaneous pacing is more readily available and can be applied expeditiously. Transcutaneous pacing will be painful, and patients will likely need to be sedated.

38. Describe Wolff-Parkinson-White syndrome and its management.

WPW is a specific type of AV reentrant tachycardia because of a congenital accessory pathway (bundle of Kent) from the atrium to the ventricle. Patients usually lack symptoms of WPW unless their heart rate is elevated. It has the following ECG characteristics (Fig. 28.10):

- Short PR interval less than 120 ms
- Long QRS interval greater than 110 ms
- Delta waves (an early rise of the QRS complex)

Wolff–Parkinson–White Preexcitation

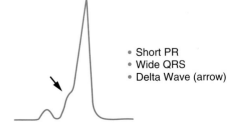

Fig. 28.10 Wolff-Parkinson-White (*WPW*) syndrome. The electrocardiogram pattern for WPW includes the following triad: (1) short PR, (2) wide QRS, (3) delta waves. (From Goldberger A, Goldberger Z, Shvilkin A. Atrioventricular (AV) conduction disorders, part II: preexcitation (Wolff–Parkinson–White) patterns and syndromes. In: Goldberger A, Goldberger Z, Shvilkin A, eds. Goldberger's Clinical Electrocardiography: A Simplified Approach. 9th ed. Philadelphia: Elsevier; 2018:184.)

- Short PR
- Wide QRS
- Delta Wave (arrow)

Preexcitation occurs when the atrial impulse bypasses the AV node through the accessory pathway and depolarizes the ventricle causing a decreased PR interval. This inefficient transmission through the ventricular myocardium bypasses the AV node, bundle of His, and PF causing a larger QRS complex (slower depolarization).

The delta wave, caused by ventricular preexcitation, is most readily apparent for slow heart rates (i.e., low sympathetic tone states) because the delay through the AV node is longer. When the sympathetic tone is high (e.g., sinus tachycardia), the conduction delay via the AV node decreases, which may rival the accessory pathway, making preexcitation less apparent on ECG.

SVT caused by WPW is classified as an AV reentrant tachycardia. Treatment usually begins by attempting vagal maneuvers and when not effective, pharmacological agents (i.e., procainamide, amiodarone). AV nodal blockers should be avoided because they will exacerbate conduction via the accessory pathway. This is particularly problematic in patients that have both atrial fibrillation and WPW because AV nodal blocking agents may cause an extremely rapid ventricular heat rate.

39. What is Brugada syndrome and how does it appear on ECG?

Brugada syndrome is the result of a mutation in the cardiac sodium channel gene causing sudden cardiac death (SCD) because of VF or polymorphic VT. It is most common in Southeast Asian populations and the average age of sudden death is around 41 years. Diagnosis requires both characteristic ECG finding and clinical criteria. Clinical criteria include the following: history of VT/VF, family history of SCD, agonal respirations during sleep, syncope. Brugada syndrome ECG findings are dynamic and might not always be apparent. Brugada syndrome is most apparent during episodes of high vagal tone (e.g., sleeping) because most SCD events occur while sleeping. Definitive treatment requires an implantable cardioverter-defibrillator.

The ECG criteria for Brugada syndrome is the following (Fig. 28.11):

- Coved ST segment elevation over 2 mm in at least two of V1–V3, followed by a negative T wave. The pattern resembles the rSR' morphology of an RBBB but with ST elevation.

40. How is atrial fibrillation treated in the operating room? What medications should be considered?

First, does the patient have a history of atrial fibrillation and are they taking medicine for it? Many patients are in "rate-controlled" atrial fibrillation. Rate control usually refers to achieving an average heart rate of less than 110 beats per minute in patients who do not feel any symptoms of their atrial fibrillation. For patients, who are symptomatic from atrial fibrillation, a heart rate of less than about 85 beats per minute is the target. These patients will likely tolerate atrial fibrillation fine, unless their heart rate is significantly increased above baseline.

Brugada Pattern

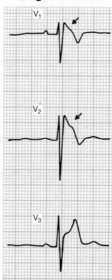

Fig. 28.11 Brugada syndrome. Brugada syndrome electrocardiogram findings include an rSR' pattern similar to a right bundle branch block but includes ST elevation in leads V1, V2, and V3. (From Goldberger A, Goldberger Z, Shvilkin A. Sudden cardiac arrest and sudden cardiac death syndromes. In: Goldberger A, Goldberger Z, Shvilkin A, eds. Goldberger's Clinical Electrocardiography: A Simplified Approach. 9th ed. Philadelphia: Elsevier; 2018:224.)

Second, and just as important as the patient's history of atrial fibrillation, is the patient stable? In other words, does the patient have an adequate cardiac output despite the arrhythmia? The loss of the efficient and appropriately timed atrial kick at end diastole can cause up to a 30% loss of left ventricular end-diastolic volume and a commensurate decrease in stroke volume.

Atrial fibrillation management consists of optimization of electrolytes (Mg > 2 mg/dL and K > 4 mEq/L) and minimization of atrial stretch (e.g., diuresis, correction of mitral valve regurgitation, or stenosis). Acute medical management of atrial fibrillation includes calcium-channel blockers, β1 blockers, digoxin, or amiodarone. Fast acting intravenous (IV) medications will be favored in the operating room: diltiazem 0.25 mg/kg IV bolus, esmolol 30 to 50 mg IV bolus, or amiodarone 75 to 150 mg IV bolus. Esmolol has the advantage of a short half-life in case of side effects. The most common side-effect of all three is hypotension, although amiodarone will be the least likely to drop the blood pressure and may be best tolerated by patients with reduced cardiac function.

The treatment of unstable atrial fibrillation is synchronized cardioversion at 100 to 200 joules.

41. **How is ventricular tachycardia and ventricular fibrillation treated?**
Both VT and VF are life-threatening dysrhythmias that require immediate management. Cardiac arrest because of VT or VF requires the initiation of cardiopulmonary resuscitation (CPR), early defibrillation, and medications (e.g., epinephrine, lidocaine, amiodarone).

Stable VT may also require synchronized cardioversion, but may be managed with vagal maneuvers, medications like adenosine (if narrow complex, regular, monomorphic), amiodarone, or procainamide. As with each instance of ACLS, continue to search for underlying causes of debility (e.g., H's and T's).

42. **How is the management of pulseless electrical activity different?**
Pulseless electrical activity (PEA) is different because there exists organized electrical activity in the heart, but that electrical activity is not translating into a life-sustaining stroke volume or a pulse. First, be sure to confirm the true lack of a pulse and the presence of electrical activity by ECG. The treatment is ACLS without electrical defibrillation because the electrical activity is already organized. CPR and medication administration (e.g., epinephrine) should be continued until a pulse is confirmed (i.e., until mechanical activity matches the electrical activity of the heart). As with each instance of ACLS, continue to search for underlying causes of debility (e.g., H's and T's).

KEY POINTS: DYSRHYTHMIAS AND OTHER ECG ABNORMALITIES

1. Disorders that impair the electrical conduction system cause mechanical dyssynchrony between the chambers of the heart and impair cardiac output.
2. A prolonged QT interval can increase the risk of an "R-on-T," which can occur if a PVC or asynchronous pacing causes the ventricle to depolarize during the T wave, when the ventricle is in a partially depolarized and repolarized state. This may lead to a lethal rhythm, such as torsade de pointes or VF.
3. Electrolyte derangements are a common and easily correctable source of ECG abnormalities.
4. Anesthesiologists must be facile with all facets of dysrhythmia and ACLS management.

SUGGESTED READINGS

Antzelevitch C, Brugada P, Borggrefe M, et al. Brugada syndrome: report of the second consensus conference. Circulation 2005;111:659–670.

Antzelevitch C, Brugada P, Brugada J, Brugada R, Towbin JA, Nademanee K. Brugada syndrome: 1992–2002: A historical perspective. J Am Coll Cardiol. 2003;41;1665–1671.

Colucci RA, Silver MJ, Shubrook J. Common types of supraventricular tachycardia: diagnosis and management. Am Fam Physician. 2010;82 (8):942–952.

Goldberger A, Goldberger Z, Shvilkin A, eds. Goldberger's Clinical Electrocardiography: A Simplified Approach. 9th ed. Philadelphia: Elsevier; 2018.

Mattu A & Brady W. ECGs for the Emergency Physician. London: BMJ Publishing Group; 2003.

Zipes DP, Libby P, Bonow RO, Mann DL, Tomaselli GF. Braunwald: Heart Disease: A Textbook of Cardiovascular Medicine. 6th ed. W.B. Saunders Company; 2001.

CHAPTER 29

PACEMAKERS AND INTERNAL CARDIOVERTER DEFIBRILLATORS

Richard Ing, MBBCh, FCA(SA), Johannes von Alvensleben, MD, Manchula Navaratnam, MBChB

1. **What are the common indications for placement of a permanent pacemaker?**
   Common indications are as follows: symptomatic bradycardia that is not reversible, third-degree heart block (sometimes referred to as *complete heart block*) is a problem of the atrioventricular (AV) node and requires permanent pacing, second-degree type II heart block (even in an asymptomatic patient), as it can progress to third-degree heart block.

2. **What is the origin of the NBG coding system for permanent pacemakers? What do positions I, II, III, IV, and V in the NBG code stand for?**
   The North American Society of Pacing and Electrophysiology and the British Pacing and Electrophysiology Group combined to produce the Generic (NBG) code. Positions I, II, and III define the chamber in which pacing or sensing occurs and the mode of the response to the sensed or triggered event. Position IV indicates the presence (R) or absence (O) of an adaptive-rate mechanism and whether it is simple (P) or multiprogrammable (M). Position V refers to multisite and antitachycardiac permanent pacemaker (PM) functions (Table 29.1).

3. **What are asynchronous pacing modes and how would you describe them in the NBG code?**
   The asynchronous pacing modes are often used for temporary pacing. The PM will be programmed to pace at a fixed rate, without the ability to sense or react to any underlying intrinsic cardiac activity. The NBG codes are AOO, VOO, or DOO. In these modes, the atrium, ventricle, or both are paced, and the PM has no sensing capability.

4. **When is it advantageous to use asynchronous pacing?**
   A PM may be reprogrammed into an asynchronous mode perioperatively to allow for the safe use of surgical electrocautery. If not reprogrammed, electrocautery used during surgery could be sensed by the PM and misinterpreted as underlying intrinsic cardiac activity, thereby inhibiting the pacing function and possibly resulting in bradycardia or even asystole in a PM-dependent patient.

5. **Define DDD pacing.**
   From the NBG code, DDD describes a situation in which the atria and ventricles are paced, the atrial and ventricular response to the pacing is sensed, and the dual mode of the response is both inhibited and triggered. This form of pacing is common and allows for an underlying sensed event from the atria to occur, and if it does not, for the atrium to be paced. An appropriately set AV delay will then be allowed to occur, and if no ventricular sensed event occurs within a preset time interval, the ventricle will be also paced. DDD mode is sometimes referred to as *physiological pacing* because it allows for AV synchrony that closely approximates normal cardiac function.

6. **What are the advantages and disadvantages of DDD pacing?**
   There is reduced incidence of atrial fibrillation with the use of DDD pacing. In addition, maintaining AV-synchrony with DDD pacing reduces atrial pressures and increases ventricular end-diastolic volumes, resulting in increased stroke volume, better cardiac output, and improved arterial blood pressure and coronary perfusion. DDD pacing has also been shown to decrease thromboembolic events, which may be related to the reduction in atrial fibrillation seen.

   However, if used too frequently, chronic right ventricular pacing in DDD mode results in adverse left ventricular (LV) remodeling, LV dysfunction, congestive heart failure, and increased incidence of atrial fibrillation.

7. **Many DDD PMs are now programmed in managed ventricular pacing mode. What does this mean?**
   Several manufacturers have developed pacing modes that give preference to intrinsic cardiac conduction when there is still some degree of native AV-conduction. This is done in an attempt to minimize unnecessary right ventricular pacing. One of these modes, managed ventricular pacing (MVP), automatically switches between AAI (R) and DDD (R) mode depending on the degree of native AV conduction.

8. **What are some of the disadvantages of unipolar versus bipolar PM systems?**
   In unipolar systems, one electrode (the cathode) is at the tip of the lead and the other (the anode) is the PM generator. Sensing can occur at either the lead or the generator. Because of the greater distance between anode and cathode in

Table 29.1 NBG Coding System for Pacemakers

I	II	III	IV	V
Chamber(s) Paced	Chamber(s) Sensed	Mode(s) of Response	Programmable functions	Antitachycardia Functions
V = Ventricle	V = Ventricle	T = Triggered	0 = None	0 = None
A = Atrium	A = Atrium	I = Inhibited	P = Simple programmable	P = Paced
D = Dual (A&V)	D = Dual (A&V)	D = Dual triggered/ inhibited	M = Multiprogrammable	S = Shocks
0 = None	0 = None	0 = None	C = Communicating	D = Dual (P&S)
			R = Rate modulated	

unipolar systems, unipolar sensing necessitates a larger electrical potential difference, resulting in decreased battery life. In addition, unipolar PM systems may be more vulnerable to skeletal muscle myopotential oversensing (skeletal muscle depolarization being sensed as cardiac electrical activity) and inappropriate far-field source sensing from pulsed electromagnetic fields (such as airport security systems, faulty microwave ovens, radios, television, some dental equipment, magnetic resonance imaging, and other sources of electromagnetic radiation). Cellular phones generally are not problematic but should not be carried directly over the PM. In addition, cross talk during dual-chamber unipolar pacing can lead to severe, life-threatening arrhythmias.

In contrast, bipolar transvenous PMs contain both the cathode and anode at the tip of the lead. The bipolar epicardial system has two small leads implanted close together on the surface of the heart. Bipolar systems result in a much smaller distance between the anode and cathode, limiting oversensing and far-field source sensing and therefore reduced sensitivity to electromagnetic interference. In addition, bipolar systems require less energy to produce the smaller electrical potential difference resulting in longer battery life.

In addition, bipolar transvenous leads have a c-axial design which enables continued functioning (as a unipolar system) if the lead fracture were to occur. In unipolar systems, lead fracture will result in the system becoming nonfunctional. Most modern PMs have bipolar leads.

9. What are the different approaches to cardiac implantable electronic device placement?
   Cardiac implantable electronic devices (CIEDs; PMs and implantable cardioverter defibrillators [ICDs]) can be placed using either a transvenous or epicardial approach, with the vast majority of devices placed transvenously. Transvenous placement entails accessing the right atrium and/or ventricle via the subclavian or axillary veins. The leads are then connected to a pulse generator located in an infraclavicular or axillary subcutaneous pocket. However, some patients either lack suitable vasculature and/or their cardiac anatomy precludes an endovascular system. This scenario is most common in patients with single ventricle physiology (from congenital heart disease), where the systemic venous system communicates directly with the systemic arterial system. For these patients, an epicardial approach is necessary to avoid the development of systemic thromboemboli.

   The epicardial approach entails performing a sternotomy and sewing the leads directly onto the myocardium overlying the chamber(s) of interest. Unlike the transvenous approach, leads can be placed onto either the right or left atria or ventricle. The pulse generator is then placed in a submuscular pocket, located either just inferior to the sternal incision or in a separate preperitoneal pocket in the abdomen.

10. What complications are associated with CIED insertion?
    Patient factors include: bleeding, hematoma, surgical site infection, myocardial damage, cardiac perforation and tamponade, pneumothorax from subclavian vein access attempts, venous thrombosis and pectoral, diaphragmatic or intercostal muscle stimulation. CIED factors include: lead fracture, lead dislodgement, lead insulation breach, and battery depletion.

11. Why do some patients require an implantable cardioverter defibrillator?
    An ICD is a battery powered, dual function PM device that has all the usual capabilities of a PM, but can also deliver an internal cardiac shock if a tachyarrhythmia is detected. They are placed in patients who are at risk for life-threatening arrhythmias to decrease the risk of sudden cardiac death. Common indications for an ICD include: symptomatic ventricular arrhythmia, prior myocardial infarction, survivor of sudden cardiac arrest, low cardiac ejection fraction, known cardiac channelopathies (e.g., long QT and Brugada syndrome) and the presence of congenital heart disease or another condition prone to sudden cardiac arrest (e.g., severe obstructive hypertrophic cardiomyopathy).

12. **What is electromagnetic interference and how does it affect PM or ICD function in the operating room?**

    PMs and ICDs are designed to detect and respond to electromagnetic signals that arise from cardiac tissue. As previously described, these signals may include normal cardiac depolarization or those arising from potentially life-threatening arrhythmias. Electromagnetic interference (EMI) arises from sources other than cardiac tissue and may interference with normal device function.

    EMI comes in two forms, *conducted* and *radiated*, with conducted sources resulting from direct contact with the body and radiated sources resulting from the body entering an electromagnetic field. Common sources of *conducted* interference in the operating room include electrocautery and defibrillation. Electrocautery uses a high voltage current that passes through the tissue to allow for cutting or coagulation and can be either unipolar or bipolar in their design. Unipolar cautery, with the current beginning at the instrument tip and passing through the tissue to the grounding patch, is most common. EMI will be found along the path of this current, making surgical site and grounding patch location important in planning whether EMI may affect PM or ICD function.

    The effect of EMI on the PM or ICD depends on the particular device and on the underlying cardiac diagnosis of the patient. The use of electrocautery may result in *oversensing* by the device, leading to inhibition of necessary pacing, or the false detection of an arrhythmia and the delivery of inappropriate defibrillation by an ICD.

13. **How can one predict if EMI is likely to be problematic during a procedure using electrocautery?**

    The path of EMI follows a course from the electrocautery instrument to the grounding patch. If the pulse generator and/or leads (pacing or ICD) are within the path of this circuit, then EMI is possible and precautions to prevent abnormal device behavior will be necessary.

    For example, a patient with a transvenous PM and pulse generator located in a left infraclavicular location is scheduled to have a thyroidectomy. If the grounding patch is placed on the lower-back, then the path of EMI will pass directly over the pacing leads within the heart. If the grounding patch is instead placed on the upper back, then the risk of interference is significantly lower. Similarly, when the surgical site involves a remote extremity, such as the leg, and the patch is placed on the lower back, then the EMI course does not include either the pacing or ICD components.

    Understanding the location of all leads, as well as the pulse generator, is important in making these assessments.

14. **If EMI is unavoidable, what precautions can be taken?**

    When patients with a pacing indication need surgery, and there is a high risk of encountering EMI, they should have their device reprogrammed into an asynchronous mode (AOO, VOO, DOO) such that all electromagnetic signals (including cardiac) are ignored and pacing occurs regardless. Although these modes are not considered physiological and should not be used for chronic pacing, they prevent the possibility of oversensing, and subsequent failure to pace. Asynchronous pacing modes can also be achieved with the placement of a magnet over the pulse generator. This will automatically result in a PM converting to VOO pacing mode for as long as the magnet remains over the pulse generator. The device reverts back to its original programming once the magnet is removed.

    An ICD should be programmed such that all therapies are turned off so that inappropriate shocks are not delivered during the procedure. This can be achieved with specific device reprogramming before the procedure or by placing a magnet over the pulse generator. Unlike a PM, placing a magnet over the ICD only suspends its ability to detect arrhythmias and deliver defibrillation therapies. It does not affect PM programming.

15. **What are the dangers of placing a magnet over a CIED before anesthesia?**

    Magnets were historically used to test PM battery life and to reprogram a PM into an asynchronous mode to avoid external EMI or cautery interference during surgery. In the 2011 Practice Advisory for CIEDs, the American Society of Anesthesiologists (ASA) advises against the routine use of a magnet over an implantable CIED. The ASA recommends interrogation of the PM to assess function before anesthesia and the development of a perioperative plan for the management of a patient with a CIED.

    In patients with an ICD and pacing indications, placement of a magnet does not affect the bradycardia pacing programming. Therefore interrogation is required with specific programming to address both aspects of the device. Furthermore, the magnet response is variable between device manufactures, particularly in the rate of asynchronous pacing. Finally, typically only found in older devices, the duration of asynchronous pacing with magnetic application may be temporary.

16. **Describe some other common factors that may increase or decrease the pacing threshold perioperatively.**

    Pacing threshold refers to the amplitude and duration of the stimulus that is applied to the myocardium. An increase in pacing threshold can be seen: during the first few weeks after device insertion, with myocardial scaring and fibrosis s/p myocardial infarction, with hypothermia, hyperkalemia, hypoxia, hypoglycemia, in the presence of a high dosage of local anesthetics or inhalation anesthetic agents. Decreased pacing thresholds can be seen with sympathomimetic amines, anticholinergic medications, and in the presence of anxiety.

17. **Can patients with CIEDs receive magnetic resonance imaging?**

An estimated 75% of patients who currently have a CIED will need magnetic resonance imaging (MRI) during their lifetimes. In the past, MRI was contraindicated in all patients with CIEDs because of concerns that the powerful magnetic and radiofrequency fields generated during imaging might damage device components, inhibit PM function, trigger rapid pacing, or deliver inappropriate shocks. More recently, however, device manufacturers have developed "MRI conditional devices" and sought retrograde clearance for previously manufactured models.

Although patients with these devices may safely undergo MRI, careful consideration and preprocedural planning is necessary to ensure appropriate device function. Devices should also be interrogated before and after MRI to ensure that no programming changes have occurred. In addition, providers comfortable in device programming should be readily available.

18. **What recommendations can be made for the operating room team caring for a patient with a PM?**

Ideally, all CIEDs should be interrogated before surgery. The dispersive electrode of the electrocautery device should be placed as close to the surgical site as possible and as far away from the PM as possible. Limit the bursts of electrocautery if possible. Have an external defibrillator in the operating room throughout the case. Use an electrocardiogram monitor with pacing mode to recognize pacing spikes. If central access is required, consider the groin to avoid dislodgement or shorting of an intravascular pacing electrode in the right side of the heart.

KEY POINTS: PACEMAKERS AND INTERNAL CARDIOVERTER DEFIBRILLATORS

1. Common indications for permanent PM placement are as follows: symptomatic bradycardia that is not reversible, second-degree type II heart block, and third-degree heart block.
2. Positions I, II, and III of the NBG PM code define the chamber in which pacing occurs, the chamber in which sensing occurs, and the mode of the response to the sensed or triggered event, respectively.
3. Asynchronous pacing modes are used most commonly for temporary pacing and to allow for the safe use of surgical electrocautery.
4. An ICD is a battery powered, dual function PM device that has all the usual capabilities of a PM, but can also deliver an internal cardiac shock if a tachyarrhythmia is detected.
5. EMI arises from sources other than cardiac tissue and may interference with normal device function.
6. Ideally, all CIEDs should be interrogated before surgery.

SUGGESTED READINGS

Arora L, Inampudi C. Perioperative management of cardiac rhythm assist devices in ambulatory surgery and nonoperating room anesthesia. Curr Opin Anaesthesiol. 2017;30(6):676–681.

Atlee JL. Cardiac pacing and electroversion. In: Kaplan JA, ed Cardiac Anesthesia, 4th edition Philadelphia: WB Saunders; 1999: p. 959–989.

Chakravarthy M, Prabhakumar D, George A. Anaesthetic consideration in patients with cardiac implantable electronic devices scheduled for surgery. Indian J Anaesth. 2017;61(9):736–743.

Crossley GH1, Poole JE, Rozner MA, et al. The Heart Rhythm Society (HRS)/American Society of Anesthesiologists (ASA) Expert Consensus Statement on the perioperative management of patients with implantable defibrillators, pacemakers and arrhythmia monitors: facilities and patient management this document was developed as a joint project with the American Society of Anesthesiologists (ASA), and in collaboration with the American Heart Association (AHA), and the Society of Thoracic Surgeons (STS). Heart Rhythm. 2011; 8(7):1114–1154.

Rooke GA, Bowdle TA. Perioperative management of pacemakers and implantable cardioverter defibrillators: it's not just about the magnet. Anesth Analg. 2013;117(2):292–294.

Yildiz M, Yilmaz Ak H, Oksen D, Oral S. Anesthetic management in electrophysiology laboratory: a multidisciplinary review. J Atr Fibrillation. 2018;10(5):1775.

CHAPTER 30

BLOOD PRESSURE DISTURBANCES

Brennan McGill, MD, Martin Krause, MD

1. **What blood pressure value is considered hypertensive?**
   The definitions for blood pressure (BP) categories changed in 2017 according to the guidelines released by the American Heart Association/American College of Cardiology. A normal BP is less than 120/80 mm Hg. An elevated BP is a systolic BP of 120 to 129 mm Hg and a diastolic BP less than 80 mm Hg. Stage 1 hypertension (HTN) is a systolic BP of 130 to 139 mm Hg or a diastolic BP of 80 to 89 mm Hg. Stage 2 HTN is a systolic BP of at least 140 mm Hg or a diastolic BP of at least 90 mm Hg. A hypertensive crisis is defined as a systolic BP greater than 180 mm Hg or a diastolic BP greater than 120 mm Hg. A hypertensive crisis is considered hypertensive urgency if there is no evidence of end-organ damage or a hypertensive emergency if there is evidence of end-organ damage. End-organ damage involves the development of posterior reversible encephalopathy syndrome, acute kidney injury, heart failure, and subsequent pulmonary edema among others. BP changes throughout the day and can be affected by posture, exercise, medications, smoking, caffeine ingestion, and mood. HTN cannot be diagnosed on the basis of one abnormal BP reading but an average of at least two measurements on at least two different occasions.

2. **What causes hypertension?**
   - Primary (or essential) HTN: unknown cause; more than 90% of all cases fall into this category
   - Medications: oral contraceptives, weight-loss medications, stimulants, corticosteroids
   - Endocrine: Cushing syndrome, hyperaldosteronism, pheochromocytoma, thyrotoxicosis, acromegaly
   - Renal: chronic pyelonephritis, renovascular stenosis, glomerulonephritis, polycystic kidney disease
   - Neurogenic: increased intracranial pressure, autonomic hyperreflexia
   - Miscellaneous: obesity, hypercalcemia, preeclampsia, acute intermittent porphyria, obstructive sleep apnea, pain, anxiety, illicit drugs

3. **What are the consequences of chronic HTN?**
   Chronically hypertensive patients are at risk for developing end-organ disease, including left ventricular hypertrophy, systolic and diastolic heart failure, coronary artery disease with increased risk of myocardial infarction, chronic renal failure, retinopathy, ischemic stroke, and intracerebral hemorrhage (ICH).

4. **Why should most antihypertensives be taken up until the time of surgery?**
   A well-controlled hypertensive patient has less intraoperative BP lability (either HTN or hypotension). Acute withdrawal of antihypertensives, specifically β blockers and α_2 agonists, may precipitate rebound HTN or myocardial ischemia. With a few exceptions, it is recommended to continue antihypertensive therapy until the time of surgery and restart therapy as soon as possible after surgery (Table 30.1).

5. **Which antihypertensives should be held on the day of surgery?**
   Although there is no universal agreement, many believe renin-angiotensin system antagonists (angiotensin-converting-enzyme [ACE] inhibitors and angiotensin II receptor blockers [ARBs]) should be held the day of surgery. Diuretics may be withheld when depletion of intravascular volume is a concern.

6. **Why does administration of renin-angiotensin system antagonists result in hypotension in the periinduction period? How might the hypotension be treated?**
   ACE inhibitors decrease the concentration of angiotensin II, which leads to reduced secretion of aldosterone and a loss of sympathetic tone. In the operating room, the sympatholytic effects are exacerbated by most anesthetic agents. For the same reason, catecholaminergic pressor agents, such as phenylephrine and ephedrine, may prove insufficient. The vasopressin system is the only remaining pathway to maintain BP; however, its effects on BP are slower compared with the sympathetic nervous system. Refractory hypotension that does not respond to fluids and other commonly used agents (e.g., phenylephrine) can usually be treated by administering vasopressin.

7. **Are hypertensive patients undergoing general anesthesia at increased risk for perioperative cardiac morbidity?**
   It is well documented that patients with uncontrolled HTN are at risk for intraoperative BP lability (HTN or hypotension). Apart from that, it remains unclear whether delaying surgery to achieve BP control reduces perioperative cardiac morbidity. Many advocate delaying elective surgical operations in patients who present in hypertensive crisis (systolic BP > 180 mm Hg or diastolic BP > 120 mm Hg).

Table 30.1 Commonly Prescribed Antihypertensive Medications

CLASS	EXAMPLES	SIDE EFFECTS
Thiazide diuretics	Hydrochlorothiazide	Hypokalemia, hyponatremia, hyperglycemia, hypomagnesemia, hypocalcemia
Loop diuretics	Furosemide	Hypokalemia, hypocalcemia, hyperglycemia, hypomagnesemia, metabolic alkalosis
β Blockers	Propranolol, metoprolol, atenolol	Bradycardia, bronchospasm, conduction blockade, myocardial depression, fatigue
α Blockers	Terazosin, prazosin	Postural hypotension, tachycardia, fluid retention
α_2 Agonists	Clonidine	Postural hypotension, sedation, rebound hypertension, decreases MAC
Calcium channel blockers	Verapamil, diltiazem, nifedipine	Cardiac depression, conduction blockade, bradycardia
ACE inhibitors	Captopril, enalapril, lisinopril, ramipril	Cough, angioedema, fluid retention, reflex tachycardia, renal dysfunction, hyperkalemia
Angiotensin receptor antagonists	Losartan, irbesartan, candesartan	Hypotension, renal failure, hyperkalemia
Vascular smooth muscle relaxants	Hydralazine, minoxidil	Reflex tachycardia, fluid retention

ACE, Angiotensin-converting enzyme; *MAC,* minimal alveolar concentration.

8. Provide a differential diagnosis for intraoperative hypertension.
   See Table 30.2.
9. How is perioperative hypertension managed?
   Pain and inadequate anesthesia are the most common causes of perioperative HTN. If deepening the anesthetic and administration of analgesics do not address HTN sufficiently, consider an alternative etiology. These include hypercarbia, hypoxia, hyperthyroidism, pheochromocytoma, malignant hyperthermia, elevated intracranial pressure, autonomic dysreflexia or iatrogenic causes, such as medication errors, fluid overload, or aortic cross-clamping. If the patient is still hypertensive, despite addressing the aforementioned causes, the patient might have preexisting essential HTN, and you should consider administering a primary antihypertensive agent.
10. Provide differential diagnoses and treatment of perioperative hypotension.
    See Table 30.3.
11. What is the first-line treatment for hypotension with general anesthesia?
    Most general anesthetic agents (e.g., volatile agents, propofol) cause decreased systemic vascular resistance and decreased contractility. In general, first-line treatment for mild hypotension with general anesthesia is with α_1 agonist (i.e., phenylephrine) or α_1/β_1 agonists (i.e., ephedrine) to restore systemic vascular resistance and contractility back to normal. Judicious fluid administration can also be helpful as many patients are nothing by mouth (NPO)

Table 30.2 Differential Diagnosis of Intraoperative Hypertension

Related to preexisting disease	Chronic hypertension, increased intracranial pressure, autonomic hyperreflexia, aortic dissection, early acute myocardial infarction
Related to surgery	Prolonged tourniquet time, postcardiopulmonary bypass, aortic cross-clamping, postcarotid endarterectomy
Related to anesthetic	Pain, inadequate depth of anesthesia, catecholamine release, malignant hyperthermia, shivering, hypoxia, hypercarbia, hypothermia, hypervolemia, improperly sized (too small) blood pressure cuff, intraarterial transducer positioned too low
Related to medication	Rebound hypertension (from discontinuation of clonidine, β blockers, or methyldopa), systemic absorption of vasoconstrictors, intravenous dye (e.g., indigo carmine)
Other	Bladder distention, hypoglycemia

Table 30.3 Differential Diagnosis of Perioperative Hypotension and Treatment

CAUSES	TREATMENT
Decreased Preload	
Hypovolemia resulting from nothing by mouth (NPO) status, hemorrhage, insensible losses, gastrointestinal losses or severe burns	Increase circulating volume by blood transfusion or intravenous fluid (IVF) administration, surgical control of hemorrhage
Decreased venous return because of venodilation, increased intrathoracic pressure, decreased skeletal muscle tone	Reverse causes of increased intrathoracic pressure, IVF administration, vasopressors
Decreased Contractility	
Cardiac ischemia, nonischemic cardiomyopathy, hypocalcemia, acidosis, acute myocarditis	Optimize myocardial oxygen supply, correct electrolyte disturbances, correct acidosis, inotropes
Arrhythmias	
Atrial arrhythmias, such as atrial fibrillation with rapid ventricular response or paroxysmal supraventricular tachycardia preventing atrial kick and causing decreased diastolic filling time	Pharmacologically or electrically convert to normal sinus rhythm
Ventricular fibrillation (Vfib), ventricular tachycardia (VT)	Stable VT: amiodarone or electrical cardioversion, unstable VT or Vfib: Advanced cardiac life support, including epinephrine and defibrillation
Bradycardia and heart block	Atropine, transvenous or transcutaneous pacing, dopamine or epinephrine infusion
Decreased Afterload	
Anesthetic medications, anaphylaxis, high neuraxial blockade/neurogenic shock, sepsis	Decrease intravenous or volatile anesthetic dose, IVF administration, vasopressors, epinephrine for anaphylaxis
Obstructive	
Cardiac tamponade	IVF administration, inotropes, preferably epinephrine until definitive treatment with pericardiocentesis
Tension pneumothorax	Immediate needle thoracostomy or chest tube
Massive pulmonary embolism	Inotropes to support myocardial contractility until more definitive treatment with systemic heparinization, systemic fibrinolysis, open surgical embolectomy or catheter directed thrombectomy
Aortocaval compression syndrome	Place the parturient in the left lateral recumbent position, IVF administration
Impaired ventricular filling because of mitral/tricuspid stenosis or outlet obstruction because of pulmonary/aortic stenosis	Surgical repair or replacement of valves

for more than 8 hours. However, in most situations the main disturbance is caused by vasodilation and decreased contractility, not hypovolemia.

12. **What is the problem with treating hypotension in hemorrhagic or cardiogenic shock with α_1 agonists?**
Recall that MAP = SVR $\times$ CO + CVP where CO = stroke volume (SV) $\times$ heart rate (HR) and SV is a function of preload, afterload, and contractility. Although administering an α_1 agonist to increase SVR may restore a normal BP, it does not correct the underlying pathophysiology in the setting of cardiogenic or hemorrhagic shock. Patients in hemorrhagic shock have hypotension because of decreased preload, and treatment should primarily surround volume resuscitation to restore preload back to normal. Cardiogenic shock is caused by decreased cardiac output, usually from decreased contractility. Pure α_1 agonists should be avoided in these patients, as any increase in afterload will reduce stroke volume and hence cardiac output. Management of cardiogenic shock usually requires vasoactive agents with positive inotropy (e.g., epinephrine, dobutamine, or milrinone). These patients are often hypervolemic, which overdistends the myosin-actin filaments, which itself can also contribute to decreased contractility and stroke volume. Treatment, therefore should include diuretics to restore preload back to normal, thereby improving contractility and

reducing ventricular pressure ($P_{ventricle}$), which overall improves coronary perfusion. Recall, the equation for coronary perfusion pressure (CPP): $CPP = P_{aorta} - P_{ventricle}$.

13. **How does neuraxial anesthesia cause hypotension?**
Spinal, and to a lesser extent epidural anesthesia, produce hypotension through sympathetic blockade and vasodilation. Block levels lower than the fifth thoracic dermatome are less likely to cause hypotension given the compensatory vasoconstriction of the upper extremities. Block levels higher than the fourth thoracic dermatome may affect cardioaccelerator nerves, resulting in bradycardia and diminished cardiac output.

14. **What is the most appropriate treatment for hypertension in the setting of intracerebral hemorrhage?**
The rationale for acutely lowering BP in the setting of ICH is to attenuate progression of the hematoma. An optimal BP target in this setting is controversial, given the concern for inadequate cerebral perfusion but studies to date suggest a target systolic BP less than 140 mm Hg is safe. Excessive reduction in BP may increase the risk of compromising cerebral perfusion pressure (CPP), defined as $CPP = MAP - ICP/CVP$ (the higher of CVP or intracerebral pressure [ICP]). For example, if ICP is greater than CVP, then $CPP = MAP - ICP$.
  Nitroglycerin and nitroprusside should be avoided in this setting as both cause cerebral venodilation with a subsequent increase in cerebral blood volume and ICP. The increase in ICP can both decrease CPP and potentially lead to herniation leading to devastating neurological sequelae. Therefore hydralazine, nicardipine, labetalol, and esmolol are the preferred agents, with nicardipine the most commonly used agent.

15. **What is the most appropriate treatment for a patient with neurogenic shock?**
Hypotension develops after traumatic or immune-mediated spinal cord injury or high spinal anesthesia because of disruption of sympathetic tracts and unopposed parasympathetic tone. Bradyarrhythmias can develop if the T1–T4 sympathetic nerves are involved, as these contain the cardioaccelerator fibers. Volume administration is first-line therapy if the patient is deemed hypovolemic, otherwise direct acting vasoactive medications (i.e., phenylephrine, norepinephrine, and epinephrine) should be administered. Indirect vasoactive agents (e.g., ephedrine) are ineffective in neurogenic shock.

KEY POINTS: BLOOD PRESSURE DISTURBANCES

1. Except for patients in hypertensive crisis (systolic BP > 180 mm Hg), there is insufficient evidence to say whether delaying surgery to achieve BP control reduces perioperative cardiac morbidity.
2. Renin-angiotensin system antagonists (ACE inhibitors and ARBs) if continued on the day of surgery can cause profound refractory hypotension that usually responds well to vasopressin administration.
3. Perioperative BP disturbances (hypotension or HTN) have a broad differential that requires accurate diagnosis to treat the problem effectively.

SUGGESTED READINGS

Matei VA, Haddadin A. Systemic and pulmonary arterial hypertension. In: Stoelting's Anesthesia and Co-Existing Disease. 6th ed. Philadelphia: Elsevier; 2012:104–119.
Nadella V, Howell SJ. Hypertension: pathophysiology and perioperative implications. Continuing Education Anaesthesia Crit Care Pain. 2015;15(6):275–279.
Salmasi V, Maheshwari K, Yang D, et al. Relationship between intraoperative hypotension, defined by either reduction from baseline or absolute thresholds, and acute kidney and myocardial injury after noncardiac surgery. Surv Anesthesiol. 2017;61(4):110.

CHAPTER 31

PULMONARY COMPLICATIONS

Annmarie Toma, MD, Brittany Reardon, MD, Alison Krishna, MD

ASPIRATION

1. **What is aspiration?**

   Aspiration is the passage of material from the pharynx into the trachea. Aspirated material can originate from the stomach, esophagus, mouth, or nose. The materials involved can be particulate matter (e.g., food), a foreign body, fluid (e.g., blood, saliva) or gastrointestinal contents. Aspiration can cause a pneumonitis or a pneumonia, with the former occurring most often as a complication on induction of anesthesia.

2. **What differentiates aspiration pneumonitis from aspiration pneumonia?**

   The primary pathophysiology of aspiration pneumonitis is *acute inflammation* because of chemical irritation of the tracheobronchial tree, caused by sterile, acidic, gastric contents containing digestive enzymes and bile acids. Aspiration pneumonia, however, is primarily *infectious* because of aspiration of bacteria in patients who are frail, elderly, and/or immunocompromised, and is associated with poor dentition and dysphagia. A key differentiating factor between aspiration pneumonitis and aspiration pneumonia is the acidity and source of the vomitus. Aspiration of acidic gastric contents not only irritates the tracheobronchial tree directly, but also activates digestive enzymes (i.e., pepsinogen), which may contribute to aspiration pneumonitis. The source of the vomitus in aspiration pneumonitis is the stomach, whereas aspiration pneumonia is often caused by bacteria from the oropharynx. Aspiration pneumonia, however, can be caused by the aspiration of gastric contents particularly if patients are on proton-pump inhibitors or histamine-2 (H2) antagonist, which increases the gastric pH, leading to gastric colonization of bacteria. The presentation of aspiration pneumonitis is more acute than aspiration pneumonia and is more commonly associated with anesthesia.

3. **How is aspiration pneumonitis and aspiration pneumonia treated?**

   Aspiration pneumonitis is treated with supportive care and aspiration pneumonia with antibiotics. It is important to note that there is a degree of overlap between aspiration pneumonia and aspiration pneumonitis, and some patients with aspiration pneumonitis can develop a pneumonia.

4. **What is Mendelson syndrome?**

   Mendelson syndrome was the first description of aspiration pneumonitis in the literature. An obstetrician named Curtis Mendelson described this syndrome as dyspnea, cyanosis, and tachycardia in obstetric patients who had aspirated while receiving general anesthesia. He also described the immediate complications of aspiration pneumonitis as asthma-like (bronchospasm, wheezing, hypercapnia, etc.), which occurred if the gastric contents were acidic, whereas if the aspiration volume was large and not acidic, the respiratory pathology was caused by obstruction of the airways leading to atelectasis and hypoxemia. He distinguished the pathology of aspiration pneumonitis as irritative as opposed to aspiration pneumonia, which is infectious. This landmark paper shaped our current preoperative fasting guidelines to reduce gastric volumes and improved our anesthetic techniques for patients at risk for aspiration, such as giving preoperative medications to neutralize gastric pH and performing rapid sequence induction and intubation (also known as rapid sequence induction [RSI]).

5. **What are the specific risk factors for a vomitus to cause aspiration pneumonitis?**

   The two primary risk factors for the development of aspiration pneumonitis are the following:
   1) pH of gastric contents under 2.5
   2) Gastric volumes over 25 mL

   Aspiration of gastric contents containing small volumes (<25 mL) and low acidity (pH > 2.5) are less likely to cause clinically significant aspiration pneumonitis.

6. **How often does aspiration occur with anesthesia, and what is the morbidity and mortality rate?**

   The incidence of significant aspiration is 1 per 10,000 anesthetics. Studies of anesthetics in children demonstrate about twice that occurrence. The average hospital stay after aspiration is 21 days, much of which may be in intensive care. Complications range from bronchospasm, pneumonia, and acute respiratory distress syndrome (ARDS), lung abscess, and empyema. The average mortality rate is 5%.

7. **What are risk factors for aspiration with anesthesia?**

   It is important to emphasize that aspiration risk is not binary and that a continuum exists between low and high risk. Risk factors for aspiration include the following:
   • Extremes of age
   • Emergency operations

- Type of surgery (most common in cases of esophageal, upper abdominal, or emergent laparotomy operations)
- Recent meal
- Delayed gastric emptying (narcotics, diabetes, trauma, pain, intraabdominal infections, and end-stage renal disease)
- Gastroesophageal reflux disease (GERD; decreased lower esophageal sphincter tone, hiatal hernia)
- Trauma
- Pregnancy
- Depressed level of consciousness (i.e., Glasgow Coma Scale < 8)
- Morbid obesity (higher incidence of hiatal hernia)
- Difficult airway
- Neuromuscular disease (impaired ability to protect their airway)
- Esophageal disease (e.g., scleroderma, achalasia, diverticulum, Zenker diverticulum, prior esophagectomy/gastrectomy)

8. **What precautions can be undertaken before anesthetic induction to prevent aspiration or mitigate its sequelae?**
The main precaution is to recognize which patients are at risk. Patients having elective surgical procedures should be fasted per American Society of Anesthesiologists guidelines. Before anesthetic induction, oral nonparticulate antacids, such as sodium citrate can be administered to patients at risk for aspiration (e.g., severe uncontrolled GERD). This functions to raise the gastric pH and lessen the severity of the pneumonitis if aspiration were to occur. H2-receptor antagonists (e.g., cimetidine, ranitidine, and famotidine) can be used to raise the gastric pH as well, but must be administered approximately 30 to 60 minutes before induction of anesthesia to be effective. The use of proton-pump inhibitors in place of, or in concert with, H2 antagonists has not proven to be more efficacious. The use of orogastric or nasogastric drainage before induction is most effective in patients with intestinal obstruction. In situ nasogastric tubes should be suctioned before induction in this patient population.

9. **How should anesthesia be induced in patients at risk for aspiration?**
RSI and intubation is the gold standard in rapidly securing an airway in patients at risk of aspiration. This process involves administering rapid acting neuromuscular blocking agents, cricoid pressure, and the avoidance of mask ventilation. Discussions on the efficacy and potential hazards of cricoid pressure continue, but to date it continues to be recommended for RSI and intubation. A regional anesthetic with little to no sedation is a potential alternative in patients at risk of aspiration, such as obstetric patients undergoing a cesarean section with a spinal anesthetic. Patients with difficult airways may require an awake intubation; however, overly sedating or topicalization of the patient's airway with local anesthetic may compromise the patient's ability to protect their airway. Therefore patients at risk for aspiration undergoing an awake intubation should remain awake with little to no sedation given and topical local anesthetic should only be applied above the glottis to preserve airway reflects below this anatomic level.

10. **Review the clinical signs and symptoms after aspiration.**
Fever occurs in over 90% of aspiration cases, with tachypnea and rales in at least 70%. Cough, cyanosis, and wheezing occur in 30% to 40% of cases. Aspiration may occur silently—without the anesthesiologist's knowledge—during anesthesia. Any of the previous clinical deviations from the expected course may signal an aspiration event. Radiographic changes may take hours to occur and may be negative, especially if radiographic images are taken soon after an event.

11. **When is a patient suspected of aspiration believed to be out of danger?**
The patient who shows none of the previously mentioned signs or symptoms and has no increased oxygen requirement at the end of 2 hours is likely to recover completely.

12. **Describe the treatment for aspiration.**
Immediate suctioning should be instituted through the endotracheal tube, immediately after intubation, before the initiation of positive pressure ventilation. Any patient who is thought to have aspirated should receive a chest radiograph and, at a minimum, several hours of observation. Supportive care remains the mainstay for aspiration pneumonitis. Supplemental oxygen and ventilatory support should be initiated if respiratory failure is a problem. Patients with respiratory failure often demonstrate atelectasis with alveolar collapse and may respond to noninvasive positive pressure ventilation (continuous positive airway pressure or bilevel positive airway pressure). Patients with particulate aspirate may need bronchoscopy to remove the larger obstructing particulate matter. Antibiotics should not generally be administered unless there is a high likelihood that gram-negative or anaerobic organisms (i.e., bowel obstruction) have been aspirated. However, a worsening clinical course over the following days suggests pneumonia and that a broad-spectrum antibiotic may be indicated. Routine bronchial alveolar lavage of the trachea after aspiration has not been shown to be helpful and may worsen the patient's condition. More aggressive treatments for severe aspiration usually occur in the critical care setting (e.g., prone positioning, lung protection ventilation strategies, bronchoscopy).

KEY POINTS: ASPIRATION

1. There are two types of aspiration: aspiration pneumonitis and aspiration pneumonia. The former is primarily irritative and obstructive in pathology, whereas the latter is primarily infectious.
2. Aspiration pneumonitis is most commonly seen on induction of anesthesia, whereas aspiration pneumonia is more common in patients who are elderly, immunocompromised, have impaired cognition or levels of consciousness, have poor dentition, and have dysphagia.
3. Aspiration risk is not binary, and a continuum exists between low and high risk.
4. Risk factors for aspiration include patients presenting for emergent operations, recent or unknown oral intake, bowel obstruction, conditions associated with delayed gastric emptying (diabetes, opioids, intraabdominal infections, severe pain), uncontrolled GERD, obesity, trauma, pregnancy, and patients who cannot protect their airway.
5. Risk factors for aspiration pneumonitis include large gastric volumes (>25 mL) and acidic gastric contents (pH < 2.5).
6. Patients at elevated aspiration risk may require prophylaxis to decrease the severity of aspiration should it occur (nonparticulate antacids, H2 blockers, etc.). Patients with bowel obstruction should receive gastric decompression with a nasogastric tube before induction of anesthesia.
7. RIS and intubation with cricoid pressure and a fast-acting neuromuscular blocking agent (e.g., succinylcholine) is the gold standard for patients at high risk for aspiration who need to be intubated. Regional anesthesia is also a reasonable option in motivated patients who can tolerate little to no sedation.
8. Treatment for aspiration pneumonitis is supportive, whereas patients with aspiration pneumonia need antibiotics.

LARYNGOSPASM

1. **What is laryngospasm?**
   Laryngospasm is a sudden, sustained closure of the vocal cords caused by a primitive airway reflex meant to prevent aspiration. In the awake state, closure of the vocal cords in response to potential aspiration can be overcome by higher cortical centers, but in light planes of anesthesia (i.e., stage 2), this reflex can be triggered without an opposing force. Oxygenation and ventilation are not possible because of the closed glottis.

2. **What are the potential causes of laryngospasm?**
   Laryngospasm typically occurs during emergence when the patient is in a light plane of anesthesia (i.e., stage 2). Stimulation of the vocal cords by excess secretions, foreign matter, or the endotracheal tube during extubation can trigger this primitive reflex. Patients who smoke, have copious secretions, had a recent upper respiratory tract infection (URI) (i.e., <4–6 weeks), or undergoing upper airway operations (e.g., tonsillectomy) are at higher risk.

3. **What should you do when a patient is in laryngospasm?**
   During a laryngospasm episode, the priority is reopening the closed glottis so that the patient can be ventilated and oxygenated. Continuous positive pressure with a facemask along with jaw thrust and chin lift should be applied. This maneuver is often sufficient to break the laryngospasm. If this is not successful, anesthetic should be deepened and a small bolus of succinylcholine (10–20 mg intravenous [IV]) should be administered. Of note, if laryngospasm occurs during induction of anesthesia before establishment of IV access (more common with pediatric patients), an intramuscular injection of succinylcholine (4–5 mg/kg) should be given. After resolution of laryngospasm, ventilation should be continued with 100% oxygen. The decision to reintubate should be made on a case by case basis and should be considered if oxygenation is borderline, aspiration or pulmonary edema is suspected, or if prolonged ventilatory support is expected.

4. **What are the potential complications associated with laryngospasm?**
   Hypoxia and hypercapnia result from lack of oxygenation and ventilation during laryngospasm but should resolve once the airway is reestablished. Prolonged hypoxia after laryngospasm may be caused by aspiration or negative pressure pulmonary edema.

5. **What is negative pressure pulmonary edema?**
   Negative pressure pulmonary edema is a transudative edema produced by the negative intrathoracic pressure, generated by patient inspiratory effort against a closed glottis (i.e., laryngospasm) or other forms of obstruction (i.e., patient biting down on the endotracheal tube causing it to kink).

6. **Describe the mechanism of negative pressure pulmonary edema? What will be found on the chest x-ray and the arterial blood gas?**
   The pressure gradient between the pulmonary capillaries (positive pressure) and the alveoli ("negative" pressure) increases causing fluid to move down the pressure gradient, from the capillaries into the alveoli. The large negative intrathoracic pressure also enhances venous return to the right heart and pulmonary circulation, increasing the pulmonary capillary pressure and worsening the pulmonary edema. Although invasive monitoring is typically not used for diagnosis, patients will have a normal central venous pressure and pulmonary capillary wedge pressure, as the cause is not cardiogenic. A chest x-ray will show bilateral fluffy pulmonary infiltrates similar to

noncardiogenic (i.e., ARDS) and cardiogenic pulmonary edema. Patients may have pink frothy airway secretions and the arterial blood gas would show a decreased arterial partial oxygen pressure.

7. **The patient is biting on the endotracheal tube on emergence from anesthesia and you are concerned the patient may develop negative pressure pulmonary edema. What can you do?**
The best way to prevent this problem is to always have a bite block in place before emergence; however, sometimes the bite block may get dislodged by the patient. If this were to occur, and the patient is biting on the endotracheal tube, the most common recommended treatment options include deepening the anesthetic and/or administering a short-acting neuromuscular blocking agent. One method that the editor (Ryan Laterza) finds helpful is to immediately deflate the cuff of the endotracheal tube, as this will allow the patient to breathe around the endotracheal tube, alleviating the obstruction. A small bolus of an IV amnestic agent (e.g., propofol) can then be given, the endotracheal cuff reinflated, and the bite block replaced.

8. **What is the recommended treatment for negative pressure pulmonary edema?**
Treatment for negative pressure pulmonary edema is supportive. Supplemental oxygen should be provided, as well as positive pressure ventilation if needed. Although furosemide may be considered, it is often not necessary as the etiology is not cardiogenic. The condition often resolves within 24 to 48 hours.

KEY POINTS: LARYNGOSPASM

1. Laryngospasm is an emergent situation caused by a primitive reflex, leading to glottic closure and the inability to ventilate. Patients at risk include those with preexisting reactive airways (i.e., asthma, smoking, and recent URIs) and upper airway operations or procedures associated with increased secretions (e.g., laryngoscopy, tonsillectomy, bronchoscopy).
2. Treatment of laryngospasm is aimed at reestablishing ventilation and includes an escalating algorithm of positive pressure, jaw thrust, deepening of the anesthetic, and succinylcholine.
3. Negative pressure pulmonary edema is a transudative edema that can result from negative intrathoracic pressure during laryngospasm. The condition is generally self-limited and treatment is supportive.

BRONCHOSPASM

1. **What is bronchospasm and how is it recognized in the operating room?**
Bronchospasm is the reversible reflex spasm of the smooth muscle lining the pulmonary bronchioles, causing increased lower airway resistance. It can be recognized under anesthesia as the inability to ventilate a patient with a properly placed endotracheal tube, in the setting of a rapidly increasing peak inspiratory pressures. Physical examination may yield diffuse wheezing. This is typically more common in patients with asthma and usually occurs during airway instrumentation (intubation and extubation) but may occur at any point throughout the anesthetic. Bronchospasm may also be the initial presentation of an anaphylactic or anaphylactoid reaction. Capnography will reveal a typical "shark fin" appearance with loss of the expiratory plateau (Fig. 31.1). Bronchospasm is an intraoperative emergency and prompt recognition and treatment is critical.

2. **How is bronchospasm treated?**
Patients with risk factors (i.e., asthma, chronic obstructive pulmonary disease, recent URI <4–6 weeks) should be treated preoperatively with an inhaled β_2 agonist (i.e., albuterol) before the induction of anesthesia. If bronchospasm occurs intraoperatively, the following sequence of events should take place. The fraction of inspired oxygen should be increased to 100% and the volatile anesthetic should be increased because of their bronchodilator properties and ideally switched to sevoflurane. Next, an attempt to manually ventilate the patient should be undertaken to evaluate pulmonary compliance. Medication treatment includes inhaled β2 agonists via the breathing circuit and consideration for IV magnesium. In severe bronchospasm, small doses (e.g., 10–20 mcg IV) of IV epinephrine should be administered, as inhaled medications may not be effectively delivered to the distal airways. Systemic corticosteroids can be given to decrease airway inflammation and prevent the recurrence of bronchospasm. Consideration should also include changing the ventilator settings to prolong the expiratory time (inspiratory:expiratory ratio set to 1:3 or 1:4) to prevent autopositive end expiratory pressure.

KEY POINTS: BRONCHOSPASM

1. Bronchospasm is the reversible constriction of bronchiolar smooth muscle, which increases airway resistance and impairs alveolar ventilation.
2. Patients with asthma are at a higher risk for bronchospasm, especially during laryngoscopy and intubation.
3. Treatment of bronchospasm includes administering bronchodilator medications, such as inhaled albuterol and, in severe cases, small doses of IV epinephrine.

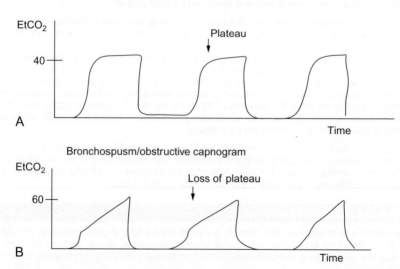

Fig. 31.1 Changes in capnography that can be seen in bronchospasm include a "shark fin" appearance with a loss of the expiratory plateau. This pattern may also be seen in asthma and chronic obstructive pulmonary disease. In severe bronchospasm, the capnography waveform may decrease or even disappear if alveolar ventilation proves impossible. *EtCO₂,* End tidal carbon dioxide.

EXTUBATION

1. **What are the criteria for extubating a patient in the operating room?**
   Extubation of the trachea is a complex process that requires careful thought and consideration before action. Important factors to consider before extubation include the following: (1) Will the patient's airway be difficult to manage with mask ventilation? (2) Was laryngoscopy and intubation difficult? (3) Has the status of the airway changed either secondary to surgery, fluid shifts, or trauma (e.g., multiple laryngoscopy attempts)? Once the decision has been made to proceed with extubation, one must ensure that the patient has met extubation criteria. Extubation criteria include adequate oxygenation, adequate ventilation, hemodynamic stability, full reversal of neuromuscular blockade, appropriate acid-base status and normothermia.

   In other words, the criteria for extubation is essentially the converse for the criteria to intubate. A patient should not be extubated if they are still meeting criteria for intubation: (1) cannot protect their airway, (2) hypercarbic respiratory failure, (3) hypoxemic respiratory failure.

2. **What pharmacological interventions should be considered in a patient who is not meeting extubation criteria or requires immediate reintubation after extubation?**
   Medications given to patients during anesthesia can be a factor in the inability to extubate at the end of surgery. These medications include neuromuscular blocking agents, opioids, and benzodiazepines.

   Residual neuromuscular blockade is one of the most common pharmacological causes of failed extubation. This is because residual neuromuscular blockade may impair a patient's ability to protect their airway, cause hypercarbic respiratory failure, and in severe cases hypoxemic respiratory failure. Reversal of neuromuscular blockade is achieved with neostigmine, which is a competitive antagonist of nondepolarizing neuromuscular blocking agents. In addition, patients may have an adequate minute ventilation, while intubated, but residual blockade may cause relaxation of pharyngeal muscles after the patient is extubated, leading to upper airway obstruction. Residual neuromuscular blockade presents as rapid shallow breathing, weak hand grip/head lift, and worsening hypercarbia after extubation. Additional reversal with neostigmine or with sugammadex should be considered and some patients will need to be reintubated.

   Opioids decrease minute ventilation by causing a small increase in tidal volume but bigger decrease in respiratory rate. A patient that has received excessive opioid will have pinpoint pupils (miosis) and may not initiate breaths on their own. Naloxone is a competitive mu-opioid receptor antagonist used for the reversal of opioid overdose. It can be titrated in small doses (40–80 mcg IV), until the patient begins spontaneous ventilation, while keeping in mind that it will reverse the analgesia as well. Because the half-life of naloxone is shorter than that of most opioids, patients should be carefully monitored in postanesthesia care unit for several hours and the initiation of a naloxone infusion should strongly be considered. Finally, flumazenil can be given to reverse the effects of benzodiazepines with its main side effect being seizures.

3. **What other factors contribute to failed extubation, following emergence of anesthesia?**
Aside from the pharmacological reasons explained earlier there are other considerations for the inability to extubate. During surgery, the status of the airway may change secondary to bleeding, edema, or trauma. Edema most commonly occurs in patients with prolonged prone or Trendelenburg positioning. Airway trauma can be caused by multiple laryngoscopy attempts in difficult airways or because of the surgery itself. Specific surgical operations that can affect the airway include the following: thyroid surgery, laryngoscopy, carotid endarterectomy, and anterior cervical spine surgery.

4. **What is the cuff-leak test?**
Surgical operations near the airway, operations associated with large volume shifts, and iatrogenic airway trauma from multiple laryngoscopy attempts may cause significant airway edema. This can present as upper airway obstruction and hypercarbic respiratory failure, following extubation, but can be avoided with a cuff-leak test. The cuff-leak test involves deflating the cuff on the endotracheal tube before extubation and assessing for leaks. The qualitative method includes listening for a leak around the endotracheal tube with positive pressure ventilation. The quantitative method requires volume-controlled ventilation, where the difference between the measured inspiratory and expiratory volume by the ventilator should be greater than 20% to 30%. Patients who do not have an adequate cuff-leak should not be extubated and transferred to the intensive care unit. Treatment for a negative cuff-leak includes placing the head of bed more than 30 degrees and scheduled steroids (i.e., dexamethasone), until the airway edema resolves.

KEY POINTS: EXTUBATION

1. Before extubation, the anesthesiologist should take into consideration the difficulty in managing the patient's airway, following induction of anesthesia, and other factors that could alter the patient's airway, increasing the odds of a failed extubation and difficult reintubation. This includes airway trauma from multiple laryngoscopy attempts and airway edema from large fluid shifts.
2. Neuromuscular blocking agents and opioids are frequently implicated in patients not meeting extubation criteria or needing to be reintubated. Neuromuscular blocking agents should always be reversed before extubation and opioid overdose can be reversed with naloxone.
3. Patients with significant airway edema (large volume shifts, airway trauma, surgical operations near the airway) should be assessed with a cuff-leak before extubation.

SUGGESTED READINGS

Alalami AA, Ayoub CM, Baraka AS. Laryngospasm: review of different prevention and treatment modalities. Paediatr Anaesth. 2008;18:281–288.

Apfelbaum JL, Caplan RA, Connis RT, et al. Practice guidelines for preoperative fasting and the use of pharmacologic agents to reduce the risk of pulmonary aspiration. Anesthesiology. 2011;114:495–511.

Cohen NH. Is there an optimal treatment for aspiration? In: Fleisher LA, ed. Evidence-Based Practice of Anesthesiology. 2nd ed. Philadelphia: Saunders; 2009:327–335.

Eikermann M, Blonbner M, Groeben H, et al. Postoperative upper airway obstruction after recovery of the train of four ratio of the adductor pollicis muscle from neuromuscular blockade. Anesth Analg. 2006;102:937–942.

Ikari T, Sasaki CT. Laryngospasm: a neurophysiological definition. Ann Otol Rhinol Laryngol. 1980;89:220–224.

Johnson RG, Arozullah AM, Neumayer L, et al. Multivariable predictors of postoperative respiratory failure after general and vascular surgery: results from the patient safety in surgery study. J Am Coll Surg. 2007;204:1188–1198.

Kluger M, Visvanathan T, Myburgh J, et al. Crisis management during anesthesia: regurgitation, vomiting and aspiration. Qual Saf Health Care. 2005;14:4–9.

Landsman IS. Mechanisms and treatment of laryngospasm. Int Anesthesiol Clin. 1997;35:67–73.

Neelakanta G, Chikyarapra A. A review of patients with pulmonary aspiration of gastric contents during anesthesia reported to the Departmental Quality Assurance Committee. J Clin Anesth. 2006;18.102–107.

Olsson GL. Bronchospasm during anaesthesia. A computer-aided incidence study of 136,929 patients. Acta Anaesthesiol Scand. 1987;31:244–252.

Olsson GL, Hallen B. Laryngospasm during anaesthesia. A computer-aided incidence study in 136,929 patients. Acta Anaesthesiol Scand. 1984;28:567–575.

Tasch M. What reduces the risk of aspiration? In: Fleisher: LA, ed. Evidence-Based Pactice of Anesthesiology Philadelphia: Saunders; 2004:118–124.

Westhorpe RN, Ludbrook GL, Helps SC. Crisis management during anaesthesia: bronchospasm. BMJ Qual Saf. 2005;14:e7.

White PF, Tufanogullari B, Sacan O, et al. The effect of residual neuromuscular blockade on the speed of reversal with sugammadex. Anesth Analg. 2009;108:846–851.

CHAPTER 32

AWARENESS DURING ANESTHESIA

Aaron Murray, MD

1. **Review the classifications of memory and awareness.**

   Memory can be classified as implicit (unconscious memory) and explicit (conscious memory). Conscious recollection of events, including intraoperative events, would fall under the category of explicit memory. Awareness with recall (AWR) during general anesthesia is referred to as *anesthetic awareness*. Although patients may speak of "remembering" certain things under general anesthesia, recall of specific *intraoperative* events is key to the concept of anesthetic awareness. The 2006 American Society of Anesthesiologists' (ASA) practice advisory for intraoperative awareness excludes dreaming as anesthetic awareness.

2. **What is the incidence of awareness?**

   Various estimates of the incidence of adult awareness exist. Overall incidence is likely on the order of one in 19,000, when large cohorts, such as National Audit Project 5 are examined. Similar studies are consistent and have reported ranges of 1:15,000 to 1:23,000. Incidence of awareness can increase, depending on the anesthetic technique or subspecialty setting. Increased incidence occurs in higher risk populations, such as obstetric, urgent/emergent surgery, and cardiothoracic cases, and is often related to depth of anesthesia. Patient characteristics, such as female gender, younger adult age, obesity, and prior awareness under anesthesia are also risk factors.

3. **Are certain techniques and clinical situations more likely to result in awareness?**

   Recognized risk factors for AWR include:
   - Light levels of anesthesia (common in hypovolemic, obstetric, and trauma patients)
   - Prior history of intraoperative awareness
   - Cardiac surgery with cardiopulmonary bypass that has historically relied on narcotic-based anesthesia which, while minimizing myocardial depression, produces unreliable amnesia
   - Use of muscle relaxants has repeatedly been shown as an independent risk factor
   - Malfunction of anesthetic administration: machine failure (e.g., empty vaporizer), intravenous (IV) anesthetic pump failure (e.g., no power, incorrect programming), infiltrated IVs, syringe swaps, and so on.
   - Unrecognized increased anesthetic requirements, such as in patients with chronic substance abuse

4. **Describe the clinical signs and symptoms of insufficient anesthesia.**

   Motor responses and sympathetic activation can indicate light levels of anesthesia. Increased respiratory effort, accessory muscle use, swallowing, grimacing, and extremity motion are all signs of insufficient anesthesia. Use of neuromuscular blockade eliminates the information that motor signs can provide regarding anesthetic depth. Sympathetic effects of light anesthesia include hypertension, tachycardia, mydriasis, tearing, and sweating. Such findings are nonspecific; thus their absence or presence may be unreliable indicators of AWR. Indeed, concomitant medications, such as β blockers and sympathetic blockade, may diminish changes in heart rate and blood pressure.

5. **What are the ramifications of AWR?**

   AWR is closely associated with patient dissatisfaction. The potential to hear operating personnel and experience weakness, paralysis, or pain can result in subsequent anxiety, a sense of helplessness, and sleep disturbances. Posttraumatic stress disorder is a common sequela that may occur in 33% to 70% of patients who experience AWR.

6. **How should a patient who may have been aware during a prior anesthetic be approached?**

   Patients may volunteer information regarding prior AWR or seem angry or sad during the perioperative interview, without a clear reason. This should prompt a more structured inquiry using open-ended questions, such as "what is the last thing you remember during your previous anesthetic?" Detailed documentation is indicated once a case has been identified. Listen to and acknowledge the patient's recollections, offer consolation, and explain the likely circumstances surrounding the situation (cardiovascular instability, trauma, etc.). Reassure the patient and offer psychological support. Notify the surgeons, nursing staff, and hospital legal counsel. The ASA Task Force on Intraoperative Awareness notes that not all patients need to be notified regarding the risk of AWR, but for high-risk patients, informed consent should include discussing the increased risk of AWR.

7. **Are there strategies to decrease the incidence of AWR?**

   Premedication with amnestic drugs, such as benzodiazepines or scopolamine, can potentially reduce the likelihood of AWR, especially in higher risk clinical situations and patient populations. Administer appropriate doses of induction agents and supplement with amnestic medications, especially if airway management is difficult or prolonged. Avoid muscle relaxants during maintenance of anesthesia if possible. Supplement nitrous-narcotic techniques with volatile anesthetics. Maintain proper functioning of anesthesia machines and ensure function of IV delivery equipment. Consider neurophysiological monitoring.

8. **Are there monitors available to assess depth of anesthesia?**
Brain electrical activity monitoring can be used to assess depth of anesthesia and includes two commonly used modalities: processed electroencephalogram (pEEG) (as opposed to multichannel EEG) and evoked responses (e.g., auditory). No single monitor can provide a definitive answer to the question of awareness and anesthetic depth. *Proprietary* pEEG technology has entered the operating room from a number of manufacturers and is the dominant technique of monitoring for awareness in this setting.

9. **How does pEEG work? What are the target levels?**
Raw EEG data, collected by electrodes placed on the forehead and temporal regions, are analyzed by microprocessors to create a dimensionless numeric representation of the degree of cortical activity, and thus serves as an indicator of anesthetic depth. Lower numbers correspond to greater anesthetic depth. One common format is the bispectral index (BIS). A BIS goal of 40 to 60 usually indicates adequate anesthetic depth. The ASA Task Force suggests that brain electrical activity monitoring is not routinely indicated but can be considered on an individualized basis for selected patients who are at high risk.

10. **Can end-tidal volatile agent monitoring be used instead of pEEG?**
Targeting end-tidal anesthetic concentration (ETAC) of 0.7 to 1.3 minimal alveolar concentration (MAC) has been shown to be an appropriate goal. The BAG-Recall and the Michigan Awareness Control Study (MACS) trials both compared large numbers of patients randomized to compare AWR with either a BIS pEEG protocol or an ETAC protocol. Neither was able to prove BIS superiority over ETAC, in reducing AWR.

11. **Should pEEG or ETAC be used to monitor for patient awareness?**
Several large studies have compared ETAC with pEEG for reducing AWR, and a trend has emerged. Most studies using volatile anesthesia have not shown any superiority for pEEG monitoring. There does appear to be an exception to this finding. Secondary posthoc analysis of three trials (MACS, B-AWARE, and Zhang et al.) showed reduction of AWR in patients receiving total IV anesthesia (TIVA). These trials strongly suggest that when TIVA is used, pEEG monitoring can reduce the incidence of AWR, whereas an ETAC protocol is sufficient when volatile anesthetics are the primary anesthesia.

KEY POINTS: AWARENESS DURING ANESTHESIA

1. Awareness is most likely to occur in cases where minimal anesthetic is administered, such as during cardiopulmonary bypass, when patients are hemodynamically unstable, during trauma, and in obstetrics.
2. Symptoms of awareness can be nonspecific, and the use of neuromuscular blockade increases the risk of unrecognized awareness.
3. The small risk of awareness should be discussed during consent if patients are deemed at higher risk.
4. Proprietary processed EEG technology can reduce awareness with recall during TIVA, whereas ETAC monitoring is sufficient during cases predominated by volatile anesthesia.

Website
American Society of Anesthesiologists: Awareness and Anesthesia Patient Education: https://www.asahq.org/~/media/sites/asahq/files/public/resources/patient-brochures/asa_awareness-anesthesia_final.pdf?la=en

Suggested Readings
ASA Task Force on Intraoperative Awareness. Practice advisory for intraoperative awareness and brain function monitoring. Anesthesiology. 2006;104:847–864.
Avidan MS, Jacobson E, Glick D, et al. Prevention of intraoperative awareness in a high risk surgical population. N Engl J Med. 2011;365:591–600.
Avidan MS, Mashour GA. Prevention of intraoperative awareness with explicit recall: making sense of the evidence. Anesthesiology. 2013;118:449–456.
Mashour GA, Orser BA, Avidan MS. Intraoperative awareness: from neurobiology to clinical practice. Anesthesiology. 2011;114:1218–1233.
Osterman JE, Hopper J, Heran W, et al. Awareness under anesthesia and the development of post-traumatic stress disorder. Gen Hosp Psychiatry. 2001;23:198–204.
Pandit JJ, et al. 5th National Audit Project (NAP5) on accidental awareness during general anaesthesia: summary of main findings and risk factors. Br J Anaesth. 2014;113:549–559.
Rampersad SE, Mulroy MF. A case of awareness despite an "adequate depth of anesthesia" as indicated by a bispectral index monitor. Anesth Analg. 2005;100:1363–1364.
Zhang C, Xu L, Ma YQ, et al. Bispectral index monitoring prevents awareness during total intravenous anesthesia: a prospective, randomized, double blinded, multicenter controlled trial. Chin Med J. 2011;124:3664–3669.

CHAPTER 33

TEMPERATURE DISTURBANCES

Abimbola Onayemi, MSc, MD, Justin N. Lipper, MD

1. **What is normal core body temperature? What is the definition of hypothermia and hyperthermia?**
   Normal core body temperature is approximately 37°C. Core body temperature is not constant and fluctuates throughout the day (± 0.5°C), with circadian rhythm, and in women with menstrual cycle. Hypothermia is defined as a core temperature less than 36°C and hyperthermia as a core temperature greater than 38°C.

2. **Should all patients under anesthesia receive continuous temperature monitoring?**
   The American Society of Anesthesiologists' Standards for Basic Anesthetic Monitoring state: "Every patient receiving anesthesia shall have temperature monitored when *clinically significant changes* in body temperature are intended, anticipated, or suspected."

   In practice, operations lasting less than 30 minutes often do not require continuous temperature monitoring, whereas operations lasting greater than 30 to 60 minutes should have continuous temperature monitoring.

3. **What sites can be used to measure core body temperature?**
   - Distal esophagus
   - Nasopharynx
   - Tympanic membrane
   - Pulmonary artery

4. **Fundamentally, what causes hypothermia?**
   Hypothermia occurs whenever heat loss exceeds heat production. Inhalational and intravenous anesthetic agents cause hypothermia because of increased heat loss (e.g., peripheral vasodilation) and decreased heat production (e.g., impaired shivering).

5. **Characterize the different stages of hypothermia in a patient not under anesthesia.**
   - **Mild hypothermia** (32°C–36°C) is associated with mild central nervous system depression, decreased basal metabolic rate, tachycardia, peripheral vasoconstriction, and shivering.
   - **Moderate hypothermia** (28°C–32°C) is associated with impaired consciousness, decreased motor activity, dysrhythmias, and cold diuresis. Patients may stop shivering with moderate and severe hypothermia.
   - **Severe hypothermia** (<28°C) is associated with coma, areflexia, and significantly depressed vital signs. Left untreated, profound hypothermia leads to cardiac arrest.

   See Table 33.1 for an overview of systemic effects resulting from hypothermia.

6. **What problems can be seen with mild intraoperative hypothermia?**
   - **Surgical site infections**. Hypothermia causes vasoconstriction, which decreases blood flow and hence oxygen and antibiotic delivery to the wound. This is particularly true following emergence of anesthesia in the postoperative care unit, as patients under general anesthesia are vasodilated. Hypothermia also has a direct immunosuppressant effect on neutrophils, whereas the corollary is true that fever or hyperthermia activates neutrophils.
   - **Coagulopathy**. Hypothermia reduces platelet function and impairs clotting factor enzyme activity. Hypothermia is associated with increased blood loss and transfusion requirements.
   - **Adverse cardiac events**. Hypothermia itself can cause dysrhythmias and increases the risk of demand ischemia because of hemorrhage and hypotension. Furthermore, shivering and increased systemic vascular resistance following the emergence of anesthesia can precipitate demand ischemia. Shivering increases oxygen consumption, causing a compensatory increased cardiac output and peripheral vasoconstriction increases afterload.
   - **Decreased drug metabolism.** This is most concerning with prolonging neuromuscular blocking agents, causing residual postoperative weakness. Furthermore, hypothermia can impair consciousness and cause delayed emergence.

7. **Which patients are at risk for hypothermia?**
   Although all patients under general anesthesia are at risk for developing hypothermia, some specific patient populations carry a greater risk. One example are patients of extreme age. Elderly patients have reduced autonomic vascular control and newborns have a large surface area-to-body mass ratio. Two other groups with increased risk are patients with burns and spinal cord injuries secondary to autonomic dysfunction.

Table 33.1 The Effects of Hypothermia on Organ Systems

SYSTEM	EFFECTS
Vascular	Increases systemic vascular resistance and peripheral hypoperfusion; plasma volume decreases because of cold diuresis
Cardiac	Decreases heart rate, contractility, and cardiac output; dysrhythmias
Pulmonary	Increases pulmonary vascular resistance; decreases hypoxic pulmonary vasoconstriction; increases ventilation-perfusion mismatching; depresses ventilatory drive; oxyhemoglobin dissociation curve shifts to the left
Renal	Decreases renal blood flow and glomerular filtration rate; impaired sodium resorption and diuresis, leading to hypovolemia
Hepatic	Decreases hepatic blood flow, metabolic and excretory functions
Central nervous system	Altered mental status, lethargy, or coma; decreases cerebral blood flow; increases cerebral vascular resistance; decreases cerebral oxygen consumption by 7%/°C; increases evoked potential latencies; decreases minimum alveolar concentration
Hematological	Decreased platelet aggregation and clotting factor activity; increased blood viscosity, impaired immune response
Metabolic	Basal metabolic rate decreases; hyperglycemia; decreased oxygen consumption and CO_2 production
Wound healing	Increased wound infections

8. Which physical processes contribute to a patient's heat loss in the operating room?
   - **Radiation:** The dissipation of energy as an electromagnetic wave caused by molecular vibration. Temperature is fundamentally a measurement of kinetic energy because of molecular movement or vibration (rapid acceleration and deacceleration). Recall, all atoms generate positive and negative electric forces and any acceleration or movement of these fields caused by molecular vibration will induce a self-propagating electromagnetic wave. Electromagnetic radiation accounts for about 60% of a patient's heat loss.
   - **Evaporation:** The energy required to vaporize liquid to gas from any surface, be it skin, serosa, or mucous membranes; accounts for 20% of heat loss. It is a function of exposed body surface area and the relative humidity.
   - **Convection:** The human body is normally surrounded by a warm "shield" of insulating air that helps maintain temperature. However, molecules with more kinetic energy (hot matter) will rise or diffuse away, whereas molecules with less kinetic energy (cold matter) will sink and replace the molecules with higher kinetic energy. This accounts for about 15% of heat loss, which can be exacerbated by high airflow over exposed surfaces (i.e., fan circulating room air over skin).
   - **Conduction:** The transfer of heat between matter; accounts for about 5% of the total heat loss and is a function of the temperature gradient, thermal conductivity, and surface contact between adjacent matter.

9. What specific factors cause hypothermia with general anesthesia?
   The initial drop of core body temperature during the first hour after induction of anesthesia is mainly because of redistribution of heat from core to periphery. The core body temperature is normally 2°C to 4°C warmer than the periphery at baseline. General anesthesia blunts thermoregulated peripheral vasoconstriction, causing increased blood flow to the extremities and redistribution of heat from core to periphery (Fig. 33.1).
   In summary, several factors can cause hypothermia in the operating room and include the following:
   - Blunted shivering response to hypothermia
   - Blunted peripheral thermoregulated vasoconstriction
   - Cool operating rooms
   - Room temperature intravenous fluids
   - Large surgical exposure to the environment (e.g., laparotomy)
   - Respiratory tract (e.g., unheated delivered breaths from the ventilator)

10. Does regional anesthesia cause hypothermia?
    Yes, regional anesthesia (e.g., epidural or spinal anesthesia) blunts afferent temperature sensory nerves, blunts efferent motor nerves responsible for shivering, and causes vasodilation promoting heat loss.

11. Describe the electrocardiographic manifestations of hypothermia.
    Mild hypothermia (32°C–36°C) is often associated with normal sinus rhythm or sinus tachycardia. Moderate hypothermia (28°C–32°C) can result in sinus bradycardia and a J wave (formerly called *Osborn wave*), which is a

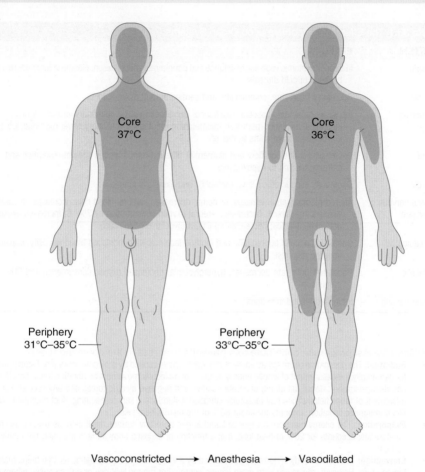

Vascoconstricted $\longrightarrow$ Anesthesia $\longrightarrow$ Vasodilated

Fig. 33.1 Normally, the core temperature is 2°C to 4°C warmer than the periphery because of thermoregulated peripheral vasoconstriction. General anesthesia (and regional anesthesia) blunts this response, causing peripheral vasodilation and a redistribution of heat from core to periphery. (From Sessler D. Temperature regulation and monitoring. In: Miller RD, ed. Miller's Anesthesia. 8th ed. Philadelphia: Elsevier Saunders; 2015:1628.)

positive deflection between the QRS complex and the ST segment. Severe hypothermia (<28°C) can cause premature ventricular contractions, atrioventricular blocks, and spontaneous atrial or ventricular fibrillation.

12. **What is unique about managing cardiac arrest in a patient with severe hypothermia?**
    Atrial fibrillation, ventricular fibrillation, and severe bradycardia below 30°C is relatively unresponsive to atropine, epinephrine, defibrillation, or pacing. Resuscitation (i.e., chest compressions, extracorporeal membrane oxygenation, cardiopulmonary bypass) should continue until the patient is rewarmed (e.g., >32°C) before terminating the code. A common school of thought is "Nobody is dead until they are warm and dead."

13. **How does hypothermia affect the actions and metabolism of drugs used in the operative environment?**
    Both metabolism and clearance of medications are decreased in hypothermia because of the decrease in blood flow to the liver and kidneys, causing a prolonged duration of action. The minimum alveolar concentration of inhalational agents is decreased by about 5% to 7% per degree centigrade decrease in core temperature. In terms of neuromuscular blockade, hypothermia may prolong the duration of action of these agents. Hypothermia can delay discharge from the postanesthetic care unit because of the prolonged effects of residual neuromuscular blocking agents and increased time of rewarming (i.e., takes approximately 1 hour to increase core body temperature by 1°C).

14. **Discuss methods of rewarming.**
    - **Passive rewarming** uses the body's ability to generate heat, provided continued heat loss is minimized by covering exposed areas

- **Active rewarming** is readily performed in the operating room and includes increasing the ambient room temperature, administering warm intravenous fluids, and using force-air warming devices. Of these modalities, forced-air warming devices are most often used and are superior to circulating water blankets. Their effect is maximal when a large surface area is exposed to active rewarming. Administration of warm inspired gases have no utility as the heat content of gases is minimal. The practice has been discontinued.

15. Review shivering and nonshivering thermogenesis.

Shivering is the spontaneous, asynchronous, random contraction of skeletal muscles that increases basal metabolic rate and releases energy. Shivering is modulated through the hypothalamus and can increase the body's production of heat by up to 300% in young, muscular individuals. It increases oxygen consumption and carbon dioxide production and can place high demands on cardiac function, which is undesirable in patients with coronary artery disease.

Infants younger than 3 to 6 months of age cannot shiver and mount a caloric response by nonshivering thermogenesis, which increases metabolic heat production, without producing mechanical work. Brown fat is the major energy source for this process.

16. How can shivering be treated following emergence from anesthesia?

All opioids reduce the shivering threshold and contribute to hypothermia. Meperidine is an opioid that is particularly efficacious in lowering the shivering threshold and is the first-choice opioid to treat shivering. It is important to emphasize that using opioids to treat shivering is only treating symptoms and can delay rewarming. Primary treatment for clinically significant hypothermia should also include actively rewarming the patient with forced-air devices.

17. Describe the manifestations of hyperthermia.

Hyperthermia is a hypermetabolic state associated with increased oxygen consumption, increased minute ventilation, sweating, tachycardia, and vasodilation. An awake patient may experience general malaise, nausea, and light-headedness. With prolonged hyperthermia, the patient may develop heat exhaustion or heat stroke. In the anesthetized patient, signs and symptoms include tachycardia, hypertension, increased end-tidal carbon dioxide, increased drug metabolism, rhabdomyolysis, oliguria, and hypovolemia. Heart rate generally increases by 10 bpm per degree centigrade increase in temperature.

18. What conditions are associated with hyperthermia?

- Malignant hyperthermia
- Hypermetabolic states, including sepsis, thyrotoxicosis, and pheochromocytoma
- Hypothalamic lesions secondary to trauma, anoxia, or tumor
- Neuroleptic malignant syndrome and serotonin syndrome
- Transfusion reaction
- Medications

19. What drugs increase the risk of hyperthermia?

Sympathomimetic drugs, cocaine, amphetamines, tricyclic antidepressants, typical antipsychotic medications, selective serotonin reuptake inhibitors including the recreational drug ecstasy (MDMA) can increase basal energy production and cause hyperthermia. Anticholinergic medications and antihistamines may also elevate temperature by suppressing sweating.

20. What are the pharmacological effects of hyperthermia?

Increases in basal metabolic rate and hepatic metabolism decrease the half-life of anesthetic drugs. Anesthetic requirements may be increased.

21. What is the treatment for hyperthermia in the operating room?

Expose skin surfaces, use cooling blankets, and administer cold intravenous fluids. Correctable causes of hyperpyrexia should be evaluated and treated. For example, administer dantrolene for malignant hyperthermia or neuroleptic malignant syndrome and cyproheptadine for serotonin syndrome.

KEY POINTS: TEMPERATURE DISTURBANCES

1. Normal body temperature is 37°C, hypothermia is less than 36°C, and hyperthermia is greater than 38°C.
2. Heat is fundamentally transferred from one source to another by radiation, convection, conduction, and evaporation.
3. Hypothermia is an extremely common problem in the operating room. Even mild hypothermia has a negative influence on patient outcomes, by increasing wound infection rates, increasing blood loss, and cardiac adverse events.
4. Hypothermia prolongs the duration of action of neuromuscular blocking agents and can increase the risk of postoperative residual weakness.
5. Mild hypothermia is treated primarily by using forced-air warming blankets. Other options include warming all fluids and blood products.
6. Malignant hyperthermia is the most concerning life-threatening cause for hyperthermia in the perioperative domain and should be treated with dantrolene.

Suggested Readings

American Society of Anesthesiologists. Standards for Basic Anesthetic Monitoring. 2015. Retrieved from https://www.asahq.org/standards-and-guidelines/standards-for-basic-anesthetic-monitoring.

Bindu B, Bindra A, Rath G. Temperature management under general anesthesia: compulsion or option. J Anaesthesiol Clin Pharmacol. 2017;33(3):306–316.

Sessler D. Temperature regulation and monitoring. In: Miller RD, ed. Miller's Anesthesia. 8th ed. Philadelphia: Elsevier Saunders; 2015: 1622–1646.

CHAPTER 34

POST-ANESTHETIC CARE

David Abts, MD

1. **Which patients should be cared for in the postanesthetic care unit?**
   According to American Society of Anesthesiologists standards, all patients who have received an anesthetic of any kind shall receive postanesthetic management of some kind. Postanesthetic care unit (PACU) care is traditionally divided into phase 1, which is functionally analogous to an intensive care unit, and phase 2, wherein transition is made from intensive observation to preparation for care on a surgical ward or at home.

   Fast-track recovery is emerging because of fast-offset anesthetic agents and adjunctive drugs. Most patients who have sedation and/or extremity regional anesthesia should be appropriate for fast-track recovery, in which phase 1 care is bypassed. Coexisting disease, the surgical procedure, and pharmacological implications of the anesthetic agents used, ultimately determine the most appropriate sequence of postoperative care for each patient.

2. **Review the important considerations for the immediate postanesthetic phase of care.**
   Transport from the operating room (OR) to the PACU can be a dangerous time for patients. Anesthetics conducted remote from the PACU (e.g., radiology) are also a site of potential instability. For this reason, it is standard practice for patients to be transported by a member of the anesthesia care team who has knowledge of the patient and can continuously assess their condition. Before transport to the PACU from remote locations, a patient should have oxygen administered, and be able to maintain a patent airway with spontaneous respirations. The use of supplemental oxygen for transport is recommended. Patients with hemodynamic or respiratory instability will require the use of a transport monitor and ventilatory equipment.

3. **Describe the process for PACU admission**
   A report is given by the anesthesia caregiver to the PACU nurse, reviewing the patient's prior health status, surgical procedure, intraoperative events, agents used, and anesthetic course.

   The use of muscle relaxants and their reversal, interventions for analgesia, and intraoperative fluids, and blood products administered guide PACU care.

   Initial assessment of the patient by the PACU nurse includes vital signs, baseline responsiveness, adequacy of ventilation, and adequacy of analgesia. Various scoring systems have been used to allow numeric scoring of subjective observations as an indicator of progress toward discharge. The Aldrete scoring system (Table 34.1) tracks five observations: activity, respiratory effort, circulation, consciousness, and oxygenation. Scales for each are 0 to 2, and a total score of 8 to 10 indicates readiness to move to the next phase of care. Regression of motor block in the case of regional anesthesia is also an important determinant of readiness for discharge, particularly when discharge home is planned.

4. **What monitors should be routinely used in the PACU?**
   Pulse oximetry and periodic blood pressure monitoring should be used routinely on all patients. Routine electrocardiogram (ECG) monitoring should be done in most patients. Finally, temperature, urine output, and surgical drainage require monitoring as appropriate.

5. **What problems should be resolved during postanesthetic care?**
   - **Hypoventilation:** The patient should be breathing easily and able to cough on command. Oxygenation status should return to near preanesthetic levels.
   - **Hemodynamic stability:** Blood pressure should be within 20% of preanesthetic measurements, with a stable heart rate and rhythm.
   - **Attenuated sensorium:** The patient should be fully awake and voluntarily move all extremities.
   - **Postoperative pain:** Pain management should no longer require continuous nursing intervention.
   - **Postoperative nausea and vomiting (PONV):** PONV should be treated aggressively, because it is associated with prolonged length of stay in the PACU and decreased patient satisfaction with the perioperative experience.

6. **Describe the appearance of a patient with residual neuromuscular blockade.**
   Residual neuromuscular blockade (NMB), opioid effects, and lingering effects of inhalational anesthesia all can result in postoperative hypoventilation (Table 34.2). Patients with residual NMB are frequently described as appearing floppy, exhibiting poorly coordinated and ineffective respiratory muscle activity. The patient may complain that breathing is restricted and efforts to deliver supplemental oxygen are suffocating. Oftentimes, they are unable to sustain a head lift or hand grasp. In the worst case scenario, weakness of the pharyngeal muscles results in upper airway collapse and airway obstruction. Of note, neither a good response to train-of-four testing in the OR nor spontaneous rhythmic ventilation before extubation rules out residual NMB.

Table 34.1 The Aldrete Scoring System

Activity	Able to move four extremities	2
	Able to move two extremities	1
	Not able to move extremities voluntarily or on command	0
Respiration	Able to breathe and cough	2
	Dyspnea or limited breathing	1
	Apneic	0
Circulation	BP ± 20% of preanesthetic level	2
	BP ± 21%–49% of preanesthetic level	1
	BP ± 50% of preanesthetic level	0
Consciousness	Fully awake	2
	Arousable on calling	1
	Not responding	0
O_2 saturation	Maintain O_2 saturation >92% in room air	2
	Needs O_2 to maintain O_2 saturation >90%	1
	O_2 saturation <90% with O_2 supplement	0

BP, Blood pressure.
Modified from Aldrete AJ, Krovlik D. The postanesthetic recovery score. Anesth Analg. 1970;49:924–933.

Table 34.2 Ventilation Problems in the Postanesthetic Care Unit

PROBLEM	SYMPTOMS	TREATMENT
Residual neuromuscular blockade	Uncoordinated, ineffectual respiratory effort	Neostigmine, 0.05 mg/kg IV
Opioid narcosis	Slow ventilation, sedated and difficult to arouse	Respiratory support, naloxone, 0.04–0.4 mg IV
Residual inhalation anesthesia	Sleepy, shallow breathing	Encourage deep breathing

IV, Intravenous.

7. **How do opioids and residual volatile anesthetics affect breathing?**
Slow rhythmic breathing or apneic pauses in a patient who is hard to arouse suggest the presence of residual opioids and/or volatile anesthetics. In contrast to patients with residual NMB, these patients are often unconcerned about ventilation despite obvious hypoxia. In fact, surprising degrees of hypercapnia may be found, even while the pulse oximetry values remain relatively normal. This phenomenon is usually observed when patients are hypoventilating, while receiving supplemental oxygen, thereby enabling their pulse oximetry (SpO_2) values to remain normal (see later).

8. **How should these causes of hypoventilation be treated?**
Hypoventilation resulting from residual NMB should be treated urgently and aggressively. Additional reversal agents may be given in divided doses up to the usual dose limitations. Treatment decisions for residual narcotic may prove to be more problematic. Indicated procedures include continuous stimulation, until spontaneous ventilation improves, placement of an oral/nasal airway to relieve airway obstruction and provide stimulation, or moving patient into a chair. Other supportive measures include increasing inspired oxygen concentrations (FiO_2). However, increasing FiO_2 does not reverse hypoventilation; it only masks it (Table 34.3).

9. **A patient has been delivered to the PACU. Oxygen saturation is noted to be in the upper 80s. How should this patient be managed?**
Fortunately, most hypoxemia in the PACU is caused by atelectasis, which is treated by sitting the patient upright, asking him or her to breathe deeply or cough, and encouraging incentive spirometry. If a patient is obtunded or unarousable, or is in respiratory distress, the following steps should be taken:
- Move to establish a patent airway (chin lift, jaw thrust) and administer supplemental oxygen.
- Suction the patient's airway if needed.

Table 34.3 Predicted FiO_2 With Supplemental Oxygen Delivery

SYSTEM	DELIVERY FLOW (L/min)	FiO_2 PREDICTED
Nasal cannula	2	0.28
Nasal cannula	4	0.36
Facemask	6	0.50
Partial rebreathing mask	6	0.6
Total rebreathing mask	8	0.8

FiO_2, Fractional inspired oxygen concentration.

- Once the airway is patent, observe and auscultate the chest. Is the patient hypoventilating? Reversal of opioid or benzodiazepines may be necessary.
- Does the abdomen distend and the chest retract with inspiration (paradoxical respirations), suggesting airway obstruction or inadequate reversal of NMB.
- Assess the patient's strength by hand grip and sustained head lift. Could there be increased ventilation/perfusion mismatch, or presence of shunt physiology?
- Assess the patient for wheezes or rales. It is possible the patient would benefit from β-agonists if you suspect bronchospasm, or diuresis if pulmonary edema is a potential etiology.
- If stridorous breath sounds are caused by laryngeal edema, administration of nebulized racemic epinephrine and intravenous steroids may be indicated.
- Finally, palpate pulses and listen to the heart because circulatory depression causes oxygen desaturation. Ultimately, the patient may require assisted ventilation or reintubation.

10. **A patient develops stridorous breath sounds upon their arrival to PACU. Describe the likely cause and appropriate management.**
   A common cause of stridorous breath sounds in the early postextubation period is laryngospasm, an upper airway reflex, which normally protects the glottis from foreign matter. Laryngospasm may be precipitated by extubation during light planes of anesthesia, when upper airway reflexes are hyperactive, or blood and/or secretions falling on the vocal cords. If laryngospasm is incomplete, the patient will have stridorous breath sounds. If laryngospasm is complete, little air movement is possible and breath sounds will be absent. Note that other causes of upper airway obstruction (e.g., postextubation croup, expanding hematoma, soft-tissue swelling) should be considered during assessment as well.

11. **How is laryngospasm treated?**
   The treatment for laryngospasm is to support ventilation. Call for an assistant, provide a jaw thrust, and assist the patient's inspiratory efforts with positive-pressure ventilation, using 100% oxygen. If this proves unsatisfactory, administer succinylcholine, 0.15 to 0.30 mg/kg (about 10–20 mg in adults), to relax the vocal cords. If the patient continues to experience difficulty with ventilation, reintubation may be necessary. Once intubation is completed and end-tidal CO_2 has been verified, the patient should receive assisted ventilation. Sedation may also be needed at this point.

12. **Following an episode of laryngospasm, chest auscultation reveals bilateral rales. What is the most likely cause?**
   Although congestive heart failure, fluid overload, adult respiratory distress syndrome, and aspiration of gastric contents need to be considered, negative-pressure pulmonary edema (NPPE) is the most likely cause. NPPE results from the generation of high negative intrapleural pressures when the patient inspires against a closed or obstructed glottis. Whereas intrapleural pressures usually vary between -5 and -10 cm H_2O during a normal respiratory cycle, inspiration against a closed glottis may generate between approximately -50 and -100 cm H_2O pressure. Such pressures increase venous return to the thorax and pulmonary vasculature and increase transcapillary hydrostatic pressure gradients, resulting in pulmonary edema. The onset of edema has been noted from 3 to 150 minutes after the inciting event.
   Some authorities refer to this syndrome as negative-pressure pulmonary injury because pink or frankly bloody pulmonary secretions suggest that some alveolar injury has taken place during attempts to breathe against a closed glottis.

13. **How is NPPE treated?**
   Once the airway obstruction is relieved, treatment is supportive. The pulmonary edema usually resolves between 12 and 24 hours. Continue oxygen therapy; note that continuous positive airway pressure and mechanical ventilation, with positive end-expiratory pressure, may occasionally be needed, depending on the severity of gas exchange impairment. Diuretics should be administered only if the patient has intravascular fluid overload or perhaps in the most severe cases. Lastly, it should be noted that these patients frequently require overnight hospital observation.

14. How are patients with undiagnosed obstructive sleep apnea identified?

The presence of obstructive sleep apnea (OSA) is associated with increased morbidity and mortality in the postoperative period. Occult, undiagnosed OSA is common in the general population. Hence, screening is indicated to identify at-risk patients. Events that manifest postoperatively and suggest the presence of OSA include hypopnea, apnea, oxygen desaturation and pain-sedation mismatch (excessive sedation relative to the patient's level of pain). These events may go undiagnosed and lead to hypoxemia, hypercarbia, and even cardiopulmonary arrest.

A popular preoperative screening tool is the STOP-BANG questionnaire. **S** (snoring: loud enough to wake a partner, or be heard in another room), **T** (tired: daytime drowsiness), **O** (observed: has anyone observed the patient stop breathing while sleeping), **P** (pressure: does the patient have high blood pressure), **B** (BMI: body mass index >35 kg/m^2), **A** (age: age >50 years), **N** (neck size: men >17 inch circumference, women >16 inch circumference), **G** (gender: is the patient a male?). In general, if the patient is a "yes" to more than 5 to 8 questions, then they are considered to be at the highest risk of having undiagnosed OSA. Proper preoperative identification of these patients helps to establish a plan of care that minimizes their risk of adverse events after surgery.

15. Describe an approach to the evaluation of postoperative hypertension and tachycardia.

Frequently observed and readily treatable causes of hypertension and tachycardia in the postoperative period include pain, hypoventilation, hypercarbia, hypothermia with shivering, bladder distention, and essential hypertension. Also consider hypoxemia, hyperthermia and its causes, anemia, hypoglycemia, tachydysrhythmias, withdrawal (e.g., drug and alcohol), myocardial ischemia, prior medications administered, and coexisting disease. In rare cases, this hyperdynamic state may reflect hyperthyroidism, pheochromocytoma, or malignant hyperthermia.

16. What might cause hypotension in the postoperative period?

Prior or ongoing blood loss, third-space sequestration of fluid, and inadequate volume replacement can all manifest as hypotension. In addition, myocardial ischemia or heart failure may present as hypotension, as can sepsis and anaphylaxis.

17. How should it be treated?

Consider the surgical procedure, intraoperative events, medications, and past medical history. Evaluate blood loss and urine output. Review the ECG rhythm strip and consider a 12-lead ECG. Volume expansion with balanced crystalloid solutions is first-line therapy. Elevation of legs and Trendelenburg positioning may help transiently. Circumstances may require administration of colloid or packed red blood cells. Should volume expansion prove inefficacious, vasopressors or inotropes may be necessary, but these suggest the need for more intensive evaluation.

18. Under what circumstances is a patient slow to awaken in the PACU?

A good initial assumption is that such patients are displaying residual drug effects. Should decreased awareness persist beyond a reasonable period of observation, ventilatory, metabolic, and central nervous system (CNS) etiologies must be considered. Does the patient have a seizure history and is the patient currently postictal? Has the patient had documented CNS ischemic events or strokes? Laboratory analysis should include arterial blood gases, as well as measurements of serum sodium and glucose. If these are normal, a computed tomographic scan of the brain may be indicated.

19. Discuss the issues surrounding postoperative nausea and vomiting.

PONV remains a significant, troublesome postanesthetic problem. It results in delayed PACU discharge and occasional unplanned hospital admission and is a recurring cause of patient dissatisfaction. Patients often say that pain is preferable to nausea and vomiting. Procedural risk factors include laparoscopic surgery; surgery on genitalia and breasts; craniotomies; and shoulder, middle ear, or eye muscle procedures. Patient risk factors include female sex, prior PONV or motion sickness history, and school-age children. Anesthetic agents associated with PONV include opioids, volatile inhalation agents, and nitrous oxide. Of note, propofol has the lowest incidence of any of the induction agents and has been used effectively as a rescue medication. Risk assessment should be made on the basis of the aforementioned factors, and prophylactic treatment or alteration of the anesthetic plan should be determined based on evidence of efficacy.

PONV rescue (treatment once PONV has ensued) requires balancing potential benefits with side effects and cost. All patients should receive PONV prophylaxis, and those at highest risk should be identified and treated aggressively.

20. Should ambulatory patients be treated differently in the PACU?

The goal of postanesthetic care of the ambulatory patient is to render the patient street ready. Pain should be treated with nonnarcotic analgesics when possible, and nerve blocks should be used whenever possible. Oral analgesics should be used in phase 2 recovery, as prescribed for postoperative care. After regional anesthesia, extremities should be protected, while the patient is mobilized, and ambulation should be assisted if transient segmental paresthesia makes movement unsteady. No ambulatory surgery patient should be discharged after receiving any sedating medication without a companion to ensure safe transportation to a place of residence.

21. Should patients be required to tolerate oral intake before PACU discharge?

Requiring the ingestion of clear liquids before discharge can increase length of stay in the PACU, and is not recommended for discharge at present. However, patients are instructed that continued oral intake is important for their recovery, and that if they are unable to tolerate food or liquids postoperatively, they should call the nurse line or return to the hospital and/or healthcare facility.

22. A patient has undergone a general anesthetic for an outpatient procedure. Recovery has been uneventful, yet the patient has no ride home. How should this be handled?
Patients should be required to have a responsible party accompany them home after anesthesia. It has been shown to decrease adverse events. The patient in this case should be kept at the healthcare facility, possibly under 24-hour observation, or until a responsible party is available.

23. What is the reasonable minimal PACU stay?
The American Society of Anesthesiologists has no recommendation for the minimal length of stay in the PACU. Length of stay should be determined on a case-by-case basis. A discharge protocol should be designed that allows patients to reach postoperative goals that will direct them toward discharge. Regardless of whether a discharge protocol is in place or not, the anesthesiologist is ultimately responsible for discharge of the patient from the PACU.

KEY POINTS: POSTANESTHETIC CARE AND COMPLICATIONS

1. Postanesthetic care is part of the continuum of perioperative care and the responsibility of the anesthesiologist.
2. Loss of normal respirations and airway obstruction are regular events that result in hypoxemia and require management.
3. Adequate oxygenation, controlled postoperative pain, and resolved PONV are requirements for PACU discharge.
4. Patients with suspected sleep apnea should be managed in the same way as patients with diagnosed sleep apnea. Supplemental oxygen, SpO_2 monitoring, and regular checks are the best standards for treatment.

Website
American Society of Anesthesiologists Standards for Postanesthesia Care: http://www.asahq.org/

SUGGESTED READINGS

An Updated Report by the American Society of Anesthesiologists Task Force on Postanesthetic Care: Practice Guidelines for Postanesthetic care. Anesthesiology. 2013;118:291–307.

Gali B, Whalen FX, Schroeder DR, et al. Identification of patients at risk for postoperative respiratory complications using a preoperative obstructive sleep apnea screening tool and postanesthesia care assessment. Anesthesiology. 2009;110:869–77.

Gan TJ, Meyer T, Apfel CC, et al. Consensus guidelines for managing postoperative nausea and vomiting. Anesth Analg. 2003;96:62–71.

Gross JB, Bachenberg KL, Benumof J, et al. Practice guidelines for the perioperative management of patients with obstructive sleep apnea, Anesthesiology. 2006;104:1081–93. Updated report available at http://www.ncbi.nlm.nih.gov/pubmed/24346178.

CHAPTER 35

CORONARY ARTERY DISEASE AND PERIOPERATIVE MYOCARDIAL INFARCTION

S. Andrew McCullough, MD

1. **What are the known risk factors for the development of coronary artery disease?**
   Age, male gender, and positive family history (first-degree relative with coronary artery disease [CAD], male <55 years or female <65 years) are risk factors that cannot be modified. Smoking, hypertension, diet, dyslipidemia, physical inactivity, obesity, and diabetes mellitus are modifiable risk factors.

2. **Describe the normal coronary blood flow.**
   The resting coronary blood flow (CBF) averages about 225 mL/min, which is 4% to 5% of the total cardiac output (CO) in normal adults. The CBF increases up to four fold to supply the extra nutrients needed by the heart at maximum coronary vasodilation, also known as *hyperemia*. The driving force for CBF is determined by the coronary perfusion pressure (CPP), which is the gradient between the aortic pressure (P_{aorta}) and the ventricular pressure ($P_{ventricle}$). There are phasic changes in CBF to the left ventricle, during systole and diastole. The CBF to the left ventricle significantly decreases in systole as the left ventricular pressure equals or exceeds the pressure in the aorta, causing the CPP to essentially equal zero. It is important to appreciate that in the case of left ventricular outflow obstruction (i.e., hypertrophic cardiomyopathy or aortic stenosis), the left ventricular intracavitary pressure may significantly exceed that of the aortic pressure during systole. In diastole, the cardiac muscle fibers relax, allowing blood to flow through the left ventricular capillaries. Further, the aortic valve closes, which creates a natural pressure gradient between the higher aortic pressure and the lower left ventricular diastolic pressure. This increases the CPP, which is the main driving force for CBF.

3. **What happens to CBF during systole and diastole?**
   The left heart is only perfused during diastole, as the aortic pressure (P_{aorta}) is greater than the ventricular pressure ($P_{ventricle}$). Therefore it is important to avoid tachycardia to maintain coronary perfusion to the left heart. The right heart, however, is perfused during systole and diastole, as the aortic pressures are generally higher than the right ventricular pressure in both systole and diastole.

4. **What is the equation for coronary perfusion pressure?**
   Coronary perfusion pressure (CPP) can be explained by the following equation:

   $$CPP = P_{aorta} - P_{ventricle}$$

   CPP, coronary perfusion pressure; P_{aorta}, aortic pressure; $P_{ventricle}$, intraventricular pressure

   Although this equation is true for the right heart for both systole and diastole, the left heart is only perfused during diastole where the equation can be simplified to the following:

   $$CPP = dBP - LVEDP$$

   CPP, coronary perfusion pressure; dBP, aortic diastolic blood pressure; LVEDP, left ventricular end-diastolic pressure.

5. **Describe the coronary anatomy.**
   The right coronary artery system is dominant in that it supplies blood to the inferior left ventricular wall via the posterior descending artery (PDA) in about 85% of people. The right coronary also supplies the sinoatrial node (SA), atrioventricular (AV) node, and right ventricle. Right-coronary artery occlusion can result in bradycardia, heart block, myocardial infarction (MI) of the right ventricle and/or inferior left ventricular wall.

   The left main coronary artery (LMCA) gives rise to the left circumflex artery (LCx) and the left anterior descending (LAD) artery. The LAD and the PDA provide blood flow to the interventricular septum via septal branches. The LAD supplies the anterior left ventricular wall directly, and the lateral left ventricular wall via diagonal branches. When the circumflex gives rise to the PDA, the circulation is termed *left dominant*, where the left coronary circulation then supplies the entire septum and the AV node. In 40% of patients, the circumflex supplies the SA node. Because the LMCA and the LAD supplant much of the blood flow to the left ventricle, occlusion of these arteries, with resultant ischemia, can result in severely depressed left ventricular function, and in the prognostically worst case, cardiogenic shock.

6. Describe the determinants of myocardial oxygen supply and their relationship.

Oxygen delivery to the myocardium is the product of CBF and the oxygen content of arterial blood (CaO_2):

$$Myocardial\ O_2\ Supply = CBF \times CaO_2$$

Recall, that oxygen content (CaO_2) is determined by the following:

$$CaO_2 = 1.36 \times [Hg] \times SaO_2 + 0.003 \times [PaO_2]$$

CBF is governed with the same relationship as Ohm's law, $I = \triangle V/R$, where "$\triangle V$" represents the coronary perfusion pressure and "I" represents CBF:

$$CBF = (P_{aorta} - P_{ventricle})/CVR$$

P_{aorta}, aortic root pressure; $P_{ventricle}$, ventricular chamber pressure; CVR, coronary vascular resistance

Therefore myocardial oxygen supply can be rewritten as the following:

$$Myocardial\ O_2\ Supply = \frac{P_{aorta} - P_{ventricle}}{CVR}\ CaO_2$$

7. How can you increase myocardial oxygen supply and delivery?

From the earlier equation, the myocardial oxygen supply can be increased by the following:
1) Increase hemoglobin concentration [Hg] by transfusing red blood cells
2) Maintain an oxygen saturation (SaO_2) of 100% with supplemental oxygen
3) Maintain an adequate coronary perfusion pressure ($P_{aorta} - P_{ventricle}$) with vasopressors (i.e., phenylephrine) to increase P_{aorta}
4) Reduce ventricular pressure ($P_{ventricle}$) with diuretics and/or venodilators (e.g., nitroglycerin)
5) Avoid tachycardia as ventricular pressure ($P_{ventricle}$) increases during systole decreasing CBF

8. How can this be used to understand myocardial ischemia? How does this pertain to coronary artery disease, aortic stenosis, and right heart failure caused by a pulmonary embolism?

In referring to the earlier equations for CBF, anything that decreases aortic blood pressure, increases ventricular pressure, increases coronary resistance (e.g., coronary stenosis or thrombosis), or decreases oxygen delivery (e.g., anemia) can cause myocardial ischemia.

In patients with CAD, it is important to avoid tachycardia, as again the left heart is only perfused during diastole. Further, any medical condition associated with an excessively high ventricular filling pressure (e.g., congestive heart failure, end-stage renal disease, aortic stenosis, pulmonary embolism) can decrease coronary perfusion. Recall, if $P_{ventricle}$ increases, then coronary perfusion pressure decreases, where $CPP = P_{aorta} - P_{ventricle}$. Therefore management of patients with these conditions include strategies to optimize coronary perfusion (e.g., diuretics or venodilators to decrease $P_{ventricle}$ or vasopressors to increase P_{aorta}).

9. What are the clinical manifestations of CAD?

Angina pectoris, defined as pressure like retrosternal chest pain radiating to the jaw, arms, or neck during physical exertion that resolves with rest, is the classic manifestation of myocardial ischemia. However, myocardial ischemia may present as ventricular failure or arrhythmias without angina or may remain clinically silent, especially in females or patients with diabetes mellitus. Angina worsens with worsening degree of stenosis, which is often described as reduced exercise tolerance. When patients develop acute chest pain at rest or with exertion, it implies that the patient has developed an acute coronary syndrome, which includes unstable angina, a non-ST elevation myocardial infarction (NSTEMI), or an ST-elevation myocardial infarction (STEMI). These syndromes are distinct from stable CAD because they are related to the rupture of an atherosclerotic plaque, with overlying thrombus formation, resulting in total or subtotal coronary occlusion. No data to date have indicated that revascularizing patients with stable CAD reduces the rate of MI. Similarly, no data to date have revealed that revascularizing patients (including high-risk patients) preoperatively, either with percutaneous coronary intervention or coronary artery bypass grafting (CABG), reduces the rate of perioperative MI.

10. Describe the pathogenesis of a perioperative MI.

A type I MI is caused by atherosclerotic plaque rupture, exposing the thrombotic subendothelium, which results in platelet aggregation, vasoconstriction, and thrombus formation. A type II MI, also known as *demand ischemia*, is caused by oxygen supply-demand mismatch, such as from a sudden increase in myocardial oxygen demand (tachycardia, hypertension) or decrease in oxygen supply (hypotension, hypoxemia, anemia, tachycardia). Complications of MI include atrial and ventricular arrhythmias, hypotension, congestive heart failure, acute mitral regurgitation, pericarditis, ventricular thrombus formation, ventricular rupture, and death.

11. What is the revised cardiac risk index?

The revised cardiac risk index (RCRI) is a well-known, validated screening tool to quickly assess a patient's risk for perioperative cardiac complications (MI, pulmonary edema, ventricular fibrillation or primary cardiac arrest, and complete heart block) and is useful in determining if further testing and medical optimization are necessary before surgery. Patients with an RCRI of 1 or higher (>2 in older studies) have an elevated risk of cardiac complications (Table 35.1).

Table 35.1 Revised Cardiac Risk Index
1. History of ischemic heart disease
2. History of congestive heart failure
3. History of cerebrovascular disease
4. History of diabetes requiring preoperative insulin use
5. History of chronic kidney disease (creatinine >2 mg/dL)
6. Undergoing suprainguinal vascular, intraperitoneal, or intrathoracic surgery

Risk for cardiac death, nonfatal myocardial infarction, and nonfatal cardiac arrest: 0 predictors = 3.9%, 1 predictor = 6%, 2 predictors = 10.1%, ≥3 predictors = 15%.

12. **What surgical operations are at high risk for a cardiac event?**
High-risk operations, per the RCRI, include intraperitoneal, intrathoracic, and suprainguinal vascular operations. Patients undergoing these operations, particularly large, suprainguinal vascular operations, are likely the most at risk in developing a perioperative cardiac complication.

13. **How can you assess a patient's functional or exercise capacity?**
A patient's exercise capacity is often assessed using metabolic equivalents (METs), where one MET equals 3.5 mL/kg/min of oxygen consumption. For example, a 70-kg adult would have an oxygen consumption at rest of approximately 250 mL/min. Note, this concept and these numbers should be memorized; this concept is emphasized in other chapters (i.e., pulmonary physiology) because it pertains to the duration of time a patient can safely undergo apnea. A person is said to have good exercise capacity if their METs are greater than 4, which is the equivalent of stating that the patient's cardiac function has the capacity to delivery 1000 mL/min of oxygen to the body, where 4 METs = 4 × (250 mL/min) of oxygen consumption. The ability to climb two to three flights of stairs without significant symptoms (i.e., angina, dyspnea, syncope) is usually an indication of adequate functional capacity greater than 4 METs. Patients with good exercise capacity (METs >4) are at low risk of perioperative cardiac events. Poor exercise tolerance (METs <4), in the absence of pulmonary or other systemic disease, indicates an inadequate cardiac reserve and elevates the patient's risk category. Patients undergoing high-risk operations should be questioned about their ability to perform daily activities.

14. **When would you consider noninvasive stress testing before noncardiac surgery?**
The guidelines integrate indication (emergency vs. elective), exercise capacity, and the risk of the surgical procedure itself in the decision-making process. Stress testing is not warranted in patients who are undergoing an emergent operation, a low-risk operation (cataract operation, sinus surgery, bunion surgery, etc.), or who have good exercise capacity (METs >4) irrespective of the risk of surgery itself. Only patients undergoing nonemergent, high-risk operations (i.e., large vascular operations), who have poor exercise capacity (i.e., METs <4) need consideration for stress testing.
It is important to understand that stress testing is not performed to identify significant coronary atherosclerosis (as revascularization has no proven benefit), but to identify the functional capacity of a patient who is otherwise sedentary. If one cannot glean a patient's functional capacity from their history alone, or they have a physical functional limitation (e.g., a prior amputation), then stress testing can be considered for high-risk, nonemergent surgical operations.

15. **What is considered an emergent operation per the guidelines?**
The American College of Cardiology (ACC)/American Heart Association (AHA) guidelines define emergency as a "threat to life or limb" if surgery is delayed beyond 6 hours. This is in contrast with time sensitive operations (e.g., oncology operations) versus truly elective operations (e.g., cosmetic operations), where further medical workup and optimization is feasible.

16. **What tests performed by medical consultants can help further evaluate patients with known or suspected CAD?**
Exercise electrocardiogram (ECG) is a noninvasive test that attempts to produce ischemic symptoms by having the patient exercise to maximum capacity. Information obtained relates to the thresholds of heart rate and blood pressure that can be tolerated. Maximal heart rates, blood pressure response, and clinical symptoms guide interpretation of the results. This is usually performed in a sedentary patient who can exercise, but their functional capacity is unknown.
Exercise thallium scintigraphy increases the sensitivity and specificity of the exercise ECG. The isotope thallium is injected at peak exercise, is taken up from the coronary circulation by the myocardium, and can be visualized radiographically. This helps identify an amount of myocardium at risk from coronary atherosclerosis.
Dipyridamole thallium imaging is useful in patients who are unable to exercise. This testing is frequently required in patients with peripheral vascular disease, who are at high risk for CAD, and the exercise test is limited by

claudication or physical impairment. Dipyridamole is a potent coronary vasodilator that causes differential flow between normal and diseased coronary arteries detectable by thallium imaging.

Echocardiography can be used to evaluate left ventricular and valvular function and to measure ejection fraction. Stress echocardiography (dobutamine echo) is similar to the aforementioned stress tests, and is used to identify at-risk myocardium.

Coronary angiography is the gold standard for defining the coronary anatomy. As coronary angiography is invasive, and it is now accepted that preoperative coronary revascularization does not reduce the rate of perioperative MI, its use has fallen out of favor.

17. **What are the main indications for coronary revascularization before noncardiac surgery?**
    - Patients with stable angina who have significant (>50%) left main coronary artery stenosis.
    - Patients with stable angina who have three-vessel disease and reduced left ventricular ejection fraction.
    - Patients with high-risk unstable angina or STEMI.
    - Patients with acute STEMI.
    - Note that coronary revascularization includes CABG or percutaneous coronary intervention (PCI).

18. **A patient who has undergone PCI is scheduled for surgery. What is your concern?**
    After PCI, patients need to be on dual-antiplatelet therapy (aspirin and clopidogrel). Discontinuation of this therapy for surgical procedure poses a high risk for stent thrombosis and MI in the perioperative period. The appropriate timing of surgery is still under investigation, but the following guidelines are accepted:
    - After plain old balloon angioplasty (POBA), nonurgent surgery can be performed with aspirin only after 14 days, but ideally these patients should be on dual-antiplatelet therapy for 4 to 6 weeks.
    - After bare-metal or drug-eluting stent (DES) placement, nonurgent surgery can be performed with aspirin monotherapy after 30 days or more than 365 days, respectively. In newer generation drug eluting stents, dual antiplatelet therapy can be safely stopped early (i.e., 6 months); however, if the stent was placed in the setting of an MI, it is more prudent to wait 1 year.

19. **Why do patients with drug-eluting stents need significantly longer dual-antiplatelet therapy?**
    DES are statistically superior to bare-metal stents for treatment of coronary artery occlusions having lower rates of target vessel revascularization. The drugs (sirolimus, paclitaxel, everolimus, zotarolimus) released from the DES inhibit endothelium surface formation inside the stent and the patient will require long-duration dual-antiplatelet therapy, as there is exposed von Willebrand factor in the coronary vessel and is at risk for thrombosis.

20. **Should all cardiac medications be continued throughout the perioperative period?**
    Patients with a history of CAD are usually taking medications intended to decrease myocardial oxygen demand by decreasing the heart rate, preload, afterload, or contractile state (β-blockers, calcium-channel antagonists, nitrates) and to increase the oxygen supply by causing coronary vasodilation (nitrates). These drugs are generally continued throughout the perioperative period. In addition, lipid-lowering therapy, namely statins, should be continued perioperatively. For patients undergoing vascular surgery, it is reasonable to initiate lipid-lowering therapy with a statin before surgery.

21. **Should preoperative β-blocker therapy be continued into the perioperative period?**
    Yes, patients receiving preoperative β-blocker therapy before surgery should continue their β-blockers into the perioperative period to reduce the incidence of cardiac complications. This contrasts with the initiation of β-blocker therapy on the day of surgery, which has a higher incidence of stroke and death in β-blocker naïve patients.

22. **What ECG findings support the diagnosis of CAD?**
    The resting 12-lead ECG remains a low-cost, effective screening tool in the detection of CAD. It should be evaluated for the presence of horizontal ST-segment depression or elevation, T-wave inversion, old MI, as demonstrated by Q waves, and disturbances in conduction and rhythm. Upsloping ST depression and ST segment flattening are benign findings.

23. **When is resting 12-lead ECG recommended?**
    The most recent guidelines from the ACC and AHA have noted that there is no class I (recommended) indication for a preoperative ECG in any patient, but instead place emphasis on assessing each individual patient's functional capacity. The guidelines state the ECG could be useful in the following settings:
    - It is reasonable to perform an ECG preoperatively in patients with known CAD or significant structural heart disease undergoing moderate or high-risk surgery.
    - It may be considered to perform an ECG in patients with no clinical risk factors who are undergoing vascular surgical procedures.

24. **How long should elective surgery be delayed if a patient had a recent MI?**
    Elective surgery should be delayed by at least 2 months at a minimum following an MI. It is important to note that perioperative complications further decrease over time (e.g., 6 months after an MI) albeit to a much lesser degree than the first 2 months.

25. **What are the hemodynamic goals of induction and maintenance of general anesthesia in patients with coronary artery disease.**

    The main goal is to reduce myocardial oxygen demand, maintain myocardial oxygen supply, and reduce the physiological response to stress of surgery. This includes maintaining a normal to high diastolic blood pressure with an α_1 agonist, such as phenylephrine, and a normal ventricular end-diastolic pressure (e.g., venodilator administration, such as nitroglycerin, and avoiding hypervolemia) to optimize the CPP gradient. A lower threshold to transfuse red blood cells may be considered to optimize oxygen content in the blood. High-dose opioids and/or β-blockers may be considered as the left ventricle is only perfused during diastole and both reduce the heart rate. Regional anesthesia should strongly be considered to blunt the physiological stress response to surgery by avoiding hypertension and tachycardia. Further, some evidence indicates epinephrine may potentiate platelet activation and regional anesthesia may reduce the catecholamine response to surgery. Lastly, hypothermia should be avoided, as shivering in the immediate postoperative period can greatly increase oxygen delivery demands on the heart.

26. **What monitors are useful for patients with coronary artery disease?**

    The V_5 precordial lead is the most sensitive single ECG lead for detecting ischemia and should be monitored routinely in patients at risk for CAD. An arterial line may be considered in high-risk patients and/or high-risk operations; however, their routine use is not recommended. Transesophageal echocardiography to assess wall change abnormalities (hypokinesia or akinesia) is not indicated, unless the patient is hypotensive and not responsive to vasoactive agents. Pulmonary artery catheters may be considered if the patient is in cardiogenic shock; however, their routine use is not indicated.

KEY POINTS: CORONARY ARTERY DISEASE AND PERIOPERATIVE MYOCARDIAL INFARCTION

1. Clinical predictors, the risk of the surgical procedure, and exercise capacity should be integrated in the decision-making process to avoid adverse perioperative cardiac events.
2. Patients with active cardiac conditions (acute coronary syndrome, recent MI) should be determined and treated before elective noncardiac surgery.
3. The risk of the surgical procedure also should be considered. Patients who are undergoing vascular surgery are likely at the greatest risk for perioperative ischemic events.
4. Patients with excellent exercise capacity, even in the presence of ischemic heart disease, will be able to tolerate the stresses of noncardiac surgery.
5. The ability to climb two or three flights of stairs (METs $\geq$4), without significant symptoms (angina, dyspnea), is usually an indication of adequate cardiac reserve. Such patients can undergo high-risk surgical operations without further cardiac testing.
6. Emergent surgical operations should not be delayed for cardiac testing, regardless of the patient's medical comorbidities, exercise capacity, or risk of surgery.
7. The type of acute revascularization (e.g., bare-metal stents vs. DES) should be carefully planned because patients with DES should be on dual-antiplatelet therapy for at least 1 year.

SUGGESTED READINGS

Feher J. Quantitative Human Physiology: An Introduction. 2nd ed. Cambridge, MA: Elsevier Academic Press; 2017:516–524.

Fleisher LA. Ischemic heart disease. In: Sweitzer BJ, ed. Handbook of Preoperative Assessment and Management. Philadelphia: Lippincott Williams & Wilkins; 2000:39–62;

Fleisher LA, Fleischmann KE, Auerbach AD, et al; American College of Cardiology; American Heart Association. 2014 ACC/AHA guideline on perioperative cardiovascular evaluation and management of patients undergoing noncardiac surgery: a report of the American College of Cardiology/American Heart Association Task Force on practice guidelines. J Am Coll Cardiol. 2014;64(22):e77–e137.

Patel AY, Eagle KA, Vaishnava P. Cardiac risk of noncardiac surgery. J Am Coll Cardiol. 2015;66(19):2140–2148.

Stafford JA, Drusin RE, Lalwani AK. When is it safe to operate following myocardial infarction? Laryngoscope. 2016;126(2):299–301.

CHAPTER 36

HEART FAILURE

S. Andrew McCullough, MD

1. **What is heart failure?**

   Heart failure (HF) is a complex clinical syndrome that can result from any structural or functional cardiac disorder that impairs the ability of the ventricle to fill or eject blood. The cardinal manifestations of HF are dyspnea, fatigue, and lower extremity edema, all of which may limit exercise tolerance. These symptoms are usually secondary to fluid retention, which in turn leads to pulmonary congestion and peripheral edema. Some patients have exercise intolerance, with little evidence of fluid retention, whereas others complain primarily of edema and report few symptoms of dyspnea or fatigue. The differences in symptoms from patient to patient are a result of which ventricle is more involved in the disease process—the failing left ventricle results in dyspnea, whereas the failing right ventricle results in edema. Because not all patients have volume overload (congestion) at the time of initial or subsequent evaluation, the term *HF* is preferred over the older term *congestive HF*.

2. **Name the causes of HF.**

   The most common causes of HF in the United States are coronary artery disease (CAD), systemic hypertension (HTN), dilated cardiomyopathy, and valvular heart disease (Box 36.1).

3. **Describe the staging of HF.**

   - **Stage A:** Asymptomatic patients with CAD, HTN, diabetes mellitus, or other risk factors who do not yet demonstrate impaired left ventricular (LV) function, LV hypertrophy, or geometric chamber distortion.
   - **Stage B:** Patients who remain asymptomatic but demonstrate LV hypertrophy, geometric chamber distortion, and/or impaired LV systolic or diastolic function.
   - **Stage C:** Patients with current or past symptoms of HF associated with underlying structural heart disease.
   - **Stage D (also termed *advanced HF*):** Patients with HF refractory to medical therapy who might be eligible for specialized, advanced treatment strategies, such as mechanical circulatory support, continuous inotropic infusions, cardiac transplantation, or palliative care.
   - This classification recognizes that there are established risk factors and structural prerequisites for the development of HF (stages A and B) and that therapeutic interventions introduced even before the appearance of LV dysfunction or symptoms can reduce the morbidity and mortality of HF.

4. **How is the severity of HF classified?**

   Typically, the clinical status of patients with HF is classified on the basis of symptoms and lifestyle impairment. The New York Heart Association (NYHA) classification is used to assess symptomatic limitations of HF and response to therapy:
   - **Class I:** Ordinary physical activity does not cause symptoms. Dyspnea occurs with strenuous or rapid prolonged exertion at work or recreation.
   - **Class II:** Ordinary physical activity results in mild symptoms. Dyspnea occurs while walking or climbing stairs rapidly or walking uphill. Walking more than two blocks on the level and climbing more than one flight of ordinary stairs at a normal pace also result in symptoms.
   - **Class III:** Less than ordinary activity results in symptoms. Dyspnea occurs while walking one to two blocks on the level or climbing one flight of stairs at a normal pace.
   - **Class IV:** Dyspnea occurs at a low level of physical activity or at rest.

   The NYHA classification describes the functional status of patients with stage C or D HF. The severity of symptoms characteristically fluctuates even in the absence of changes in medications, and changes in medications can have either favorable or adverse effects on functional capacity, in the absence of measurable changes in ventricular function. Some patients may demonstrate remarkable recovery associated with improvement in structural and functional abnormalities. Medical therapy associated with sustained improvement should be continued indefinitely.

5. **What major alterations in the heart occur in patients with HF?**

   Normal heart function can be characterized by the pressure-volume curve showing the end-diastolic volume (*B or C*) and end-systolic volume (*D or A*) and pressure, stroke volume (SV) (*C–D*), and ejection fraction (EF) ((*C–D*)*/C*) (Fig. 36.1, *loop 1*). It is important to understand that the pressure for propelling the SV from the heart is generated mostly during isovolumetric contraction *(BC)*, and the relaxation preceding diastolic filling occurs mostly during isovolumetric relaxation *(DA)* (see Fig. 36.1, *loop 1*). LV dysfunction begins with injury of the myocardium. The myocardial injury can be initiated by hypoxia, infiltration, or infection, and is generally a progressive process causing systolic dysfunction, with increasing end-systolic volume, and thus increasing intracavitary pressures. The left ventricle dilates with increasing end-diastolic volume and becomes more spherical—a process called *cardiac remodeling* (see Fig. 36.1, *loop 3*). Specific patterns of ventricular remodeling occur in response to augmentation in workload. In pressure overload, the increased

Box 36.1 Causes of Heart Failure

Mechanical Abnormalities

Pressure overload
Aortic stenosis, systemic hypertension, aortic coarctation
Volume overload
Valvular regurgitation, circulatory shunts, congenital heart disease
Restriction of ventricular filling
Mitral stenosis, constrictive pericarditis, left ventricular hypertrophy

Myocardial Disease

- Primary
  Cardiomyopathies, hypertrophic/restrictive/dilated cardiac disease
- Secondary
  Coronary artery disease: ischemic cardiomyopathy
  Metabolic: alcoholic cardiomyopathy, thyroid disorders, pheochromocytoma, uremic cardiomyopathy
  Drugs: doxorubicin, heroin, cocaine, methamphetamine
  Metals: iron overload, lead poisoning, cobalt poisoning
  Myocarditis: bacterial/viral/parasitic/mycotic disease
  Connective tissue diseases: rheumatic arthritis, systemic lupus erythematosus, scleroderma
  Neurological diseases: myotonic dystrophy, Duchenne muscular dystrophy
  Inherited diseases: glycogen storage diseases, mucopolysaccharidoses
  Other diseases: amyloidosis, leukemia, irradiation to heart

wall tension during systole initiates parallel addition of new myofibrils causing wall thickening and concentric hypertrophy (see Fig. 36.1, *loop 2*). In volume overload, the wall tension is increasing during diastole, which initiates new sarcomeres resulting in chamber enlargement and eccentric hypertrophy (see Fig. 36.1, *loop 3*). Ventricular dilation allows the chamber to eject an adequate SV with less muscle shortening, but wall stress is increased, as described by LaPlace's law:

$$Wall\ tension = P \times R/2h$$

P, intracavital pressure; R, radius of the chamber; h, thickness of the chamber wall

Increasing wall tension accompanies higher oxygen demand. Myocardial hypertrophy with increasing wall thickness allows the heart to overcome pressure overload with decreasing wall tension.

6. **What is the Frank-Starling law?**

The Frank-Starling law states that the force or tension developed in a muscle fiber depends on the extent to which the fiber is stretched. When increased volume of blood flows into the heart (increased preload), the tension will increase in the walls of the heart. The result of this increased stretch of the myocardium is that the cardiac muscle contracts, with increased force, and empties the expanded chambers, with increasing SV. There is an optimal sarcomere length and thus an optimal fiber length at which the most forceful contraction occurs. Any stretch below or above this

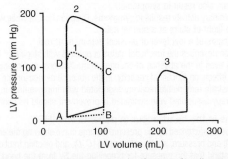

Fig. 36.1 Left ventricular *(LV)* pressure-volume loops illustrating normal performance *(loop 1)*, pressure overload *(loop 2)*, and systolic dysfunction or volume overload *(loop 3)*. Loop 1: The phases of the heart cycle in normal heart. *AB,* Diastolic filling; *BC,* isovolumic contraction; *CD,* ejection; *DA,* isovolumic relaxation. Loop 2: This loop represents the pressure-volume relationship in chronic hypertension or aortic stenosis with concentric LV hypertrophy. The stroke volume and ejection fraction are normal. The high LV end-diastolic pressure suggests diastolic dysfunction, based on decreased LV compliance. Loop 3: In systolic dysfunction, the LV end-diastolic and end-systolic volumes are enlarged with normal or less than normal stroke volume. The end-diastolic pressure can be normal or higher than normal (secondary diastolic dysfunction), depending on the compliance of the left ventricle. This loop may represent dilated cardiomyopathy or eccentric LV hypertrophy in volume overload.

optimal sarcomere length will cause a decrease in the force of contraction. The clinical implication is that SV decreases in hypovolemia and in hypervolemia, with the idea that euvolemia can be defined as the optimal position on the Frank-Starlin curve, where sarcomere stretch is optimized. In systolic HF, the myocardial contractility is decreased and the heart is often "congested," which is characterized as an elevated end-diastolic volume (i.e., excessive preload), which can further impair contractility, increase wall tension, and decrease coronary perfusion (CPP $= P_{aorta} - P_{ventricle}$).

7. **What is the role of cardiac output in patient evaluation?**
Cardiac output is the amount of blood that the heart can pump in 1 minute. The main determinants of the cardiac output are as follows:

$$CO = SV \times HR$$

CO, cardiac output; SV, stroke volume; HR, heart rate where SV is affected by preload, afterload, and contractility
   Cardiac output varies with the level of physical activity. The average value for resting adults is about 5 L/min. For women, this value is 10% to 20% less. Cardiac output increases in proportion to the surface area of the body. To compare the cardiac output of people of different sizes, the term of *cardiac index* (CI) was introduced, which is the cardiac output per square meter of body surface area. The normal CI for adults is more than 2.5 L/min/m^2. Sympathetic stimulation increases heart rate, contractility, and preload through venous vasoconstriction, which together can raise the cardiac output up to 25 L/min. Patients with systolic HF are unable to generate appropriate cardiac output to the exercise level, and in patients with severe HF, the cardiac output may decrease with exercise. This results in fatigue, dyspnea, and presyncope.

8. **What is the connection between exercise and cardiac output?**
Exercise increases the oxygen consumption ($\dot{V} O_2$) and is matched by an increase in oxygen delivery ($\dot{D}O_2$) by increasing cardiac output:

$$\dot{D}O_2 = CO \times \text{Blood oxygen content}$$

   Oxygen consumption and cardiac output increase in a parallel manner. HF results in a mismatch between tissue oxygen consumption and oxygen delivery, based on the inappropriate cardiac output to match oxygen consumption demands. The mismatch provokes tissue hypoxemia, acidosis, and inability to exercise at the level where the mismatch occurs.

9. **What is systolic dysfunction?**
The symptoms and signs of HF can be caused by either a decreased ability of the heart muscle to contract, resulting in a decreased EF and systolic dysfunction, or a decreased ability of the heart to relax, resulting in impaired ventricular filling and diastolic dysfunction.
   Systolic dysfunction results from decreased ejection of blood from the left ventricle. The EF is thus reduced, the end-systolic and end-diastolic volumes are enlarged, the intracavitary pressures are abnormally high, and the left ventricle is dilated. It is important to understand that the actual SV may be close to normal in some patients, despite a decrease in EF because of the increased end-diastolic volume. However, this compensatory mechanism will be at the expense because of increased wall tension and oxygen consumption (see LaPlace's law earlier). In this pathological condition, the left ventricle has less reserve capacity to overcome pressure or volume overload causing the symptoms of HF (see Fig. 36.1, *loop 3*).

10. **How can we identify systolic dysfunction and HF?**
The classic characteristic physiological abnormalities for systolic dysfunction are increased end-systolic and end-diastolic volume, decreased EF, and decreased SV. These parameters can be obtained by echocardiography. In general, the decreased SV with decreased cardiac output causes fatigue and dyspnea. Systolic (and diastolic) dysfunction lead to an increased end-diastolic left ventricle and left atrial (LA) pressure, causing cardiogenic or hydrostatic mediated pulmonary edema. Further, the decreased cardiac output leads to a decreased oxygen delivery ($\dot{D}O_2$) and a compensatory increase in the body's oxygen extraction ratio, leading to a decrease in mixed venous oxygen in the pulmonary artery. This contributes to hypoxemia when this blood mixes from Zone 3 of the lung (i.e., ventilation/perfusion mismatch region) with oxygenated blood in the left atrium. Together, pulmonary edema and decreased mixed venous oxygen may lead to hypoxemia and contribute to dyspnea. These abnormalities may only become apparent with mild HF with exertion; however, in severe HF or cardiogenic shock these physiological abnormalities may be apparent at rest.
   Patients that have clinical symptoms of HF, in addition to reduced EF, are given the diagnosis of HF with reduced ejection fraction (HFrEF). However, it is important to remember that to diagnose *HF*, an echocardiogram is not necessary, as the entity is a clinical diagnosis.

11. **What is diastolic dysfunction?**
Normally, the left ventricle fills with blood at low (<12 mm Hg) LA pressure. The LA pressure stays low, even with a high cardiac output during strenuous exercise. This low-pressure filling is largely dependent on the LV diastolic function. As the left ventricle relaxes, blood is drawn into the low pressure, empty LV cavity by two prominent flows. *Early* diastolic filling starts with isovolumetric relaxation after the mitral valve opens and continues during the early filling of the left ventricle. It is energy-dependent (recall that adenosine triphosphate is necessary for actin/myosin uncoupling) and relies

on the reuptake of calcium from the cytosol into the sarcoplasmic reticulum of the myocytes. This active relaxation generates about 80% of the diastolic volume. Late diastolic filling is secondary to atrial contraction and is dependent on both LA contractility and LV compliance. Diastolic dysfunction is always present with impaired systolic function but can also occur with normal systolic function, if there is impaired relaxation or reduced LV compliance. Ischemia, myocardial hypertrophy, pericardial constriction, fibrosis, or myocardial diseases may impair the diastolic filling process. Systolic dysfunction primarily causes an increase in LV volume and pressure, whereas diastolic dysfunction leads to decrease in LV relaxation and compliance and an increase in LV pressure for a given volume. Patients with a normal EF, but with clinical symptoms of HF, likely have diastolic HF better known as *HF with preserved ejection fraction (HFpEF)*.

12. **What are the presenting symptoms of HF?**
Exertional dyspnea and fatigue are most often the primary chief complaints of patients with HF. Paroxysmal nocturnal dyspnea, nocturia, coughing, wheezing, right upper quadrant pain, and anorexia are also associated. Although HF is generally regarded as a hemodynamic disorder, many studies have indicated that there is a poor relation between measures of cardiac performance and the symptoms produced by the disease. Patients with a very low EF may be asymptomatic (stage B), whereas patients with preserved EF may have severe disability (stage C).

13. **What physical examination findings suggests HF?**
Cardiac palpation may reveal an expanded point of maximal impulse (ventricular dilation) or a forceful sustained impulse with LV hypertrophy. Auscultation reveals a gallop rhythm with S_3 or S_4, secondary to impaired LV filling or forceful atrial contraction, respectively. Murmurs of valvular diseases should be investigated. Pulmonary examination often reveals rales located most prominently over the lung bases. Decreased breath sounds, secondary to pleural effusions, occur more often in patients with chronic HF. Patients may also have elevated jugular venous pressures; however, it takes much practice to reliably identify this finding.

14. **What diagnostic studies are useful in evaluating the patient with HF?**
The chest radiograph may detect an enlarged cardiac silhouette or evidence of pulmonary vascular congestion, including perihilar engorgement of the pulmonary veins, cephalization of the pulmonary vascular markings, or pleural effusions.
The electrocardiogram (ECG) is often nonspecific, but ventricular or supraventricular dysrhythmias, conduction abnormalities, and signs of myocardial hypertrophy, ischemia, or infarction are frequently present.
Echocardiography is arguably the most important study for the assessment of HF. It characterizes chamber size, wall motion, valvular function, and LV wall thickness. SV can be measured using Doppler methods. EF can be calculated by measuring the end-diastolic and end-systolic volumes. Diastolic function can be evaluated by studying the flow pattern through the mitral valve and the left upper pulmonary vein using the Doppler technique.

15. **What laboratory findings are often abnormal in HF?**
Serum electrolytes, arterial blood gases, liver function tests (LFTs), and blood cell counts are frequently evaluated. Many patients with HF are hyponatremic from the activation of the vasopressin system or from the treatment with angiotensin-converting enzyme (ACE) inhibitors. Treatment with diuretics often lead to hypokalemia and hypomagnesemia. Some degree of prerenal azotemia, hypocalcemia, and hypophosphatemia is often present. Hepatic congestion may result in elevated bilirubin levels and elevated LFTs.
Elevated brain natriuretic peptide levels may aid in the diagnosis of HF or trigger consideration of HF when the diagnosis is unknown.

16. **How can we diagnose diastolic dysfunction?**
Diastolic function can be quantified using echocardiography. Intraoperative transesophageal echocardiography (TEE) can aid in identifying diastolic dysfunction in the operating room. The diagnosis is made based on the Doppler study of the mitral valve inflow, pulmonary vein inflow, and tissue Doppler measurement of the velocity of the mitral valve annulus. Specifically, we identify early diastolic filling (the E flow), atrial contraction (the A flow), and the motion of the mitral valve annulus during filling (if filling is normal, the annulus should move briskly). By assessing the velocity of these flows, we can determine the filling characteristic of the LV filling pressures.
- **Mitral inflow:** The E wave represents the velocity curve of early diastolic filling, and the A wave is the velocity curve of atrial contraction (late diastolic filling). A normal E/A ratio is usually greater than 0.8, indicating that the ventricle fills more in early diastole than from the atrial contraction. The time from the peak to zero velocity of the E wave is the deceleration time of E (DecT), which is normally 160 to 200 ms, and it represents effective early relaxation and normal LV compliance (Fig. 36.2).
- **Pulmonary vein inflow:** During systole, blood flows from the pulmonary vein into the left atrium, resulting in the systolic wave or S wave. During early diastole, the flow increases again from the pulmonary vein into the left atrium, resulting in the D wave. During late diastole, during the atrial contraction there is a negligible reversal of flow into the pulmonary vein: A reversal (Ar). Usually, the S/D ratio is close to 1 and the Ar is less than 35 cm/sec (Fig. 36.3).
- **Tissue Doppler:** The mitral valve and pulmonary vein inflow velocity curves are volume-dependent parameters that can vary depending upon the patient's volume status. To minimize variability because of volume status changes, the motion of the mitral valve annulus using Doppler echocardiography is different measurement that can be useful. The mitral valve annulus velocities (E_m) during early diastole at the septum, and the lateral wall, are sensitive parameters of diastolic dysfunction and less sensitive to volume changes. In normal conditions,

Mitral valve inflow

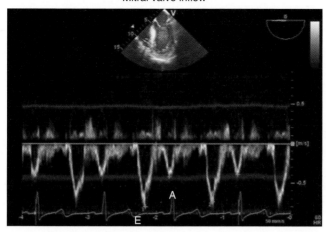

Fig. 36.2 Pulsed-wave Doppler detection of mitral valve inflow. In the small segment of the upper part of the picture, the echo image of the four-chamber view can be seen. In this view, the Doppler probe detects the flow velocity through the mitral valve during the heart cycle. The Doppler probe is in the tip of the segment. The flow is going from the left atrium to the left ventricle, away from the transducer during diastole; thus two negative velocity waves can be seen. The electrocardiogram helps to determine the phase of systole and diastole. The first wave is the E wave, which represents early diastolic filling, and the second wave is the A wave, which represents the atrial contraction.

Pulmonary vein inflow

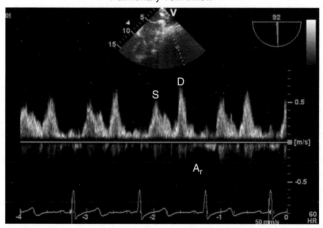

Fig. 36.3 Pulsed-wave Doppler detection of pulmonary vein inflow. The small segment on the upper part of the figure represents the echo image of the two-chamber view. In this view, the left upper pulmonary vein can be visualized just above the left atrial appendage. The flow is going from the pulmonary vein to the left atrium toward the transducer, during systole and early diastole, and a small flow can be detected during the atrial kick back to the pulmonary vein. The first wave is the S wave, which represents the inflow during systole; the D wave represents the inflow during early diastole; and the small A_r (A reversal) is the flow back to the pulmonary wave during atrial contraction.

the septal annulus velocity is more than 8 cm/sec and the lateral annulus velocity is more than 10 cm/sec (Fig. 36.4). Note that these velocities parallel the mitral inflow pattern.

17. **What treatment strategies are used in the different stages of HF?**
    See Table 36.1.

18. **How would you plan anesthetic management of patients with HF?**
    Patients with that good exercise capacity or functional status in that they can walk at least two flights of stairs, without dyspnea (i.e., METs >4), can generally undergo surgery without further intervention. Patients that have poor exercise

Tissue Doppler velocity

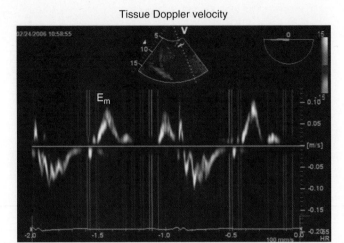

Fig. 36.4 Tissue Doppler velocity measurement. The small segment of the upper part of the picture represents the echo image of the four-chamber view in tissue Doppler mode. The pulsed-wave Doppler probe is placed on the mitral valve annulus at the lateral wall, and it shows the movement during systole and two waves during diastole. The electrocardiogram helps to differentiate between systole and diastole. The wave at early filling is the E_m velocity curve, which is a relatively volume-independent diastolic parameter.

capacity (i.e., METs <4) and/or are in decompensated HF, undergoing nonemergent surgery, need further intervention for medical optimization, to better assess the benefit-risk of surgery, and to facilitate an anesthetic plan.

19. **What are the physiological goals in managing patients with systolic heart failure?**
    Patients with impaired contractility, such as in systolic HF may present with excess preload (i.e., hypervolemia) and afterload (i.e., increased systemic vascular resistance), in part because of their elevated sympathetic tone causing venous and arterial vasoconstriction and fluid retention by the kidneys. Both excessive preload and afterload can decrease SV and cardiac output. Vasodilators, in addition to diuretics, can help in "unloading the heart" by reducing both preload and afterload to a more optimal physiological state, thereby improving SV or forward flow.

20. **How would you manage a patient with decompensated HF?**
    In general, patients in decompensated HF are not candidates for elective procedures. In emergent circumstances, invasive monitoring (arterial-line, pulmonary artery catheter, central line, etc.) is indicated to guide fluid therapy and assess response to anesthetic agents and inotropic or vasodilator therapy. A pulmonary artery catheter is helpful for titrating inotropic agents, using mixed venous oxygen saturation and cardiac output. Note that routine pulmonary artery catheterization is generally more harmful than helpful and should only be used in selected patients (i.e., cardiogenic shock or mixed shock states, e.g., septic shock with severe HF). The TEE is also helpful to evaluate systolic and diastolic function, evaluate the effect of fluid therapy on the heart, and to measure and monitor SV and cardiac output.

21. **Which anesthetic agents can be used in decompensated HF?**
    Avoidance of myocardial depression remains the goal of anesthetic management. Propofol can cause profound depression of cardiac function and hypotension. Etomidate produces only small aberrations in cardiovascular status, although hypotension may still. Ketamine administration may result in elevated cardiac output and blood pressure, secondary to increased sympathetic activity. However, in patients with increased sympathetic activation caused by decompensated HF, ketamine can act as a negative inotropic agent and may cause hypotension and cardiac failure. Although all volatile anesthetic agents are myocardial depressants, they are usually well tolerated at low doses. For patients with severely compromised myocardial function, narcotic-based anesthesia, with or without a low-dose volatile agent, is useful. Remifentanil as a short-acting opioid can be well suited especially for short surgical procedures.

22. **Is regional anesthesia contraindicated in patients with HF?**
    No. Regional anesthesia, when prudently administered, is an acceptable anesthetic technique. In fact, modest preload and afterload reduction (venous and arterial vasodilation) may enhance cardiac output when using a neuraxial technique. However, it is recommended to "slowly titrate" the epidural with small boluses to facilitate a gradual loss of sympathetic tone that may be treated with vasoactive drugs, to maintain "normal" vascular tone.

23. **How would you support the heart in decompensated HF during anesthesia?**
    Patients with HF often require circulatory support intraoperatively and postoperatively. After optimization of preload and afterload, inotropic drugs, such as dobutamine, have been shown to be effective in low-output states.

Table 36.1 Management of Heart Failure

STAGE	RECOMMENDATIONS
A) Patients at high risk for HF	• Control comorbidities: hypertension, lipid disorders, thyroid disorders, and diabetes mellitus • Advise patients to avoid smoking, excessive alcohol consumption, and illicit drug use • Patients who have known atherosclerotic vascular disease should be followed for secondary prevention • ACE inhibitors or ARBs in combination with β-blockers[a]
B) Asymptomatic HF	• Apply all recommendations for stage A • β-blockers[a] and ACE inhibitors should be used in all patients with a recent or remote history of MI, regardless of EF or presence of HF • β-blockers[a] and ACE inhibitors are indicated in all patients who have a reduced EF, despite no HF symptoms
C) Symptomatic HF with normal EF	• Apply all recommendations for stage A/B including β-blockers[a] and ACE inhibitor medications for all patients • Coronary revascularization in patients with CAD that is likely to have an adverse effect on cardiac function • Ventricular rate control in patients with atrial fibrillation • Diuretics to control pulmonary congestion and peripheral edema
C) Symptomatic HF with reduced EF	• Apply all recommendations for stage A/B including β-blockers[a] and ACE inhibitor medications for all patients • Diuretics and salt restriction for patients with edema • Addition of an aldosterone antagonist should be considered • Consider addition of combination neprilysin inhibitors/angiotensin receptor blockers • Automatic implant cardioverter defibrillator (AICD) therapy and cardiac resynchronization therapy (CRT) with dual-chamber pacemaker can be instituted in high-risk patients (i.e., AICD for patients with LVEF <35% and/or CRT for patients with left bundle branch block)
D) End-stage HF	• Apply all recommendations for stage A/B including β-blockers[a] and ACE inhibitor medications for all patients • β-blockers [a] may need to be withheld in patients in cardiogenic shock • Consider mechanical circulatory support, continuous intravenous positive inotropic therapy, and referral for cardiac transplantation • Emphasize goals of care with consideration for hospice

[a]Use only one of the three β-blockers proven to reduce mortality. Specifically, bisoprolol, carvedilol, or sustained-release metoprolol succinate.

ACE, Angiotensin-converting enzyme; *ARBs*, angiotensin-receptor blockers; *CAD*, coronary artery disease; *EF*, ejection fraction; *HF*, heart failure; *LVEF*, left-ventricular ejection fraction; *MI*, myocardial infarction.

Phosphodiesterase III inhibitors, such as milrinone, possessing inotropic and vasodilating properties may also improve hemodynamic performance. Note that these therapies are not vasopressors, but vasodilators. SV is inversely related to afterload in the failing ventricle, and the reduction of LV afterload, with selective vasodilating drugs, such as nitroprusside, is also effective in increasing cardiac output. Patients under anesthesia are vasodilated by most of the anesthetic agents. Epinephrine and dopamine have positive inotropic and vasoconstrictive properties and can be used alone or in combination with a vasodilating agent (i.e., nitroprusside). Dobutamine and milrinone cause vasodilation and may need to be combined with vasoconstrictive agents, such as vasopressin, epinephrine, or norepinephrine.

24. Why should phenylephrine be avoided in patients with severe heart failure?
    Vasopressors, such as phenylephrine, vasoconstrict both venous vasculature (increase preload) and arterial vasculature (increase afterload) through α_1 mediated venous and arterial vasoconstriction. Healthy patients with normal cardiac contractility generally tolerate the increase in afterload and, depending upon the situation, venoconstriction may improve preload and cardiac output. For most patients undergoing surgery, with either general anesthesia or neuraxial anesthesia, phenylephrine is often a good choice to counteract the anesthetic-induced vasodilation. However, in patients with decreased contractility, simultaneously increasing preload and afterload with vasopressors can "overload" the heart's physiological reserve, leading to a decrease in cardiac output; therefore careful administration should be used to strike the appropriate balance.

25. **What are percutaneous LV assist devices?**

    In patients with severe HF or in cardiogenic shock, percutaneous LV assist devices can be used to stabilize patients during recovery. They are available for short-term use only. It is important to understand the hemodynamic conditions in the presence of these devices to plan the anesthetic management and additional inotropic support. As a general concept, although these devices support the LV function, it is important to keep the right ventricular function optimal to match the cardiac output generated by the devices.

26. **Why can we not use positive inotropic medications for long-term treatment of HF?**

    Patients with HF are treated with β-blockers, ACE inhibitors, and diuretics for long-term therapy. The effects of these medications are often antagonistic to the β_1 and α_1 receptor agonist medications we often use in the operating room. Outcome studies show that patients with HF have optimal long-term survival on β-blockers and ACE-inhibitor therapy and increased mortality on medications with positive inotropic properties. This phenomenon can be explained by the protective effect of β-blockers and ACE inhibitors on adverse cardiac remodeling. Fundamentally, the goals of outpatient care are on long-term survival, whereas the goals in the acute setting (i.e., intensive care unit or operating room) is more on short-term survival. In life-threatening situations, this may require using β_1 and α_1 agonist medications; otherwise, in general, the goal of care should be what is in the best long-term interest for the patient, which means continuing their outpatient medications in the perioperative period.

KEY POINTS: HEART FAILURE

1. The symptoms and signs of HF can be caused by either an abnormality in systolic function that leads to a diminished EF or an abnormality in diastolic function that leads to impaired ventricular filling.
2. Diastolic dysfunction can cause HF with preserved EF, and is always present in systolic HF. Different types of diastolic dysfunction need different types of fluid and hemodynamic management as outlined earlier.
3. Patients in decompensated HF are not candidates for elective procedures and may require a few days of treatment to optimize cardiac performance. However, in urgent cases, intravenous inotropic support and/or percutaneous LV assist device placement can be considered to perform anesthesia and surgery.
4. In emergent circumstances, invasive monitoring (arterial line, pulmonary artery catheter, and TEE) is indicated to guide fluid therapy and assess response to anesthetic agents, inotropic, or vasodilator therapies.
5. Patients with decreased myocardial reserve are more sensitive to the cardiovascular depressant effects caused by anesthetic agents, but careful administration with close monitoring of hemodynamic responses can be accomplished with most agents.
6. Noncardiac surgery for patients with a percutaneous or implanted LV assist device requires an understanding of the hemodynamic effect of the device, and of the monitoring options to maintain patient stability. As a general concept, the right ventricular function should be optimized to keep up with the cardiac output generated by the device.

SUGGESTED READINGS

Falk S. Anesthetic considerations for the patient undergoing therapy for advanced heart failure. Curr Opin Anesthesiol. 2011;243:314–319.

Fleisher LA, Fleischmann KE, Auerbach AD, et al. American College of Cardiology; American Heart Association. 2014 ACC/AHA guideline on perioperative cardiovascular evaluation and management of patients undergoing noncardiac surgery: a report of the American College of Cardiology/American Heart Association Task Force on Practice Guidelines. J Am Coll Cardiol. 2014;64(22):e77–e137.

Yancy CW, Januzzi JL Jr, Allen LA, et al. 2017 ACC Expert Consensus Decision Pathway for Optimization of Heart Failure Treatment: Answers to 10 Pivotal Issues About Heart Failure With Reduced Ejection Fraction: A Report of the American College of Cardiology Task Force on Expert Consensus Decision Pathways. J Am Coll Cardiol. 2018;71(2):201–230.

Yancy CW, Jessup M, Bozkurt B, et al. Colvin MM, et al. 2017 ACC/AHA/HFSA Focused Update of the 2013 ACCF/AHA Guideline for the Management of Heart Failure: A Report of the American College of Cardiology/American Heart Association Task Force on Clinical Practice Guidelines and the Heart Failure Society of America. J Am Coll Cardiol. 2017;70(6):776–803.

Yancy CW, Jessup M, Bozkurt B, et al. American College of Cardiology Foundation; American Heart Association Task Force on Practice Guidelines. 2013 ACCF/AHA guideline for the management of heart failure: a report of the American College of Cardiology Foundation/American Heart Association Task Force on Practice Guidelines. J Am Coll Cardiol. 2013;62(16):e147–e239.

CHAPTER 37

VALVULAR HEART DISEASE

Stephen Spindel, MD

1. **Discuss the basic pathophysiology of valvular heart diseases.**

   Valvular heart diseases cause chronic volume or pressure overload, where each evokes a characteristic ventricular response causing ventricular hypertrophy. Ventricular hypertrophy is an increase in left ventricular (LV) mass. Pressure overload produces concentric ventricular hypertrophy, which is characterized by an increase in ventricular wall thickness with a relatively normal cardiac chamber size. Volume overload, however, leads to eccentric hypertrophy, which is characterized by normal wall thickness, with an enlarged cardiac chamber.

2. **Describe common findings on history and physical examination in patients with valvular heart disease.**

   Most systolic heart murmurs do not signify cardiac disease and are caused by physiological increases in blood flow velocity. Diastolic and continuous murmurs, however, virtually always represent pathological conditions and require further cardiac evaluation.

   A history of rheumatic fever, intravenous drug abuse, embolization in different organs, genetic diseases such as Marfan syndrome, heart surgery in childhood, or known heart murmur should alert the examiner to the possibility of valvular heart disease. Exercise tolerance is frequently decreased, and patients may exhibit signs and symptoms of heart failure, including dyspnea, orthopnea, fatigue, pulmonary rales, jugular venous congestion, hepatic congestion, and dependent edema. Enlargement or hypertrophy of the left ventricle may be associated with angina, whereas enlargement of the atria may cause atrial fibrillation.

3. **Which tests are useful in the evaluation of valvular heart disease?**

   Echocardiography with doppler technology is a fundamental diagnostic method in the evaluation of valvular heart disease. The size and function of the heart chambers can be measured and assessed and the pressure gradients across the valves, including valve areas, can be calculated to determine disease severity.

   Echocardiography is recommended for:
   - Asymptomatic patients with diastolic murmurs, continuous murmurs, holosystolic murmurs, mid-peaking systolic murmurs, late systolic murmurs, murmurs associated with ejection clicks, or murmurs that radiate to the neck or back.
   - Patients with heart murmurs and symptoms or signs of heart failure, myocardial ischemia, syncope, thromboembolism, infective endocarditis, or other clinical evidence of structural heart disease.

   A standard 12-lead electrocardiogram (ECG) should be obtained and examined for evidence of ischemia, dysrhythmias, atrial enlargement, and ventricular hypertrophy. A chest radiograph can also be helpful and may show enlargement of cardiac chambers, suggest pulmonary hypertension, or reveal pulmonary edema and pleural effusions. Cardiac catheterization is often used in the evaluation of such patients before surgery, mostly for diagnosing coronary artery disease to determine if coronary artery bypass surgery is also indicated. Cardiac catheterization also allows direct measurement of pressure within various heart chambers, which can be used to directly calculate pressure gradients across different valves.

4. **How is echocardiography helpful in the surgical management of valvular disease?**

   Transesophageal echocardiography (TEE) can be used in the operating room during the surgical management of valvular diseases. The severity of the valvular disease and accompanying structural or functional changes can be reevaluated. Evaluation of valve repair and function of artificial valves are important parts of postcardiopulmonary bypass assessment. Systolic and diastolic function of the left and right ventricles before and after cardiopulmonary bypass can be analyzed to better guide management of inotropes and volume resuscitation.

5. **Which other monitors aid the anesthesiologist in cardiac surgery?**

   Besides standard American Society of Anesthesiologists monitors, an arterial catheter provides real-time blood pressure measurement and continuous access to the bloodstream that can be sampled to perform laboratory tests (e.g., arterial blood gas, electrolytes). Pulmonary artery catheters allow measurement of cardiac output, mixed venous saturation, central venous and pulmonary artery pressures, as well as pulmonary capillary wedge pressure. These are important indices of biventricular function and filling (i.e., preload) and are useful for guiding intravenous fluid and inotropic therapy.

6. **What is a pressure-volume loop?**

   A pressure-volume loop plots LV pressure against volume through one complete cardiac cycle. Each valvular lesion has a unique profile that suggests compensatory physiological changes by the left ventricle.

7. **How does a normal pressure-volume loop appear? What does the area under this loop mean?**
See Fig. 37.1 to review a normal cardiac pressure-volume loop. The area under the pressure-volume loop represents the amount of "work" done by the heart in one cardiac cycle. Recall from physics, the following equation for work:

$$Work\,(joule) = Force\,(newton) \times Distance\,(meter)$$

which can be calculated for the heart as the following:

$$Cardiacwork\,(joule) = Pressure\,(newton/meter^2) \times Strokevolume\,(meter^3)$$

Note that the aforementioned equation is simplified. The true equation would involve an integral to calculate the area under the curve and would need to subtract the work done on the heart during diastole (i.e., preload).

The clinical implication means that any valve disease, which increases either pressure (valvular stenosis) or volume (valvular insufficiency), will increase the amount of work for the affected cardiac chamber in one cardiac cycle. This implies the heart will need to consume more energy (joules) to do more work (joules), which makes the heart susceptible to oxygen supply-demand mismatch (i.e., demand ischemia) and other pathophysiological changes (i.e., eccentric and concentric LV hypertrophy).

8. **What is meant by the terms *preload* and *afterload* in managing patients with valvular heart disease? What are some of the caveats in targeting these parameters?**
Preload and afterload can be thought of as the wall tension on a particular cardiac chamber during diastole and systole, respectively. Although blood pressure is typically thought of as the primary determinant of afterload, valvular heart disease can also affect afterload. For example, aortic stenosis (AS) increases LV afterload, whereas mitral regurgitation (MR) decreases LV afterload. However, most commonly, afterload is modified by increasing or decreasing systemic vascular resistance using vasoactive agents.

When targeting physiological endpoints for patients with valvular heart disease (Table 37.1), it is important to emphasize that care should be individualized. For example, patients with mitral stenosis may need "increased" preload; however, excessive fluid administration may precipitate pulmonary edema and right heart failure. The concept of "increased" or "normal" preload is a bit of a misnomer and reflects the difference between using pressure versus volume to assess preload. Ideally, adequate preload should reflect optimal myosin-actin overlap such that patients are on the optimal position of the Frank-Starling curve. Patients with a noncompliant ventricle (e.g., AS) may need a "higher" pressure to obtain this. Excessive preload, however, can be counterproductive and could decrease contractility by placing patients on the opposite, downsloping side of the Frank-Starling curve and cause other sequela, such as pulmonary edema and right heart failure.

9. **Discuss the pathophysiology of AS.**
AS is classified as valvular, subvalvular, or supravalvular obstruction of the LV outflow tract. Concentric hypertrophy (thickened ventricular wall with normal chamber size) develops in response to the increased intraventricular systolic pressure and wall tension necessary to maintain forward flow. Ventricular relaxation decreases, causing

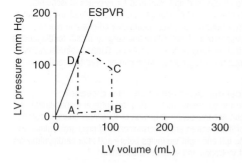

Fig. 37.1 Pressure-volume loop for a normal heart. *LV*, Left ventricle; *AB*, diastolic filling; *BC*, isovolumic contraction; *CD*, ejection; *DA*, isovolumic relaxation. *A*, Mitral valve opening; *B*, mitral valve closing; *C*, aortic valve opening; *D*, aortic valve closing. Stroke volume through the aortic valve is the distance between points *C* and *D*. End-systolic volume can be measured at point *D* and end-diastolic volume can be measured at point *B*. The end-systolic pressure–volume relationship (*ESPVR*) curve is a load-independent index of myocardial contractility. If the contractility is increasing, the ESPVR curve is moving counterclockwise. The pressure-volume loop is an excellent tool to characterize the performance of the heart in different pathological conditions.

Table 37.1 Generalized Physiological Goals for Valvular Heart Disease			
	PRELOAD	**AFTERLOAD**	**HEART RATE**
Aortic stenosis	↑	↑	↓
Aortic insufficiency	↔	↓	↑
Mitral stenosis	↑	↔ or ↑	↓
Mitral regurgitation	↔	↓	↑

diastolic dysfunction. Decreasing LV compliance accompanies elevated LV end-diastolic pressure. Contractility and ejection fraction are usually maintained until late in the disease process. Atrial contraction may account for up to 40% of ventricular filling (normally 20%). In developing countries, rheumatic valve disease is still the most common cause of AS. In North America and Europe, AS is primarily caused by calcification of a native trileaflet or a congenital bicuspid valve. Patients often present with angina, syncope, or congestive heart failure. Angina with exertion can occur in the absence of coronary artery disease, because the thickened myocardium is susceptible to ischemia, and the elevated LV end-diastolic pressure reduces the coronary perfusion pressure. Life expectancy with symptoms of angina is about 5 years. Once syncope appears, the average life expectancy is 3 to 4 years. Once congestive heart failure occurs, the average life expectancy is 1 to 2 years. An easy acronym to help remember the symptoms of AS is "SAD" where "S" is syncope, "A" is angina, and "D" is dyspnea or heart failure.

10. **What are the indications for surgical aortic valve replacement in aortic stenosis?**
The indications for aortic valve replacement (AVR) in AS according to the 2014 and 2017 (focused update) American Heart Association (AHA)/American College of Cardiology (ACC) guidelines are the following:
- Symptomatic patients with severe AS
- Asymptomatic patients with severe AS and an ejection fraction less than 50%
- Patients with severe AS undergoing other cardiac surgery
- AVR is reasonable for:
  - Patients with moderate AS undergoing other cardiac surgery
  - Asymptomatic patients with very severe AS

11. **How are the compensatory changes in the left ventricle represented by a pressure-volume loop?**
Because of AS, the left ventricle is working against a higher intraventricular pressure to generate a normal stroke volume. The higher systolic wall tension initiates myocardial thickening and LV hypertrophy, which is a pathophysiological adaptation to reduce wall tension (see *LaPlace's law* in Chapter 36 on Heart Failure). The hypertrophied left ventricle allows the heart to increase its contractility to generate the necessary pressure (Fig. 37.2) to maintain cardiac output. As the stenosis gets tighter, LV systolic pressure increases to a level where LV hypertrophy can no longer reduce wall tension. At this point, the heart starts dilating, causing congestive heart failure symptoms because of systolic and diastolic dysfunction, and a commensurate decrease in cardiac output. Thus life expectancy drops to 1 to 2 years after congestive heart failure symptoms develop.

12. **What are the hemodynamic goals in the anesthetic management of patients with aortic stenosis?**
Patients must have adequate intravascular volume to fill the noncompliant ventricle. Contractility should be maintained to overcome the high-pressure gradient through the aortic valve. Reduction in blood pressure or systemic vascular resistance does little to decrease LV afterload relative to the already increased afterload because of AS. Further, a normal to high blood pressure is necessary for coronary perfusion as a result of the increased LV end-diastolic pressure. Hypotension, such as on induction of anesthesia, can result in cardiac ischemia and cardiac arrest if the blood pressure is not immediately corrected. In addition, bradycardia and tachycardia should be avoided. Bradycardia leads to a decrease in cardiac output in patients with relatively fixed stroke volume. Tachycardia may produce ischemia with a limited diastolic time for coronary perfusion. Maintenance of low normal sinus rhythm, as opposed to atrial fibrillation, is imperative to ensure adequate time for ventricular filling and because of the importance of atrial contraction in LV filling, which can provide up to 40% of LV filling in patients with severe AS. Emergent cardioversion is indicated if a patient suffers severe hemodynamic compromise because of a dysrhythmia. External defibrillator pads should be attached to patients with severe AS undergoing any procedure that may result in either decreased systemic vascular resistance (i.e., most anesthetic induction agents) or dysrhythmias (wire manipulation during central line or pulmonary artery catheter placement; see Table 37.1).

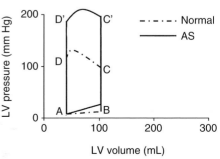

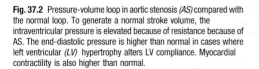

Fig. 37.2 Pressure-volume loop in aortic stenosis *(AS)* compared with the normal loop. To generate a normal stroke volume, the intraventricular pressure is elevated because of resistance because of AS. The end-diastolic pressure is higher than normal in cases where left ventricular *(LV)* hypertrophy alters LV compliance. Myocardial contractility is also higher than normal.

13. Discuss the postoperative management of patients with aortic stenosis after AVR.
    Postoperatively, LV end-diastolic pressure decreases and stroke volume increases, but the hypertrophied LV often still requires an elevated preload to function adequately. Depressed myocardial function may suggest inadequate myocardial protection during cardiac surgery because of difficulty in perfusing the hypertrophied left ventricle. Inotropic agents (milrinone, dobutamine, epinephrine) can improve LV performance in this situation.

14. Describe the role of transcatheter aortic valve replacement in the treatment of severe aortic stenosis.
    Although surgical AVR has been the gold standard for treatment of AS, transcatheter aortic valve replacement (TAVR) is a relatively new procedure that has a significant role in treating symptomatic severe AS in high risk patient populations. The procedure involves a fully collapsible stented aortic valve, which is delivered to the native stenotic valve via a catheter technique, through the femoral artery (most common), subclavian artery, LV apex, or directly through the ascending aorta. These collapsible valves are either self-expanding or require a balloon to expand the stent into the native aortic valve annulus. According to the 2017 ACC/AHA guidelines, treatment of symptomatic severe AS with TAVR has a class I indication ("should perform the procedure") in high-risk patients and a class II indication ("reasonable to perform the procedure") in intermediate-risk patients. Both indications depend upon patient-specific risks and preferences and are discussed by a heart valve team comprised of cardiologists and cardiac surgeons. The surgical risk for each patient is computed via the Society of Thoracic Surgeons' risk model (STS score), which uses patient demographics and clinical variables to calculate morbidity and mortality. The STS score is the likelihood of mortality for a given cardiac surgical procedure. The risks of TAVR compared with surgical AVR are the following: higher major vascular complications (6.0% vs. 1.1%), higher paravalvular aortic regurgitation rates (5.3% vs. 0.6%), and significantly higher need for permanent pacemaker implantations (8.5%–25.9% vs. 6.6%–6.9%). In addition, the longevity of transcatheter aortic valves is questionable, whereas for surgical aortic valves, numerous studies show that freedom from reoperation at 15 years is 77% to 88%. Therefore high importance is emphasized on the selection of patients undergoing TAVR instead of traditional surgical AVRs.

15. Describe the special characteristics of the anesthetic management of TAVR.
    This procedure is generally performed in an elderly patient population with severe AS and significant comorbidities. Two large-bore intravenous lines, a central line with a transvenous pacing catheter, and an intraarterial catheter are required. Either general anesthesia with endotracheal intubation or monitored anesthesia care (MAC) administered by an anesthesiologist can be used for the procedure, with higher risk patients often undergoing the former. Intraoperative transesophageal or transthoracic echocardiogram is essential for evaluating the stenotic and the implanted valve, as well as monitoring the ventricular function and assessing cardiac perforation (i.e., tamponade). Anesthetic management is based on using medications with minimal effect on hemodynamics (e.g., etomidate). Hemodynamic stability can be maintained with infusion of phenylephrine, vasopressin, norepinephrine, or epinephrine with cautious titration. The goal is to keep the blood pressure in a normal range to prepare for the rapid ventricular pacing period. During rapid ventricular pacing, a transvenous pacemaker generates heart rates of 160 to 180 beats per minute. At these heart rates, the mean arterial pressure will be low with minimal pulsation, so the valve placement can be performed without the heart dislodging the new aortic prosthesis before its fixation against the aortic annulus. After placement, the new valve is evaluated, and the ECG is analyzed. If there are no signs indicating a need for permanent pacemaker implantation, the transvenous pacer and central line may be removed.

16. What complications can be expected during the TAVR procedure?
    - Annular rupture (<1%): a life-threatening complication, particularly concerning in patients with heavily calcified aortic annuli. Requires emergent aortic root replacement.
    - Cardiogenic shock (1.1%): especially in patients with low ejection fractions because the rapid ventricular pacing period results in transient cardiac ischemia.
    - Cardiac perforation (1.7%): usually caused by wire manipulation and can result in cardiac tamponade, treated with pericardiocentesis or open surgery.
    - Stroke (5.5%): in the early TAVR trials, the incidence of stroke was greater in TAVR patients than in surgical AVR patients, but recent studies now show that the rates are similar.
    - Vascular complications (6%): usually because of rupture or dissection of the vessels accessed during delivery of the valve, mainly the femoral, iliac, and subclavian arteries, as well as the aorta.
    - Permanent pacemaker implantation (8.5%–25.9%): high-risk patients include preoperative bundle branch block and first- or second-degree atrioventricular block.
    - Paravalvular regurgitation: a common complication, with mild regurgitation in 22.5% and moderate or severe regurgitation in 3.7% of patients. The presence of more than mild aortic regurgitation is associated with increased risk of late mortality.

17. Discuss the pathophysiology of aortic insufficiency.
    In developed countries, acute aortic insufficiency (AI) is most often because of aortic dissection and endocarditis, whereas chronic AI is most commonly because of aortic root or ascending aortic dilation and congenital bicuspid aortic valve. Chronic AI is associated with LV diastolic volume overload because a fraction of the stroke volume regurgitates

Fig. 37.3 Pressure-volume loops in aortic insufficiency compared with the normal loop. In acute aortic insufficiency *(AI)*, the end-diastolic and end-systolic volume is increased. The stroke volume can be increased, normal, or decreased depending on the severity of AI. The left ventricular *(LV)* volume is increasing during the isovolumic relaxation period (*DA* segment) because of regurgitant flow through the aortic valve. The end-diastolic pressure (*AB* segment, *B* point) is high. Contractility is decreased because the myocardium is overstretched. In chronic AI, the end-diastolic, end-systolic, and stroke volumes are enlarged. Cardiac output is normal because of the increased stroke volume and the contractility is decreased. The LV volume is increasing during the isovolumic relaxation period also (*DA* segment), but the end-diastolic pressure (*AB* segment, *B* point) is normal because of ventricular remodeling, which increases ventricular compliance (i.e., eccentric hypertrophy).

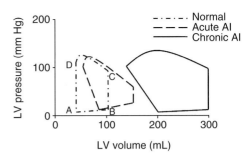

across the incompetent aortic valve in diastole. Patients generally have large end-diastolic volumes and stroke volumes. The volume overload generates high wall tension in diastole, initiating eccentric hypertrophy (dilated left ventricle, with normal or slightly thickened wall). Increasing regurgitant orifice area (area of incompetent valve), slow heart rate (relatively more time spent in diastole), and increased systemic vascular resistance increase the amount of regurgitant flow. Compliance and stroke volume may be markedly increased in chronic AI, whereas contractility gradually diminishes (Fig. 37.3). Patients with chronic AI should undergo valve replacement surgery before the onset of irreversible myocardial damage. In acute AI, the left ventricle is subjected to rapid, massive volume overload with elevated end-diastolic pressure, which can result in acute heart failure and cardiogenic shock. Treatment often requires emergent AVR.

18. **What are the indications for AVR in aortic insufficiency?**
    The indications for AVR in AI according to the 2014 and 2017 (focused update) AHA/ACC guidelines are the following:
    - Symptomatic patients with severe AI
    - Asymptomatic patients with severe AI and an ejection fraction <50%
    - Patients with severe AI undergoing other cardiac surgery
    - AVR is reasonable for:
      - Patients with moderate AI undergoing other cardiac surgery
      - Asymptomatic patients with severe AI and severe LV dilatation.

      Because of the dilated aortic annulus (i.e., aortic root aneurysm), oval-shaped annulus (i.e., bicuspid aortic valve), or noncalcified annulus (i.e., endocarditis, aortic dissection), the use of TAVR is contraindicated for the treatment of AI. Surgical AVR or (less often) aortic valve repair remain the gold standard.

19. **What does the pressure-volume loop look like in acute and chronic aortic insufficiency?**
    See Fig. 37.3.

20. **What are the hemodynamic goals in the anesthetic management of patients with AI?**
    Appropriate preload is necessary for maintenance of forward flow. Modest tachycardia reduces ventricular volumes and limits the time available for regurgitation. Contractility must be maintained with β adrenergic agonists if necessary. Dobutamine can be useful because it does not increase the afterload. Afterload reduction augments forward flow, but additional intravascular volume may be necessary to maintain preload. Increases in afterload result in increasing LV end-diastolic pressure and pulmonary hypertension. In acute AI, the goal is to achieve the lowest tolerable systemic blood pressure to increase the stroke volume and cardiac output (see Table 37.1).

21. **Discuss the hemodynamic changes in patients with AI after AVR.**
    After surgery, LV end-diastolic volume and pressure decrease. Preload may need to be increased by volume administration to maintain filling of a dilated left ventricle. The decreased myocardial contractility may necessitate inotropic support.

22. **What is the pathophysiology of mitral stenosis?**
    Mitral stenosis is usually secondary to rheumatic disease (80%–90%), infective endocarditis (3.3%), and mitral annular calcification (2.7%). Symptoms (fatigue, dyspnea on exertion, lower extremity edema) can be exacerbated when increased cardiac output is needed, as with exercise, pregnancy, illness, and anemia. Critical stenosis of the valve occurs 10 to 20 years after the initial rheumatic disease. As the orifice of the mitral valve narrows, the left atrium experiences pressure overload and enlarges. Left atrial enlargement results in atrial fibrillation and blood stasis, and can cause thrombus formation and systemic embolization. In contrast to other valvular lesions, the left ventricle in patients with mitral stenosis shows relative volume underload because of the obstruction of forward blood flow from the atrium. The elevated atrial pressure may be transmitted to the pulmonary circuit and thus lead to pulmonary edema, pulmonary hypertension, and right-sided heart failure. When the enlarged atrium converts to atrial fibrillation, there is loss of atrial systole, leading to reduced ventricular filling and decreased cardiac output.

23. **What are the indications for mitral valve surgery in mitral stenosis?**
The indications for mitral valve repair or replacement in mitral stenosis according to the 2014 and 2017 (focused update) AHA/ACC guidelines are the following:
- Symptomatic patients with severe mitral stenosis plus:
  - Moderate or severe MR
  - *Or* presence of left atrial thrombus
  - *Or* unfavorable valve morphology for percutaneous mitral balloon valvuloplasty
- Asymptomatic patients with severe mitral stenosis undergoing other cardiac surgery
- Mitral valve repair or replacement is reasonable for:
  - Patients with moderate mitral stenosis undergoing other cardiac surgery

In general, percutaneous mitral balloon valvuloplasty is the treatment of choice for symptomatic moderate or severe mitral stenosis patients (except for the earlier exclusions) because of the slow progression of valvular disease.

In patients who undergo mitral valve surgery, repair of the valve is generally preferred over replacement; however, many stenotic mitral valves are not anatomically suitable for valve repair. In addition, when advanced and/or extensive repair techniques are required to fix a valve with unfavorable anatomy, the long-term results have been questionable and mitral valve replacement may provide improved longevity.

24. **How is the pressure-volume loop changed from normal in mitral stenosis?**
See Fig. 37.4.

25. **What are the anesthetic considerations in mitral stenosis?**
The intravascular volume must be adequate to maintain flow across the stenotic valve. In other words, the pressure in the left atrium needs to be sufficiently high to overcome the resistance of mitral valve stenosis to ensure adequate ventricular filling. However, excessive fluid administration may lead to pulmonary edema, increased pulmonary artery pressure, and increased right ventricular afterload. A lower heart rate is beneficial in allowing more time for blood to flow across the mitral valve into the ventricle. Sinus rhythm should be maintained for adequate filling of the left ventricle, as atrial contraction contributes up to 40% of the stroke volume. Chronic underfilling of the left ventricle leads to depressed ventricular contractility, even after the restoration of normal filling. Negative inotropic agents should be avoided. Any increase in pulmonary vascular resistance because of hypoxemia, hypercarbia, and acidosis should be avoided. This is because the "fragile" right heart might not tolerate any further increase in pulmonary artery pressure, which could lead to right heart failure. For this reason, the respiratory depressant effects of preoperative medications (i.e., midazolam, fentanyl) may be particularly deleterious (see Table 37.1).

26. **Discuss the postoperative management of patients with mitral stenosis after mitral valve surgery or percutaneous mitral balloon valvuloplasty.**
Decline of left atrial pressure decreases pulmonary artery pressure, which decreases right heart afterload, leading to an increase in cardiac output. However, LV function can be depressed because of the chronic underfilling of the left ventricle, especially after cardiopulmonary bypass. Preload augmentation and LV afterload reduction may help improve forward blood flow. Inotropic support may be necessary to improve the systolic performance of the left ventricle.

After balloon valvuloplasty, the gradient through the mitral valve, as well as MR should be evaluated. Severe acute MR is an indication for immediate surgical management.

27. **Describe the pathophysiology of MR.**
Acute MR is most often because of endocarditis, ischemia (papillary muscle rupture caused by myocardial infarction), or, less commonly, trauma. Chronic MR can be primary or secondary and the valvular dysfunction can have normal leaflet motion, excessive leaflet motion, or restricted leaflet motion, all causing MR. Chronic MR with normal leaflet motion can be caused by annular dilation (as in chronic atrial fibrillation and dilated cardiomyopathy) or leaflet perforation (as in endocarditis). Chronic MR with excessive leaflet motion can be caused by elongated or ruptured chordae or leaflets (as in degenerative valve disease, which includes fibroelastic deficiency, Barlow disease, and Marfan syndrome). Chronic MR with restricted leaflet motion can be caused by restriction during both systole and

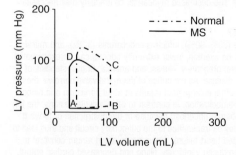

Fig. 37.4 Pressure-volume loop in mitral stenosis *(MS)* compared with the normal loop. The end-diastolic volume, end-systolic volume, and stroke volume are small because of the limited flow into the left ventricle *(LV)*. The LV is at risk for being underfilled (i.e., decreased preload), leading to a decrease in contractility and stroke volume, which generates a lower blood pressure.

diastole (as in rheumatic heart disease and carcinoid heart disease) or restriction during systole alone (as in ischemic or dilated cardiomyopathies).

In acute MR, the left atrium is small and noncompliant and suddenly experiences a marked increase in volume because of the acutely regurgitant mitral valve. This abrupt elevation in left atrial pressure is reflected into the pulmonary circulation, resulting in suddenly increased pulmonary artery pressure and right ventricular pressure. This may precipitate acute pulmonary hypertension, pulmonary edema, and right ventricular failure. In addition, acute MR reduces the afterload for the left ventricle, causing a large portion of the "stroke volume" generated by a nondilated left ventricle to be ejected back into the left atrium, and subsequently a reduced proportion of the LV ejection fraction to be delivered into the aorta. This results in a decrease in cardiac output and possibly cardiogenic shock.

In chronic MR, the left ventricle and atrium become volume overloaded, leading to increased LV end-diastolic volume, with normal end-diastolic pressure. LV end-systolic volume is normal so the stroke volume is high, but part of the stroke volume escapes through the incompetent valve into the left atrium. Ejection fraction is usually high because of the low resistance through the mitral valve. An ejection fraction of 50% or less may indicate significant LV dysfunction. A large compliant left atrium can maintain near-normal left atrial pressure despite large regurgitant volumes. Similar to AI, regurgitant flow in chronic MR depends on regurgitant orifice size, time available for regurgitant flow (i.e., bradycardia), and transvalvular pressure gradient.

28. **What are the indications for mitral valve surgery in mitral regurgitation?**
The indications for mitral valve surgery in MR according to the 2014 and 2017 (focused update) AHA/ACC guidelines are the following:
- Symptomatic patients with severe MR and an ejection fraction greater than 30%.
- Asymptomatic patients with severe MR and an ejection fraction less than 60%.
- Patients with severe MR undergoing other cardiac surgery.
- Mitral valve surgery is reasonable for:
  - Symptomatic patients with severe MR and an ejection fraction of 30% or under.
  - Asymptomatic patients with severe MR and new onset atrial fibrillation or pulmonary hypertension.
  - Patients with moderate MR undergoing other cardiac surgery.
  - Asymptomatic patients with severe MR and preserved LV function, and the likelihood of a successful repair is greater than 95% with an expected mortality rate under 1%.
- MV repair is recommended over MV replacement in patients with primary severe chronic MR who meet the aforementioned indications.
  - However, MV replacement instead of MV repair is reasonable in patients with severe chronic ischemic MR.

29. **How is the pressure-volume loop in mitral regurgitation changed from normal?**
See Fig. 37.5.

30. **What are the hemodynamic goals in anesthetic management of mitral regurgitation?**
The intravascular volume needs to be sufficient to fill the dilated left ventricle. Bradycardia should be avoided, as it increases the regurgitant volume and decreases the ejected volume into the aorta. A normal or a slightly elevated heart rate helps to decrease the regurgitant flow volume. Afterload reduction helps to augment forward flow and to decrease regurgitation. An inotropic agent, such as dobutamine or milrinone, can help maintain contractility and reduce afterload to maintain forward flow. As in mitral stenosis, drugs and maneuvers that increase pulmonary vascular resistance should be avoided (see Table 37.1).

31. **Discuss the postoperative management of patients with mitral regurgitation after mitral valve surgery.**
Once the valve is working appropriately (either repaired or replaced), the left ventricle has to eject the full stroke volume into the aorta. This immediate pressure load increases LV tension and may compromise the ejection fraction. Therefore inotropic support may be necessary, until the left ventricle can adjust to the new hemodynamic condition. Preload should be augmented to fill the dilated left ventricle.

Fig. 37.5 Pressure-volume loop in mitral regurgitation *(MR)* compared with the normal loop. In acute MR, the end-diastolic volume increases with a higher end-diastolic pressure. Total overall stroke volume (SV) is increased, but the actual SV ejected into the aorta is decreased because of a fraction of the left ventricular *(LV)* volume regurgitating into the left atrium during the isovolumic contraction period *(BC* segment). This causes the end-systolic volume to be less than normal because part of the SV is flowing back into the low-pressure left atrium. In chronic MR, the end-diastolic volume is high with normal end-diastolic pressure because of the chronic myocardial remodeling process, causing the LV to be more compliant. The end-systolic volume is larger than normal. The markedly increased SV preserves forward cardiac output, despite significant regurgitation. Contractility is decreased.

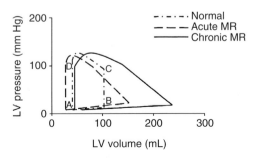

32. Describe the role of transcatheter mitral valve procedures in the treatment of mitral valve regurgitation.

Currently, the only US Food and Drug Administration approved transcatheter treatment for mitral valve disease is the MitraClip. This procedure is performed via a catheter through the femoral vein, which punctures the interatrial septum and places one or more clips, securing a portion of the anterior leaflet of the mitral valve to the posterior leaflet, reducing the degree of regurgitation. Results of MitraClip studies show an acute decrease in MR in most patients; however, a large portion of these patients return with moderately severe or severe regurgitation by 30 days postprocedure. The major difficulty with transcatheter treatment of mitral disease is the higher complexity of the mitral valve apparatus versus the aortic valve. Therefore numerous transcatheter devices and strategies are currently undergoing testing in trials, but it is unclear if these will have the success that TAVR has earned.

The indication for transcatheter mitral valve repair in MR according to the 2014 and 2017 (focused update) AHA/ACC guidelines is the following:

- Severely symptomatic patients with severe MR who have a reasonable life expectancy, but a prohibitively high surgical risk because of severe comorbidities.

33. Discuss the valve replacement options for aortic and mitral valve diseases.

For both aortic and mitral diseases, mechanical prostheses and bovine or porcine stented prostheses are the most commonly used valves. Traditionally, mechanical valves are used more often in younger patients (<60 years old) and biological valves are used in older patients (>70 years old), but each valve has its advantages and disadvantages. Patients with mechanical valves require anticoagulation and have a higher risk of bleeding, as well as thromboembolic events; however, the likelihood of undergoing another valve replacement is less than that in patients with biological valves. Overall, long-term survival for either valve replacement option is similar and the choice in prosthesis is decided by the patient.

KEY POINTS: VALVULAR HEART DISEASE

1. Hemodynamic goals in AS include maintaining intravascular volume, contractility, systemic vascular resistance, normal sinus rhythm, and a slightly lower heart rate. Dysrhythmias associated with hypotension, such as atrial fibrillation require emergent cardioversion.
2. Hemodynamic goals in AI include augmenting preload, maintaining contractility, maintaining normal or elevated heart rate, and reducing afterload.
3. Hemodynamic goals in mitral stenosis include maintaining intravascular volume, afterload, sinus rhythm, and a slower heart rate. Avoid hypoxemia, hypercarbia, and acidosis because they may increase pulmonary vascular resistance. This includes avoiding preoperative respiratory depressant medications (e.g., opioids, benzodiazepines).
4. Hemodynamic goals in MR include maintaining intravascular volume, contractility, and elevated heart rate, while reducing afterload. As in mitral stenosis, avoid situations that will increase pulmonary vascular resistance.
5. Anesthetic management in patients undergoing TAVR is similar to that of patients having aortic valve surgery. A unique part of the procedure is the rapid pacing, which generates a low output state for the valve placement.

Website
Online STS risk calculator: http://riskcalc.sts.org

SUGGESTED READINGS

Nishimura RA, Otto CM, Bonow RO, et al. AHA/ACC focused update of the 2014 AHA/ACC guideline for the management of patients with valvular heart disease: a report of the American College of Cardiology/American Heart Association Task Force on Clinical Practice Guidelines. Circulation 2017;135(25):e1159–e1195.

Nishimura RA, Otto CM, Bonow RO, et al. AHA/ACC guideline for the management of patients with valvular heart disease: a report of the American College of Cardiology/American Heart Association Task Force on Practice Guidelines. J Thorac Cardiovasc Surg. 2014;148(1): e1–e132.

Leon MB, Smith CR, Mack MJ, et al. Transcatheter or surgical aortic-valve replacement in intermediate-risk patients. N Engl J Med. 2016;374(17):1609–1620.

David TE, Armstrong S, Maganti M. Hancock II bioprosthesis for aortic valve replacement: the gold standard of bioprosthetic valves durability? Ann Thorac Surg. 2010;90(3):775–781.

Reardon MJ, Van Mieghem NM, Popma JJ, et al. Surgical or transcatheter aortic-valve replacement in intermediate-risk patients. N Engl J Med. 2017;376(14):1321–1331.

Whitlow PL, Feldman T, Pedersen WR, et al. Acute and 12-month results with catheter-based mitral valve leaflet repair: the EVEREST II (Endovascular Valve Edge-to-Edge Repair) High Risk Study. J Am Coll Cardiol. 2012;59(2):130–139.

CHAPTER 38

PULMONARY HYPERTENSION

Samuel Gilliland, MD, Nathaen Weitzel, MD

1. **Define pulmonary hypertension and pulmonary artery hypertension.**
   - Pulmonary hypertension (PH) refers to a mean pulmonary arterial pressure ($>$25 mm Hg) from any cause.
   - Pulmonary artery hypertension (World Health Organization [WHO] group 1) was previously referred to as *primary pulmonary hypertension*. Pulmonary artery hypertension (PAH) is defined by a mean pulmonary artery pressure (PAP) over 25 mm Hg at rest, with a pulmonary capillary wedge pressure (PCWP) of 15 mm Hg or lower, and a pulmonary vascular resistance (PVR) greater than 3 Wood units.

2. **List the WHO classifications of pulmonary hypertension**
   See Table 38.1.

3. **How is PVR calculated? What are normal values?**

$$PVR = (mPAP - PCWP)/CO$$

   PCWP reflects the left atrial pressure, which reflects the left ventricular end-diastolic pressure. The cardiac output (CO) is used as substitute for pulmonary blood flow in the aforementioned equation. Note, that the mean PAP (mPAP) is used to calculate PVR. A PVR greater than 3 Wood units (or $>$240 dyn $\cdot$ sec/cm^5) is abnormal and consistent with a diagnosis of PAH (WHO group I). Pulmonary and systemic vascular resistance is often given with the units of dyn $\cdot$ sec/cm^5, where 1 Wood unit equals 80 dyn $\cdot$ sec/cm^5.

4. **What is cor pulmonale?**
   Cor pulmonale is right ventricular (RV) failure as a result of elevated PAP.

5. **What is Eisenmenger syndrome?**
   Eisenmenger syndrome is the result of a chronic left-to-right shunt inducing PAH from remodeling, with eventual reversal of shunt flow (right-to-left). It may also be seen in arterial or ventricular septal defects, patent ductus arteriosus, or truncus arteriosus. Eisenmenger syndrome implies a fixed PVR.

6. **What is hypoxic pulmonary vasoconstriction?**
   Hypoxic pulmonary vasoconstriction (HPV) is the diversion of blood flow to segments of the lung, which are better oxygenated by constriction of pulmonary vessels supplying poorly oxygenated segments, thereby optimizing ventilation/perfusion ($\dot{V}/\dot{Q}$) matching. This is in contrast to tissues elsewhere in the body, where vasodilation occurs in the presence of hypoxemia. HPV reduces intrapulmonary shunt and increases the oxygen content of blood exiting the lung into the left atrium. PAP increases when many lung segments vasoconstrict because of HPV, which is the mechanism by which hypoxemia increases PVR.

7. **Discuss the pathophysiology and natural history of pulmonary hypertension.**
   Endothelial cell injury leads to an imbalance between vasodilator and vasopressor molecules. This is characterized as a reduction in endogenous vasodilators (nitric oxide [NO] and prostacyclin [PGI$_2$]) and an increase in vasoconstrictors (thromboxane and endothelin). Vasoconstriction appears to be only part of the answer; however, because thrombosis, inflammation, free radical generation, and smooth muscle hyperplasia are also common features found in PH. Vascular remodeling is a prominent feature of PH. The pulmonary circulation normally has high flow and low resistance. Changes in CO, airway pressure, and gravity affect the pulmonary circulation more than the systemic circulation. The right ventricle is thin walled and accommodates changes in volume better than changes in pressure. To accommodate increases in flow, for example during exercise, unopened vessels are recruited, patent vessels distended, and PVR may decrease. Normal adaptive mechanisms can accommodate a 3- to 5-fold increase in flow without significant increases in PAPs.

   Early in the evolution of PH, the pressure overload results in hypertrophy of the right ventricle, without significant changes in CO or RV filling pressures. As the disease progresses, the vessel walls thicken, and smooth muscle cells proliferate. Vessels become less distensible, and the actual cross-sectional area of the pulmonary circulation decreases. The CO eventually declines, despite modest increases in RV end-diastolic pressure (RVEDP). Mechanisms for enhancing contractility are limited, because the right ventricle is highly compliant and easily distensible, it is susceptible to overdistention causing the right ventricle to operate on the opposite, downsloping side of the Frank-Starling curve. RV failure worsens and patients become symptomatic even at rest. RV myocardial blood flow becomes compromised. Tricuspid regurgitation often develops secondary to right ventricle distention worsening RV failure. In addition, left ventricular (LV) filling may be compromised by excessive septal incursion into the left ventricle, with a resultant decrease in CO.

Table 38.1 WHO Classification of Pulmonary Hypertension (PH)

I	Idiopathic pulmonary artery hypertension (IPAH)—formerly primary pulmonary hypertension
	Familial (FPAH)
	Associated (APAH)—secondary or associated with connective tissue disorders, congenital systemic to pulmonary shunts, portal hypertension, human immunodeficiency virus infection, drugs, toxins, metabolic disorders, including thyroid disorders, glycogen storage disease, Gaucher disease, hereditary hemorrhagic telangiectasia, hemoglobinopathies, chronic myeloproliferative disorders, splenectomy, chronic hemolytic anemia
	Associated with significant venous or capillary involvement
	Persistent PH of the newborn
II	PH with left-sided heart disease—left atrial, ventricular systolic or diastolic dysfunction, aortic or mitral valvular disease, restrictive cardiomyopathy, constrictive pericarditis, left atrial myxoma
III	PH associated with lung diseases—chronic obstructive pulmonary disease, interstitial lung disease, obstructive sleep apnea, alveolar hypoventilation disorders, chronic high-altitude disease
IV	PH caused by chronic thromboembolic disease—thrombotic pulmonary embolism, tumor, infection
V	Miscellaneous—myeloproliferative disorders, sarcoidosis, histiocytosis X, lymphangiomatosis, exterior compression of pulmonary, sickle cell disease

8. What symptoms suggest pulmonary hypertension?
   - Dyspnea
   - Angina (50% of patients)
   - Fatigue (20% of patients)
   - Weakness
   - Syncope

9. What signs suggest pulmonary hypertension?
   Cyanosis, clubbing, peripheral venous insufficiency, edema, rales, hepatomegaly, ascites, increase in the pulmonic component of S2 (pulmonic valve closure), RV S3 or S4 heart sound (RV hypertrophy), holosystolic murmur louder with inspiration (tricuspid regurgitation), RV heave, jugular V waves (tricuspid regurgitation), jugular A waves (decreased RV compliance).

10. What are some electrocardiographic and radiological features of the disease?
    The electrocardiogram commonly shows right axis deviation, RV hypertrophy (tall R waves in V1–V3), RV strain (T-wave inversion in V1–V3), S wave in V6, and enlarged P waves in II, III, and aVF. Dysrhythmias, such as atrial fibrillation, are problematic because the right ventricle loses atrial kick.
    Abnormalities on chest radiograph include prominence of the right ventricle, right atrium, increased right-sided heart border and the hilar pulmonary artery (PA) trunk, rapid tapering of vascular markings, a hyperlucent lung periphery, peripheral hypovascularity, and decrease in the retrosternal air space.

11. What is the gold standard for evaluating pulmonary hypertension?
    Right-sided heart catheterization, using a PA catheter, is the gold standard for confirming the diagnosis of PH, because it directly measures the pulmonary pressure, the wedge pressure, and CO, which are all needed to calculate PVR. An elevated wedge pressure is an indication for further testing to rule out left-sided heart pathology as a cause of PH. Vasoreactivity tests can be performed during right-sided heart catheterization to determine which drug therapies are effective.

12. What are echocardiographic signs of pulmonary hypertension?
    Echocardiographic features of PH include RV dilation and/or hypokinesis, small LV dimension, abnormal septal motion, thickened interventricular septum, RV pressure overload (paradoxical bulging/flattening of septum into LV, RV hypertrophy), right atrial (RA) dilation, and tricuspid regurgitation (TR) secondary to RV dilation.

13. How do you calculate the PAP using echocardiography?
    See Figs. 38.1 and 38.2.
    - The right ventricular systolic pressure (RVSP) is calculated, which is essentially the equivalent of systolic pulmonary artery pressure (sPAP).
    - The RVSP can be calculated as follows: $RVSP = 4 \times TRV^2 + RA$.
    - This equation is derived from the Bernoulli equation, which states the pressure gradient is equal to the velocity squared multiplied by four: $\triangle P = 4 \times Velocity^2$
    - TRV is tricuspid regurgitant jet velocity.

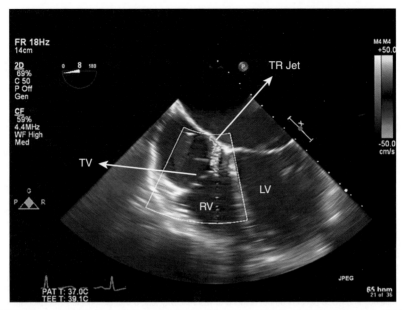

Fig. 38.1 Midesophageal four-chamber view with color Doppler on the tricuspid valve. *LV,* Left ventricle; *RV,* right ventricle; *TR Jet,* tricuspid regurgitant jet; *TV,* tricuspid valve.

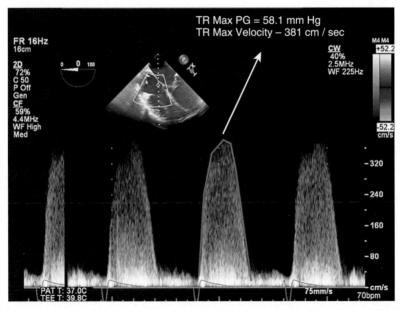

Fig. 38.2 Continuous wave Doppler tracing of tricuspid regurgitant *(TR)* jet and measured tricuspid regurgitant velocity (TRV). To calculate the right ventricular systolic pressure (RVSP), use the Bernoulli equation: RVSP = 4 × TRV^2 + RAP. In this example, convert the 381 cm/sec to 3.81 m/sec and use this value for the velocity. Assuming a normal right atrial pressure (RAP) of 10 mm Hg, the calculated RVSP (or sPAP) would be 68 mm Hg.

- RAP is RA pressure (estimated on echo by inferior vena cava diameter, by examination using jugular venous pressure, or taken from direct hemodynamic measurement).
- An RVSP over 40 means PH is likely and depending upon the situation may warrant further evaluation (i.e., right heart catheterization).
- The RVSP is an indirect not a direct measurement and is susceptible to error (e.g., inaccurate RAP assessment, Doppler interrogation beam angle not correctly aligned with tricuspid jet, small errors measuring TRV produce large errors when squared, it assumes sPAP = RVSP).
- This method cannot be used if there is no tricuspid regurgitation present.

14. **What are the possible treatments for PH (WHO group 1–5)?**
Treatment depends on the cause of PH. Treatment for idiopathic PAH (WHO group 1) is different from treatment of PH with an underlying cause. The following are examples of treatments considered for all WHO groups:
- Anticoagulation is controversial for PH and depends on the underlying cause. Anticoagulation is used more commonly in patients with drug-induced PH or thromboembolic PH (WHO group 4). Note, that data also support its use in idiopathic PAH (WHO group I).
- Diuretics are considered for symptomatic control of RV failure, hepatic congestion, and peripheral edema in patients with PH (WHO groups 1–5). However, excessive diuresis may decrease RV preload and CO.
- Cardiac glycosides (digoxin) are used when there are signs of RV failure and in patients who have developed atrial dysrhythmias (e.g., multifocal atrial tachycardia, atrial fibrillation, or atrial flutter). Serum electrolytes must be closely followed when digoxin is administered to a patient on diuretics.

15. **Discuss therapies for patients suffering from PAH (WHO group 1).**
There is no treatment for the underlying cause of PAH (WHO group 1), so therapies are focused on dilating the pulmonary vasculature to reduce PVR. Patients often undergo right-sided heart catheter vasoreactivity tests to assess for responsiveness of potential treatments. Therapies tested include calcium channel blockers (CBBs), epoprostenol, and NO. If patients do not respond to vasoreactivity test, a trial of endothelin receptor antagonists (bosentan or ambrisentan) or phosphodiesterase (PDE)-5 inhibitors (sildenafil, tadalafil, or vardenafil) may be considered.

16. **Discuss therapies for patients suffering from pulmonary hypertension in WHO groups 2 through 5.**
In PH (WHO groups 2–5), therapy is first directed at the underlying cause to prevent progression of PH. Therapies that improve PAH (WHO group 1) are not always beneficial for PH from other known causes. For example, epoprostenol improves survival for WHO group 1, but may increase mortality for WHO groups 2 and 3 by causing $\dot{V}/\dot{Q}$ mismatch, worsening left-sided heart failure, increased hypoxemia, or pulmonary edema.
- WHO group 2: Medical and surgical treatment of underlying left-sided heart disease is helpful in reducing PAP (e.g., mitral valve repair).
- WHO group 3: Patients with severe chronic obstructive pulmonary disease causing PH, oxygen therapy to raise arterial partial oxygen pressure (PaO_2) is correlated with improved survival. It is administered to maintain oxygen saturation greater than 90%.
- WHO group 4: Treatment includes anticoagulation and surgical thromboendarterectomy
- WHO group 5: Treat underlying causes

17. **What are some surgical therapies for patients suffering from pulmonary hypertension?**
- Thromboendarterectomy
- Atrial septostomy: Creation of right-to-left interatrial shunt that relieves right-sided heart filling pressures. Creating a shunt decreases systemic arterial saturation but improves CO. It is reserved for treating critically ill PAH patients and is often a bridge to transplant. It is associated with a high morbidity and mortality.
- RV assist device: Various models of assist devices can be used in RV failure and should be considered a bridge to transplant. There are no mechanical support devices currently approved for destination therapy in right-sided heart failure.
- Extracorporeal membrane oxygenation: A bridge to transplant.
- Bilateral lung or heart-lung transplantation is the final treatment option for selected patients with PH. Three-year survival is approximately 50%.

18. **Describe calcium channel blocker use in PAH.**
Examples of CCBs include nifedipine, diltiazem, and amlodipine. Some patients with PAH respond with PA vasodilation in response to CCB in right-sided heart catheterization vasoreactivity tests. Those patients tend to have long-term functional improvement and survival in observational studies. Potential side effects include systemic hypotension and worsening hypoxemia from blunting HPV and worsening $\dot{V}/\dot{Q}$ mismatch.

19. **What are endothelin receptor antagonists?**
Endothelin-1 is a vasoconstrictor and causes PA vasoconstriction. Common endothelin receptor antagonists include bosentan and ambrisentan. Endothelin receptor antagonists have been shown to improve symptoms of PH, but have not been proven to decrease mortality. Adverse effects include hepatotoxicity and peripheral edema.

20. **What are prostanoids and their therapeutic counterparts?**
Patients with PAH have low levels of prostacyclin synthase and prostacyclin. Prostacyclin is a strong vasodilator, and decreased levels cause decreased vasodilation. Prostacyclin also has antiproliferative effects.
   A prostanoid (synthetic prostacyclin analog) acts like prostacyclin and causes vasodilation in the PA and prevents platelet aggregation. Examples of prostanoids include epoprostenol, treprostinil, beraprost, and iloprost. They have been shown to decrease PAP and increase CO. Prostanoids can be inhaled or administered intravenously, subcutaneously, or enterally. Intravenous administration causes more systemic vasodilation and $\dot{V}/\dot{Q}$ mismatch than does the inhalational route. For this reason, the inhalational route is generally preferred in the operating room and the intensive care unit (ICU).
   Epoprostenol is the most studied and commonly used prostanoid. When administered by continuous intravenous infusion, epoprostenol (PGI_2) has a half-life of 2 to 3 minutes. Intravenous prostanoids lack pulmonary selectivity. It can cause systemic hypotension and decreased RV coronary perfusion. Epoprostenol has been shown to prolong survival and improve functional status in patients with PAH (WHO group 1). Epoprostenol may cause increased mortality in PH WHO groups 2 and 3.

21. **Discuss the properties of nitric oxide.**
Nitrous oxide (NO) is a small molecule produced by the vascular endothelium that stimulates guanylate cyclase, which is an enzyme that catalyzes the conversion of guanosine-5′-triphosphate to cyclic guanosine monophosphate (cGMP). The cGMP levels increase, which activates protein kinase G, which acts to decreases intracellular calcium, causing smooth muscle relaxation and vasodilation.
   NO can be administered by inhalation and crosses the alveolar membrane into the vascular endothelium, producing smooth muscle relaxation. In the circulation, it rapidly binds to hemoglobin (with an affinity 1500 times greater than carbon monoxide) and is deactivated; thus it has no systemic vasodilator effect. Because it is only delivered to ventilated alveoli, it increases perfusion to those areas and improves $\dot{V}/\dot{Q}$ matching.

22. **What are phosphodiesterase-5 inhibitors?**
Because PDE-5 degrades cGMP, inhibiting PDE-5 acts to increase cGMP, which causes vasodilation (see previous question). The PDE-5 inhibitors are orally administered vasodilators that potentiate the effect of NO. Currently available PDE inhibitors include sildenafil, tadalafil, and vardenafil. They are synergistic when used in conjunction with NO or prostanoids. PDE-5 inhibitors have not been shown to affect mortality but do improve the functional status of patients with PAH.

23. **What is the concern with PDE-5 inhibitors (e.g., sildenafil) and nitrovasodilators (i.e., nitroglycerin and nitroprusside)?**
Administering nitroprusside or nitroglycerin in patients taking PDE5 inhibitors, such as sildenafil (Viagra), tadalafil (Cialis), and vardenafil (Levitra) should be avoided because this can lead to severe hypotension. This is thought to occur because both nitrovasodilators and PDE5 inhibitors converge on the same pathway through different mechanisms to increase cGMP, an important secondary messenger in promoting vasodilation.

24. **How should a patient with pulmonary hypertension be monitored intraoperatively?**
Intraarterial pressure monitoring is commonly used for patients with moderate to severe PH. It allows real time assessment of blood pressure and allows frequent blood gas analysis. Arterial systolic or pulse pressure variation can be used to assess volume status, although its accuracy has not been validated in PH.
   PA catheters directly monitor PAP and RAP. They allow indirect measurement of LV filling pressure (i.e., preload) by measuring wedge pressures. PA catheters help in differentiating causes of systemic hypotension when PH is present. Patients with PH are at increased risk for PA rupture from PA catheters, and Eisenmenger patients are at even higher risk of rupture. Many consider PA catheter use in patients with Eisenmenger syndrome to be contraindicated.
   Transesophageal echocardiography is useful in assessing volume status, LV and RV performance, valvular regurgitation, and early detection of segmental wall motion abnormalities, secondary to myocardial ischemia.

25. **How do you manage systemic hypotension with pulmonary hypertension using a PA catheter?**
   - Decreased SVR (increased CO, normal CVP, normal or decreased PCWP, normal or increased PAP): Treat the cause of decreased SVR, administer vasopressors and volume.
   - Decrease RV preload (decreased CO, decreased CVP, decreased PCWP, decreased PAP, normal or increased SVR): Treatment is volume.
   - Increased PVR (decreased CO, increased CVP, decreased PCWP, normal or increased PAP): Treat cause of increased PVR (e.g., acidosis, hypercarbia, hypoxia), administer pulmonary vasodilators.
   - Decreased RV contractility (decreased CO, increased CVP, normal PCWP, increased SVR): Reverse cause of decreased contractility, administer inotropes.

26. **What is the concern with excessive RV afterload and preload? How does this cause right heart failure?**
High RVEDP causes the intraventricular septum to shift into the left ventricle, with a subsequent decrease in LV stroke volume. It is important to note that unlike the left ventricle, coronary perfusion to the right ventricle occurs during both systole and diastole. If RV pressure increases during either systole or diastole, perfusion from the coronary

arteries decreases worsening RV contractility. Impaired RV contractility causes the RV diastolic pressure to increase and impairs CO, leading to more hypotension and subsequent decreased RV perfusion from the coronary arteries. Thus a vicious, lethal cycle develops. Further, increased RVEDP can overdistend the right ventricle, causing the right ventricle to operate on the opposite, downsloping side of the Frank-Starling curve, further worsening contractility. Thus too much preload to the "fragile" right ventricle is poorly tolerated, particularly in PH (high afterload).

27. **What is the potential morbidity and mortality for noncardiac surgery on patients with PH?**
    - Mortality (1%–10%)
    - Morbidity (15%–42%)
    - Postoperative respiratory failure (7%–28%)
    - Heart failure (10%–13%)
    - Hemodynamic instability (8%)
    - Dysrhythmias (12%)
    - Renal insufficiency (7%)
    - Sepsis (7%–10%)
    - Ischemia/myocardial infarction (4%)
    - Delayed tracheal extubation (8%–21%)
    - Longer ICU/hospital stay

28. **What intraoperative measures may decrease pulmonary hypertension?**
    - Patients on chronic PH medication should take their PH medication up to and including the day of surgery. Prostaglandin infusions must be continued intraoperatively.
    - Avoid hypoxia, hypercarbia, and acidosis. In contrast to systemic vessels, pulmonary vessels constrict with hypoxia, hypercarbia, and acidosis. Essentially, the role of the systemic circulation is to deliver O_2 and receive CO_2, and this role is reversed in the pulmonary circulation. HPV, which serves to optimize ventilation and flow in the lungs can increase PAP in the presence of hypoxemia, hypercarbia, and acidosis.
    - Assess myocardial performance; increasing PA pressures may be secondary to a failing left ventricle. In the setting of a failing LV, supportive measures for optimizing myocardial oxygen supply and demand should be used, such as reducing heart rate, increasing the diastolic pressure, and providing coronary vasodilation if ischemia is suspected.
    - Inotropic drugs, such as milrinone or dobutamine can improve contractility, provide moderate pulmonary vasodilation, and improve CO. The effects of acidosis on increasing PVR are worse in the presence of hypoxia. Moderate hyperventilation (a $PaCO_2$ of about 30 mm Hg) is suggested to decrease PVR.
    - Ensure adequate preload. Patients with PAH have a fixed afterload and are more preload dependent. However, RV volume overload can shift the intraventricular septum into the left ventricle, decreasing CO, and cause overdistention of the right ventricle, impairing its contractility.
    - Avoid spinal anesthesia, because it can cause a sudden decrease in SVR and preload.
    - Catecholamine release will increase PAP, so adequate depth of anesthesia is needed.
    - If systemic hypotension and coronary perfusion are problematic, vasopressin should be considered as it does not increase PVR, unlike phenylephrine. Norepinephrine increases SVR more than PVR, thereby promotes RV coronary perfusion and is easier to titrate compared with vasopressin because of its short half-life (~90 seconds).
    - Consider the use of direct-acting pulmonary vasodilators, such as inhaled NO (iNO) and epoprostenol for PAH. Recent data suggest these medications are equally efficacious.

29. **What effect does positive end-expiratory pressure have in PH?**
    Recruitment maneuvers decrease atelectasis and improve V̇/Q̇ matching. However, high levels of positive end-expiratory pressure (PEEP) may constrict blood vessels in well-ventilated areas of the lungs, causing increased shunting and decreased PaO_2. Increasing PEEP causes increased intrathoracic pressure and decreases RV preload by decreasing venous return. It also increases RV afterload, which can exacerbate PH. Thus PEEP must be carefully optimized in these patients, and increasing fraction of inspired oxygen may be better than high PEEP to improve PaO_2, in patients with PAH.

30. **Discuss the effect of volatile anesthetics and nitrous oxide on the pulmonary pressure.**
    Volatile anesthetics (isoflurane, desflurane, sevoflurane) cause vasodilation and decreased PAP. High concentrations of volatiles can cause V̇/Q̇ mismatch by blunting HPV and can lead to hypoxemia. Volatile anesthetics should be titrated carefully, because impaired RV function is a risk with higher concentrations. Nitrous oxide can increase PVR because of its effect in worsening hypoxemia, also known as *diffusion hypoxia*.

31. **What are the effects of intravenous anesthetics on PAP?**
    - Etomidate does not change SVR, PVR, or contractility, so it is often used for patients with PH. Etomidate is associated with adrenal suppression and must be used with caution, especially in the critically ill.
    - Propofol infusions have been shown to decrease PVR, SVR, and contractility.

- Opioids do not have a direct vasodilator effect but may attenuate the vasoconstrictor effect of noxious pain stimuli, preventing increased PAP. Respiratory depression can lead to hypercapnia and cause increased PAP in spontaneously breathing patients.
- Ketamine increases PVR and is not ideal for PH. In children with intracardiac shunts, ketamine may prevent reversal of left-to-right shunts because it increases systemic vascular resistance to a greater extent than PVR.

32. **Is neuraxial anesthesia an option?**

Epidural anesthesia has been used safely in patients with PH. Acute changes in SVR associated with spinal anesthesia suggest that epidural anesthesia is preferred. Invasive monitoring is still suggested. Loss of cardioaccelerator fibers from T1 to T4 may result in undesirable bradycardia. Ensure adequate preload before neuraxial anesthesia and have medications to treat acute decreases in SVR or heart rate immediately available.

Many PH patients take anticoagulants, so this must be taken into account when performing regional anesthesia. Regional anesthesia is a useful adjunct for postoperative pain control and avoids the use of narcotics.

33. **List potential surgeries that pose the risk of increasing pulmonary hypertension.**

- Liver transplantation: microembolization and large volume infusion may overwhelm the right side of the heart and cause increased PH.
- Hip replacement: bone cement implantation syndrome occurs when many small pulmonary embolisms of cement, bone, and air occur during placement of prosthesis.
- Laparoscopic procedures: inflation of CO_2 can cause hypercapnia, as well as a rapid decline in RV preload.

34. **What is the role of vasopressors and inotropes in managing pulmonary hypertension?**

The goal is to maintain systemic pressures above pulmonary pressures to ensure coronary artery perfusion to the right ventricle. The right coronary artery perfuses the right ventricle during systole and diastole; therefore elevated preload or afterload can impair right heart perfusion. A decrease in the normal coronary perfusion pressure gradient to the right heart can cause ischemia to the right ventricle, with a subsequent increase in RVEDP, leading into a downward spiral (Table 38.2).

35. **Why is it recommended to avoid pregnancy in pulmonary hypertension?**

The mortality rate during pregnancy with PH is 30% to 50%. Avoiding pregnancy is commonly recommended to patients with PH. Pregnancy is associated with a significant increase in circulating blood volume and CO, which are poorly tolerated with PH. This is especially true during the peripartum period, which includes several months after delivery.

Table 38.2 Vasoactive Agents in Pulmonary Hypertension

AGENT	MECHANISM OF ACTION	NOTES
Norepinephrine	$\alpha_1 > \beta_1$ agonist	An effective vasopressor in acute RV failure, increases SVR > PVR and so favors RV perfusion, while supporting CO More pronounced increase in PVR at higher doses, >0.5 mcg/kg/min in animal studies
Phenylephrine	α_1 agonist	Increases PVR, leading to increased RV afterload
Vasopressin	V_1 agonist	Increases SVR with no change in PVR, thus decreasing PVR/SVR ratio Vasopressin is useful in vasodilatory shock with PH
Dopamine	$D_1, D_2, \beta_1, \alpha_1$ agonist	Increases CO, without increasing PVR. Side effects include tachycardia and dysrhythmias that preclude its use in cardiogenic shock
Dobutamine	$\beta_1 > \beta_2$ agonist	Increases contractility and CO, while decreasing PVR and SVR. Less chronotropic effect than dopamine
Milrinone	PDE III Inhibitor	Decreases PVR, SVR, and increases CO
Epinephrine	$\beta_1 \geq \beta_2 \geq \alpha_1$	Increases CO. Decreases PVR/SVR ratio
Isoproterenol	$\beta_1 = \beta_2$ agonist	Used as a chronotrope in denervated hearts (cardiac transplant). Also associated with dysrhythmias

CO, Cardiac output; *PDE*, phosphodiesterase; *PH*, pulmonary hypertension; *PVR*, pulmonary vascular resistance; *RV*, right ventricular; *SVR*, systemic vascular resistance.

KEY POINTS: PULMONARY HYPERTENSION

1. Milrinone is an effective drug in decreasing PVR and increasing CO.
2. Epoprostenol and nitric oxide are effective intraoperative medications to decrease PVR.
3. Hypoxia, hypercarbia, and acidosis increase PVR.
4. Vasopressin increases SVR without increasing PVR. Norepinephrine increases SVR > PVR and is thus also useful in PAH.
5. Nonselective vasodilators (e.g., CCBs, nitroglycerine, nitroprusside, volatile anesthetics) can cause hypoxemia by blunting HPV.
6. Unlike the left ventricle, coronary perfusion to the right ventricle occurs during both systole and diastole. Therefore elevations in afterload or preload to the right ventricle can decrease coronary perfusion, which can cause ischemia and right heart failure.

Suggested Readings

Gille J, Seyfarth HJ, Gerlach S, et al. Perioperative anesthesiological management of patients with pulmonary hypertension. Anesthesiol Res Pract. 2012(2012):356982.

McLaughlin VV, Archer SL, Badesch DB, et al. Accf/Aha 2009 Expert Consensus Document on Pulmonary Hypertension: a report of the American College of Cardiology Foundation Task Force on Expert Consensus Documents and the American Heart Association: Developed in Collaboration with the American College of Chest Physicians, American Thoracic Society, Inc., and the Pulmonary Hypertension Association. Circulation. 2009;119(16):2250–2294.

Minai OA, Yared JP, Kaw R, et al. Perioperative risk and management in patients with pulmonary hypertension. Chest. 2013;144(1):329–340.

Pilkington SA, Taboada D, Martinez G. Pulmonary hypertension and its management in patients undergoing non-cardiac surgery. Anaesthesia. 2015;70(1):56–70.

Westerhof BE, Saouti N, van der Laarse WJ, et al. Treatment strategies for the right heart in pulmonary hypertension. Cardiovasc Res. 2017;113(12):1465–1473.

CHAPTER 39

OBSTRUCTIVE LUNG DISEASE: ASTHMA AND CHRONIC OBSTRUCTIVE PULMONARY DISEASE

Alma N. Juels, MD, Howard J. Miller, MD

1. **Define reactive airway disease.**

   The term *reactive airway disease (RAD)* is used to describe a family of diseases that share the common characteristic of airway sensitivity to physical, chemical, or pharmacological stimuli. This sensitivity results in a bronchoconstrictor response throughout the tracheobronchial tree and is seen in patients with asthma, chronic obstructive pulmonary disease (COPD), emphysema, viral upper respiratory illness, and some other respiratory disorders.

2. **What is asthma and what are the different types of asthma?**

   Asthma is airway hyperactivity and inflammation. There are two subgroups that respond well to bronchodilator treatment, allergic and idiosyncratic. Allergic asthma is thought to result from an immunoglobulin E–mediated response to antigens, such as dust and pollen. Among the mediators released are histamine, leukotrienes, prostaglandins, bradykinin, thromboxane, and eosinophilic chemotactic factor. Their release leads to inflammation, airway capillary leakage, increased mucus secretion, and bronchial smooth muscle contraction. Idiosyncratic asthma is mediated by nonantigenic stimuli, including exercise, cold, pollution, and infection. Bronchospasm results from increased parasympathetic (vagal) tone. Although the primary stimulus differs, the same mediators as those in allergic asthma are released (also note: some patients with allergic asthma have enhanced vagal tone).

   Asthmatic bronchitis can develop from the progression of asthma or chronic bronchitis, where the patient always has some degree of airway obstruction and is less responsive to bronchodilator treatment.

3. **What are the important historical features of an asthmatic patient?**
   - Duration of disease
   - Frequency, initiating factors, and duration of attacks
   - Does the patient cough at night?
   - Has the patient ever required inpatient therapy? Did the patient ever require intensive care unit admission or intubation?
   - What are the patient's medications, including daily and as-needed usage, over-the-counter medications, and steroids?

4. **What symptoms and physical findings are associated with asthma?**

   Common symptoms include coughing, shortness of breath, and tightness in the chest. The most common physical finding is expiratory wheezing. Wheezing is a sign of obstructed airflow and is often associated with a prolonged expiratory phase. As asthma progressively worsens, patients use accessory respiratory muscles. A significantly symptomatic patient, with quiet auscultatory findings, may signal impending respiratory failure because not enough air is moving to elicit a wheeze. Patients may also be tachypneic and probably are dehydrated; they prefer an upright posture and demonstrate pursed-lip breathing. Cyanosis is a late and ominous sign.

5. **Describe the mainstays of therapy in asthma patients (Table 39.1).**

   The mainstay of therapy remains inhaled β-adrenergic agonists. Selective short-acting β2 agonists, such as albuterol and terbutaline, offer greater β2-mediated bronchodilation and fewer side effects (e.g., β1-associated tachydysrhythmias and tremors). Albuterol can be nebulized, administered orally or by metered-dose inhaler (MDI). Terbutaline is effective via nebulizer, subcutaneously, or as a continuous intravenous (IV) infusion. Note that β2 agonists may result in hypokalemia, lactic acidosis, and cardiac tachydysrhythmias, particularly with IV use. Patients with coronary artery disease may have particular difficulty with tachycardia and need β2- specific agents given via the inhaled route. Long-acting β2 agonists, such as salmeterol and formoterol, are used for chronic dosing and are sometimes paired with a steroid. Lastly, epinephrine is available for subcutaneous use in severely asthmatic patients.

6. **What other medications and routes of delivery are used in asthma (see Table 39.1)?**
   - Corticosteroids: reverse airway inflammation, decrease mucus production, and potentiate β-agonist–induced smooth muscle relaxation. Steroids are strongly recommended in patients with moderate to severe asthma or in

Table 39.1 Agents Used to Treat Reactive Airway Disease

CLASS AND EXAMPLES	DOSE	ACTIONS
β-Adrenergic agonists: albuterol, metaproterenol, fenoterol, terbutaline, epinephrine	2.5 mg in 3 mL of normal saline for nebulization, or 2 puffs by MDI Terbutiline dose is 0.3–0.4 mg subcutaneously Epinephrine dose is 0.3 mg subcutaneously, 5–10 mcg IV	Increases adenylate cyclase, increasing cAMP and decreasing smooth muscle tone (bronchodilation); short-acting β-adrenergic agonists (e.g., albuterol, terbutaline, and epinephrine) are the agents of choice for acute exacerbations
Methylxanthines: aminophylline, theophylline	5 mg/kg IV over 30 minutes as a loading dose	Phosphodiesterase inhibition increases cAMP; potentiates endogenous catecholamines; improves diaphragmatic contractility; central respiratory stimulant
Corticosteroids: methylprednisolone, dexamethasone, prednisone, cortisol	Methylprednisolone, 60–125 IV every 6 hours; or prednisone 30–50 mg orally daily	Antiinflammatory and membrane stabilizing; inhibits histamine release; potentiates β agonists
Anticholinergics: atropine, glycopyrrolate, ipratropium	Ipratropium, 0.5 mg by nebulization or 4–6 puffs by MDI; Atropine, 1–2 mg per nebulization	Blocks acetylcholine at postganglionic receptors, decreasing cGMP, relaxing airway smooth muscle
Cromolyn sodium		Also a membrane stabilizer, preventing mast cell degranulation, but must be given prophylactically
Antileukotrienes: zileuton, montelukast		Inhibition of leukotriene production and/or zafirlukast, leukotriene antagonism; antiinflammatory; used in addition to corticosteroids; however, may be considered first-line antiinflammatory therapy for patients who cannot or will not use corticosteroids

cAMP, Cyclic adenosine monophosphate; *cGMP*, cyclic guanosine monophosphate; *IV*, intravenously; *MDI*, metered-dose inhaler.

patients who have required steroids in the past 6 months. Onset of action is 1 to 2 hours after administration. Methylprednisolone is popular because of its strong antiinflammatory but weak mineralocorticoid effects. Side effects include hyperglycemia, hypertension, hypokalemia, and mood alterations, including psychosis. Long-term steroid use is associated with myopathy. Steroids may be given orally, via MDI, or intravenously.
- Anticholinergic agents: produce bronchodilation by blocking muscarinic cholinergic receptors in the airway, therefore attenuating bronchoconstriction resulting from inhaled irritants (and, occasionally, β-blocker therapy). They are commonly prescribed to patients with severe airway obstruction (predicted forced expiratory volume in 1 second [FEV_1] <25%) and in COPD. Ipratropium, glycopyrrolate, and atropine may be given via nebulizer, and ipratropium is available in an MDI.
- Leukotriene receptor antagonists: act by inhibition of the 5-lipoxygenase pathway or antagonism of the cysteinyl-leukotriene type 1 receptors. They are commonly prescribed and may be used in conjunction with inhaled steroids.
- Cromolyn sodium: a mast cell stabilizer useful for long-term maintenance therapy. Patients younger than 17 years of age and with moderate to severe exercise-induced asthma appear to benefit the most. Administered via MDI, side effects include some minimal local irritation on delivery. Cromolyn sodium is not indicated for acute asthmatic attacks.

7. **What preoperative tests, if any, should be ordered?**
The patient's history guides the judicious ordering of preoperative tests. A mild asthmatic patient maintained on as-needed medication and currently healthy will not benefit from preoperative testing. Symptomatic patients with no recent evaluation may merit closer attention.

The most common test is a pulmonary function test (PFT), which allows simple and quick evaluation of the degree of obstruction and its reversibility. A comparison of values obtained from the patient with predicted values aids assessment of degree of obstruction. Severe exacerbation correlates with a peak expiratory flow rate (PEFR) or FEV_1 of less than 30% to 50% of predicted. In most adults, this is a PEFR of less than 120 L/min and an FEV_1 of less than 1 L. Tests should be repeated after a trial of bronchodilator therapy to assess reversibility and response to treatment.

Arterial blood gases are usually not helpful. Electrocardiograms, chest radiographs, and blood counts are rarely indicated for evaluation of asthma, unless particular features of the patient's presentation suggest alternative diagnoses (e.g., fever and rales, suggesting pneumonia).

8. **What induction agents are indicated for asthmatic patients?**
IV induction agents used in asthmatic patients include propofol and ketamine. Ketamine has well-known bronchodilatory effects secondary to release of endogenous catecholamines, with β2-agonist effects. Ketamine also has a small, direct relaxant effect on smooth muscle. Propofol decreases both airway resistance and airway reflexes after administration. IV lidocaine is a useful adjunct for blunting the response to laryngoscopy and intubation.
Mask induction with sevoflurane is an excellent method to block airway reflexes and to relax airway smooth muscles directly. This agent is much more palatable to the airway than isoflurane or desflurane.

9. **What are the complications of intubation in asthmatic patients?**
The stimulus of intubation (and the presence of the endotracheal tube) causes significant increases in airway resistance and, in severely asthmatic patients, may precipitate a bronchospastic crisis. As a result, deep extubation (removal of the endotracheal tube, while the patient is breathing spontaneously, but still under general anesthesia) is a commonly used strategy to facilitate a smooth emergence. Deep extubations should be avoided in patients with difficult airways, who are morbidly obese, or who may be at risk for aspiration.

10. **Define COPD.**
COPD encompasses a spectrum of diseases that includes emphysema, chronic bronchitis, and asthmatic bronchitis. It is characterized by progressively increased resistance to breathing. Airflow limitation may result from loss of elastic recoil or obstruction of small or large (or both) conducting airways. This increased resistance may have some degree of reversibility. Cardinal symptoms are cough, dyspnea, and wheezing.

11. **Describe chronic bronchitis and emphysema.**
   - Chronic bronchitis: Characterized by cough, sputum production, recurrent infection, and airway obstruction for a period of many months to several years. Patients with chronic bronchitis have mucous gland hyperplasia, mucus plugging, inflammation and edema, peribronchiolar fibrosis, airway narrowing, and bronchoconstriction. Decreased airway lumina caused by mucus and inflammation increase resistance to flow of gases.
   - Emphysema: Characterized by progressive dyspnea and variable cough. Destruction of the elastic and collagen network of alveolar walls without resultant fibrosis leads to abnormal enlargement of air spaces. In addition, the loss of airway support leads to airway narrowing and collapse during exhalation (known as *air trapping*).

12. **What features distinguish pink puffers from blue bloaters?**

Pink Puffers (Emphysema)	Blue Bloaters (Chronic Bronchitis)
Usually older (>60 years)	Relatively young
Pink in color	Cyanotic
Thin	Heavier in weight
Minimal cough	Chronic productive cough; frequent wheeze

13. **List contributory factors associated with the development of COPD.**
   - **Smoking:** Smoking impairs ciliary function, depresses alveolar macrophages; leads to increased mucous gland proliferation and mucus production, increases the inflammatory response in the lung, leads to increased proteolytic enzyme release, reduces surfactant integrity, and causes increased airway reactivity.
   - **Occupational and environmental exposure:** Animal dander, toluene and other chemicals, various grains, cotton, and sulfur dioxide and nitrogen dioxide in air pollution.
   - **Recurrent infection:** Bacterial, atypical organisms (mycoplasma), and viral (including human immunodeficiency virus, which can produce an emphysema-like picture).
   - **Familial and genetic factors:** A hereditary predisposition to COPD exists and is more common in men than women. α_1-Antitrypsin deficiency is a genetic disorder resulting in autodigestion of pulmonary tissue by proteases and should be suspected in younger patients with basilar bullae on chest x-ray film. Smoking accelerates its presentation and progression.

14. **List the common pharmacologic agents used to treat COPD and their mechanisms of action.**
See Table 39.1.

15. **What historical information should be obtained before surgery in patients with COPD?**
   - Smoking history: number of packs per day and duration in years. Use of vape pens and marijuana should be included in the history. Smoking marijuana tends to be worse than cigarettes because it is usually not filtered.
   - Dyspnea, wheezing, productive cough, and exercise tolerance.
   - Prior hospitalizations for RAD, including the need for IV steroids, intubation, and mechanical ventilation.
   - Medications, including home oxygen therapy and steroid use, either systemic or inhaled.
   - Recent pulmonary infections, exacerbations, or change in character of sputum.

- Recent weight loss that may be caused by end-stage pulmonary disease or lung cancer.
- Symptoms of right-sided heart failure, including peripheral edema, hepatomegaly, jaundice, and anorexia, secondary to liver and splanchnic congestion.

16. What laboratory examinations are useful?
    - White cell count and hematocrit: Elevation suggests infection and chronic hypoxemia, respectively.
    - Basic metabolic panel: Bicarbonate levels are elevated to buffer a chronic respiratory acidosis if the patient retains carbon dioxide. Hypokalemia can occur with repeated use of β-adrenergic agonists.
    - Arterial blood gas: Hypoxemia, hypercarbia, and acid-base status, including compensations, can be evaluated.
    - Chest x-ray: Look for lung hyperinflation, bullae or blebs, flattened diaphragm, increased retrosternal air space, atelectasis, cardiac enlargement, infiltrate, effusion, masses, or pneumothorax.
    - Electrocardiogram: Look for decreased amplitude, signs of right atrial (peaked P waves in leads II and V_1) or ventricular enlargement (right axis deviation, R/S ratio in $V_6 \leq 1$, increased R wave in V_1 and V_2, right bundle-branch block), and arrhythmias. Atrial arrhythmias are common, especially multifocal atrial tachycardia and atrial fibrillation.

17. What abnormal physical findings are common in patients with COPD?
    - Tachypnea and use of accessory muscles
    - Distant or focally diminished breath sounds, wheezing, or rhonchi
    - Jugular venous distention, hepatojugular reflux, and peripheral edema suggest right-sided heart failure

18. How does a chronically elevated arterial partial pressure of carbon dioxide affect respiratory drive in a person with COPD?
    Chronically elevated arterial partial pressure of carbon dioxide ($PaCO_2$) results in elevated cerebrospinal fluid (CSF) bicarbonate concentration, increasing CSF pH, and effectively "resetting" the medullary respiratory chemoreceptors to a higher concentration of CO_2. This results in diminished ventilatory drive to elevated CO_2 concentration. In these patients, ventilatory drive may be more responsive to partial pressure of oxygen (PO_2) than $PaCO_2$.

19. How can administering supplemental oxygen lead to hypoxemia in COPD patients?
    Yes. Inhalation of 100% oxygen may increase ventilation-perfusion mismatch by inhibiting hypoxic pulmonary vasoconstriction (HPV) in certain regions of the lung. HPV is an autoregulatory mechanism in the pulmonary vasculature that decreases blood flow to poorly ventilated areas of the lung, ensuring that more blood flow is available for gas exchange in better ventilated areas. Inhibition of HPV results in increased perfusion of poorly ventilated areas, thus contributing to hypoxemia (and hypercarbia). In COPD patients, it is prudent to always administer the minimum amount of supplemental oxygen necessary to achieve the desired pulse oximetry (SpO_2).

20. Explain why the CO_2 may rise when a patient with COPD is given supplemental oxygen.
    - Decreased ventilatory drive, resulting in diminished minute ventilation.
    - Impairment of HPV, decreasing the efficiency of CO_2 elimination.
    - The Haldane Effect. Deoxygenated hemoglobin (Hb) is better at carrying CO_2 than oxygenated Hb. More specifically, reduced (deoxygenated) Hb binds the H^+ ions produced when carbonic acid dissociates, thereby promoting the formation of more carbonic acid from CO_2 and H_2O. Conversely, providing supplemental oxygen increases the amount of oxygen bound to Hb, thereby allowing for more free H^+, which in turn binds HCO_3-, producing CO_2 and H_2O.

21. How do general anesthesia and surgery affect pulmonary mechanics?
    Vital capacity is reduced by up to 25% to 50%, following many general anesthetics and surgical procedures, and residual volume increases. Thoracotomy and upper abdominal incisions affect pulmonary mechanics the greatest, followed by lower abdominal incisions and sternotomy. Atelectasis and hypoventilation are common after surgery, and the incidence of pulmonary infection increases because of decreased mucociliary clearance. Many of these changes take weeks to months to return to their baseline function.

22. What factors are associated with increased perioperative morbidity and/or mortality?
    Increased morbidity results from postoperative hypoxemia, hypoventilation, pulmonary infection, prolonged intubation, and mechanical ventilation. Patients may be risk stratified according to their planned surgery and preoperative PFTs (Table 39.2).

23. What therapies are available to reduce perioperative pulmonary risk?
    - Smoking cessation
        - Cessation for 48 hours before surgery decreases carboxyhemoglobin levels. The oxyhemoglobin dissociation curve shifts to the right, allowing increased tissue oxygen availability.
        - Maximum benefit is obtained if smoking is stopped at least 8 weeks before surgery, with some studies suggesting that cessation less than 8 weeks before surgery is associated with increased risk of postoperative complications. These benefits result from improved pulmonary mechanics and ciliary function, and reduced sputum production.
    - Optimize pharmacologic therapy. Continue medications even on the day of surgery.

Table 39.2 Pulmonary Function Values Associated With Increased Perioperative Mortality/Morbidity

PFT	ABDOMINAL SURGERY	THORACOTOMY	LOBECTOMY/PNEUMONECTOMY
FVC	<70%	<70%	<50% or <2 L
FEV$_1$	<70%	<1 L	<1 L
FEV$_1$/FVC	<50%	<50%	<50%
FEF$_{25-75}$	<50%	<50%	
RV/TLC	40%		
PaCO$_2$	>45–55 mm Hg	>45–50 mm Hg	

Percentages are of predicted values.
FEF$_{25-75}$, Forced expiratory flow in the midexpiratory phase; *FEV$_1$,* forced expiratory volume in 1 second; *FVC,* forced vital capacity; *PaCO$_2$,* arterial partial pressure of carbon dioxide; *PFT,* pulmonary function test; *RV,* residual volume; *TLC,* total lung capacity.

- Recognize and treat underlying pulmonary infections.
- Maximize nutritional support, hydration, and chest physiotherapy.
- Institute effective postoperative analgesia, allowing the patient to cough effectively, take large tidal volumes, and ambulate early after surgery.

24. **Do advantages exist with regional anesthesia techniques in patients with COPD?**
   Yes. Regional anesthesia may obviate the need for general anesthesia in certain procedures. However, spinal or epidural blockade above the T10 dermatome may reduce effective coughing secondary to abdominal muscle dysfunction and lead to atelectasis and decreased sputum clearance. Regional anesthesia of the brachial plexus can result in blockade of the phrenic nerve, resulting in hemidiaphragmatic paralysis. It is estimated that approximately 15% to 20% of FVC will be lost with unilateral phrenic nerve paralysis.

25. **What agents can be used for induction and maintenance of general anesthesia in patients with COPD?**
   All of the standard induction agents can be used safely. Ketamine produces bronchodilation secondary to its sympathomimetic effects by direct antagonism of bronchoconstricting mediators, but secretions increase remarkably. Anecdotal evidence exists of the bronchodilating properties from propofol. IV lidocaine given before intubation can help blunt airway reflexes.
   All volatile anesthetics are bronchodilators. Desflurane has been demonstrated to produce increased airway resistance and bronchoconstriction, and is best avoided in these patients.
   Nitrous oxide increases the volume and pressure of pulmonary blebs or bullae, thereby increasing the risk of barotrauma and pneumothorax. In addition, it may increase pulmonary vascular resistance and pulmonary artery pressures. This would be especially deleterious in patients with coexisting pulmonary hypertension or cor pulmonale. For these reasons, nitrous oxide also should be avoided in patients with COPD.

26. **Discuss the particular concerns regarding muscle relaxation (and reversal) in patients with COPD.**
   Atracurium (but not cisatracurium) produces histamine release and should be avoided. Succinylcholine also produces histamine release, and the benefits and risks of rapid paralysis and endotracheal intubation must be evaluated when considering its use.
   Anticholinesterases (neostigmine and edrophonium) may precipitate bronchospasm and bronchorrhea secondary to stimulation of postganglionic muscarinic receptors. However, bronchospasm is rarely seen after administration of these agents, possibly because anticholinergic agents (atropine or glycopyrrolate) are concurrently administered.

27. **Discuss the medication choices for postoperative pain in patients with COPD.**
   Opioids may help with coughing because they blunt airway reflexes. However, it is important to remember their respiratory depressant effects. Morphine produces histamine release and should be used with caution.
   Hydromorphone, fentanyl, sufentanil, and remifentanil do not cause histamine release. Other analgesic options include regional analgesia, nonsteroidal aniiinflammatory drugs, acetaminophen, ketamine, gabapentin, pregabalin, lidocaine, and oral narcotics.

28. **Define auto-positive end-expiratory pressure.**
   Auto-positive end-expiratory pressure ([PEEP]; also known as air-trapping) results from the "stacking" of breaths that occurs when full exhalation is interrupted during mechanical ventilation. This can lead to an impairment of oxygenation and ventilation and ultimately, hemodynamic compromise, by decreasing preload and increasing pulmonary vascular resistance. Patients with COPD are particularly susceptible to auto-PEEP given their baseline pulmonary pathology.

Increasing expiratory time reduces the likelihood of auto-PEEP. This can be accomplished by increasing the expiratory phase of ventilation and decreasing the respiratory rate.

29. **Form a differential diagnosis for intraoperative wheezing.**
    - Bronchoconstriction (but remember, all that wheezes is not asthma)
    - Mechanical obstruction of the endotracheal tube by secretions or kinking
    - Aspiration of gastric contents or of a foreign body (e.g., a dislodged tooth)
    - Endobronchial intubation (most commonly right mainstem intubation)
    - Inadequate anesthesia
    - Pulmonary edema (cardiogenic and noncardiogenic)
    - Pneumothorax
    - Pulmonary embolus

30. **How would you treat intraoperative bronchospasm?**
    - Administer 100% oxygen and manually ventilate, allowing sufficient expiratory time. Identify and correct the underlying conditions.
    - Administer therapy:
        - Relieve mechanical obstructions.
        - Increase the volatile anesthetic agents and/or administer IV lidocaine, ketamine, or propofol.
        - Administer β-adrenergic agonists: aerosolized via the endotracheal tube (e.g., albuterol), subcutaneously (e.g., terbutaline), or IV (e.g., epinephrine or terbutaline).
        - Administer anticholinergic bronchodilators: aerosolized via the endotracheal tube (e.g., ipratropium) or IV (e.g., atropine or glycopyrrolate).
        - IV aminophylline and corticosteroids are also suggested therapies.
        - Consider magnesium.
    - Although controversial, extubation may be beneficial because the endotracheal tube itself may be a stimulus for bronchoconstriction.

KEY POINTS: CHRONIC OBSTRUCTIVE PULMONARY DISEASE

1. Patients with a significant reactive (and reversible) component to their lung disease require thorough preoperative preparation, including inhaled β-agonist therapy and possibly steroids.
2. Consider alternatives to general anesthesia in patients with a significant reactive component. An actively wheezing patient is not a good candidate for an elective surgical procedure.
3. All that wheezes is not asthma. Also consider mechanical airway obstruction, congestive failure, allergic reaction, pulmonary embolus, pneumothorax, aspiration, and endobronchial intubation.
4. Patients with chronic bronchitis may require antibiotic therapy, inhaled β agonists, and measures to mobilize and reduce sputum before surgery to improve outcome. Smoking cessation is very beneficial in the long term.
5. Patients for planned pulmonary resections absolutely require PFTs to ensure that more lung is not resected than is compatible with life. Injudicious resections may create a ventilator-dependent patient.

SUGGESTED READINGS

American Academy of Allergy, Asthma and Immunology: http://www.aaai.org

Qaseem S, Snow V. Risk assessment for and strategies to reduce perioperative pulmonary complications for patients undergoing noncardiothoracic surgery: a guideline from the American College of Physicians. Ann Intern Med 2006;144:575–580.

Rabe KF, Wedzicha JA. Controversies in treatment of chronic obstructive pulmonary disease. Lancet 2011;378:1038–1047.

Stoller JK. Clinical practice. Acute exacerbations of chronic obstructive pulmonary disease. N Engl J Med 2002;346:988–994.

Sutherland ER, Cherniack RM. Management of chronic obstructive pulmonary disease. N Engl J Med 2004;350:2689–2697.

Wedzicha JA, Seemungal TA. COPD exacerbations: defining their cause and prevention. Lancet 2007;370:786–796.

CHAPTER 40

ACUTE RESPIRATORY DISTRESS SYNDROME

Deepa Ramadurai, MD, Mark Kearns, MD

1. **How would you define acute respiratory distress syndrome?**

   The most commonly used definition for acute respiratory distress syndrome (ARDS), known as the Berlin definition (Table 40.1), was described in 2012. The Berlin definition describes ARDS as: (1) the development of respiratory failure that occurs within 7 days of a known clinical insult and represents new or worsening respiratory symptoms that are associated with (2) the presence of bilateral opacities consistent with pulmonary edema on either chest x-ray or computed tomography (CT) scan that is complicated by (3) hypoxemia requiring mechanical ventilation with a minimum positive end expiratory pressure (PEEP) or continuous positive airway pressure (CPAP) of 5 cm H_2O.

   The respiratory failure should not be fully explained by cardiac failure or fluid overload (e.g., end-stage renal disease). In other words, the pulmonary edema in ARDS is caused by an increase in capillary permeability (i.e., noncardiogenic pulmonary edema) and not because of an increase in hydrostatic pressure (i.e., cardiogenic pulmonary edema). The Berlin criteria further characterizes the severity of disease into mild, moderate, or severe categories based on the ratio of partial pressure of arterial oxygen (PaO_2) to the fraction of inspired oxygen (FiO_2) (P/F ratio) with a minimum PEEP of 5 cm H_2O.

2. **What are the risk factors for ARDS?**

   ARDS is an acute diffuse inflammatory reaction of the pulmonary parenchyma, resulting in increased pulmonary vascular permeability that occurs in response to a variety of insults (Box 40.1). Frequently, risk factors for ARDS are organized, as to whether the inciting event results in either a direct or indirect insult to the lung. Notably, ARDS develops in only a minority of all patients with common risk factors, such as pneumonia and sepsis. As such, inferences have been made to genetic susceptibility playing a role in the pathogenesis of ARDS, although attempts to associate specific genes have yielded limited results. Chronic alcohol abuse is a known, modifiable risk factor for the development of ARDS.

3. **What is the most common cause of ARDS, and what is the mortality rate for ARDS?**

   Pneumonia, sepsis, and aspiration are the most common risk factors for the development of ARDS. In the LUNG SAFE trial, pneumonia was the risk factor for 59.4% of patients who developed ARDS; extrapulmonary sepsis and aspiration were each identified as the risk factor in approximately 15% of cases. It is important to note that patient population, environmental exposures, and temporal factors can substantially impact the relative frequency of causes of ARDS.

   The LUNG SAFE trial also assessed mortality in patients who met the Berlin definition for ARDS, with reported in-hospital mortality rates of 34.9%, 40.3%, and 46.1% for patients with mild, moderate, and severe ARDS, respectively.

4. **What is the pathogenesis of ARDS?**

   Common to all inciting risk factors is an initial inflammatory insult that triggers resident alveolar macrophages to activate and release proinflammatory cytokines, resulting in recruitment of neutrophils and circulating macrophages to the alveolar space. These recruited inflammatory cells produce cytokines, proteases, reactive oxygen species, phospholipids, and eicosanoids that induce epithelial and endothelial cell injury and death, and further perpetuate the inflammatory response. The alveolar space becomes flooded with proteinaceous, neutrophil-predominant exudate. This impairs gas exchange through both ventilation-perfusion ($\dot{V}/\dot{Q}$) mismatch and shunt, results in decreased functional lung volume and compliance, and can result in pulmonary hypertension. Additional contributors to ARDS pathophysiology include activation of the ubiquitin proteasome system, inactivation and depletion of surfactant proteins, and formation of neutrophil extracellular traps.

5. **Describe the stages of ARDS.**

   The clinical, radiographic, and histopathologic abnormalities of ARDS are classically described in three phases: an acute or exudative phase, a proliferative phase, and finally a fibrotic phase. Although they are classically described as distinct phases, animal studies have demonstrated the overlapping nature of these pathophysiologic stages.

   1. The initial phase, known as the exudative phase, is characterized clinically by symptoms of respiratory distress, hypoxemia, and development of bilateral radiographic infiltrates. The classic histologic correlate, known as *diffuse alveolar damage* (DAD), is characterized by intraalveolar protein-rich edema fluid and inflammatory cells, alveolar epithelial cell injury, and hyaline membrane formation. Notably in an autopsy study of ARDS patients, only 45% of patients who met the Berlin definition of ARDS demonstrated DAD.

   2. The proliferative phase is characterized by cellular processes that aim to restore tissue structure and function. Within the alveolus, recruited macrophages and apoptotic neutrophils are cleared. There is proliferation of airway

Table 40.1 Berlin Criteria Definition of Acute Respiratory Distress Syndrome

CRITERIA	
Timing	Onset of new respiratory failure within 7 days of related clinical insult
Radiographic findings	Bilateral opacities on x-ray or CT scan not explained by effusion, collapse, or nodules
Edema	Type of pulmonary edema is not explained by cardiac failure or fluid overload. If no clinical risk factor for ARDS identified, objective assessment of cardiac function is required
PEEP/CPAP	Minimum PEEP or CPAP of 5 cm H_2O
Categorization of severity	*Mild* $PaO_2:FiO_2$ of 201–300 mm Hg *Moderate* $PaO_2:FiO_2$ of 101–200 mm Hg *Severe* $PaO_2:FiO_2$ of $\leq$100 mm Hg

ARDS, Acute Respiratory Distress Syndrome; *CPAP*, continuous positive airway pressure; *CT*, computed tomography; *FiO_2*, fraction of inspired oxygen; *PaO_2*, arterial oxygen partial pressure; *PEEP*, positive end-expiratory pressure.

Box 40.1 Inciting Events Associated With Acute Respiratory Distress Syndrome

Direct Lung Injury	Indirect Lung Injury
Pneumonia	Sepsis
Bacterial	Trauma
Fungal	Massive hemorrhage
Viral	Transfusion related
Opportunistic	Drug overdose
Aspiration of gastric contents	Burn injury
Inhalational injury	Acute pancreatitis
Near drowning	Cardiopulmonary bypass
Pulmonary contusion	Ischemia-reperfusion injury after lung transplant

progenitor cells and type II alveolar epithelial cells, which subsequently differentiate into new type I alveolar epithelial cells. Fibroblasts transiently proliferate in the interstitium to form a provisional matrix. In addition, a variety of distinct mechanisms restore alveolar epithelial and vascular endothelial function, resulting in restoration of barrier function and clearance of alveolar-interstitial edema.

3. The third phase, known as the *fibrotic phase*, does not occur in all patients and is associated with poor outcomes. Clinically, pulmonary opacities persist, lung compliance remains markedly decreased, and patients typically require prolonged ventilatory support. Histopathologic abnormalities include extensive basement membrane damage, widespread collagen deposition related to the proliferation of fibroblasts, with subsequent differentiation into highly synthetic myofibroblasts, which results in interstitial and intraalveolar fibrosis along with destruction of the capillary network.

6. How do patients who develop ARDS typically present?

ARDS patients present with respiratory distress, hypoxemia, and presence of bilateral pulmonary opacities on imaging studies. Approximately 40% of patients will develop ARDS within the first 24 hours of onset of their inciting event. The remainder will typically have onset of ARDS within the following 48 to 72 hours. By definition, patients who have ARDS will have hypoxemia refractory to supplementary oxygen that requires advanced respiratory support in the form of heated high flow nasal cannula, CPAP, or invasive mechanical ventilation. The extent of hypoxemia cannot be predicted but may be influenced by the patient's baseline pulmonary function, intravascular volume status, adequacy of cardiac output, and severity of the inciting risk factor. Auscultation of the lungs is often normal and, with the exception of ARDS associated with pneumonia, secretions are minimal.

7. Do any pulmonary diseases mimic ARDS?

There are a number of noninfectious disorders characterized by the acute onset of diffuse parenchymal lung disease, with resultant gas exchange abnormalities (Box 40.2). These imitators of ARDS often present with symptoms that might suggest an infectious disorder, including fever, cough, and leukocytosis. This is further compounded by the large percentage of patients with infectious pneumonia in which a microbe is not able to be identified. Patients in whom there is concern for an imitator of ARDS should undergo bronchoalveolar lavage to assist in diagnosis. In some

Box 40.2 Acute Respiratory Distress Syndrome Mimics

Acute interstitial pneumonia
Acute eosinophilic pneumonia
Cryptogenic organizing pneumonia
Diffuse alveolar hemorrhage
Acute hypersensitivity pneumonia
Drug induced pneumonitis
Acute exacerbation of interstitial lung disease
Collagen vascular disease related pneumonitis
Acute fibrinous organizing pneumonia

cases, an open lung biopsy may assist in making the diagnosis of the etiology. Ensuring the correct diagnosis is critical as many of the ARDS mimicking disorders can respond to early, appropriate treatment.

8. **Are any drug therapies available to treat ARDS?**
   Despite multiple high-quality clinical trials, no definitive effective drug therapy has been identified that improves survival in ARDS. Thromboxane synthetase inhibitors, nitric oxide (NO), corticosteroids, surfactant, *N*-acetylcysteine, beta-agonists, statins, inhaled prostacyclin, liquid ventilation, activated protein C, and other agents have been trialed without definitive benefit. The only therapies that definitively improve survival in ARDS are ventilation strategies, including low tidal volume (V_t) ventilation in all ARDS patients and early prone positioning in patients with moderate-severe ARDS.

9. **Does that mean that medical therapy has no role in patients with refractory ARDS?**
   Because no pharmacological agent has demonstrated a reduction in mortality does not mean that an individual patient may not respond favorably to a targeted drug therapy. For example, inhaled NO, once considered a promising therapy because of its ability to provide selective pulmonary vasodilation and improve $\dot{V}/\dot{Q}$ mismatch, has not improved mortality outcomes but does transiently improve oxygenation, which may allow time for other therapies used to treat the underlying disorder to become effective. Early administration of systemic glucocorticoids may be beneficial, if the etiology of ARDS is a steroid-responsive condition but is not recommended for all ARDS patients. Late administration of steroids in ARDS is relatively well-documented as harmful. Neuromuscular blocking agents also represent a class of drugs that may improve outcomes when appropriately applied (i.e., severe ARDS). Given the marked heterogeneity of patients with ARDS, decisions regarding advanced pharmacologic therapies must be evaluated in light of the patient's pathophysiology.

10. **Is there an optimal fluid strategy in ARDS?**
    The Fluids and Catheters Treatment Trial demonstrated that a conservative fluid management protocol, including conservative fluid resuscitation strategy followed by early use of diuretics, resulted in more ventilator-free days, and less intensive care unit days without increase in nonpulmonary organ failure. With regard to type of fluid, albumin does not provide appreciable benefit over crystalloid in ARDS patients.

11. **Does mechanical ventilation produce a uniform effect on the lung regions affected by ARDS?**
    Although ARDS is a diffuse process, there is marked heterogeneity in regional distribution of aeration. Early CT scan images from patients with ARDS demonstrated preferential aeration in nondependent lung regions (zone I), with dense consolidation, and lack of aeration in dependent areas (zone III). This observation led to the conceptual description of the pulmonary system in ARDS as the *baby lung*. The baby lung concept relates to the observation that the aerated lung volume in adult ARDS patients is comparable in size to a healthy baby's lungs. This concept informs our therapeutic use of low Vt ventilation because the volume of distribution for the delivered V_t is significantly decreased in ARDS patients, relative to normal patients. Furthermore, the delivered V_t is preferentially delivered to the most compliant lung, which can result in regional overdistension, resulting in ventilator-induced lung injury (VILI) to the previously healthy, aerated lung regions. In addition to the lung regions described earlier, there are also areas of partially flooded alveoli, which can potentially be recruited and become involved in gas exchange, dependent on ventilator settings and patient positioning.

12. **Can mechanical ventilation hurt the lung affected by ARDS?**
    Mechanical ventilation can perpetuate damage to injured lungs and initiate injury in previously healthy lung. This process, known as VILI can occur by a variety of mechanisms, including maldistribution of V_ts, causing excessive alveolar stretch (volutrauma), high alveolar pressures causing overdistension (barotrauma), and cyclic alveolar opening and collapse (atelectrauma). VILI can initiate lung inflammation and injury, as well as systemic inflammation and multiorgan failure.

13. **So how should patients with ARDS be ventilated?**
    The mainstay of mechanical ventilation strategy in ARDS patients is the application of a V_t of 6 mL/kg of ideal body weight (IBW) with a targeted plateau pressure of less than 30 cm H_2O. Studies have shown decreased mortality

including less pulmonary complications in patients ventilated at lower tidal volumes (V_t of 6 mL/kg IBW) compared to the traditional, larger tidal volume (V_t of 10 to 12 mL/kg IBW) used in the past. Studies impacting the importance of enhancing lung recruitment and minimizing atelectrauma through use of have been less definitive. Applying PEEP of at least 5 cm H_2O is recommended to prevent atelectrauma with many hospitals using an FiO_2/PEEP ladder defined by the ARDS Net to guide PEEP titration. The optimal PEEP to use is not clearly defined. However, recent data suggests using "driving pressure" as a method to titrate PEEP may be beneficial in reducing mortality and pulmonary complications. Recruitment maneuvers, in which high levels of positive pressure are applied intermittently to the respiratory system to enhance lung recruitment, have also been hypothesized to be beneficial in ARDS. Given the lack of clarity regarding the potential benefits of high PEEP and recruitment maneuvers, the "open lung approach," which incorporated recruitment maneuvers, along with application of higher titrated PEEP to optimize lung recruitment, was assessed in the Alveolar Recruitment for Acute Respiratory Distress Syndrome Trial (ART). The ART trial demonstrated significantly increased mortality in patients that received the "open lung approach."

14. What is "driving pressure"? How can it be used as a ventilator strategy to minimize ventilator-induced lung injury in ARDS?

To attempt to parse out the impact of Vt, plateau pressure management, and optimal PEEP strategies on ARDS outcomes, a group of investigators hypothesized and confirmed by posthoc analysis of multiple ARDS trials that the driving pressure (ΔDP), which is calculated as $\Delta DP = P_{pl} - PEEP$, was the ventilation variable that best stratified risk of death in ARDS. Titrating the PEEP such that ΔDP is minimized is essentially a method to titrate PEEP, where the lung is most compliant. Recall, Compliance = ΔVolume/ΔPressure, where ΔVolume = Vt and ΔPressure (or driving pressure) = $P_{pl} - PEEP$. Therefore titrating PEEP to make the ΔDP minimized is essentially titrating PEEP such that Vts are delivered when the lung is most compliant on the pulmonary pressure-volume curve. This is contrast to the more empirical method used by the FiO_2/PEEP ladder defined by the ARDS Net to guide PEEP titration. The concept of driving pressure is relatively new and further studies are needed before widespread acceptance of this ventilator strategy.

15. Is high-frequency oscillatory ventilation or extracorporeal membrane oxygenation useful for patients with ARDS?

High-frequency oscillatory ventilation (HFOV) was used with increased frequency during the 2009 H1N1 influenza pandemic to manage ARDS with refractory hypoxemia, but when subjected to randomized control trial testing, was associated with a higher risk of mortality.

Extracorporeal membrane oxygenation (ECMO) has also been used in patients with severe ARDS. Similar to HFOV, use of ECMO grew during the 2009 H1N1 pandemic both because of large number of patients with severe ARDS with refractory hypoxemia, but also related to significant recent technologic advances in the ECMO venous access catheters and circuits. Although the clinical experience in this setting demonstrated the feasibility of venovenous ECMO, the benefit and risk could not be quantified. At present, ECMO remains a treatment strategy for severe ARDS with refractory hypoxemia but is not the standard of care for all patients with severe ARDS.

16. What is a lung recruitment maneuver? How is it done?

A recruitment maneuver (RM) is a process in which high levels of PEEP are administered with the goal of recruiting atelectatic lung. Although there are many ways to perform an RM, the most rigorously studied protocols have used pressure control ventilation. In the ART trial, the RM began by applying a PEEP of 25 cm H_2O and an inspiratory ΔDP of 15 cm H_2O above the PEEP, with uptitration to a maximal PEEP of 35 cm H_2O. This was followed by a return to volume control ventilation and stepwise down-titration of PEEP every 3 minutes with measurement of respiratory system static compliance at each step. The PEEP associated with the highest compliance was considered the optimal PEEP. RMs were interrupted when uptitration of PEEP induced hypotension or worsening hypoxemia. Although commonly accepted as part of an open lung strategy for ARDS, protocolized care, including RMs with associated PEEP titration, is associated with increased mortality in moderate to severe ARDS patients. As such, RMs are best served to improve oxygenation in patients with refractory hypoxemia not responsive to other evidence-based strategies, but not in standard ventilator management protocols.

17. How does prone ventilation improve oxygenation?

CT scans of supine patients with ARDS demonstrate opacification of the dependent areas of the lung because of atelectasis and consolidation. In addition to alveolar flooding, mechanical imbalances caused by cephalic displacement of the diaphragm, decreased thoracic and abdominal compliance, increased pleural pressure in dorsal lung regions, and the weight of the heart causing compression of the left lower lobe, all act in concert to worsen atelectasis and promote $\dot{V}/\dot{Q}$ mismatching in the supine position. Notably, gravity plays only a minor role in distribution of blood flow throughout the lung. Therefore the dorsal caudal lung regions, regardless of supine or prone positioning, receive preferential perfusion. Improvements in oxygenation by using the prone position result from enhanced $\dot{V}/\dot{Q}$ matching because of:
- Recruitment of collapsed dorsal lung by a redistribution of edema to ventral regions
- Increased diaphragm motion
- Elimination of the compressive effects of the heart on the left lower lobe

18. **Does prone ventilation offer a survival benefit in patients with ARDS?**
Early initiation of prone ventilation in patients with severe ARDS by Berlin definition (specifically with P/F ratio <150 mm Hg requiring an FiO_2 of $\geq$60%) reduces mortality and is now a guideline recommendation.

19. **What is the role of neuromuscular blockade in ARDS?**
Neuromuscular blocking agents should not be routinely administered for patients with moderate-to-severe ARDS. Large randomized controlled studies have not shown a mortality benefit compared to usual sedative strategies. However, neuromuscular blocking agents may be considered in patients who are intubated (e.g., severe ARDS) for the following indications: 1) to reduce the risk of VILI caused by ventilator dyssynchrony that cannot otherwise be managed, 2) to treat refractory hypoxemia, or 3) to correct profound acid-base derangements.

KEY POINTS: ADULT RESPIRATORY DISTRESS SYNDROME

1. The pulmonary edema found in ARDS is caused by increased capillary permeability (i.e., noncardiogenic pulmonary edema) and is not caused by increased hydrostatic pressure (i.e., cardiogenic pulmonary edema). This is an important distinction because both can present similar on imaging (i.e., bilateral opacities).
2. Historically, sepsis has been identified as the most common risk factor for ARDS.
3. VILI can be caused by volutrauma, barotrauma, and atelectrauma.
4. Mechanical ventilation settings for patients with ARDS includes Vt at 6 mL/kg of IBW and limiting plateau pressures to less than 30 cm H_2O.
5. PEEP should be adjusted to prevent end-expiratory collapse and cyclic reopening.
6. Early prone positioning in patients with moderate-severe ARDS improves mortality.

SUGGESTED READINGS

Bellani G, Laffey JG, Pham T, et al. Epidemiology, patterns of care, and mortality for patients with acute respiratory distress syndrome in intensive care units in 50 countries. JAMA. 2016;315:788–800.
Fan E, Brodie D, Slutsky AS. Acute respiratory distress syndrome: advances in diagnosis and treatment. JAMA. 2018;319:698–710.
Guerin C, Reignier J, Richard J-C, et al. Prone positioning in severe acute respiratory distress syndrome. N Engl J Med. 2013;368:2159–2168.
The ARDS Definition Task Force. Acute respiratory distress syndrome: the Berlin definition. JAMA. 2012;307:2526–2533.
Thompson BT, Chambers RC, Liu KD. Acute respiratory distress syndrome. N Engl J Med. 2017;377:562–572.
Schwarz MI, Albert RK. "Imitators" of the ARDS: implications for diagnosis and treatment. Chest. 2004;125:1530–1535.
Slutsky AS, Ranieri VM. Ventilator-induced lung injury. N Engl J Med. 2013;369:2126–2136.

HEPATIC DYSFUNCTION AND LIVER TRANSPLANTATION

Natalie K. Smith, MD, Alan J. Sim, MD, Samuel DeMaria, Jr, MD

1. **Describe normal liver anatomy. How is blood supply provided to the liver?**
   The human liver consists of four anatomic lobes (left, right, caudate, quadrate) and eight surgical lobes (I–VIII). The liver receives approximately 20% to 25% of the cardiac output and contains 10% to 15% of the total blood volume. Its blood supply is provided by the portal vein (75%) and hepatic artery (25%), where each vessel provides 50% of the liver's oxygen requirements. Hepatic blood flow is regulated by the hepatic artery buffer response, which is mediated by adenosine and modulated by hypoxemia, hypercarbia, and acidosis. Sympathetic stimulation decreases hepatic blood flow.

2. **What are the normal physiological functions of the liver?**
   Almost all plasma proteins are synthesized in the liver. These include albumin, α_1-acid glycoprotein, pseudocholinesterase, most coagulation factors, and anticoagulant proteins (i.e., protein C, S, and antithrombin III). Factor VIII is not synthesized by the liver. The liver is also involved in carbohydrate, lipid, and cholesterol metabolism, glucose homeostasis, and bile synthesis. The liver produces 20% of the body's heme. The liver also possesses immune function in that hepatic Kupffer cells filter splanchnic venous blood of bacteria. The liver serves as the main organ of drug metabolism and detoxification. Through three hepatic reactions (phases I, II, and III), drugs are metabolized to a more water-soluble form and excreted in the urine or bile. The liver metabolizes nitrogen-containing compounds to urea and ammonia.

3. **Review the most common cause of parenchymal liver disease.**
   The most common causes of liver disease include viral hepatitis from hepatitis B virus (HBV) and hepatitis C virus (HCV), alcoholism, and nonalcoholic steatohepatitis (NASH). NASH will likely become the most common indication for liver transplantation in the United States because of advancements in treatment for viral hepatitis, including the HBV vaccine and antiviral treatments for HCV. Other causes of liver disease include viruses, such as Epstein-Barr virus and cytomegalovirus, autoimmune hepatitis, hemochromatosis, primary biliary cholangitis (PBC), primary sclerosing cholangitis (PSC), and drug-induced liver injury (DILI). DILI can mimic acute viral hepatitis and is most commonly caused by alcohol, acetaminophen, antibiotics, and nonsteroidal antiinflammatory drugs.

4. **What is cirrhosis?**
   Cirrhosis is the sequela of long-term liver disease characterized by diffuse hepatocyte death, with resultant fibrosis and nodular hepatocellular regeneration. Distortion of hepatic circulation further propagates cellular damage and results in progressive reduction of hepatocytes, eventually manifesting as impaired organ function. Hepatic synthetic failure, indicated by a prolonged prothrombin time (PT), hypoalbuminemia, and impaired detoxification mechanisms causing hepatic encephalopathy, is often termed *end-stage liver disease* (ESLD).

5. **Describe the neurologic derangements in patients with cirrhosis.**
   Several neurologic complications are associated with cirrhosis. Hepatic encephalopathy, ranging from confusion to coma is a common sequela of cirrhosis. Factors associated with encephalopathy include ammonia, blood-brain barrier alterations, and changes to central nervous system (CNS) neurotransmission. Although increased ammonia levels do not directly correlate with the degree of encephalopathy, treatment consists of lactulose to reduce ammonia absorption, and rifaximin to reduce ammonia production by urease-producing bacteria in the gut.

   Acute liver failure, formerly called *fulminant hepatic failure*, often causes severe cerebral edema, leading to intracranial hypertension. It must be appreciated that one of the more common causes of death in acute liver failure is brain stem herniation. In contrast, cerebral edema in patients with chronic liver disease is less severe and generally does not cause intracranial hypertension, unless they develop acute or chronic liver failure.

6. **Is cirrhosis a risk factor for sepsis?**
   Yes, and sepsis is a major cause of mortality in patients with cirrhosis. Patient with cirrhosis are immunocompromised and although the exact mechanism is complex, both the innate and adaptive immune systems are affected. Specifically, the liver is the main source of the complement system and secreted pattern-recognition receptors (toll-like receptors, etc.). The synthesis of these crucial proteins is impaired in cirrhosis. This is also complicated by the fact that the liver is the first organ in direct contact with translocated gut bacteria via the portal vein.

Note that there are frequently other factors contributing to immunodeficiency in this patient population because of the higher prevalence of malnutrition (alcohol abuse, ulcerative colitis, etc.) and immunosuppressive medications for autoimmune disorders (PBC, PSC, etc.).

7. **Describe the cardiovascular changes in patients with cirrhosis. Why do these patients have a "hyperdynamic" circulation?**

Cirrhosis causes increased vascular resistance within the hepatic circulation causing portal hypertension, which results in nitric oxide (a potent vasodilator) to be released from the splanchnic circulation. This leads to increased nitric oxide within the systemic circulation, causing venous and arterial vasodilation. Blood is sequestered primarily into the splanchnic circulation because of venodilation, causing a decrease in circulating blood volume. The decrease in circulating blood volume (venodilation) and decrease in systemic vascular resistance (SVR) (arterial vasodilation) activates the sympathetic nervous system, renin-angiotensin-aldosterone system (RAAS), and, in severe cases, the nonosmotic release of antidiuretic hormone (ADH). This compensatory response increases total blood volume by retention of salt and water, leading to hypervolemia, ascites, and in severe disease, hyponatremia. The decrease in SVR reduces cardiac afterload, which facilitates a compensatory, sympathetic-mediated increase in cardiac output (i.e., hyperdynamic circulation). Note, that the increase in cardiac output is necessary to prevent severe hypotension and organ failure from decreased perfusion. Mixed venous oxygen saturation is higher than normal in ESLD because of increased cardiac output and shunting from vasodilation.

8. **Is coronary artery disease a common comorbidity in chronic liver disease?**

Coronary artery disease (CAD), with impaired myocardial function (previously thought uncommon in patients with liver disease), may be present, especially when the patient has NASH. CAD in liver transplant patients older than 50 years of age occurs in the range of 5% to 27%. Abnormalities in both systolic and diastolic function (cirrhotic cardiomyopathy) may be present and may be masked by reduced cardiac afterload and high cardiac output. This is especially true in patients with a history of alcohol abuse.

9. **What is hepatopulmonary syndrome?**

Arterial hypoxemia with compensatory hyperventilation may be secondary to atelectasis from ascites/hydrothorax or from hepatopulmonary syndrome (HPS). HPS occurs in the setting of portal hypertension and is caused by pulmonary vasodilation, which leads to intrapulmonary arteriovenous (AV) shunting and hypoxemia. The features of HPS include platypnea (shortness of breath while standing), orthodeoxia (decreased saturation when upright), cyanosis, and finger clubbing. HPS can be diagnosed by preforming an agitated saline study on transthoracic echocardiography (TTE); saline microbubbles appearing in the left atrium within 3 to 6 cardiac cycles indicates HPS. The only definitive treatment that can HPS is liver transplantation.

10. **What is portopulmonary hypertension?**

Portopulmonary hypertension (PoPH), defined as a mean pulmonary artery pressure (PAP) greater than 25 mm Hg and pulmonary vascular resistance (PVR) over 240 dyn · sec/cm^5, is seen in 3% to 5% reverse of patients with cirrhosis. PoPH is caused by intimal proliferation, smooth muscle hypertrophy, and fibrosis in the pulmonary arterial circulation, leading to an increase in PVR. PoPH is subdivided by severity (mild: 25–34 mm Hg, moderate: 35–44 mm Hg, severe: ≥45 mm Hg). Mild to moderate PoPH may be reversible with liver transplant; however, more severe PoPH may be irreversible and is associated with high intraoperative and postoperative mortality, secondary to right ventricular dysfunction. Severe PoPH is a contraindication to liver transplantation because it is associated with a high mortality rate.

Vasodilators reduce PAP and prolong survival in some patients with PoPH. Inhaled prostacyclin (iloprost) and inhaled nitric oxide (iNO) may be used to acutely reduce PAP and is more frequently used in the operating room or in the intensive care unit. Phosphodiesterase inhibitors, such as sildenafil or an infusion of prostaglandin I2 (epoprostenol), can be used to bridge patients to transplantation.

11. **What is hepatorenal syndrome (HRS)? How does it differ from acute kidney injury (AKI) in patients with ESLD?**

Both HRS and AKI can occur in cirrhotic patients and are characterized by oliguria and increases in serum creatinine. The etiology in both cases is renal hypoperfusion. Differentiation is important because treatment and prognosis vary.

HRS occurs in cirrhotic patients with portal hypertension and ascites. HRS is defined as a plasma creatinine of more than 1.5 mg/dL in patients with acute or chronic liver disease who do not improve with volume expansions in the absence of other renal disease. The etiology is thought to be renal hypoperfusion from decreased SVR and profound splanchnic sequestration of blood. RAAS and sympathetic stimulation increase salt and water retention to maintain blood pressure and, in severe cases, nonosmotic secretion of ADH, leading to hyponatremia.

AKI in cirrhosis is often caused by prerenal pathology. Prerenal AKI results from decreased blood flow to the kidneys from hypovolemia, such as hemorrhage (e.g., ruptured varices), splanchnic sequestration of blood, ascites formation, or dehydration. In contrast to HRS, restoring blood volume typically corrects prerenal AKI.

12. **What are the gastrointestinal derangements that occur with cirrhosis?**

Gastrointestinal (GI) complications result from portal hypertension (>10 mm Hg). Portal hypertension leads to the development of portosystemic venous collaterals, including esophagogastric varices. Ruptured varices with hemorrhage account for a third of patient mortality. Ascites results from fluid sequestration because of portal hypertension. Patients with decompensated cirrhosis and ascites are prone to spontaneous bacterial peritonitis from translocation of bacteria from the GI tract.

13. **What are the hematological derangements that occur with cirrhosis?**
Hematological disorders include anemia, thrombocytopenia, and coagulopathy. Anemia is secondary to GI bleeding, malnutrition, and bone marrow suppression. Thrombocytopenia is caused by splenic sequestration attributed to portal hypertension, bone marrow suppression caused by alcohol abuse, malnutrition, and so on, and decreased platelet production resulting from decreased synthesis of thrombopoietin by the liver. Coagulopathy is caused by derangements in both pro- and anticoagulant protein synthesis, accelerated fibrinolysis (liver metabolizes tissue plasminogen activator [tPA]), and thrombocytopenia. Most clotting factors, except for Factor VIII, are made in the liver and are decreased in liver cirrhosis, causing the international normalized ratio (INR)/PT and partial thromboplastin time (PTT) to increase. Natural anticoagulants, such as protein C, S, and antithrombin III, are also synthesized in the liver and are also reduced. It is important to note that the prolongation of PT/INR and PTT does not correlate with the risk of bleeding because these tests do not reflect the natural anticoagulant proteins. In fact, patients with cirrhosis can be hypercoagulable because of decreased anticoagulant protein levels. Patients with cirrhosis are at risk of thrombotic complications, such as deep vein thrombosis, pulmonary embolism, and portal venous thrombosis. Therefore the coagulation status in patients with cirrhosis is complex, as they are at risk for both hemorrhagic and thrombotic complications. Viscoelastic testing, such as thromboelastography (TEG) or rotational thromboelastometry (ROTEM), should strongly be considered instead of INR/PTT, when assessing the overall coagulation status in this patient population.

14. **Describe the laboratory tests used to assess hepatic synthetic function.**
Reduction in clotting factor synthesis may prolong PT/INR and PTT. However, these tests only measure procoagulant factors and do not measure the natural anticoagulant proteins (i.e., protein C, S, and antithrombin III). Therefore these tests should only be used to assess liver function and to aid in prognosis. They should not be used to assess for coagulopathy in patients with cirrhosis.

Albumin is synthesized in the liver and reflects hepatic function. However, renal and GI losses, malnutrition, and changes in vascular permeability can also affect albumin levels. A reduction in synthesis caused by liver disease may require 20 days to detect because of the long plasma half-life of albumin. Therefore low serum albumin levels are more useful indicators of *chronic* liver disease.

15. **Which liver function tests are used to detect hepatic cell damage?**
The enzymes alanine aminotransferase (ALT) and aspartate aminotransferase (AST) are released into the blood as a result of increased membrane permeability or cell necrosis. They tend to rise and fall in parallel. AST is cleared more rapidly from the circulation by the reticuloendothelial system. AST and ALT levels are not affected by changes in renal or biliary function. In contrast with ALT, which is mainly confined to hepatocytes, AST is found in heart and skeletal muscle, pancreas, kidney, and red blood cells. Therefore AST lacks specificity as a single diagnostic test. ALT is more specific, but less sensitive for detection of hepatic disease.

16. **Can a patient with cirrhosis have normal liver function tests?**
Yes, recall liver function tests (LFTs) reflect liver injury and not liver function. Patients with cirrhosis may have decreased liver function (i.e., elevated INR, decrease albumin), but normal LFTs, and patients with hepatitis may have normal liver function but elevated LFTs.

17. **What is the most common cause of mildly elevated LFTs?**
The most common cause of mildly elevated LFTs is fatty liver, either from alcohol use or nonalcohol fatty liver disease.

18. **What laboratory tests are used to diagnose cholestatic liver disease?**
Alkaline phosphatase (ALP), γ-glutamyltransferase (GGT), and 5′-nucleotidase are commonly used to assess biliary tract function. These enzymes are located in the biliary epithelial cell membranes. ALP occurs in a wide variety of tissues and is elevated in several conditions, including bone disease and pregnancy. The hepatic origin of an elevated ALP is often suggested by the clinical context and simultaneous elevations of GGT and 5′-nucleotidase.

19. **What scoring systems are used to predict short-term mortality in patients with cirrhosis?**
The Child-Pugh score and the Model for End-Stage Liver Disease (MELD) are two commonly used scoring systems for patients with chronic liver disease. These scoring systems are used to predict short-term mortality and to prioritize liver transplantation (i.e., MELD score). The Child-Pugh scoring system uses a combination of objective data measurements and subjective clinical examination findings. Specifically, it uses bilirubin, albumin, and INR, in addition to the degree of encephalopathy and ascites found on clinical examination. One of the main criticisms of the Child-Pugh scoring system is its overreliance on subjective clinical examination findings, which can vary depending upon the clinician and treatment (i.e., diuretics, lactulose, rifaximin). The MELD score was developed to serve as a more objective scoring system because it only includes objective, laboratory measurements and does not depend upon clinical assessment. The MELD score has been well-validated in multiple studies to predict 90-day mortality (Table 41.1) and can be readily calculated (Box 41.1). Only the MELD score, and not the Child-Pugh score, is used to prioritize liver transplant recipients.

Table 41.1 Model of End-Stage Liver Disease Score: Estimated 90-Day Mortality

SCORE	MORTALITY
>40	71.3%
30–39	52.6%
20–29	19.6%
10–19	6.0%
<9	1.9%

Box 41.1 Model for End-Stage Liver Disease Equation

First, calculate the initial Model of End-Stage Liver Disease (MELD) score:

$$MELD(i) = 3.8 \times \ln[Bili\,(mg/dL)] + 11.2 \times \ln[INR] + 9.6 \times \ln[Cr\,(mg/dL)] + 6.43$$

Bili, total bilirubin; INR, international normalized ratio; Cr, creatinine
If the initial MELD(i) >11, then recalculate MELD using the patient's sodium (Na) level:

$$MELD = MELD(i) + 1.32 \times (137 - Na) - [0.033 \times MELD(i) \times (137 - Na)]$$

Rules
- Patient ≥12 years old
- If Cr or INR <1.0, use 1.0
- If Cr >4.0 or recent hemodialysis, then Cr = 4.0
- If Na <125, then Na = 125; if Na >137, then Na = 137

Table 41.2 Risk Factors for Liver Disease

RISK FACTOR	EXAMPLE
Viral hepatitis	Intravenous drug abuse, transfusion, tattoos, contact with infected person
Drugs	Alcohol, prescription medications (e.g., acetaminophen, haloperidol, tetracycline, isoniazid, hydralazine, captopril, and amiodarone)
Autoimmune disease	Systemic lupus erythematosus, sarcoidosis, mixed connective tissue disorder
Metabolic disease	Hemochromatosis, Wilson disease, cystic fibrosis, α_1-antitrypsin deficiency, glycogen storage disease
Inflammatory bowel disease	Crohn disease and ulcerative colitis/primary sclerosing cholangitis

20. **What risk factors and characteristics of liver disease can be identified by history and physical examination?**
    See Table 41.2. Stigmata of chronic liver disease include ascites, hepatosplenomegaly, spider angiomata, caput medusae, gynecomastia, asterixis, and jaundice.

21. **What is jaundice?**
    Jaundice is a visible yellow or green discoloration, usually first observed in the sclera, caused by elevation of serum bilirubin. Bilirubin levels greater than 2.5 mg/dL (normal 0.5–1 mg/dL) result in jaundice.

22. **Distinguish between unconjugated and conjugated hyperbilirubinemia.**
    The distinction is essential to the differential diagnosis of jaundice. Unconjugated (indirect) hyperbilirubinemia is usually prehepatic in etiology (e.g., hemolysis) because of increased production of bilirubin (Table 41.3). Conjugated (direct) hyperbilirubinemia is usually posthepatic in etiology (e.g., cholestasis) and typically signifies obstructive pathology (Table 41.4).

23. **What are the main causes of hepatocyte injury?**
    See Table 41.5.

Table 41.3 Causes of Unconjugated Hyperbilirubinemia

CAUSE	EXAMPLE
Hemolysis	Incompatible blood transfusion, arterial/venous bypass circuit, congenital, or acquired defects (e.g., autoimmune and drug-induced hemolytic anemia, glucose-6-phosphatase deficiency)
Hematoma resorption	Retroperitoneal or pelvic hematoma
Enzymatic deficiencies	Congenital deficiency (Gilbert syndrome) to complete absence (Crigler-Najjar syndrome) of hepatic uridine diphosphate glucuronyl transferase

Table 41.4 Causes of Conjugated Hyperbilirubinemia

EXTRAHEPATIC OBSTRUCTION	INTRAHEPATIC OBSTRUCTION
Tumor (bile duct, pancreas, and duodenum)	Primary biliary cholangitis
Cholecystitis	Drugs (estrogens, anabolic steroids, tetracycline, and valproic acid)
Biliary stricture	Total parenteral nutrition
Ascending cholangitis	Pregnancy
Sclerosing cholangitis	

Table 41.5 Causes of Hepatocyte Injury

CAUSE	EXAMPLE
Infection	Hepatitis A, B, and C; cytomegalovirus; Epstein-Barr virus
Drugs	Acetaminophen, isoniazid, phenytoin, hydralazine, α-methyldopa, sulfasalazine
Sepsis	Pneumonia
Total parenteral nutrition (TPN)	Abnormal liver function tests in 68%–93% of patients given TPN for longer than 2 weeks
Hypoxemia	Lower arterial oxygen or interference with peripheral use, as in cyanide and carbon monoxide poisoning
Ischemia	Increased venous pressure (e.g., congestive heart failure, pulmonary embolus, and positive-pressure ventilation) Decreased arterial pressure (e.g., hypovolemia, vasopressors, and aortic cross-clamp)

24. **Do volatile anesthetics produce hepatic dysfunction?**
Rarely, inhalational agents can cause inflammation or death of hepatocytes because of their metabolic products. In general, the degree of metabolism of the agents is halothane >sevoflurane >isoflurane >desflurane. Halothane, the most extensively metabolized agent, is associated with mild hepatic dysfunction in up to 30% of individuals exposed and manifests as asymptomatic transient elevation of hepatic AST and ALT. Modern volatile anesthetics including isoflurane, sevoflurane, and desflurane are safe for use in patients with cirrhosis.

25. **Do inhalational agents alter hepatic blood flow?**
These agents dilate the hepatic artery and preportal blood vessels, decreasing mean hepatic artery pressure, and increasing splanchnic blood pooling. Portal flow decreases. Overall, the result is suboptimal hepatic perfusion. However, at levels below 1 minimum alveolar concentration, isoflurane, sevoflurane, and desflurane only minimally decrease hepatic blood flow.

26. **What adjustment in intravenous anesthetics should be made in a patient with liver disease?**
CNS dysfunction, metabolic derangements, and an increased volume of distribution can lead to changes in the response to anesthetic agents that is difficult to predict. Propofol, etomidate, and ketamine have high hepatic extraction ratios, and their pharmacokinetic profile is relatively unchanged in mild to moderate cirrhosis. Although pseudocholinesterase levels are decreased in patients with liver disease, the clinical prolongation of succinylcholine is not significant. Intermediate-acting steroidal nondepolarizing muscle relaxants, such as vecuronium and rocuronium, display a prolonged effect in patients with cirrhosis. Benzylquinolinium neuromuscular blockers, such as

atracurium and cisatracurium, undergo organ-independent elimination, and their duration is not affected by liver disease. Benzodiazepines should be dosed judiciously in patients with liver disease and should be avoided in patients with encephalopathy.

All opioids, except for remifentanil, are metabolized in the liver. Morphine and meperidine have a prolonged half-life in patients with liver disease and can precipitate hepatic encephalopathy. Fentanyl, although completely metabolized by the liver, does not have a prolonged clinical effect in cirrhosis. Therefore fentanyl and remifentanil are the opioids of choice in liver disease.

27. **What are the preoperative management goals in a patient with liver disease?**
The type and severity of liver disease should be determined. The benefit of surgery must outweigh the risk, as patients with decompensated cirrhosis (MELD > 14) are at high risk of morbidity and mortality from large, invasive operations. If surgery is deemed necessary, a complete organ system review should be performed, specifically looking for encephalopathy, ascites, portal hypertension, varices, and renal insufficiency. A complete laboratory evaluation should be performed, including transaminases, bilirubin, albumin, basic metabolic profile, complete blood count with platelet count, and a coagulation profile. TEG or ROTEM may be useful in guiding component therapy when correcting coagulopathy.

28. **What are the intraoperative management goals in a patient with liver disease?**
Hypoxemia, hemorrhage, hypotension, and sympathetic stimulation may all reduce hepatic blood flow; and should be avoided. Hypotension occurs in the setting of low SVR and hypovolemia and can be treated with vasoconstrictors and judicious volume resuscitation. Rapid sequence induction should be considered for patients with large ascites or delayed gastric emptying.

29. **Describe some indications and contraindications for liver transplantation.**
Indications for liver transplantation include the following:
- ESLD (e.g., viral hepatitis, alcohol cirrhosis, and NASH)
- Cholestatic disease (e.g., PBC, primary sclerosis cholangitis, and biliary atresia)
- Metabolic disease (e.g., hemochromatosis and Wilson disease)
- Hepatic malignancy (e.g., hepatocellular carcinoma and neuroendocrine tumors)
- Acute liver failure (e.g., acetaminophen toxicity)

    Over time, relative and absolute contraindications for liver transplantation have evolved (Table 41.6). Because MELD predicts 3-month survival, those with higher scores are more likely to die from liver disease and thus have the best risk-benefit ratio for undergoing transplantation; as such organs are preferentially offered to sicker patients with higher MELD scores.

30. **What are some anesthetic considerations in a liver transplant patient?**
Optimal anesthetic management of these complex, critically ill patients requires management of the pathophysiologic changes of liver disease, comorbid conditions, and the physiologic changes associated with the surgery. Prior abdominal surgeries, episodes of spontaneous bacterial peritonitis, and encephalopathy are important features to note. Coagulopathy can be evaluated by PT/INR, platelet count, and viscoelastic testing. Recall, PT/INR may be elevated but does not necessary imply coagulopathy, as these tests do not reflect the natural anticoagulant proteins (i.e., protein C, S, and antithrombin III). A decrease in anticoagulant proteins because of ESLD may cause these patients to be hypercoagulable. Ideally, viscoelastic testing (i.e., TEG or ROTEM) should be used because these tests allow for simultaneous measurement of clot kinetics (pro- and anticlotting factor function), clot strength (platelet and fibrin function), and clot durability (fibrinolysis). Recall, patients with ESLD may be coagulopathic as a result of decreased clotting factor synthesis, decreased platelets, and increased fibrinolysis because tPA is metabolized by the liver.

Table 41.6 Contraindications to Liver Transplantation

ABSOLUTE CONTRAINDICATIONS	RELATIVE CONTRAINDICATIONS
Uncontrolled sepsis	Advanced age
Extrahepatic malignancy	Severe obesity or severe malnutrition
Advanced cardiopulmonary disease	Severe pulmonary hypertension
Active substance or alcohol abuse	Severe hepatopulmonary syndrome
AIDS	Severe hepatorenal syndrome
Anatomic abnormality precluding transplant	Severe cardiomyopathy
Intrahepatic cholangiocarcinoma	HIV with high viral load
	Psychosocial conditions

AIDS, Acquired immunodeficiency syndrome; *HIV,* human immunodeficiency virus.
Modified from Martin P, DiMartini A, Feng S, et al. Evaluation for liver transplantation in adults: 2013 practice guidelines by the American Association for the Study of Liver Diseases and the American Society of Transplantation. Hepatology. 2014 Mar;59(3):1147–1165.

Electrolytes should be evaluated because abnormalities are common. Hypokalemia is commonly seen in earlier stages of liver disease because hepatic injury leads to hyperaldosteronism. Hyperkalemia can also be seen especially if patients with ascites are being treated with potassium-sparing diuretics. Hyponatremia may result from diuretic use, hyperaldosteronism, or from nonosmotic release of ADH because of renal hypoperfusion.

In acute liver failure, cerebral cytotoxic edema is a common complication, and there must be aggressive preoperative control of intracranial pressure to prevent brainstem herniation and death. Patients with cerebral edema may benefit from intracranial pressure monitoring.

All potential transplant candidates should undergo cardiac testing, including electrocardiogram, TTE, and cardiac stress test. TTE should assess left and right ventricular function, valvular abnormalities, pulmonary arterial pressures, and intrapulmonary shunting. If Doppler-derived pulmonary arterial pressures are elevated or right ventricular function is decreased on transesophageal echocardiography (TEE), a right-sided heart catheterization may be indicated. Other preoperative testing should include a chest x-ray for baseline pulmonary status and an upper endoscopy to evaluate for varices.

31. What monitoring tools, vascular access, and special equipment are indicated for liver transplant?

Monitoring should include invasive arterial pressure, central venous pressure, and PAP monitoring. In the absence of contraindications, intraoperative TEE is often used to monitor volume status and cardiac function. Access should include large bore intravenous peripheral and central access. Blood products should be prepared. A rapid infusion system should be available as massive volume resuscitation is often necessary.

32. Describe the three stages of liver transplantation.

- **Stage 1 or preanhepatic stage:** This involves surgical incision, drainage of ascites, dissection, and hepatic mobilization. Surgeons identify the hepatic artery, portal vein, the inferior vena cava (IVC), and the biliary tree. Also referred to as *the dissection stage.*
- **Stage 2 or anhepatic stage:** This includes isolating the liver from the circulation and occluding the hepatic artery, portal vein, suprahepatic IVC, and infrahepatic IVC. After the liver is isolated from circulation, the liver is surgically removed. The donor liver is then inserted into the circulation by anastomoses to the patient's vena cava and portal vein. The preservative solution is flushed out of the graft before reperfusion. The anhepatic stage concludes with removal of the vascular clamps, resulting in reperfusion of the donor liver graft.
- **Stage 3 or reperfusion stage:** This begins with hepatic reperfusion and extends to the conclusion of the operation. Hepatic artery anastomosis, biliary reconstruction, and assessment of neohepatic function occurs during this phase.

33. What are the major surgical techniques for liver transplantation?

Conventional caval replacement was the first liver transplant technique used. It involves total vascular isolation where clamps are placed on the supra- and infrahepatic IVC, and the porta hepatis, followed by anastomosis of the liver graft. Complete caval cross-clamping leads to a large decrease in preload and hemodynamic derangements that may not be tolerated by all patients. The piggyback technique was designed to avoid complete IVC clamping. The piggyback technique uses a side clamp on the IVC, at the level of the hepatic veins, which allows partial flow to continue through the IVC during the anhepatic phase and leads to less hemodynamic instability. The piggyback technique is the most common method used for liver transplantation. A third technique involves venovenous bypass (VVB), allowing venous return from the lower body to bypass the IVC clamps. During VVB, a cannula is placed into the femoral vein and drains blood from the lower extremities. Blood is returned to the superior vena cava via the internal jugular or subclavian vein. VVB is associated with complications, including thromboembolic events, gas embolism, hypothermia, coagulopathy, and fibrinolysis, and is only used if hypotension during initial IVC clamping does not respond adequately to volume, vasopressors, and inotropes.

34. List some of the anesthetic concerns during the stage 1 (preanhepatic).

- Maintaining normothermia is important because the metabolic activity of a healthy liver contributes significantly to maintaining body temperature. Early hypothermia is difficult to correct and potentiates coagulation disturbances.
- Hyperkalemia during the preanhepatic stage may be caused by the administration of blood products and/or impaired excretion caused by HRS. This may result in hyperkalemic cardiac arrest during reperfusion if not adequately treated. The donor organ preservative solution contains 150 mEq/dL of potassium. On reperfusion, much of this potassium reaches the patient's circulation. Therefore it is important to control potassium from the beginning of surgery, maintaining serum levels at approximately 3.5 mEq/dL.
- Hyponatremia in patients with liver disease should not be corrected rapidly because fluctuations in the serum sodium during transplantation can produced central pontine myelinolysis.
- Citrate toxicity from transfusion of blood products because the liver may not be able to metabolize citrate, leading to hypocalcemia.
- In addition to preexisting coagulopathies, portal hypertension can cause excessive bleeding. A splanchnic vasoconstrictor, such as vasopressin, may be started in an attempt to return the splanchnic blood to the systemic circulation.

35. **What are some anesthetic concerns that arise during stage 2 (anhepatic)?**
At the end of dissection, volume status should be adequate to tolerate IVC clamping. Vasopressors and inotropes may be necessary to maintain blood pressure during stage 2. Cross-clamping the IVC leads to an abrupt decrease in preload. Most therapy in this phase is directed toward achieving hemodynamic stability and preparing for reperfusion.
    As previously discussed, serum potassium must be aggressively lowered to prevent hyperkalemia-induced arrhythmia and asystole during reperfusion. Sodium bicarbonate, calcium, and insulin are effective interventions. Note, hyperventilation is not effective in treating hyperkalemia.

36. **Define reperfusion syndrome and its implications.**
Reperfusion syndrome is characterized by either a decrease of 30% or more in mean arterial pressure from baseline, for more than 1 minute, and occurring within the first 5 minutes of reperfusion, or a mean arterial pressure less than 60 mm Hg under the same circumstances. Following portal vein unclamping, approximately 30% of patients will exhibit profound cardiovascular collapse on reperfusion, irrespective of attentive management during stage 2. The bradycardia, myocardial depression, and systemic vasodilation noted during reperfusion are secondary to rapid increases in serum potassium, decreases in temperature, acute acidosis, and release of vasoactive substances by the grafted liver. Increased age, larger donor organs, longer cold ischemic time, presence of renal disease, and acute liver failure are risk factors.
    Treatment with calcium, atropine, and/or epinephrine improves cardiovascular function. Fluid administration should be judicious because it can aggravate the already increased filling pressures (secondary to myocardial depression), resulting in impaired hepatic perfusion. When pulmonary hypertension, elevated central venous pressure, and hypotension persist, an inotropic infusion may be necessary to maintain cardiac output. Vasopressor infusions, such as vasopressin and norepinephrine, may be necessary to combat persistent vasodilation.

37. **Describe some of the major anesthetic management issues during stage 3 (reperfusion).**
    - Wide swings in blood pressure and arrhythmias can be expected. Hypertension may be caused by a large increase in preload, following caval unclamping. More frequently, release of the portal vein clamp directs blood through the liver graft to the heart, and products of cell death and residual preservation fluid can cause severe hypotension, bradycardia, supraventricular and ventricular arrhythmias, electromechanical dissociation, and occasionally cardiac arrest. A defibrillator should be immediately available in the event advanced cardiovascular life support is required. Hypotension may also result from surgical bleeding, because the anastomotic sites are exposed to venous pressure for the first time.
    - After venous reperfusion, the hepatic artery anastomosis is completed and reperfused. At this stage induction of immunosuppression takes place with steroid administration.
    - Coagulation defects are commonly observed during stage 3 because the new liver requires time to resume its synthetic functions. Viscoelastic testing should guide treatment.
    - Urine output typically improves, even in patients with prior HRS.
    - The procedure is completed after biliary reconstruction.

38. **What are indicators of graft function during stage 3 (reperfusion)?**
An important part of the neohepatic phase is the evaluation of graft function. The patient should have the ability to maintain normocalcemia, without supplementation, as the liver is now metabolizing citrate; elevated lactate levels should decrease, implying hepatic lactate clearance; achieve normothermia; produce bile; synthesize clotting factors, as noted by less bleeding.
    Signs suggestive of poor graft function include unexplained acute deterioration in urinary output, prolonged hypotension requiring pressor support, and increasing lactate. If bleeding persists despite fresh frozen plasma and platelet transfusions, then prothrombin complex concentrate (Factors II, VII, IX, X, C, and S) should be considered.

KEY POINTS: PERIOPERATIVE HEPATIC DYSFUNCTION AND LIVER TRANSPLANTATION

1. The portal vein supplies up to 75% of total hepatic blood flow, but only 50% of the liver's oxygen requirements.
2. Because of liver's large physiologic reserve, significant impairment of function must occur before clinical signs and symptoms of liver failure become evident.
3. Patients with ESLD have a hyperdynamic circulation characterized by decreased systemic vascular resistance and increased cardiac output.
4. Liver synthetic function can be assessed with INR/PT, PTT, and albumin but these laboratory tests do not reflect coagulopathy, as the natural anticoagulation proteins (protein C, S, antithrombin III) are also decreased.
5. Patients with ESLD may be coagulopathic or hypercoagulable, depending upon the ratio of pro- and anticoagulation proteins.
6. Common comorbidities include hepatorenal syndrome, hepatopulmonary syndrome, and portopulmonary hypertension. Patients with ESLD are at risk of death because of hemorrhage, venous thromboembolism, sepsis, and multiorgan failure.
7. Patients with acute liver failure are also at risk of severe cerebral edema and brainstem herniation.

Continued

KEY POINTS: PERIOPERATIVE HEPATIC DYSFUNCTION AND LIVER TRANSPLANTATION *(Continued)*

8. The Model of End-Stage Liver Disease (MELD) score predicts 90-day mortality and is used to prioritize recipients for organ transplant.
9. Concerns during the preanhepatic stage of liver transplantation include aggressive rewarming; monitoring serum potassium, sodium, and calcium levels; replacing significant blood losses; treating coagulation disturbances; and restoring effective arterial blood volume.
10. Concerns during the anhepatic stage include correction of hyperkalemia, hypocalcemia, and metabolic acidosis and restoration of intravascular volume in anticipation of vascular unclamping and reperfusion syndrome.
11. Wide swings in blood pressure and arrhythmias can be expected during the postanhepatic stage. Surgical bleeding and impaired coagulation are common. Urine output typically improves, the biliary tree is reconstructed, and graft function must be assessed.

Website
United Network for Organ Sharing: http://www.unos.org

SUGGESTED READINGS

Ge PS, Runyon BA. Treatment of patients with cirrhosis. N Engl J Med. 2016;375:767–777.
Hall TH, Dhir A. Anesthesia for liver transplantation. Semin Cardiothorac Vasc Anesth. 2013;17(3):180–194.
Kalra A, Wedd JP, Biggins SW. Changing prioritization for transplantation: MELD-Na, hepatocellular carcinoma exceptions, and more. Curr Opin Organ Transplant. 2016;21:120–126.
Martin P, DiMartini A, Feng S, Brown R, Fallon M. Evaluation for liver transplantation in adults: 2013 practice guideline by the American Association for the Study of Liver Diseases and the American Society of Transplantation. BMJ. 2013;59(3):1144–1165.

CHAPTER 42

RENAL FUNCTION AND ANESTHESIA

Khalil Chaibi, MD, Stephane Gaudry, MD, PhD

1. Describe the anatomy of the kidney.
   The kidneys are paired organs lying retroperitoneally against the posterior abdominal wall. Although their combined weight is only 300 g (about 0.5% of total body weight), they receive 20% to 25% of the total cardiac output. That means that within 5 minutes, the body's entire blood volume has circulated through the kidneys. This exceeds skeletal muscle perfusion, even during heavy exercise by 8-fold and makes the kidney the most highly perfused major organ in the body. The renal arteries are branches of the aorta and originate just inferior to the superior mesenteric artery. The renal veins drain directly into the inferior vena cava. Nerve supply is abundant; sympathetic constrictor fibers are distributed via celiac and renal plexuses. Pain fibers, mostly from the renal pelvis and upper ureter, enter the spinal cord via splanchnic nerves.

   The kidney can be divided into two zones: cortex and medulla. The medulla can further be subdivided into the outer and inner medulla (Fig. 42.1). Each kidney contains about 1 million nephrons, which can be categorized as short, cortical nephrons or long, juxtamedullary nephrons. The short, cortical nephrons predominate and make up 85% of all nephrons in the kidney. All nephrons originate within the cortex with their loop of Henle contained in the medulla.

   The glomerulus and Bowman capsule are known collectively as the renal corpuscle. Each Bowman capsule connects to a proximal convoluted tubule within the renal cortex which, as the name suggests, takes on the form of a "convoluted" structure, before it straightens and descends into the outer medulla, where it becomes the loop of Henle. The loop of Henle, for cortical nephrons, is short in that it only descends to the intermedullary junction where it makes a hairpin turn, becomes thick limbed, and ascends back into the cortex, where it becomes the distal convoluted tubule and comes into contact with the glomerulus and other cellular structures, known as the *juxtaglomerular apparatus*. Distal convoluted tubules then merge together to form collecting tubules within the cortex. The juxtamedullary nephrons (remaining ~15% of nephrons) are different from cortical nephrons in that they have a longer loop of Henle that descend deep into the medullary tissue. Juxtamedullary nephrons, in part because of their longer loop of Henle, play a significant role in the conservation of water.

   About 5000 tubules join to form collecting ducts. Collecting ducts merge to form minor calyces, which then merge to form major calyces. The major calyces join and form the renal pelvis, the most cephalic aspect of the ureter.

2. List the major functions of the kidney.
   - Regulation of body fluid volume and its composition
   - Acid-base balance
   - Detoxification and excretion of waste products, including drugs
   - Secretion of renin (involved in extrarenal regulatory mechanisms)
   - Endocrine and metabolic functions, such as erythropoietin secretion, vitamin D conversion, and calcium and phosphate homeostasis

3. Discuss glomerular and tubular function.
   Glomerular filtration results in production of about 180 L of glomerular fluid each day. Filtration does not require the expenditure of metabolic energy and is mediated by a balance of hydrostatic and oncotic forces. The glomerular filtration rate (GFR) is the most important index of intrinsic renal function. A normal GFR is 125 mL/min in males and is slightly less in females.

   Normal tubular function reduces 180 L/day of filtered fluid to about 1 L/day of excreted fluid, altering its composition through active and passive transport. Transport is passive when it is the result of physical forces, such as electrical or concentration gradients. When transport is undertaken against an electrical or concentration gradient, metabolic energy is required, and the process is termed active.

   Substances may be reabsorbed or secreted from the tubules and may move bidirectionally, taking advantage of both active and passive transport. The direction of transit for reabsorbed substances is from tubule to interstitium to blood, whereas the direction for secreted substances is from blood to interstitium to tubule. Secretion is the major route of elimination for drugs and toxins, especially when they are plasma protein bound.

4. Review the site of action and significant effects of commonly used diuretics.
   See Table 42.1.

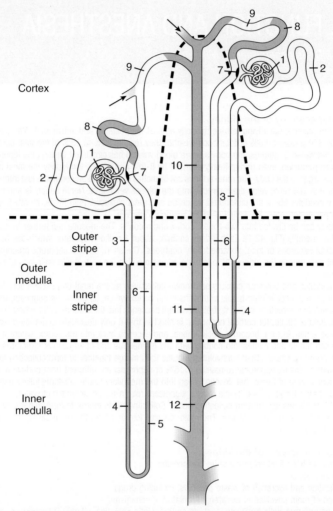

Fig. 42.1 This figure depicts a "long" juxtamedullary and a "short" cortical nephron, together with the collecting system (not drawn to scale). Within the cortex, a medullary ray is delineated by a *dashed line*. (*1*) Renal corpuscle, including Bowman capsule and the glomerulus (glomerular tuft), (*2*) proximal convoluted tube, (*3*) proximal straight tubule, (*4*) descending thin limb, (*5*) ascending thin limb, (*6*) distal straight tubule (thick ascending limb), (*7*) macula densa located within the final portion of the neck of the thick ascending limb, (*8*) distal convoluted tube, (*9*) connecting tubule of the juxtamedullary nephron that forms an arcade, (*10*) cortical collecting tubule, (*11*) outer medullary collecting duct, (*12*) inner medullary collecting duct. (From Kriz W, Bankir I. A standard nomenclature for structures of the kidney. Am J Physiol. 1988;254:F1, with permission.)

5. Describe the unique aspects of renal blood flow and control.
    The renal blood flow (RBF) is about 1200 mL/min and is maintained at a constant flow for a mean arterial pressure ranging from 80 to 180 mm Hg because of autoregulation. The cortex requires about 85% of RBF to achieve its excretory and regulatory functions, the outer medulla about 15%, and the inner medulla about 1% of total RBF. The inner medulla only needs a small percentage of blood flow, as a higher flow would wash out the solutes that are needed to maintain the high tonicity (1200 mOsm/kg) of the inner medulla. Without this hypertonicity, urinary concentration would not be possible.
    The principal goal of RBF autoregulation is to maintain a normal GFR, which is mediated by afferent and efferent arterioles, sympathetic tone, and hormonal influences. The euvolemic, nonstressed state has little baseline sympathetic tone. Under mild to moderate stress, RBF decreases slightly, but efferent arterioles constrict, maintaining GFR. During periods of severe stress (e.g., hemorrhage, hypoxia, major surgical procedures), both RBF and GFR decrease secondary to sympathetic stimulation.

Table 42.1 Diuretics

DRUG (EXAMPLE)	SITE OF ACTION	ACTION AND SIDE EFFECTS
Carbonic anhydrase inhibitors (acetazolamide)	Proximal convoluted tubule	Inhibits sodium resorption; interferes with H^+ excretion; hyperchloremic, hypokalemic acidosis
Thiazides (hydrochlorothiazide)	Cortical diluting segment (between ascending limb and aldosterone responsive DCT)	Inhibits sodium resorption; accelerates sodium-potassium exchange (hypokalemia); decreases GFR in volume-contracted states
Potassium-sparing diuretics (spironolactone, triamterene)	Competitive inhibition of aldosterone in DCT	Inhibiting aldosterone prevents sodium resorption and sodium-potassium exchange
Loop diuretics (furosemide, bumetanide, ethacrynic acid)	Inhibit Cl^- resorption at thick ascending loop of Henle	Potent diuretic; acts on critical urine-concentrating process; renal vasodilator; hypokalemia; can produce hypovolemia
Osmotic diuretics (mannitol, urea)	Filtered at glomerulus but not reabsorbed; creates osmotic gradient in tubules; excretion of water and some sodium	Hyperosmolality reduces cellular water; limited ability to excrete sodium; renal vasodilator

With the exception of osmotic diuretics, all diuretics interfere with sodium conservation.
DCT, Distal convoluted tubule; *GFR*, glomerular filtration rate.

The renin-angiotensin-aldosterone axis also affects RBF. At the juxtaglomerular apparatus, the macula densa can sense a decrease in sodium chloride delivery, causing the juxtaglomerular cells to release renin, which catalyzes the conversion of angiotensinogen to angiotensin I. Enzymes, primarily within the lung, convert angiotensin I to angiotensin II. Angiotensin II is a potent renal vasoconstrictor (especially on the efferent arteriole) and any increase (in addition to increased sympathetic tone) will cause a decrease in RBF.

6. Describe the sequence of events associated with decreased RBF.
    The high perfusion to mass ratio of the kidney makes them highly susceptible to injury from decreased RBF. The initial response to decreased RBF is to preserve ultrafiltration by redistributing blood flow to the kidneys, selective afferent arteriolar vasodilation, and efferent arteriolar vasoconstriction. Renal hypoperfusion results in active absorption of sodium and passive absorption of water in the ascending loop of Henle. Although afferent vasodilation and efferent vasoconstriction can initially help maintain GFR, if these compensatory mechanisms are exhausted, GFR will decrease, leading to oliguria. However, the kidney is attempting to maintain intravascular volume, and from the kidney's perspective, the process described is *renal success*.
    Oliguria, itself, is a poor measure of renal function, because other factors, aside from hypovolemia or acute kidney injury (AKI), can decrease urine output, such as stress because of surgery or acute illness. For example, one physiological response to stress is to secrete antidiuretic hormone and increased sympathetic tone, where both can decrease urine output despite euvolemia, normal RBF, and normal functioning kidneys.

7. What is the equation that describes renal perfusion pressure?
    Renal perfusion pressure can be calculated using the subsequent equation:

$$RPP = MAP - (CVP \text{ or } IAP)$$

RPP, renal perfusion pressure; MAP, mean arterial pressure;
CVP, central venous pressure; IAP, intrabdominal pressure

Note that only the higher of CVP or IAP should be used. This equation (and concept) is similar to the equations for cerebral and coronary perfusion pressure, as discussed in other chapters.

8. How is the renal perfusion equation clinically relevant?
    Any disturbance in physiology that reduces renal perfusion can cause AKI. For example, any decrease in mean arterial pressure (MAP) can decrease renal perfusion, causing decreased oxygen delivery and AKI. Similar to the cerebral vasculature, the renal vasculature is also autoregulated and can shift to the right in patients who have uncontrolled, chronic hypertension, leading to poor renal perfusion despite a normal blood pressure. Further, in the setting of advanced heart failure or cardiogenic shock, the central venous pressure (CVP) rises, which decreases renal perfusion, which is exacerbated in the setting of hypotension. Administering diuretics to patients with heart

failure can reduce the CVP (and renal congestion) and improve renal perfusion and oxygen delivery. Lastly, disease states that increase intraabdominal pressure, such as abdominal compartment syndrome or excessively high intraabdominal pressure during laparoscopic surgery, can also impair renal perfusion, leading to a decrease in urine output and subsequent AKI.

9. **How would you define an AKI?**
   AKI has replaced the term *acute renal failure*. The Kidney Disease Improving Global Outcomes (KDIGO) guidelines defines AKI as an abrupt decrease of kidney function over a period of 7 days or less, based on a rise in serum creatinine (Scr) or a decrease in urine output. Specifically, the first stage of AKI is defined as an increase in Scr of 0.3 mg/dL or an increase in Scr of more than 1.5 × baseline (either within 48 hours) or a urine output of less than 0.5 mL/kg/h for longer than 6 hours.
   Note that the term *chronic kidney disease* (*CKD*) is defined as kidney dysfunction, which continues to persist after 90 days.

10. **What preoperative risk factors are associated with postoperative kidney injury?**
    Several factors are known to contribute to postoperative AKI. Underlying medical conditions, such as CKD, diabetes mellitus, hypertension, cardiovascular disease, liver disease, chronic obstructive pulmonary disease, and obesity, are well-documented risk factors predisposing a patient to postoperative AKI. Advanced age is also closely related to the development of postoperative AKI.
    Patients undergoing cardiac or aortic surgery are also at elevated risk for developing postoperative AKI, especially when the cardiopulmonary bypass machine is used during surgery.

11. **Discuss the major causes of perioperative AKI.**
    Traditionally, AKI is categorized into prerenal, intrarenal, and postrenal etiologies. Unfortunately, the pathophysiology of AKI does not always strictly obey these definitions. For example, prerenal AKI will eventually lead to intrinsic AKI, if profound and lasting in duration. Prerenal AKI is because of decreased blood flow to the kidney and accounts for about 60% of all cases of AKI. In the perioperative setting, ischemia may be because of inadequate perfusion from blood and/or volume losses or from hypotension of any cause (e.g., decreased systemic vascular resistance). In fact, studies show that the first organ to demonstrate injury to hypotension during surgery are the kidneys. Further, even mild hypotension (i.e., MAP 50–60 mm Hg) for a short duration (i.e., <5 minutes) can cause AKI.
    Intrarenal AKI accounts for about 30% of all cases of AKI. Acute tubular necrosis (ATN) is the leading cause of intrarenal AKI and may be because of either ischemia or toxins. Nephrotoxins include radiocontrast media, aminoglycosides, tacrolimus, cyclosporine, vancomycin, amphotericin, angiotensin-converting enzyme inhibitors, nonsteroidal antiinflammatory drugs (NSAIDs), and serum-free hemoglobin or myoglobin. For example, autoimmune hemolysis or transfusing old packed red blood cells releases serum-free hemoglobin and rhabdomyolysis releases myoglobin.
    Postrenal AKI is less common and accounts for about 10% of all cases of AKI. Etiologies include obstructive nephropathy, such as benign prostatic hypertrophy or other causes of ureteral obstruction, such as pelvic malignancies.

12. **What laboratory abnormalities can be observed in patients with AKI?**
    Aside from the increase of Scr, which defines AKI (per KDIGO guidelines), several other laboratory abnormalities can also be observed. The blood urea nitrogen (BUN) will increase but is tolerated in most cases. However, an extremely elevated BUN can lead to neurologic impairment (i.e., uremic encephalopathy) or pericarditis. In intensive care unit patients with multiorgan failure, it is not uncommon for AKI to be associated with hyperkalemia, hyponatremia, hyperphosphatemia, hypocalcemia, and metabolic acidosis. Patients may also show evidence of anemia, in large part because patients with CKD are at a higher risk of AKI and may have a preexisting anemia of CKD. Other complications of uremia include platelet and leukocyte dysfunction, increasing the risk of bleeding and infection.

13. **Comment on various laboratory tests and their use in detecting AKI.**
    Indices of renal function can be divided into measurements of glomerular or tubular function. Measurements of clearance (e.g., creatinine clearance) assess glomerular function, whereas the ability to concentrate urine and retain sodium (e.g., fractional excretion of sodium [FENa]) is a measurement of tubular function. The majority of renal function tests are neither sensitive nor specific in predicting perioperative renal dysfunction and are affected by many variables common to the perioperative environment.
    Ammonia is generated from amino acid metabolism in the liver and is converted to urea (measured as BUN). Urea is rapidly cleared by glomerular filtration but is also reabsorbed by the tubules. Thus a BUN level can only be used to assess for tubular function and not glomerular filtration. Creatinine is the end-product of creatinine phosphate metabolism. It is generated from muscle tissue and excreted through the kidney. The Scr level can be affected by muscle mass and other factors, such as physical activity, diet (dietary meat is a common source of creatinine), and hemodilution. Additional nonrenal factors may also be responsible for an elevation of BUN and creatinine, including increased nitrogen absorption, muscle trauma from injury, hypercatabolism, hepatic disease, diabetic ketoacidosis, hematoma resorption, gastrointestinal bleeding, hyperalimentation, and drugs (e.g., anabolic steroids).

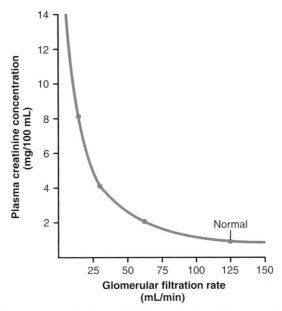

Fig. 42.2 The relationship between glomerular filtration rate (GFR) and serum creatinine (Scr) is inverse and exponential. In other words, a small increase in a previously normal Scr (0.5–1 mg/dL) represents a large decrease in GFR; however, a large increase in a previously abnormal Scr (4–8 mg/dL) represents a smaller decrease in GFR. (From John E. Hall. Renal Tubular Reabsorption and Secretion. Guyton and Hall Textbook of Medical Physiology. 13th ed. Philadelphia: Elsevier; 2016:347–369.)

The Scr rises in AKI because its half-life increases from 4 hours to 24 to 72 hours if the GFR decreases, and thus is a delayed indicator of renal insult. Recall that it takes four to five half-lives to reach steady state, so it could take up to 15 days (72 hours × 5) before creatinine levels stabilize. This fact alone greatly diminishes its utility as an accurate real-time assessment of kidney function in acutely ill patients with AKI because the GFR at a given moment in time may be much higher (or lower) than what the Scr suggests.

The relationship between Scr and GFR is inverse and exponential (Fig. 42.2). For example, an increase of Scr from 4 to 8 mg/dL does not represent a large absolute decrease in GFR, whereas at the same time an increase of Scr from 0.5 to 1 mg/dL represents a large absolute decrease in GFR.

14. **How can serum creatinine be used to estimate GFR?**
When renal function is stable, nomograms of Scr are a reasonable measure of GFR; however, the renal function of acutely ill patients is rarely stable, precluding the accuracy in assessing GFR using Scr. For example, if the patient is starting with a normal GFR, then the Scr might not become abnormally elevated until the GFR is reduced by over 50%. Also recall that the Scr does not reflect current kidney function because it takes time for the Scr level to rise. Because creatinine production is proportionate to muscle mass, cachectic patients (e.g., chronic illness, advanced age, deconditioned patients) may have a normal Scr, despite a markedly reduced GFR.

GFR also declines with age. For example, a healthy 20-year-old individual will have a GFR of about 125 mL/min, whereas an otherwise healthy 60-year-old individual will have a GFR about 60 mL/min. Recall, because of the exponential and inverse relationship between Scr and GFR, Scr does not begin to significantly increase until the GFR falls to about 50 mL/min.

GFR can be estimated using population studies based on the patient's age, Scr, sex, and weight. The method of Cockcroft and Gault uses the following formula for estimating GFR: GFR = (140 − age) × weight (kg)/(Scr × 72). This result is multiplied by 0.85 to determine the GFR for females. It is obvious that this overestimates GFR in obese patients, when total body weight, not ideal body weight, is used. This formula may also overestimate GFR in cachectic patients in whom creatinine production is low.

15. **What is creatinine clearance?**
Creatinine clearance (Ccr) is a sensitive test of renal function. Creatinine is filtered at the glomerulus and not reabsorbed. There is some secretion of creatinine with the tubules, and this results in about a 15% overestimation of Ccr. (Note that clearance of inulin, a polyfructose sugar, is the gold standard for measurement of GFR, because it is filtered at the glomerulus, and neither reabsorbed, nor secreted at the tubules.) It has been a long-held belief that measurement of Ccr requires 12- to 24-hour urine collections. In fact, if Scr is rapidly changing, calculations of Ccr, based on a 24-hour of urine collection and a single Scr measurement, may be inaccurate.

Table 42.2 Various Tests of Renal Function

TEST	NORMAL VALUES	ABNORMAL VALUES	COMMENTS
Specific gravity	1.010–1.030	Prerenal AKI >1.030; loss of concentrating ability, <1.010	Nonspecific; affected by glucose, mannitol, diuretics, endocrine disease, radiocontrast
Serum BUN	10–20	>50 definitely associated with renal impairment	Nonspecific; influenced by a wide variety of factors
Serum creatinine (mg/dL)	0.8–1.3 (men) 0.6–1.0 (women)	>1.3 (men) or >1.0 (women)	A delayed indicator of AKI; normal values reflect decreased function, as patient ages and muscle mass decreases
Urinary sodium (U_{Na}) (mEq/L)	$U_{Na} \approx 20$	ATN >60–80; prerenal AKI <20	Changes with composition of resuscitation fluid; affected by aldosterone, ADH, diuretics
Fractional of excretion of sodium (FENa)	1%–3%	Prerenal AKI, FENa <1%; ATN, FENa >3%	May not be accurate early in disease process (when most valuable); also nonspecific; affected by diuretics. Consider FEUrea if patients on diuretics
BUN/creatinine ratio	10–20:1	Prerenal AKI, >20:1; Intrarenal AKI, <10:1	Studies show test is highly inaccurate. Evidence-based medicine argues against this test
Creatinine clearance (mL/min)	100–125	Decreased renal reserve 60–100; mild renal impairment 40–60; renal failure <25 mL/min	A good test for measuring GFR; requires 24-hour urine collection but a 2-hour collection may be reasonably accurate

ADH, Antidiuretic hormone; *AKI*, acute kidney injury; *ATN*, acute tubular necrosis; *BUN*, blood urea nitrogen; *GFR*, glomerular filtration rate.

In addition, this method requires meticulous urine collection, and failure to accomplish this is a common source of laboratory error. Two-hour spot tests are thought to be reasonably accurate, and serial 2-hour spot tests may be particularly valuable when renal function is acutely deteriorating. Table 42.2 describes various tests of renal function.

16. What tests measure nephron tubular function?
As opposed to the measurement of glomerular function as previously discussed (creatinine, GFR, Ccr), tests of tubular function describe the ability of the kidney to concentrate urine and handle sodium. These tests are helpful in differentiating between prerenal AKI (i.e., dehydration, decreased renal perfusion) and intrarenal AKI (i.e., ATN).
In the setting of hypovolemia, renal tubules will retain salt and water, causing a relatively hyponatremic, concentrated urine. Conversely, this concentrating ability is lost in ATN, which results in increased volume of dilute urine high in sodium. The loss of concentrating ability in ATN may be detected 24 to 48 hours before BUN or creatinine begins to rise. Other tests of tubular function include urine-to-plasma osmolar ratio, free water clearance, urine-to-plasma creatinine ratio, urine sodium (U_{Na}), and FENa. In the setting of hypovolemia or dehydration, U_{Na} is less than 20 mEq/L. In ATN, U_{Na} exceeds 60 mEq/L. However, diuretic medications may increase U_{Na} in the setting of hypovolemia, in which case the fractional excretion of urea (FEUrea) should be used instead of FENa.

17. Discuss the utility of urine output in assessing renal function.
Urine output is easily measured by inserting an indwelling Foley catheter. A daily output of 400 to 500 mL of urine is necessary to excrete obligatory nitrogenous wastes. In adults, an inadequate urine output (oliguria) is often defined as less than 0.5 mL/kg/h. GFR is decreased by the effects of sympathetic activity, hormonal influences, and decreased perfusion. Oliguria is not uncommon during surgery because many factors can cause a decrease in urine output that does not necessarily imply AKI. For example, stress of surgery itself can increase sympathetic tone and the secretion of ADH, where both can lead to a transient decrease in urine output that does not necessarily imply AKI. Conversely, a normal urine output does not rule out AKI either.

18. What is the best way to protect the kidneys during surgery?
There are no magic bullets to prevent perioperative AKI. The best method is to maintain renal perfusion during surgery by ensuring an adequate intravascular volume, maintenance of cardiac output, avoid hypotension, avoid excessive intraabdominal pressure (e.g., during laparoscopic surgery), and avoid nephrotoxic medications (NSAIDs, certain antibiotics, etc.).

19. Does dopamine have a role in renal preservation?

There is considerable evidence that dopamine is not renal protective and should not be used to prevent or treat AKI.

20. Describe the effects of volatile anesthetics on renal function.

General anesthesia temporarily depresses renal function as measured by urine output, GFR, RBF, and electrolyte excretion. Renal impairment is usually short-lived and completely reversible. Maintenance of systemic blood pressure and preoperative hydration decreases this effect on renal function. Spinal and epidural anesthesia also depress renal function but not to the same extent as general anesthesia.

Compound A, a breakdown product because of the interaction of sevoflurane and CO_2 absorber, was thought to be a theoretical risk of nephrotoxicity particularly with low-flow (<2 L/min) anesthetic techniques. However, nephrotoxicity has only been documented in animal models, namely rats, and not in humans. Furthermore, extensive experience, including several studies, show that sevoflurane is not nephrotoxic in humans in clinically used doses. Moreover, all currently used inhalation agents are greenhouse gases, which damage the earth's ozone layer (a real, not theoretical danger to humans). Sevoflurane has the lowest atmospheric lifetime ($\sim$1 year) compared with other agents: isoflurane ($\sim$3 years), desflurane ($\sim$10–14 years), and nitrous oxide ($\sim$110–150 years). Thus the use of sevoflurane, particularly at low-flow states (<1 L/min), is not only safe but also beneficial to the environment!

21. What is the preferred neuromuscular blocking agent for patients with renal impairment? Is succinylcholine safe in this patient population?

Most neuromuscular blocking agents are renally excreted, which may cause problems with residual paralysis. However, atracurium and cisatracurium are the exception, as they undergo spontaneous degradation (i.e., Hofmann elimination) and therefore are the preferred agent in patients with AKI or end-stage renal disease (ESRD). Succinylcholine may be used if the serum potassium concentration is lower than 5.5 mEq/L. Interestingly, patients with ESRD who are adapted to higher serum potassium levels (i.e., have both high intra- and extracellular potassium levels, with a normal extracellular/intracellular potassium ratio) may tolerate succinylcholine administration better, despite a somewhat higher baseline potassium compared with patients with AKI. This implies that the rate of change in extracellular potassium or the ratio of extracellular/intracellular potassium, and not just the absolute potassium level itself, may play a large role in the pathology of hyperkalemia.

22. How are patients with CKD managed perioperatively?

Preoperative preparation is important for patients with ESRD because they have up to a 20% greater mortality for emergent surgical operations. Primary causes of death include sepsis, dysrhythmias, and cardiac dysfunction. Hemodynamic instability is common. From the standpoint of renal dysfunction, this patient population will have a decreased ability to concentrate urine, decreased ability to regulate extracellular fluid and sodium, impaired handling of acidic metabolites, and are at risk of hyperkalemia and impaired excretion of medications. CKD is also associated with anemia, uremic platelet dysfunction, dysrhythmias, pericardial effusions, myocardial dysfunction, chronic hypertension, neuropathies, malnutrition, and susceptibility to infection. Nephrotoxic agents (e.g., amphotericin, NSAIDs, aminoglycosides, vancomycin) should be avoided. If a radiocontrast study is contemplated, a risk-benefit analysis may suggest avoiding the study. If a contrast study is strongly indicated and worth the risks of subjecting the patient to contrast-induced nephrotoxicity, the patient should be well hydrated, and the contrast dose limited to the minimum amount needed.

Medications used perioperatively may have increased effects in patients with CKD. Because this patient population may have hypoalbuminemia, medications that are usually protein bound (e.g., benzodiazepines) may have increased serum levels. Both morphine and meperidine have metabolites that are renally excreted and should be avoided. Succinylcholine increases extracellular potassium (0.5–1 mEq/L), but can be used if the serum potassium is normal.

Before surgery, patients should be euvolemic, normotensive, normonatremic, normokalemic, not acidotic or severely anemic, and without significant platelet dysfunction. A recent potassium level should be checked just before surgery, particularly in patients with ESRD. Ideally, patients should undergo dialysis either the day of or the day before surgery. Dialysis usually corrects uremic platelet dysfunction and is best performed within the 24 hours before surgery, although 1-deamino-8-ᴅ-arginine vasopressin may be administered to treat bleeding caused by uremic platelet dysfunction.

23. Is it safe to give balanced salt solutions (i.e., lactated Ringer's, PlasmaLyte) to patients with ESRD?

Traditionally, it was thought that only normal saline should be used for intravenous fluids because it is free of potassium; however, studies show, perhaps counterintuitively, that the incidence of hyperkalemia is greater with normal saline than with balanced salt solutions (i.e., lactated Ringer's, PlasmaLyte), which contain potassium. This is likely because of the hyperchloremic acidosis caused by normal saline, which increases extracellular potassium. Conversely, balanced salt solutions contain buffers (i.e., acetate, gluconate, lactate), which yield a more neutral pH compared with normal saline. Further, balanced salt solutions have little potassium in their solutions (4–5 mEq/L). In other words, administering balanced salt solutions cannot raise the potassium level to a higher degree than the actual concentration of potassium for that solution.

24. What are the indications for renal replacement therapy (i.e., hemodialysis)?

The simple mnemonic **AEIOU** can be helpful in remembering general clinical indications for renal replacement therapy (RRT):

Acid-base problems
Electrolyte problems
Intoxications (e.g., overdose on drugs, toxins)
Overload (hypervolemia)
Uremic symptoms

25. How does RRT work?

Blood is removed from the patient and flows across a semipermeable membrane, the area of which is about 1 to 1.8 m^2. Across the membrane is a dialysate with normal electrolyte concentrations. Electrolytes and waste products move down their concentration gradients into the dialysate. In addition, alkali within the dialysate moves into the blood. Negative pressure within the dialysate results in excess fluid removal. The duration of intermittent RRT (also known as [aka] intermittent hemodialysis) depends on the flow rates and usually lasts from 4 to 6 hours. High-flow rates are associated with rapid changes in electrolytes and volume status, which is often poorly tolerated. Usually, patients with ESRD have intermittent hemodialysis 3 times a week. The mortality rate for patients with ESRD on intermittent hemodialysis is 5% annually.

Critically ill patients in AKI who are unstable often cannot hemodynamically tolerate intermittent RRT because of rapid fluid shifts. In such patients, continuous RRT is often a better choice compared with intermittent renal replacement because it runs at a much slower, continuous rate, causing less fluid shifts and better hemodynamic stability.

26. When should you start RRT for AKI?

The better question is not "when to start hemodialysis" but "why start hemodialysis"? RRT should be initiated emergently when life-threatening conditions occur. There are three relatively common life-threatening conditions: (1) severe hyperkalemia (potassium >6 mmol/L, or >5.5 mmol/L, despite medical treatment), (2) severe acidosis (pH <7.15), and (3) acute pulmonary edema because of fluid overload (often causing severe hypoxemia). There is no threshold of BUN concentration that indicates RRT. However, extremely high levels of uremia may be associated with neurologic impairment or bleeding complications, which may itself indicate the need for RRT. In all other situations, there is no evidence that early initiation of RRT yields better outcomes. Moreover, recent studies show that early RRT could be associated with delayed renal function recovery.

KEY POINTS: RENAL FUNCTION AND ANESTHESIA

1. Risk factors for postoperative AKI include a history of CKD, left ventricular dysfunction, advanced age, and diabetes mellitus.
2. Scr is a delayed indicator of renal insult and may take days or weeks to reach steady state.
3. The relationship between GFR and Scr is inverse and exponential.
4. Patients undergoing cardiac or aortic surgery are particularly at risk for developing postoperative AKI.
5. The majority of renal function tests are neither sensitive nor specific in predicting perioperative renal dysfunction and are affected by many variables common to the perioperative environment.
6. Compound A, a byproduct of sevoflurane and CO_2 absorber, has only shown to cause nephrotoxicity in rats, not humans.
7. Low-flow (<1 L/min) anesthetic technique with sevoflurane is safe in humans and significantly better for the environment than other inhalational agents.
8. The best way to maintain renal function during surgery is to ensure an adequate intravascular volume, maintain cardiac output, avoid hypotension, and avoid nephrotoxic agents.
9. Common indications for emergent RRT (aka dialysis) include life-threatening conditions, such as hyperkalemia, severe acidosis, hypoxemia respiratory failure because of hypervolemia, and/or complications related to uremia. Drug overdose and toxins are other indications to consider if life threatening.

SUGGESTED READINGS

Devabeye YA, Van den Berghe GH. Is there still a place for dopamine in the modern intensive care unit? Anesth Analg. 2004;98:461–468.
Khwaja A. KDIGO clinical practice guidelines for acute kidney injury. Nephron Clin Pract. 2012;120:c179–c184.
Meersch M, Schmidt C, Zarbock A. Perioperative acute kidney injury: an under-recognized problem. Anesth Analg. 2017;125:1223.
Motayagheni N, Phan S, Eshraghi C, et al. A review of anesthetic effects on renal function: potential organ protection. Am J Nephrol. 2017;46:380–389.
Park JT. Postoperative acute kidney injury. Korean J Anesthesiol. 2017;70:258–266.

CHAPTER 43

INTRACRANIAL AND CEREBROVASCULAR DISEASE

Anthony M. Oliva, MD, PhD

1. **What is normal cerebral blood flow (CBF)? At what level is CBF considered ischemic?**
   Normal CBF in humans is 40 to 60 mL/100 g/min (15% of cardiac output). The cerebral metabolic rate for oxygen ($CMRO_2$) in adults is 3 to 4 mL/100 g/min (20% of whole-body oxygen consumption). The CBF at which ischemia becomes apparent on electroencephalogram (EEG) is 18 to 20 mL/100 g/min. The threshold between reversible and irreversible ischemia depends on many factors, but most importantly on how low CBF goes and how long it stays low.

2. **Define cerebral autoregulation. How is it affected in cerebrovascular disease?**
   Cerebral autoregulation is the ability of the brain vasculature to maintain CBF in a normal range over varying mean arterial pressures (50–150 mm Hg). To illustrate in a patient with carotid stenosis, the obstruction in the internal carotid artery causes a pressure drop beyond the obstruction. In an effort to maintain CBF, the cerebral vasculature dilates. Conversely, in a patient with uncontrolled hypertension, arteries in the brain vasoconstrict to limit blood flow. Importantly, in both cases, once compensatory mechanisms reach their limits, CBF becomes passive and is linearly correlated with systemic blood pressure. Patients with cerebrovascular disease likely have dysfunctional cerebral autoregulation and blood pressure control is critically important.

3. **What is cerebrovascular insufficiency?**
   Cerebrovascular insufficiency refers to any condition resulting from inadequate blood supply to the brain. Inadequate blood flow is most often from partial or complete arterial obstruction. This leads to inadequate delivery of essential oxygen and nutrients placing the affected tissue at risk of ischemia. Cerebrovascular accidents (CVA) or transient ischemic attacks (TIA) are common outcomes and the severity depends on the extent and location of the obstruction, as well as the duration of insufficient blood flow.

4. **What are the symptoms of cerebral ischemia?**
   Cerebral ischemia presentation depends on whether the injury is global or focal in nature. Global ischemia occurs over a wide area and is severe, often leading to loss of consciousness and widespread neurologic dysfunction. Cardiac arrest is the most common cause of global ischemia. Other causes include respiratory failure, heart failure, and congenital heart defects. In contrast, focal ischemia presents in numerous ways and neurologic dysfunction is much more limited. Focal insults can impair vision, motor function, and the ability to understand or speak language. Thrombotic and embolic phenomena are the most common causes of focal ischemia. Other causes include hemorrhage, vasospasm, and trauma.

5. **What are the factors that increase the risk for cerebral ischemic events?**
   The leading cause of a CVA is uncontrolled hypertension. Other risk factors include a previous CVA or TIA, diabetes, hypercholesterolemia, sickle cell disease, coronary artery disease, atrial fibrillation, and cardiac valvular disease. Lifestyle choices also play a significant role in the long-term CVA risk. High fat and salt diets, physical inactivity, obesity, excessive alcohol intake, and tobacco use are important and modifiable risk factors. Age, gender, ethnicity, and genetics are nonmodifiable risk factors. The elderly, women, and African descent and Latino populations are at higher risk of a CVA.

6. **What are the two types of CVA?**
   Ischemic CVA occurs when a blood vessel supplying blood to the brain is obstructed. This is the most common type of CVA and accounts for nearly 90% of all cases. The obstruction is most often thrombotic and can form at atherosclerotic plaques in the cerebral arteries or can embolize from more distant locations, such as the heart and carotid arteries.

   Hemorrhagic CVA occurs when a blood vessel supplying blood to the brain ruptures. Weakened walls in cerebral aneurysms, arteriovenous malformations (AVM), and tumors lead to blood vessel rupture. Aneurysms make up the majority of hemorrhagic CVAs. Hemorrhage in the brain can be within the parenchyma, called *intracerebral hemorrhage*, or in the space surrounding the brain, called *subarachnoid hemorrhage*. Rupture is most often the result of uncontrolled hypertension.

7. **How does TIA differ from CVA?**
   TIA, or mini-stroke, mimics CVA in terms of acute onset of neurologic dysfunction. However, the difference is that symptoms resulting from TIA resolve spontaneously within one hour and patients should have no evidence of infarction on brain imaging studies. Importantly, a TIA significantly increases the likelihood of a future CVA because

nearly half of those who have a TIA will later have a CVA. In those that ultimately do have a CVA, many had a TIA in the days preceding. The risk of a future CVA is increased as age increases, and as the time for TIA symptom resolution increases. An online validated calculator called the *ABCD² (age, blood pressure, clinical features, duration of TIA, and presence of diabetes) score*, can aid in stratifying patients into various risk categories.

8. **A patient has carotid artery disease, what are their treatment options?**
Patients with significant carotid disease, greater than 70% stenosis, have two options to treat their stenotic lesions. Carotid endarterectomy (CEA) is a surgical option to remove plaque from the diseased artery. An endovascular option is angioplasty and stenting, similar to what is done for diseased cardiac vessels. In patients undergoing either type of procedure, numerous anesthetic options exist. No matter the procedure chosen, a means to assess adequate cerebral perfusion is essential. Keeping the patient awake is considered the best method to confirm adequate CBF. Using local anesthesia and titrated intravenous (IV) sedation, a patient can be kept comfortable and assessed neurologically throughout the procedure. Needless to say, the majority of procedures are done under general anesthesia, as studies show no difference in outcomes between general anesthesia versus keeping the patient awake using local anesthesia with sedation. Various modalities to monitor neurologic function and/or cerebral perfusion are used when this operation is performed under general anesthesia. Neurologic function can be assessed using intraoperative neuromonitoring, including EEG and somatosensory evoked potentials. Cerebral perfusion can be assessed using stump pressure, transcranial Doppler, and cerebral oximetry. Interestingly, regardless of what anesthetic approach is used, intraoperative stroke is rare and there is no superior approach. Importantly, if a CVA occurs, it is most often postoperatively because of cerebral hyperperfusion.

9. **What is cerebral hyperperfusion syndrome?**
Cerebral hyperperfusion syndrome can occur following carotid artery endarterectomy or carotid artery stenting. After correction of carotid artery stenosis, CBF may increase by as much as 200%. Poorly controlled hypertension contributes to this complication. Symptoms and side effects of hyperperfusion are headache, face and eye pain, cerebral edema, nausea and vomiting, seizure, and intracerebral hemorrhage. The blood pressure of such patients should be carefully controlled postoperatively to maintain a systolic blood pressure lower than 120 to 140 mm Hg, with vasodilating agents, which do not increase intracerebral pressure (ICP).

10. **A patient has a cerebral aneurysm, what are their treatment options?**
A patient with a cerebral aneurysm, either unruptured or ruptured, has either surgical or endovascular options available for treatment. Regardless of the intervention, general anesthesia is normally required. Modalities to assess neurologic function or CBF are not typically required. If surgery is chosen, a clip is placed on the aneurysm to prevent blood flow to it. This type of intervention is slowly giving way to the endovascular placement of coils into the aneurysm. A soft wire is inserted into the aneurysm until the entire cavity is filled to seal off flow from the artery. Another, newer, endovascular intervention is the placement of flow diverters. Flow diverters are simply a stent-like implant that diverts blood flow away from the aneurysm. A ruptured aneurysm can rebleed or lead to vasospasm, which further worsens a patient's condition and prognosis. Rebleeding, if it occurs, usually happens in the first 1 to 2 days after the initial rupture and may require surgical clipping.

11. **When does intracranial vasospasm occur with subarachnoid hemorrhage (SAH)? How do you treat it?**
Vasospasm occurs in up to 70% of patients with SAH, although many are not symptomatic, and is responsible for significant neurologic disability and up to 50% of deaths because of SAH. The risk of vasospasm is the highest 7 to 10 days following rupture, but can occur anywhere from 3 to 21 days postrupture. To prevent vasospasm, patients are prophylactically treated with nimodipine and the avoidance of hypovolemia. In the event of vasospasm, treatment often includes permissive hypertension and endovascular interventions, such as intraarterial vasodilators and/or angioplasty.
Hypervolemia to treat vasospasm as part of "triple-H therapy" (i.e., hypervolemia, hypertension, hemodilution) is no longer advocated because of concerns of complications, such as cerebral and pulmonary edema. Further, any benefit from CBF because of hemodilution is countered by decreased oxygen delivery in hemodiluted blood.

12. **A patient has an AVM, what are their treatment options?**
A patient with an AVM, either unruptured or ruptured, similarly has surgical and endovascular options available to them, often both in tandem. Unique to AVMs, radiosurgery is an option to induce fibrosis and to obliterate the vessels. These lesions are often complex networks of vessels that shunt blood in a high flow, low resistance manner. Over time, they increase in size. General anesthesia is normally required for surgical and endovascular interventions. Modalities to assess neurologic function or CBF are not typically used. For most lesions, endovascular embolization is attempted before surgical resection to decrease intraoperative bleeding. Similar to aneurysms, ruptured AVMs can rebleed or result in vasospasm that further worsens a patient's condition and prognosis.

13. **What interventions are undertaken when a patient suffers from an ischemic CVA?**
Guidelines from the American Heart Association and American Stroke Association, updated in 2018, delineate how to manage patients with ischemic CVA. Mechanical thrombectomy and IV tissue plasminogen activator (tPA) are the two options to treat ischemic CVA. Mechanical thrombectomy is preferred if the vessel occluded is large, the interval

time since the start of symptoms is greater than 6 hours, or the patient is ineligible for IV tPA. Otherwise, IV tPA is often the first-line of therapy and aims to promote clot breakdown.

Other interventions include starting aspirin within 24 to 48 hours, treatment of hyperthermia ($>38°C$), and hyperglycemia control (i.e., 140–180 mg/dL), as uncontrolled hyperglycemia is associated with worse outcomes.

14. **What interventions are undertaken when a patient suffers from a hemorrhagic CVA?**

Managing patients with hemorrhagic CVA requires a multifaceted approach. First, blood pressure control is critical. Patients often are hypertensive at presentation and are at high-risk of rebleeding and hematoma expansion. Typically, a systolic blood pressure less than 140 mm Hg is targeted to minimize bleeding. Second, upwards of 20% of patients presenting with a hemorrhagic CVA are taking anticoagulation agents. Reversal of these agents is necessary in these patients. Third, the seizure threshold is lowered in these patients, thus seizure prophylaxis and treatment are important. Fourth, hyperglycemia on admission is associated with worse outcomes and should be controlled (i.e., 140–180 mg/dL). The remaining management depends on the severity of symptoms. When symptoms are mild, close observation is warranted. As symptoms progress, pharmacologic interventions are aimed at reducing ICP. Osmotic diuretics, such as mannitol and hypertonic saline, are first-line agents to decrease ICP. Anesthetic agents, such as propofol and barbiturates, can be used as well. In patients who have an elevated ICP that is refractory to medical management, a decompressive craniectomy should be considered, although this intervention is not benign and may prolong life at the expense of quality of life.

15. **How do you assess CVA severity?**

Of the many tools to assess the severity of CVA, there are two scoring systems that are frequently used. The National Institutes of Health Stroke Scale (NIHSS) is perhaps the most well studied and applied in clinical practice. When this scoring system is used within the first 48 hours following a CVA, it correlates well with clinical outcomes at the 3-month and 1-year intervals. The NIHSS score can predict the likelihood of hospital discharge, the requirement of nursing home admission, the need for rehabilitation therapy, and whether the patient is likely to achieve functional independence. The Hunt and Hess Scale is used extensively for SAH to predict morbidity and mortality. This score is obtained on patient presentation to the hospital and is based on the extent of neurologic dysfunction seen on clinical examination.

16. **What factors impact neurologic outcome following a CVA?**

Patients suffering from CVA have a high rate of death. Those that survive often will have permanent neurologic dysfunction. The type and size of plaque or embolus, the site of ischemia, the extent of collateral circulation, the duration of inadequate perfusion, and the inherent response of the brain to the insult all contribute to the neurologic sequelae. Patients who are young and who have a low NIHSS score are the mostly likely to have full recovery after CVA.

17. **What are some local CBF perturbations seen in cerebrovascular disease?**

In ischemic brain tissue, arterial vessels are maximally dilated to promote as much CBF as possible. It is in this instance that local paradoxical effects to changes in arterial carbon dioxide ($PaCO_2$) are seen. A phenomenon called *steal syndrome* involves the diversion of blood flow away from ischemic areas in the setting of hypercapnia. Here, there is global dilation of cerebral arteries in response to elevated $PaCO_2$, which results in the ischemic area getting even less blood flow. On the other hand, the Robin Hood effect describes how hypocapnia results in global constriction of cerebral arteries, resulting in hyperperfusion of the ischemic tissue. Lastly, in conditions that chronically result in low local blood flow, such as AVM, some arteries may lack any ability to autoregulate. In this instance, changes in local blood flow related to AVM embolization or surgical resection can lead to hyperperfusion, cerebral edema, and intracranial hemorrhage.

KEY POINTS: INTRACRANIAL AND CEREBROVASCULAR DISEASE

1. Cerebral autoregulation is often dysregulated in patients with cerebrovascular disease. Tight blood pressure control is crucial and placement of an arterial line should be done for any procedure.
2. Atherosclerotic disease is the most common cause of ischemic CVA. Treatment requires timely IV administration of tPA and/or manual thrombectomy.
3. Uncontrolled hypertension is the most common cause of hemorrhagic CVA. Treatment includes pharmacologic and surgical interventions depending on the severity of symptoms and the cause of the bleed.
4. In patients with carotid artery disease, treatment options include CEA and angioplasty with stent placement. Intraoperative stroke is rare and no particular anesthetic technique has superior outcomes. When a stroke occurs, it is most often in the days following the procedure because of hyperperfusion.
5. In patients with cerebral aneurysm, treatment options include clipping and coiling of the aneurysm. Flow diverters are a newer type of endovascular intervention.

Continued

KEY POINTS: INTRACRANIAL AND CEREBROVASCULAR DISEASE *(Continued)*

6. In patients with AVM, treatment options include embolization and surgical resection. Most often, the lesion is embolized using an endovascular technique and then subsequently resected surgically.
7. Patients who are most likely to have a full recovery, without residual neurologic deficits, after suffering a CVA are young (<65 years old) and present with a low NIHSS score.
8. Many online validated tools exist to risk stratify patients, to assess for severity of neurologic dysfunction, and to predict outcomes.

SUGGESTED READINGS

Connolly ES, Rabinstein AA, Carhuapoma JR, et al. Guidelines for the management of aneurysmal subarachnoid hemorrhage: a guideline for healthcare professionals from the American Heart Association/American Stroke Association. Stroke. 2012;43(6):1711–1137.

Drummond JC, Patel PM, Lemkuil BP. Anesthesia for neurologic surgery. In: Miller's RD, ed. Miller's Anesthesia. 8th ed. Philadelphia, PA: Elsevier Saunders. 2015:2158–2199.

Hines, RL, Marschall, KE. Diseases affecting the brain. In: Handbook for Stoelting's Anesthesia and Coexisting Diseases. 4th Ed. Philadelphia, PA. Elsevier Saunders; 2013:122–146.

Kernan, WN, Ovbiagele, B, Black, HR, et al. Guidelines for the prevention of stroke in patients with stroke and transient ischemic attack: a guideline for healthcare professionals from the American Heart Association/American Stroke Association. Stroke. 2014;45(7):2160–2236.

Meschia, JF, Bushnell, C, Boden-Albala, B, et al. Guidelines for the primary prevention of stroke: a statement for healthcare professionals from the American Heart Association/American Stroke Association. Stroke. 2014;45(12):3754–3832.

Powers, WJ, Rabinstein, AA, Ackerson, T, et al. Guidelines for early management of patients with ischemic stroke: a guideline for healthcare professionals from the American Heart Association/American Stroke Association. Stroke. 2018;49(3):e138, e233, e234.

INTRACRANIAL HYPERTENSION AND TRAUMATIC BRAIN INJURY

Charles J. Bengson, MD, Ross Martini, MD

CHAPTER 44

1. **Define intracranial hypertension.**
   Intracranial pressure (ICP) in humans is normally between 5 and 15 mm Hg. Intracranial hypertension is defined as a sustained ICP greater than 20 mm Hg.

2. **What are the determinants of ICP?**
   The brain parenchyma, cerebrospinal fluid (CSF), and the blood perfusing the brain are all contained within the fixed volume of the cranial vault. The Monro-Kellie doctrine defines the relationship between these components where any increase in a single component must be matched by a decrease in another to maintain a stable ICP. Once compensatory mechanisms are exhausted, including translocation of CSF into the spinal cord and compression of the cerebral vascular bed, any increase in volume will increase ICP.

3. **Summarize the conditions that commonly cause intracranial hypertension.**
   See Table 44.1.

4. **What are the symptoms of intracranial hypertension?**
   Early symptoms associated with increased ICP include headache, nausea and vomiting, and lethargy. Signs of elevated ICP include papilledema, focal neurological deficits, cranial nerve palsies, progressive decerebrate/decorticate posturing, abnormal brainstem reflexes, abnormal respiratory patterns, and eventually hemodynamic instability/collapse. The constellation of signs and symptoms are related to the severity of the intracranial hypertension and the regional/global compression of brain structures.

5. **How can you monitor ICP?**
   ICP can be monitored either noninvasively or invasively. Common noninvasive methods include imaging studies and physical examination. Imaging studies may show effacement or obliteration of cistern, sulcal, or ventricle CSF spaces, midline shift, and brain herniation, depending upon etiology and severity of ICP. Physical examination with fundoscopy may reveal papilledema, as the CSF is in continuity with the optic nerve.

   Invasive methods directly measure ICP and are divided into fluid-based catheter systems (e.g., external ventricular drain) and implantable microtransducers (e.g., fiberoptic sensor). Invasive techniques require access to the intracranial compartment and carry the risk of brain tissue damage, hematoma, and infection. The external ventricular drain (EVD) is a common fluid-based catheter system, which involves placement of a small catheter into the lateral ventricle. The EVD is considered the gold standard because it is cheap, reliable, and allows therapeutic drainage of CSF to treat elevated ICP. The major risks of EVDs include overdrainage of CSF, infection, and hemorrhage. Implantable microtransducers are often placed intraparenchymal but can also be placed in the epidural, subdural, or subarachnoid space. These devices are less traumatic to brain tissue and have less infection and bleeding complications compared with an EVD. However, these devices are prone to measurement "drift," where the integrity of pressure monitoring decreases over time and cannot be corrected by recalibrating the transducer. This is because the pressure transducer is implanted invasively and cannot be "rezeroed" to atmospheric pressure in contrast to fluid-filled transducer systems (i.e., EVD), where the transducer is external to the patient, often at the level of the tragus or inner ear.

6. **Discuss the possible consequences of intracranial hypertension.**
   Intracranial hypertension can result in a decrease in cerebral perfusion pressure and cerebral blood flow, leading to ischemia. Critical elevations of ICP may precipitate herniation of brain tissue across pressure gradients between dura and bony boundaries. Unilateral brain edema can cause a pressure gradient, leading to uncal herniation, compression of the midbrain, coma, and ipsilateral pupil dilation/hemiparesis. Globally, elevated ICP may cause downward compression and herniation of the brainstem and cerebellum through the foramen magnum. Medullary compression and subsequent ischemia will cause a profound sympathetic activation known as the *Cushing reflex*: systemic hypertension, reflex bradycardia, and irregular breathing. Brain herniation may damage the cardiorespiratory centers in the medulla, causing respiratory arrest, cardiac arrest, and brain death.

7. **What are the determinants of cerebral perfusion pressure?**
   Cerebral perfusion pressure (CPP) is calculated by the following equation:

Table 44.1 Common Causes of Elevated Intracranial Pressure

INCREASED CSF VOLUME	INCREASED BLOOD VOLUME	INCREASED BRAIN TISSUE VOLUME
Communicating hydrocephalus	Intracerebral hemorrhage (aneurysm or AVM)	Tumor
Obstructing or noncommunicating hydrocephalus	Epidural or subdural hematoma	Cerebral edema (cytotoxic vs. vasogenic)
	Malignant hypertension	Cysts

AVM, Arteriovenous malformation; *CSF*, cerebrospinal fluid.

$$CPP = MAP - ICP \, (or \, CVP)$$

CPP, cerebral perfusion pressure; MAP, mean arterial pressure; ICP, intracranial pressure; CVP, central venous pressure

CPP is the difference between MAP and ICP (or CVP, whichever is higher). In an intact autoregulatory system, CBF is maintained at a constant level, despite changes in CPP, where arterial constriction occurs with increases in CPP and arterial dilation occurs with decreases in CPP. Chronic hypertension, strokes, traumatic brain injury (TBI), and brain tumors can shift or blunt cerebral autoregulation of CBF.

8. What is intracranial elastance? Why is it clinically significant?
   Intracranial elastance describes the variation in ICP in response to changes in intracranial volume (Elastance = ΔPressure/ΔVolume). Although intracranial elastance is the reciprocal of compliance (Compliance = 1/Elastance = ΔVolume/ ΔPressure), the term *elastance* better defines this relationship because the ICP change is the result of a change in volume within a closed space. Initially, ICP remains somewhat constant over a limited range of intracranial volumes because of the ability to translocate intracranial CSF and venous blood to the spinal compartments and extracranial vascular beds, respectively. However, when these compensatory mechanisms are exhausted, the intracranial elastance increases (i.e., decreased compliance) and ICP rises exponentially with the slightest increase in volume (Fig. 44.1).

9. How is CBF regulated?
   CBF is influenced by several factors, including cerebral metabolic rate, arterial O_2 and CO_2 tension, CPP, and intracranial pathology. In general, an increase in the cerebral metabolic rate for oxygen (CMRO$_2$) leads to an increase in CBF. An increase in the partial pressure of carbon dioxide in arterial blood (PaCO$_2$) is an extremely powerful cerebral vasodilator, with CBF increasing 1 to 2 mL/100 g/min for every 1 mm Hg change in PaCO$_2$. A decrease in the partial pressure of oxygen (PaO$_2$) in arterial blood increases CBF, when the PaO$_2$ falls below 50 mm Hg. Variations in MAP also may result in changes in CBF. However, with an intact autoregulation system, between a CPP of 50 to 150 mm Hg, flow is nearly constant. Chronic hypertension shifts the autoregulation curve to the right, necessitating a higher baseline MAP to adequately perfuse the brain. In addition, following a brain injury, such as stroke or trauma, autoregulation is impaired, and CBF becomes pressure dependent (Fig. 44.2).

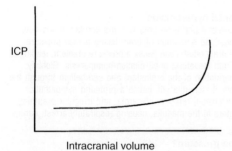

ICP

Intracranial volume

Fig. 44.1 Intracranial elastance curve. Note how small changes in intracranial volume can lead to catastrophic elevations in ICP when on the steep portion of the curve. *ICP*, Intracranial pressure.

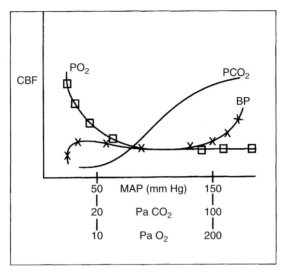

Fig. 44.2 Regulation of cerebral blood flow (*CBF*). *BP*, Blood pressure; *MAP*, mean arterial pressure; *PaCO₂*, arterial partial pressure of carbon dioxide; *PaO₂*, arterial partial pressure of oxygen; *PCO₂*, partial pressure of carbon dioxide; *PO₂*, partial pressure of oxygen.

KEY POINTS: FACTORS AFFECTING CBF

1. Cerebral autoregulation
2. CPP (particularly when cerebral autoregulation is impaired)
3. PaO_2
4. $PaCO_2$
5. $CMRO_2$

10. **What are the goals of anesthetic care for patients with intracranial hypertension?**
    Under normal physiological conditions, CBF directly changes in response to changes in $CMRO_2$, a phenomenon known as CBF-$CMRO_2$ coupling. The goal of anesthetic care is to maintain and optimize the cerebral oxygen delivery/demand ratio, while preventing secondary insults, such as ischemia. This is accomplished by reducing $CMRO_2$, decreasing intracranial volume, and avoiding situations where ICP or $CMRO_2$ may rise as a result of anesthetic/surgical stimuli.

11. **What interventions can reduce ICP?**
    - Decompressive craniectomy
    - CSF drainage (e.g., EVD)
    - Hyperosmolar agents (mannitol and hypertonic saline)
    - Hyperventilation
    - Head of bed higher than 30 degrees to facilitate venous drainage
    - Corticosteroids can reduce vasogenic edema from a tumor but can be harmful in cytotoxic edema caused by ischemia
    - Anesthetic agents (e.g., barbiturates, propofol) may reduce CBF and $CMRO_2$
    - Paralytics may reduce ventilator dyssynchrony ("bucking" or coughing)
    - Hypothermia can reduce $CMRO_2$ and cerebral edema

12. **What are some of the limitations of the interventions to reduce ICP?**
    Decompressive craniectomy, while highly effective at reducing ICP and mortality, comes at the expense of increased neurological disability and persistent vegetative state in survivors. Indications for decompressive craniectomy primarily include intracranial hypertension refractory to medical management. Strong consideration to quality of life expectations for the patient should be discussed with family members whenever possible, as this intervention may prolong life at the expense of quality of life. Hyperosmolar agents and hyperventilation are also limited, as the brain adapts to both interventions over time (brain cells increase osmoles and CSF removes bicarbonate restoring a normal pH). Further, both can lead to a rebound elevation in ICP when either is abruptly discontinued. Excessive hyperventilation can be particularly dangerous as it may decrease ICP at the expense of decreased CBF, worsening ischemic injury, especially when the $PaCO_2$ is less than 25 mm Hg. Although paralytics may be helpful to facilitate

ventilator patient synchrony, they mask the ability to perform neurological examinations, which can be detrimental to patient care because the neurological examination is an extremely important modality in assessing prognosis and treatment. Hypothermia is also limited in that it increases the risk of infection, coagulopathy, and cardiac dysrhythmias. Evidence to date emphasizes targeted temperature management to avoid hyperthermia, to maintain a normal core body temperature, and only apply hypothermia treatment in selected situations.

13. **How do commonly used intravenous induction agents affect ICP?**
Propofol and barbiturates (e.g., thiopental) are the preferred intravenous (IV) induction agents in hemodynamically stable patients because these agents reduce CBF, cerebral blood volume (CBV), ICP, and $CMRO_2$. Etomidate similarly decreases $CMRO_2$, ICP, and CBF, and is associated with significantly less hypotension than propofol. Although it is often avoided as an induction agent because it lowers the seizure threshold, causes myoclonus, and may cause adrenal insufficiency, it is important to emphasize that hypotension is associated with increased mortality in patients with intracranial hypertension. Therefore the benefits afforded by less hypotension with etomidate may outweigh these concerns, particularly in hemodynamically unstable patients. The use of ketamine in the setting of intracranial hypertension was once contraindicated because of theoretical concerns, based on weak data that it increases both $CMRO_2$ and CBF, causing an increase in ICP. However, a recent meta-analysis found that ketamine does not increase ICP and in some patients may actually decrease ICP and should be considered in hemodynamically unstable patients. Liberal administration of opioids in a spontaneously breathing patient with an elevated ICP should be avoided, as it may cause hypoventilation, hypercapnia, and an increase in CBF and ICP. Other adjuncts on induction include IV lidocaine (0.5–1 mg/kg) to blunt the sympathetic response to intubation; however, the evidence to support this is weak and mixed. Short-acting β-blockers, such as esmolol, may also be helpful in minimizing the systemic hypertension commonly encountered during laryngoscopy.

14. **What are the considerations in selecting a neuromuscular blocking agent for intubation in patients with intracranial hypertension?**
Succinylcholine, a depolarizing neuromuscular blocker (NMB), may transiently raise ICP, but the clinical significance of this is incompletely understood. Nondepolarizing NMBs (e.g., rocuronium, vecuronium, cisatracurium) have no effect on ICP and can be safely used. Previous concerns surrounding prolonged neuromuscular blockade, masking the patient's neurological examination with high doses of nondepolarizing NMBs (i.e., rapid sequence intubation [RSI] dose of rocuronium), may be mitigated by the availability of sugammadex, a selective and reliable reversal agent for nondepolarizing NMBs. However, intubating conditions during an RSI with succinylcholine may be achieved more rapidly than with rocuronium. Thus for TBI patients at high risk for aspiration or with predicted difficult airway, succinylcholine is an appropriate choice. In other situations, nondepolarizing neuromuscular blockade is preferred to avoid increasing ICP, with strong consideration in administrating sugammadex after intubation, to facilitate neurological examination.

15. **What are the effects of volatile anesthetics on CBF and $CMRO_2$?**
All of the commonly used inhaled volatile anesthetics (isoflurane, sevoflurane, and desflurane) decrease $CMRO_2$. When administered in concentrations greater than 0.5 minimum alveolar concentration (MAC), they have direct cerebral vasodilatory effects increasing CBF in a dose-dependent manner. This can potentially lead to elevated CBV and ICP. Nitrous oxide, in contrast to the volatile anesthetics, increases $CMRO_2$ and CBF, presumably because of sympathetic stimulation, which can also lead to increased ICP. Prolonged nitrous oxide should be avoided in most neurosurgical procedures because of the risk of pneumocephalus, postoperative nausea and vomiting, and the potential for neurotoxicity.

16. **How is ICP managed during the maintenance of anesthesia?**
Most intraoperative methods for controlling ICP rely on the reduction of CSF, CBV, or total brain water content. If a ventriculostomy catheter (i.e., EVD) is available, CSF can be removed in increments of 10 to 20 mL. Blood volume can be reduced by hyperventilation to a lower $PaCO_2$ (30–35 mm Hg), resulting in transient cerebral vasoconstriction, and by using anesthetic agents that lower $CMRO_2$. Halogenated volatile agents reduce $CMRO_2$ but should be limited to a dose of less than 0.6 MAC to reduce cerebral vasodilation and preserve systemic hemodynamics. Nitrous oxide is often avoided because it increases both CBF and $CMRO_2$, may be neurotoxic, and may result in tension pneumocephalus. Maintaining the patient in slight reverse Trendelenburg position promotes venous drainage and reduces intracranial blood volume. Brain water can be acutely reduced with hyperosmolar agents, such as mannitol or hypertonic saline. The use of positive end-expiratory pressure (PEEP) may elevate CVP (and ICP) by impeding venous return to the right atria and should be used with caution.

17. **Is hyperventilation a reasonable strategy for long-term ICP management?**
Hyperventilation induces cerebral vasoconstriction, reducing CBV, and lowers ICP. This effect is mediated by an elevation in cerebral pH and is effective over a period of several hours (i.e., <6 hours). However, over time, cerebral pH returns to normal by a gradual decrease in the bicarbonate concentration in the CSF because of various compensatory mechanisms. In addition, hyperventilation below a $PaCO_2$ of 25 mm Hg should be avoided, as it can exacerbate cerebral ischemia because of decreased O_2 delivery (cerebral vasoconstriction) and decreased oxygen unloading from hemoglobin (alkalosis causes leftward shift of the hemoglobin-oxygen dissociation curve). Hyperventilation is only effective in the short term (i.e., <6 hours), thus limiting its use as a temporizing measure, such as when herniation is imminent.

18. **What are the preferred intravenous fluids for intracranial hypertension?**
Hypotonic crystalloid infusions, such as half-normal saline (0.45%), should be avoided because they increase brain water content and can increase ICP. Glucose-containing solutions should also be avoided because of concerns of worsened neurological outcome in the setting of ischemia and hyperglycemia. Balanced salt solutions (Ringer's lactate, Plasma-Lyte) and normal saline (0.9%) are often used for resuscitation and maintenance IV fluids. Although both balanced salt solutions and normal saline (0.9%) are categorized as isotonic, technically, normal saline (0.9%) is slightly hypertonic (308 mOsm/L), Ringer's lactate slightly hypotonic (273 mOsm/L), and Plasma-Lyte truly isotonic (294 mOsm/L). This argues that normal saline (0.9%) is the preferred maintenance fluid in reducing cerebral edema. However, the acidosis resulting from large volume resuscitation with normal saline can be avoided with balanced use of Ringer's lactate (or Plasma-Lyte) and normal saline (alternating between normal saline and balanced salt solutions for each liter administered). Occasionally, hypertonic saline (3% or 7.5%) is used for fluid resuscitation, as it results in the movement of water from the intracellular space to the extracellular space. This may increase intravascular volume and decrease ICP, but can lead to electrolyte abnormalities and complications because of hypervolemia if not monitored closely.

19. **Is albumin safe to give to patients with TBI?**
Colloid solutions, such as albumin, can also provide acute intravascular volume expansion similar to hypertonic saline. However, albumin has been associated with increased morbidity and mortality in TBI. It is important to note that the oft-cited study (Saline versus Albumin Fluid Evaluation trial), which found this association was with hypotonic (4%) albumin and it is unknown if this is also true with isotonic (5%) or hypertonic (25%) albumin.

KEY POINTS: AGENTS TO AVOID IN THE SETTING OF ELEVATED ICP

1. Nitrous oxide
2. Hypotonic intravascular fluids
3. Glucose-containing intravascular fluids
4. High concentrations of inhalation agents (>0.5 MAC)

20. **What is the role of hyperosmolar agents in the management of intracranial hypertension?**
Hyperosmolar agents (mannitol and hypertonic saline) are effective in decreasing ICP by selectively increasing plasma osmolarity, as both are impermeable to the blood brain barrier. This creates a concentration gradient that draws water from tissues, including the brain. In addition to reducing ICP, an early effect of mannitol and hypertonic saline is decreased blood viscosity, which optimizes CBF.
Mannitol also works as an osmotic diuretic and requires an intact blood-brain barrier (BBB) for maximal effectiveness. In doses of 0.25 to 1 g/kg, mannitol decreases ICP within 30 minutes with peak effectiveness occurring within 1 to 2 hours. Hypertonic saline (HTS) can be given in intermittent boluses of 1 to 2 mL/kg of concentrations ranging from 3% to 23.4%. It has a more rapid onset (~5 minutes), lasts longer (up to 12 hours), and may be more efficacious in decreasing ICP compared with mannitol. However, studies thus far have failed to show a difference in neurological outcomes between these two agents.

21. **What are the limitations of hyperosmolar agents?**
Although both mannitol and HTS can cause acute hypervolemia, mannitol is a diuretic and can cause hypovolemia, hypotension, and related sequela (electrolyte abnormalities, acute kidney injury). Conversely, HTS can lead to hypervolemia and has a theoretical concern of central pontine myelinolysis. However, this is more likely a concern when correcting hyponatremia and not in the treatment of intracranial hypertension, provided the initial serum sodium levels are normal.
It is preferable to give hyperosmolar agents by intermittent bolus rather than by infusion, because the brain adapts to a chronic hyperosmolar state by increasing cellular osmoles. This can have two detrimental effects: (1) hyperosmolar agents will be less effective over time, and (2) rebound ICP can be seen when hyperosmolar infusions are abruptly discontinued.

22. **What is the upper limit for mannitol and hypertonic saline?**
In general, the upper limit for HTS is a serum sodium level of 155 mEq/L and for mannitol a serum osmolarity of 320 mOsm/L. Recall the equation for calculating osmolarity:

$$Serum\ osmolarity\left(\frac{mOsm}{L}\right) = 2 \times [Na] + \frac{Glucose}{18} + \frac{BUN}{2.8}$$

A serum sodium of 155 mEq/L (upper limit for HTS), with a normal glucose of 100 mg/dL and blood urea nitrogen (BUN) of 15 mg/dL will yield an osmolarity of 320 mOsm/L (upper limit for mannitol). Note that the data supporting this upper threshold are based on older, weak data, with small data sets showing decreased survival, when this limit is reached. In some situations, a higher limit may be considered (e.g., sodium limit of 160 mEq/L) because care should be individualized and the data suggesting these limits are not strong.

23. **Discuss strategies for controlling ICP at emergence from anesthesia.**

Careful consideration of the patient's likelihood to maintain a patent airway and achieve adequate spontaneous ventilation and oxygenation should be made before a decision to extubate. Coughing should be avoided, as it may increase ICP. Withdrawal of anesthetic agents at the time of emergence can increase the risk of seizure, as most anesthetic agents have anticonvulsant properties. IV opioids and lidocaine may blunt laryngeal and tracheal stimulation during extubation. β-blockers, such as esmolol and labetalol, can be titrated to attenuate the increased sympathetic tone associated with emergence from anesthesia. Additional measures include elevating the head of the bed to facilitate venous drainage and maintaining normo- to slight hypocarbia.

24. **What other options are available to decrease ICP if previous interventions fail to work?**

Barbiturate coma has been used in patients who are refractory to other methods of ICP control. Typical doses of pentobarbital are 10 mg/kg given over 30 minutes to load, followed by three hourly doses of 5 mg/kg. This regimen usually provides a therapeutic serum level of 30 to 50 mcg/mL. Maintenance is usually achieved by dosing of 1 to 2 mg/kg/h. Propofol may be used temporarily in the perioperative setting, but because of the concerns surrounding propofol infusion syndrome, caused by high doses over a long duration, limit its use in the intensive care unit, as a method to induce coma for treating elevated ICP.

KEY POINTS: INTERVENTIONS TO DECREASE ICP

1. Decompressive craniectomy (intracranial hypertension refractory to medical management)
2. CSF drainage (e.g., EVD)
3. Hyperosmolar agents (mannitol and hypertonic saline)
4. Hyperventilation ($PaCO_2$ 30–35 mm Hg)
5. Head of bed >30 degrees to facilitate venous drainage
6. Corticosteroids can reduce vasogenic edema from a tumor
7. Anesthetic agents (e.g., barbiturates, propofol) may reduce CBF and $CMRO_2$
8. Paralytics may reduce ventilator dyssynchrony ("bucking" or coughing)
9. Avoid hyperthermia
10. Avoid hypervolemia
11. Keep PEEP and ventilator pressures as low as tolerated

25. **What is the difference between primary and secondary brain injury in TBI?**

Damage to the brain after traumatic head injury can be sustained during the initial injury and as a result of secondary insults, such as elevated ICP, hypotension, hypoxemia, and hyperglycemia. The primary mechanism of injury can result in focal or global neurological damage. Focal injuries are primarily caused by penetrating trauma, contusions, or intracranial hemorrhage (ICH). Global injuries often occur because of widespread cerebral ischemia or as a result of diffuse axonal injury, a condition in which rapid deceleration and rotation cause shearing between neocortical gray and white matter. The initial brain injury may not be responsive to therapeutic interventions. However, secondary injuries from hypoperfusion or hypoxemia may be preventable.

26. **What are the anesthetic goals in a patient with TBI?**

The main anesthetic goal of managing a patient with TBI is to prevent the occurrence of secondary injury. The compromised brain is extremely susceptible to hypoperfusion and subsequent hypoxemia. The airway should be rapidly secured if the patient cannot protect their airway (i.e., Glasgow Coma Scale <8). Cerebral perfusion should be closely monitored, but the literature is unequivocal regarding specific goals for CPP or MAP. Because the cerebral autoregulation is disrupted in TBI, cerebral hypoperfusion can occur, despite a seemingly normal blood pressure (BP), and hypertension can cause hyperperfusion, worsening intracranial bleeding, and increasing ICP. Studies suggest that a target CPP of 50 to 70 mm Hg, provided an ICP monitor is available, correlates to the best outcomes, where both hypotension and hypertension are avoided.

27. **What type of monitoring is generally indicated in patients undergoing intracranial surgery?**

It is important to have reliable peripheral IV access, as large blood and evaporative losses can occur quickly during intracranial surgery. In addition to the American Society of Anesthesiologists standard monitors, an arterial catheter may be indicated for real time BP monitoring and need for frequent blood draws to assess hematocrit levels, coagulation status, electrolyte levels, and blood gases. Central venous catheterization may also be indicated for the administration of vasoactive infusions or hyperosmolar therapy (hypertonic saline).

28. **How is hypertension managed in patients with ICH?**

Control of the hypertensive response in acute ICH is critical because elevated BP has been associated with hematoma expansion, mortality, and disability. The overall goal is to maintain adequate cerebral perfusion, while balancing the risk of rebleeding against the risk of ischemia, with aggressive BP reduction. Current guidelines for treating hypertension in spontaneous ICH recommend invasive arterial monitoring and aggressive control of BP with IV agents to a goal systolic BP lower than 140 mm Hg.

29. Which medications should be used to control blood pressure in the setting of intracranial hypertension?

Commonly used antihypertensive agents include selective "arterial vasodilators," such as calcium channel blockers (i.e., nicardipine), angiotensin-converting enzyme inhibitors (i.e., enalapril), and hydralazine. β-blockers, particularly labetalol because of its α_1 antagonism properties, may also be used. Nitroprusside and nitroglycerin should be avoided because they cause cerebral "venous vasodilation," which increases ICP. An excellent first choice agent in the acute setting is nicardipine, as it can be administered intravenously, does not impair contractility or cardiac output, is a selective arterial vasodilator, and does not increase ICP.

Website
Brain Trauma Foundation: http://www.braintrauma.org

SUGGESTED READINGS

Brain Trauma Foundation. American Association of Neurologic Surgeons, Joint Section on Neurotrauma and Critical Care: Guidelines for the management of severe traumatic brain injury, 4th edition. Neurosurgery. 2017;80(1):6–15.

Hemphill JC, Greenberg SM, Anderson CS, et al. Guidelines for the management of spontaneous intracerebral hemorrhage. Stroke. 2015;46:1–29.

Maloney-Wilensky E, Gracias V, Itkin A, et al. Brain tissue oxygen and outcome after severe traumatic brain injury: a systematic review. Crit Care Med. 2009;37(6):2057–2063.

Martini R, Orfanakis A, Brambrink A. Intracranial pressure monitoring. In: Koht A, et al., ed. Monitoring the Nervous System for Anesthesiologists and Other Health Care Professionals. Cham, CH: Springer International Publishing; 2017:243–252.

Pasternak JJ, Lanier WL. Diseases affecting the brain. In: Hines, RL, Marschall KE. Stoelting's Anesthesia and Co-Existing Disease, 7th ed. Philadelphia: Elsevier; 2018:265–303.

Stocchetti N, Maas AIR. Traumatic intracranial hypertension. N Engl J Med. 2014;370:2121–2130.

CHAPTER 45

MALIGNANT HYPERTHERMIA AND OTHER MYOPATHIES

Nicole Arboleda, MD

1. **What is malignant hyperthermia (MH) and its underlying defect?**

   Malignant hyperthermia is a disastrous and sudden syndrome evoked by the administration of triggering anesthetic agents, including volatile anesthetics and depolarizing neuromuscular blocking agents. Unfortunately, there is no distinct phenotype before exposure to the triggering agent. MH is a syndrome characterized by dysregulation of excitation-contraction coupling in skeletal muscle. Patients with MH have a persistent increase in the concentration of sarcoplasmic calcium, which increases the need for adenosine triphosphate (ATP), therefore producing heat with resultant hyperthermia. This is caused by abnormal function of the skeletal muscle ryanodine receptor RyR1 in MH susceptible (MHS) patients. The gene for this receptor is found on chromosome 19 in 50% to 80% of MHS patients.

2. **What is the inheritance pattern of MH and what are the triggering agents?**

   MH is thought to be inherited via an autosomal dominance pattern, although not strictly. Over 210 mutations in RyR1 exist in MHS patients, with an additional 4 mutations discovered in Cav1 (slow inactivating calcium channel) on the *CACNL1A3* gene. The anesthesia drugs that trigger MH include volatile agents (ether, halothane, sevoflurane, isoflurane, desflurane) and depolarizing muscle relaxants (succinylcholine). Preadministration of sedatives, propofol, and nondepolarizing muscle relaxants may delay the onset of MH in MHS patients.

3. **Describe the cellular events, presentation, and metabolic abnormalities associated with MH.**

   MH syndrome as the result of abnormal RyR1 receptor is characterized by a persistent increase in calcium within the sarcoplasmic reticulum. This increases the activity of pumps and exchangers to correct the increased sarcoplasmic calcium, thereby generating ATP. As a result, excessive heat production and increased oxygen consumption occur.

   Presentation of MH is typically after normal induction of anesthesia, followed by onset of unexplained tachycardia, hypercarbia with adequate ventilation, hypoxia, a mixed metabolic and respiratory acidosis, and late increase in core body temperature over 38.8°C. Patients also develop muscle rigidity and rhabdomyolysis, hyperkalemia, and acute renal failure. In North America, any patient suspected of having an MH episode should be reported to Malignant Hyperthermia Association of the United States (MHAUS) via a hotline (800-644-9737) that is staffed 24 hours a day, 7 days a week. Outside of North America, MHAUS can be reached at 001-209-417-3722.

4. **How is MH treated?**

   - Call for assistance, as aggressive therapy requires more than one person.
   - Turn off all triggering agents and hyperventilate the patient with 100% oxygen and flows greater than10 L/min.
   - Switch to a nontriggering anesthetic, for example, propofol infusion.
   - Notify the surgeon and operating room personnel of the situation and expedite conclusion of the procedure, even if it may require that surgery go unfinished.
   - Administer dantrolene, 2.5 mg/kg; repeat every 5 minutes to a total dosage of 10 mg/kg, if needed. Dantrolene sodium inhibits calcium release via RyR1 antagonism, thereby reducing cellular hypermetabolism. Note that reconstitution of dantrolene is performed with sterile water.
   - Monitor blood gases. Administer bicarbonate, 1 to 4 mEq/kg for a pH less than 7.1.
   - Cool the patient using interventions, such as cold fluids and cooling blankets, but become less aggressive in reducing body temperature at about 38°C.
   - Promote urine output (2 mL/kg/h), principally with aggressive fluid therapy. Note that mannitol and furosemide may also be required. Administration of bicarbonate will alkalinize the urine to protect the kidneys from myoglobinuria induced renal failure.
   - Treat hyperkalemia with calcium chloride, bicarbonate, and insulin/glucose.
   - Check for hypoglycemia and administer dextrose, particularly if insulin has been administered.
   - Send coagulation studies (fibrinogen, prothrombin time, partial thromboplastin time, international normalized ratio) to monitor coagulation status.

5. **How does dantrolene work? How is it prepared?**

   Dantrolene impairs calcium-dependent muscle contraction. This rapidly halts the increased metabolism and secondarily results in a return to normal levels of catecholamines and potassium. The older preparation was prepared by mixing 20 mg of dantrolene containing 3 g of mannitol in 60 mL of sterile water. The newer formulation of dantrolene (Ryanodex) makes preparation much easier and only takes 20 seconds to reconstitute. It is supplied as 250 mg vials of dantrolene sodium with 125 mg mannitol in lyophilized powder form and is reconstituted with 5 mL sterile water.

6. **How is MH susceptibility assessed in an individual with a positive family history or prior suggestive event?**
   The diagnosis of MH is immensely difficult. There are clinical grading scales that have been developed to help determine how likely a suspected episode is a true MH episode. The gold standard for diagnosis is the caffeine-halothane contracture test (CHCT). The patient's muscle is biopsied and then exposed to incremental doses of halothane and caffeine. The muscle is then evaluated for degree of contracture. This test is offered at only five centers in the United States and two in Canada. It is 85% to 90% specific, and 99% to 100% sensitive.

   Genetic testing for the abnormal RyR1 isoform is now available in the United States and other selected countries. The role for genetic testing is expanding. It is much cheaper than muscle biopsy/CHCT and can be performed on children who are considered too young to have CHCT ($<$10 years of age or $<$40 kg). Genetic testing is especially valuable in homogeneous populations in whom the genetic defect is prevalent. However, if genetic testing is negative in a susceptible individual, a CHCT must be performed. Limitations to genetic testing include low sensitivity, secondary to diverse mutations of genes.

   Of note, exertional heat illnesses characterized by rhabdomyolysis may suggest that a patient is susceptible to MH.

7. **What are the indications for muscle biopsy and halothane-caffeine contracture testing?**
   - Definite indications: suspicious clinical history for MH, family history of MH, prior episode of masseter muscle rigidity (MMR).
   - Possible indications: unexplained rhabdomyolysis during or after surgery, sudden perioperative cardiac arrest caused by hyperkalemia, mild to moderate MMR with evidence of rhabdomyolysis during surgery, exercise-induced hyperkalemia.
   - Questionable indications: occurrence of neuroleptic malignant syndrome, sudden unexplained cardiac arrest during anesthesia or in the early postoperative period not associated with rhabdomyolysis.

8. **What is MMR, and what is its relation to MH?**
   MMR is defined as jaw muscle tightness and limb muscle flaccidity, following a dose of succinylcholine. There is a spectrum of masseter response, from a tight jaw to a rigid jaw to severe spasticity, or trismus, otherwise described as *jaws of steel*. Of concern, the mouth cannot be opened sufficiently to intubate in a patient with MMR. If jaws of steel are present, MH susceptibility is also likely to be present.

   Note there is some controversy as to the management of patients experiencing MMR. Patients with masseter spasm should be closely monitored in the hospital for at least 24 hours. Creatine kinase (CK) levels should be checked every 6 hours. CK levels greater than 20,000 have a 95% predictive value that the patient is MH susceptible.

9. **Describe the preparation of an anesthetic machine and anesthetic for a patient with known MH susceptibility.**
   Clean the anesthetic machine, remove vaporizers, and replace the CO_2 absorbent cannisters, circuit, and breathing bag. Flush the machine for 10 to 20 minutes with 10 L/min of oxygen. Place activated charcoal filters on the expiratory and inspiratory limbs of the anesthesia circuit. Have the MH cart near the operating room. Notify the postanesthesia care unit (PACU) to be prepared with an appropriate number of personnel. A nontriggering anesthetic technique, such as continuous intravenous infusion of propofol and/or regional anesthesia should be used. MHS patients should be monitored for 6 to 8 hours after surgery in PACU.

10. **Should a known MH–susceptible patient be pretreated with dantrolene?**
    Dantrolene pretreatment is not indicated, providing that a nontriggering agent and appropriate monitoring are used and an adequate supply of dantrolene is available. Dantrolene pretreatment may cause mild weakness in normal patients and significant weakness in patients with muscle disorders. MHS patients with an uncomplicated intraoperative course should be monitored for at least 6 hours after surgery.

11. **What patients are at risk for redeveloping symptoms of MH after treatment with dantrolene?**
    Review of data from the North American Malignant Hyperthermia Registry (NAMHR) suggest that about 50% of patients redevelop symptoms, known as *recrudescence*. Typically, this occurs within 6 to 7 hours. It should be mentioned that the accuracy of this data is limited by its retrospective nature. Patients identified as being at risk for recrudescence were more muscular (and thus had greater muscle mass), had an MH score of 35 or greater (meaning that MH was very likely to be present), and experienced a temperature increase to as high as 38.8°C. There was no strong relationship between the use of succinylcholine or a particular volatile anesthetic and recrudescence. It is probably true that the most severely affected patients are the ones most likely to develop recrudescence. Taken together, these findings suggest that all patients who develop MH require at least 24 hours of posttreatment management in a critical care setting.

12. **What drugs commonly administered intraoperatively are safe to use in MH-susceptible patients?**
    - Induction agents: barbiturates, propofol, etomidate, ketamine
    - Benzodiazepines and opiates
    - Amide and ester local anesthetics
    - Nitrous oxide
    - Nondepolarizing muscle relaxants
    - Calcium

13. **Of the congenital myopathies, which ones are known to have a definitive relationship with MH?**
    Although many congenital myopathies were originally believed susceptible to MH, central core disease, multiminicore disease, and King-Denborough syndrome are the only ones noted to have a definite relationship.

14. **Compare neuroleptic malignant syndrome with MH.**
    Neuroleptic malignant syndrome (NMS) is a clinical syndrome characterized by mental status changes, generalized rigidity, fever, and dysautonomia. It is caused by administration of neuroleptic medications, such as haloperidol, phenothiazines, and thioridizine that have dopamine receptor antagonist properties. The pathogenesis of NMS remains unknown. NMS is treated with dantrolene or bromocriptine (dopamine receptor agonist) and has a mortality rate of 10%. Patients with NMS are not prone to MH.

15. **What are the most common muscular dystrophies and their clinical history?**
    Duchenne muscular dystrophy (DMD) is the most common and most severe muscular dystrophy (MD) with an X-linked recessive inheritance pattern. The defect is related to the protein dystrophin, which stabilizes muscle integrity. Dysfunction of dystrophin leads to progressive leakage of intracellular components and increased CK levels. Cytotoxic T cells then destroy the muscle cells, resulting in pseudohypertrophy of the muscle with fatty infiltrates. Clinically, patients have weakness and wasting of proximal muscles, which is progressive and presents early in life. Cardiopulmonary compromise is often the cause of death with dilated cardiomyopathy and respiratory failure contributing. Often affected areas include the brain (with resulting intellectual impairment) and scoliosis.
    Patients with DMD may be sensitive to the myocardial depressant effects of inhaled anesthetics. There is weakness of respiratory muscles, and a restrictive pattern is observed on pulmonary function testing. Smooth muscle may also be affected, manifesting as gastrointestinal tract hypomotility, delayed gastric emptying, and impaired swallowing, all of which may lead to an increased risk of aspiration. Becker muscular dystrophy has similar, although milder, symptoms and a more protracted course.

16. **What are the anesthetic considerations of patients with MD?**
    Patients with MD should have a thorough preoperative evaluation, given the likelihood of cardiopulmonary comorbid conditions. Preoperative electrocardiogram (ECG) and echocardiogram are necessary, as well as prior anesthetic history and pulmonary function tests.
    Patients with MD may have decreased gastric emptying and decreased laryngeal reflexes, leading to an increased risk of aspiration. They are also likely to have masseter spasm on induction of anesthesia. Postoperative monitoring is essential given their increased risk of respiratory compromise. Succinylcholine should be avoided because of the risk of hyperkalemia and rhabdomyolysis. Patients with MD are also less likely to have successful resuscitation after a hyperkalemic cardiac arrest. Nondepolarizing muscle relaxants are acceptable but may be associated with longer recovery times. There are reports of significant elevations in CK, severe myoglobinuria, and cardiac arrest after use of volatile anesthetics. Although patients with MD are not at risk for MH, a nontriggering general anesthetic or regional anesthesia may be preferred.

17. **Are patients with MD at risk for MH?**
    After succinylcholine administration, children with MH and MD may have similar clinical pictures, including hyperkalemia, elevated CK, and even cardiac arrest, although the mechanism are different. There are also reports of children with MD exposed to inhalational agents (but not succinylcholine) that have demonstrated MH-like anesthetic events. However, it is not true that children with MD are at increased risk for MH.

18. **What is myotonic dystrophy?**
    Myotonic dystrophy is an autosomal-dominant disease that usually presents in the second or third decade and is the most common inherited myopathy in adults. It is characterized by progressive muscle weakness and wasting, myotonia, and cardiac conduction abnormalities. Clinically, there will be persistent contraction of skeletal muscle after administration of succinylcholine. The contractions are not relieved by regional anesthetics, nondepolarizing muscle relaxants, or deep anesthesia and can make mask ventilation and tracheal intubation difficult. Triggering factors, such as shivering, hypotension, and mechanical stimulation should also be avoided.

19. **How does myotonic dystrophy affect the cardiopulmonary system?**
    Heart failure is rare, but dysrhythmias and atrioventricular block are common. Mitral valve prolapse occurs in 20% of patients. Restrictive lung disease, with mild hypoxia on room air, a weak cough, and inadequate airway protective reflexes may lead to aspiration and pneumonia. These patients are also sensitive to medications that depress ventilatory drive and need close monitoring in the postoperative period.

20. **What is myasthenia gravis?**

Myasthenia gravis (MG) is an autoimmune disease of the neuromuscular junction. Antibodies to the acetylcholine receptor reduce the absolute number of functional receptors by direct destruction, blockade, or complement-mediated destruction.

21. **Describe the clinical presentation of MG.**

Myasthenic patients present with generalized fatigue and weakness that worsen with repetitive muscular use and improve with rest. Extraocular muscles are very commonly the first muscles affected, and patients may complain of diplopia or ptosis. Of particular concern are myasthenic patients who develop weakness of their respiratory muscles or the muscles controlling swallowing or airway protection. Depending on whether extraocular, airway, or respiratory muscles are affected, MG may be described as ocular, bulbar, or skeletal, respectively. There is a strong clinical correlation of MG and thymus hypertrophy.

22. **How is MG treated? What can lead to an exacerbation of symptoms?**

Cholinesterase inhibitors, corticosteroids, and other immunosuppressants are effective, as is plasmapheresis. However, in many patients, thymectomy results in complete remission. Physiological stress, such as acute infection, pregnancy, or surgery can lead to exacerbations of MG.

23. **What are some of the principal anesthetic concerns in the management of a myasthenic patient?**

Principal concerns include the degree of pulmonary impairment, the magnitude of bulbar involvement (risk of pulmonary aspiration), and adrenal suppression from long-term steroid use. Although uncommon, cardiac disease that is related to MG should be considered in the preoperative evaluation. Because symptoms are primarily related to arrhythmias, a preoperative ECG should be performed.

24. **Describe the altered responsiveness of myasthenic patients to muscle relaxants.**

Patients with MG might need larger doses of succinylcholine (2 mg/kg) to achieve intubating conditions because of the decreased number of acetylcholine receptors. They can also be very sensitive to nondepolarizing neuromuscular blockers with an often unpredictable response. Dosing nondepolarizing muscle relaxants should start at around 1/10th of the usual recommended dose. Recovery time for these reduced doses varies but may be quite prolonged. Reversal of neuromuscular blockade can be successfully accomplished with the use of Sugammadex in appropriate doses. Often, no muscle relaxant is needed for surgical cases, as these patients are already weak; if volatile anesthetics are used, suitable muscle relaxation is often achieved.

25. **What is Eaton-Lambert myasthenic syndrome? Describe its symptoms, associations, and treatment.**

This is an immune-mediated disease of the neuromuscular junction that frequently arises in the setting of malignancy, often small cell carcinoma of the lung. Other associated malignancies include lymphoma, leukemia, prostate, and bladder. Autoantibodies affect the presynaptic calcium channels and result in decreased acetylcholine release. As opposed to MG, weakness improves with motor activity, although frequently, the improvement is transient. Proximal muscles are affected more than distal muscles, and legs more than arms. Cranial nerve involvement is also less frequent when compared with MG. Weakness often precedes the cancer diagnosis, although treatment focuses on management of the underlying malignancy. Autonomic dysfunction is common and manifests as dry mouth, orthostatic hypotension, and bowel and bladder dysfunction. Plasmapheresis, immunoglobulin therapy, corticosteroids, and 3,4-diaminopyridine improve strength.

26. **Review the anesthetic concerns for patients with Eaton-Lambert myasthenic syndrome.**

Patients with Eaton-Lambert myasthenic syndrome are sensitive to both depolarizing and nondepolarizing muscle relaxants, and these medications are best avoided. If given, paralysis can last for days and is not reversible with anticholinesterase medications. Volatile anesthetics are safe and often provide the necessary degree of muscle relaxation to facilitate endotracheal intubation. When applicable, regional techniques are encouraged.

KEY POINTS: MALIGNANT HYPERTHERMIA AND OTHER MOTOR DISEASES

1. MH is a hypermetabolic disorder that presents in the perioperative period after exposure to triggering agents, such as inhalational agents or succinylcholine. Early recognition is critical, and treatment is complex and multifaceted, requiring the assistance of other experienced personnel.
2. The sine qua non of MH is an unexplained rise in end-tidal carbon dioxide in a patient with unexplained tachycardia. A temperature rise and rigidity is a late feature.
3. Patients with a history of, or susceptibility to, MH must receive anesthesia with a nontriggering agent. The anesthesiologist must have a heightened awareness of MH, have prepared the anesthetic machine, and have the MH cart with dantrolene in the room.
4. Succinylcholine must be avoided in children with muscular dystrophy and should be limited to airway emergencies in children.

Continued

KEY POINTS: MALIGNANT HYPERTHERMIA AND OTHER MOTOR DISEASES *(Continued)*

5. Patients with muscular dystrophies are prone to aspiration and respiratory insufficiency and may have dysrhythmias, conduction blockade, and dilated cardiomyopathy.
6. Nondepolarizing muscle relaxants should be used at about 1/10th of normal doses (if at all) in patients with MG.
7. Patients with Eaton-Lambert myasthenic syndrome are sensitive to both depolarizing and nondepolarizing muscle relaxants, and these medications are best avoided.

Websites

Malignant Hyperthermia Association of the United States: http://www.mhaus.org
Myasthenia Gravis Foundation of America: http://www.myasthenia.org

---

SUGGESTED READINGS

Berman B. Neuroleptic malignant syndrome: a review for neurohospitalists. Neurohospitalist. 2011;1(1):41–47.
Hirshey Dirksen SJ, Larach MG, Rosenberg H, et al. Future directions in malignant hyperthermia research and patient care. Anesth Analg. 2011;113:1108–1119.
Larach MG, Brandom BW, Allen GC, et al. Cardiac arrests and deaths associated with malignant hyperthermia in North America from 1987 to 2006. Anesthesiology. 2008;108:603–611.
Litman RS, Flood CD, Kaplan RF, et al. Postoperative malignant hyperthermia. An analysis of cases from the North American malignant hyperthermia registry. Anesthesiology. 2008;109:825–829.
Miller RD, Cohen NH, Eriksson LI, et al. Miller's Anesthesia. 8th ed. Philadelphia: Elsevier, 2015:1287–1314

DEGENERATIVE NEUROLOGICAL DISEASES AND NEUROPATHIES

Daniel J. Janik, MD, FASA

CHAPTER 46

1. **What is amyotrophic lateral sclerosis and its anesthetic considerations?**

   Also known as *Lou Gehrig disease*, amyotrophic lateral sclerosis (ALS) is a disease of both upper and lower motor neurons resulting from degeneration of alpha motor neurons in the brainstem and spinal cord. It usually affects men in the sixth through eighth decade of life. Patients with ALS develop progressive weakness, muscle atrophy, spasticity, and hyperreflexia, and eventually die (from pneumonia and pulmonary failure), often in a 3- to 5-year period. Bulbar muscles become affected, increasing the risk of aspiration. The pathogenesis is poorly understood and treatment options are limited. Tracheostomy, gastrostomy, mechanical ventilation, and other supportive treatments are common. There is no evidence that either regional or general anesthesia exacerbates the disease. Succinylcholine-induced hyperkalemia and subsequent cardiac arrest have been reported. Nondepolarizing muscle relaxants have a prolonged duration of action. One should anticipate varying degrees of autonomic dysfunction. Patients will likely need postoperative ventilatory support. Medications with respiratory depressant effects should be used with caution because of increased sensitivity.

2. **Review the clinical manifestations of Guillain-Barré syndrome.**

   Guillain-Barré syndrome (also known as *acute inflammatory demyelinating polyradiculopathy*) usually presents with sudden onset of weakness or paralysis, typically in the legs, that ascends to the trunk, arms, and bulbar muscles over several days. Bulbar involvement may be suggested by facial muscle weakness. Areflexia is also a feature. Respiratory failure requiring mechanical ventilation occurs in 20% to 30% of cases. About half of all cases are preceded by a respiratory or gastrointestinal infection. The pathogenesis is thought to be autoimmune, and recovery may occur within weeks. Mortality results from sepsis, adult respiratory distress syndrome, pulmonary embolism, or cardiac arrest.

3. **How is the autonomic nervous system affected in Guillain-Barré syndrome?**

   Autonomic dysfunction is a common finding. Patients may experience wide fluctuations in blood pressure, profuse diaphoresis, peripheral vasoconstriction, tachyarrhythmias and bradyarrhythmias, cardiac conduction abnormalities, and orthostatic hypotension. Sudden death has been described.

4. **What are the major anesthetic considerations for patients with Guillain-Barré syndrome?**

   Patients may not handle oral secretions well because of pharyngeal muscle weakness and have respiratory insufficiency secondary to intercostal muscle paralysis. Aspiration is a risk. Compensatory cardiovascular responses may be absent, and patients may become hypotensive, with mild blood loss or positive-pressure ventilation. Laryngoscopy may produce exaggerated increases in blood pressure. Responses to indirect-acting vasoactive drugs may also be exaggerated. Intraarterial blood pressure monitoring is recommended.

   Succinylcholine is contraindicated because of the potential for exaggerated potassium release, and this state may persist even after symptoms resolve. Nondepolarizing neuromuscular blockers may cause prolonged weakness. Postoperative ventilation may be necessary.

5. **Review the pathophysiological features of Parkinson disease.**

   Parkinson disease, an adult-onset degenerative disease of the extrapyramidal system, is characterized by the loss of dopaminergic neurons in the basal ganglia. With the loss of dopamine, there is diminished inhibition of the extrapyramidal motor system and unopposed action of acetylcholine.

6. **Describe the clinical manifestations of Parkinson disease.**

   Patients with Parkinson disease display increased rigidity of the extremities, facial immobility, akinesia, shuffling gait, rhythmic resting tremor, dementia, depression, diaphragmatic spasms, and oculogyric crises (a dystonia in which the eyes are deviated in a fixed position).

7. **What are the effects of levodopa therapy, particularly on intravascular volume status?**

   Levodopa, the immediate precursor to dopamine, crosses the blood-brain barrier, where it is converted to dopamine by a decarboxylase enzyme. Treatment with levodopa increases dopamine both in the central nervous system and peripherally. Increased levels of dopamine may increase myocardial contractility and heart rate. Renal blood flow increases, as do glomerular filtration rate and sodium excretion. Intravascular fluid volume decreases, the renin-angiotensin-aldosterone system is depressed, and orthostatic hypotension is a common finding. High concentrations of dopamine may cause negative feedback for norepinephrine production, which also causes orthostatic hypotension.

8. **Review the anesthetic considerations for a patient with Parkinson disease.**
   - Abrupt withdrawal of levodopa may lead to skeletal muscle rigidity, which interferes with adequate ventilation; continue administration on the day of surgery.
   - Extremes of blood pressure and cardiac dysrhythmias may occur.
   - The patient may be treated with type B monoamine oxidase inhibitor selegiline.
   - Phenothiazines (e.g., chlorpromazine, promethazine, fluphenazine, prochlorperazine) and butyrophenones (e.g., droperidol and haloperidol) may antagonize the effects of dopamine in the basal ganglia. Metoclopramide inhibits dopamine receptors in the brain. These medications should all be avoided.
   - Patients may be intravascularly volume depleted; therefore aggressive administration of crystalloid or colloid solutions may be required in the setting of hypotension.

9. **What are the clinical signs and symptoms of Alzheimer disease?**
   Alzheimer disease accounts for most of the severe cases of dementia in the United States, with progressive worsening of memory and decreased ability to care for oneself and manage the usual activities of daily life. Apraxia, aphasia, and agnosia may also be present.

10. **What is the most significant anesthetic problem associated with Alzheimer disease?**
    The inability of some patients to understand their environment or to cooperate with healthcare providers becomes an important consideration. Sedative drugs may exacerbate confusion and probably should be avoided in the perioperative period. Regional techniques may be used with the understanding that the patient may be uncooperative. Reductions in the level of volatile anesthetic or opioid administered may be of benefit, as is the use of short-acting agents to hasten return of cognitive function. Patients treated with cholinesterase inhibitors will show prolonged duration of action of succinylcholine and resistance to nondepolarizing neuromuscular blockers.

11. **What are the hallmark features of multiple sclerosis?**
    The corticospinal tract neurons of the brain and spinal cord, as well as posterior columns show random and multifocal demyelination, which slows nerve conduction, resulting in visual and gait disturbances, limb paresthesias and weaknesses, and urinary incontinence. There is increasing evidence that there is demyelination of peripheral nerves as well. The onset of disease is typically between the ages of 20 and 40 years. The cause appears to be autoimmune. The course of multiple sclerosis (MS) is characterized by symptomatic exacerbations and remissions, although symptoms eventually persist. Female patients often experience remission during pregnancy.

12. **Do steroids have a role in the treatment of MS?**
    Steroids may shorten the duration and severity of an attack but probably do not influence progression of the disease. Other therapies, such as immunosuppressive drugs, interferon, and plasmapheresis are also occasionally of benefit. Symptomatic treatment is with baclofen, benzodiazepines, anticonvulsants, β-blockers, and selective serotonin reuptake inhibitors.

13. **What factors have been associated with an exacerbation of MS?**
    Emotional or physical stress, fatigue, infections, hyperthermia, trauma, and surgery may exacerbate symptoms. It is thought that elevated temperature causes complete blocking of conduction in demyelinated neurons.

14. **Review some perioperative concerns for patients with MS. Are medications used for most general anesthetics safe?**
    Surgical stress most likely will exacerbate the symptoms of MS. Even modest increases in body temperature ($>1°C$) must be avoided. Because MS may be associated with autonomic dysfunction, pay close attention to maintain preload and afterload. There are no known unique interactions between MS and drugs selected for general anesthesia. However, severe disease is often accompanied by varying degrees of dementia. Patients with dementia will likely have an increased sensitivity to the sedative effects of anesthetic agents, and short-acting agents are recommended. Controlling the known factors associated with MS exacerbation is more important than the choice of medications for general anesthesia.

15. **Are local anesthetics especially toxic for patients with MS?**
    Above threshold concentrations, local anesthetics are neurotoxic. This potential may be amplified in the setting of MS because of the loss of the protective effect of the myelin, resulting in the spinal cord and nerves being exposed to higher local anesthetic concentrations.

16. **Are epidural and spinal anesthesia safe for patients with MS?**
    Regional anesthesia may be beneficial in patients with MS because of a decreased stress response to surgery. Epidural anesthesia is considered safe by most authorities. The safety of peripheral nerve blocks cannot be guaranteed, as evidenced by a patient with MS sustaining a severe brachial plexopathy after interscalene block (Koff et al 2008). Exacerbation of MS symptoms has been reported after spinal anesthesia. This difference in outcomes may be caused by reduced concentrations of local anesthetic at the spinal cord, when epidural is compared with spinal techniques.

When performing an epidural anesthetic or labor analgesic, use the minimum dose necessary and shorter-acting agents. Supplementation with epidural opioids will reduce the local anesthetic requirement.

17. **Are muscle relaxants safe in patients with MS?**
Because these patients (particularly the patients with severe disease) can have significant motor impairment with associated muscle wasting, succinylcholine is best avoided because of a potential hyperkalemic response. Lower doses of nondepolarizing relaxants should be used in patients with baseline motor weakness. Shorter-duration nondepolarizing relaxants may be advantageous in this situation.

18. **Describe postpoliomyelitis syndrome.**
Postpoliomyelitis syndrome is characterized by progressive weakness of the previously affected muscles that begins years after a severe attack of poliomyelitis. Muscles never affected by polio are less often affected. Common signs and symptoms include fatigue, cold intolerance, joint deterioration, muscle pain, atrophy, respiratory insufficiency, dysphagia, and sleep apnea. Patients with postpoliomyelitis syndrome, who complain of dysphagia, may have some degree of vocal cord paralysis. Some patients have decreased lung function, and considerable cardiorespiratory deconditioning may also be present.

19. **What are the anesthetic considerations for patients with postpoliomyelitis syndrome?**
Patients should be informed about the possibility of postoperative mechanical ventilation. If sleep apnea is present, the patient may have coexisting pulmonary hypertension. Dysphagia and vocal cord paralysis may place patients at increased risk for aspiration. If progressive skeletal muscle weakness is present, succinylcholine should be avoided because of the possibility of exaggerated potassium release. These patients also exhibit sensitivity to nondepolarizing neuromuscular blockers, pain, and the sedative effects of anesthetics.

20. **Review critical illness polyneuropathy and the patient subsets prone to developing it.**
As many as 50% to 70% of patients with sepsis, multiple organ dysfunction, or systemic inflammatory response syndrome hospitalized in the intensive care unit for more than 2 weeks develop generalized weakness, associated with sensory loss and other neurological findings, caused by diffuse axonal degeneration of both motor and sensory neurons. This syndrome has been termed *critical illness polyneuropathy* (CIP). The longer the duration of the underlying illness is, the more severe the weakness will be. Patients with mild or moderate underlying critical illness are likely to have improvement in strength once their primary condition improves, although death is not infrequent in those severely affected (and usually related to the primary illness). Factors that may be associated with CIP include long-term administration of muscle relaxants and steroids, plus malnutrition and hyperglycemia.

21. **Describe the clinical features of CIP.**
Failure to wean is the most common presentation, but coexistent encephalopathy often clouds the clinical picture. Severe cases may present as areflexic quadriparesis. Other clinical characteristics include predominantly distal limb weakness with muscle wasting, decreased or absent deep tendon reflexes, and variable sensory loss, often in a stocking and glove distribution. Cranial nerves are intact. Creatine kinase levels are normal or slightly elevated. Cerebrospinal fluid is normal. Biopsies of nerves show fiber loss with axonal degeneration, whereas muscle biopsies demonstrate denervation atrophy. Electrophysiological studies reveal an axonal polyneuropathy.

22. **Review the anesthetic concerns in patients with CIP.**
The response to nondepolarizing relaxants cannot be predicted. Succinylcholine should be avoided out of concerns for hyperkalemia, secondary to prolonged immobility, and a paradoxic insensitivity to nondepolarizing neuromuscular blockers. The associated medical problems are probably the greatest risk for patients with CIP.

KEY POINTS AND SECRETS: DEGENERATIVE NEUROLOGICAL DISEASES

1. Patients with neuropathies often are aspiration risks secondary to bulbar muscle weakness.
2. Similarly, orthostatic hypotension is a common finding.
3. Often these patients require postoperative mechanical ventilation.
4. Because of denervation atrophy, succinylcholine may produce severe hyperkalemia, resulting in cardiac arrest. Thus succinylcholine should be avoided.
5. The response to nondepolarizing muscle relaxants is unpredictable, but most of these patients are probably sensitive to them.
6. Spinal anesthesia should be avoided in patients with multiple sclerosis.
7. With the exception of spinal anesthesia in multiple sclerosis, neither general nor regional anesthesia exacerbates the course of disease in the neuropathies described.

SUGGESTED READINGS
Arora SS, Gooch JL, Garcia PS. Postoperative cognitive dysfunction, Alzheimer's disease, and anesthesia. Int J Neurosci. 2014; 124(4):236–242.
Brambrink AM, Kirsch JR. Perioperative care of patients with neuromuscular disease and dysfunction. Anesthesiol Clin. 2007;25:483–509.

Fleisher LA, Mythen M. Anesthetic implications of concurrent diseases. In: Miller RD, ed. Miller's Anesthesia. 8th ed. Philadelphia: Elsevier; 2015:1156–1225.

Koff MD, Cohen JA, McIntyre JJ, et al. Severe brachial plexopathy after an ultrasound-guided single-injection nerve block for total shoulder arthroplasty in a patient with multiple sclerosis. Anesthesiology. 2008;108:325–328.

Lambert DA, Giannouli E, Schmidt BJ. Postpolio syndrome and anesthesia. Anesthesiology. 2005;103(3):638–644.

Pasternak JJ, Lanier WL. Diseases affecting the brain. In: Hines RL, Marschall KE, eds. Stoelting's Anesthesia and Co-Existing Disease. 7th ed. Philadelphia: Elsevier; 2018:265–304.

Pasternalk JJ, Lanier WL. Diseases of the autonomic and peripheral nervous systems. In: Hines RL, Marschall KE, eds. Stoelting's Anesthesia and Co-Existing Disease. 7th ed. Philadelphia: Elsevier; 2018:315–326.

Pasternak JJ, Lanier WL. Spinal cord disorders. In: Hines RL, Marschall KE, eds. Stoelting's Anesthesia and Co-Existing Disease. 7th ed. Philadelphia: Elsevier; 2018:305–314.

Perlas A, Chan VW. Neuraxial anesthesia and multiple sclerosis. Can J Anaesth. 2005;52:454–458.

Wijeysundera DN, Sweitzer B. Preoperative evaluation. In: Miller RD, ed. Miller's Anesthesia. 8th ed. Philadelphia: Elsevier; 2015:1085–1155.

CHAPTER 47

DIABETES MELLITUS

Robin Slover, MD, Robert H. Slover, MD

1. **Describe the principal types of diabetes mellitus.**
   - Type 1 diabetes mellitus: An autoimmune disorder in which destruction of the insulin-producing beta cells in the pancreatic islets results in the inability to produce insulin. Onset is more common in children and young adults up to age 35 years.
   - Type 2 diabetes mellitus: A disorder in the body's ability to use insulin (insulin resistance). Early in the course of the disease, the patient may be able to make sufficient insulin, but cell-receptor impairment results in hyperglycemia, despite normal or high insulin levels. Type 2 diabetes is usually a disease of older adults; onset in the sixth decade and beyond is common. As obesity increases in the population, type 2 diabetes also increases and is now commonly seen in adolescents and young adults with obesity and a sedentary lifestyle.
   - Gestational diabetes: Seen in 2% to 5% of pregnant women. Some 40% to 60% of these women will develop type 2 diabetes mellitus later in life.

2. **What is considered ideal (target) glucose control?**
   The American Diabetes Association 2018 Clinical Practice Recommendations recommend an A_1C goal for nonpregnant diabetic adults of less than 7% ($\leq$6% is the nondiabetic A_1C goal). Acceptable preprandial glucose is 80 to 130 mg/dL, and postprandial glucose is under 180 mg/dL. Less stringent goals apply to children, patients with a history of severe hypoglycemia, and individuals with comorbid conditions. Target A_1C for the pediatric population is 7.5% or less.

3. **What comorbidities are frequently observed in patients with diabetes mellitus and to what significance?**
   - Hypertension is seen in 40% of patients with poorly controlled diabetes who undergo surgery. Hypertension is a risk factor for coronary artery disease and cardiac failure. If these patients are treated with potassium-wasting diuretic agents, there is often significant total body loss of potassium.
   - Coronary artery disease is common, occurs in younger patients, and may be silent or present atypically.
   - Autonomic neuropathy may compromise neuroreflexic control of cardiovascular and gastrointestinal function, manifesting as orthostatic hypotension, gastroparesis (increased risk of aspiration), ileus, and urinary retention. Peripheral neuropathies are common.
   - Disturbances in renal function are common, including increased blood urea nitrogen (BUN) and creatinine, protein loss, hypoalbuminemia, acidosis, and electrolyte disturbances.
   - Occult infections are present in 17% of patients with diabetes.
   - Retinal hemorrhages are seen in up to 80% of patients with diabetes over 15 years' duration and may lead to retinal detachment and vision loss.

4. **What oral medications are currently used in type 2 diabetes?**
   There are two categories of drugs used in treating type 2 diabetes: those that enhance the effectiveness of insulin and those that increase the supply of insulin to the cells. These drugs are outlined in Table 47.1.

5. **What insulins are in current use?**
   Modern intensive insulin therapy relies on newly designed insulin analogs. Insulin therapy is given using a basal-bolus construct: long-acting insulin is used to provide a steady basal platform, and rapid-acting insulin is used to provide boluses for carbohydrate intake in meals and snacks, and for correction of high glucose. This necessitates giving at least four injections per day or the use of an insulin pump. The specific insulins are outlined in Table 47.2.

6. **Describe the role of insulin on glucose metabolism and discuss the impact of surgery on this.**
   Insulin enhances glucose uptake, glycogen storage, protein synthesis, amino acid transport, and fat formation. Basal insulin secretion is essential, even in the fasting state, to maintain glucose homeostasis.
   Surgical procedures lead to increased stress and high counterregulatory hormone activity with a decrease in insulin secretion. Counterregulatory hormones, including epinephrine, cortisol, glucagon, and growth hormone, promote glycogenolysis, gluconeogenesis, proteolysis, and lipolysis. Therefore in diabetic patients, without adequate insulin replacement, the combination of insulin deficiency and excessive counterregulatory hormones can result in severe hyperglycemia and diabetic ketoacidosis, which are associated with hyperosmolarity, increases in protein catabolism, fluid loss, and lipolysis.

7. **Is there evidence that tight glucose control is beneficial in critically ill patients?**
   Until recently, it was believed that intensive insulin therapy to maintain glucose at or below 110 mg/dL reduced morbidity and mortality in critically ill patients in a surgical intensive care unit (ICU). It has subsequently been

Table 47.1 Oral Drugs Used in Type 2 Diabetes

ACTION	GENERIC NAME	BRAND NAME	DOSE	DOSING INTERVAL	SIDE EFFECTS
Enhance Insulin Effect					
Biguanide	Metformin	Glucophage	1000 mg	bid or tid	Transient gastrointestinal symptoms: Lactic acidosis[a]
Thiazolidinedione "glitazones"	Rosiglitazone Pioglitazone	Avandia Actos	Up to 600 mg Daily Used in combination	Daily or bid	Weight gain, anemia, edema, congestive heart failure,[a] hepatocellular disease[a]
α-Glucosidase inhibitors	Acarbose Miglitol	Precose Glyset	50 mg tid (acarbose) 25 mg tid (miglitol)	bid to qid	Flatulence, intestinal disease[a]
Increase Insulin Supply					
Sulfonylureas	Tolbutamide Chlorpropamide Tolazamide Glipizide Glyburide Glimepiride	Orinase Diabinese Tolinase Glucotrol DiaBeta, Micronase, Glynase Amaryl	2.5–5 mg (Glyburide)	Daily to tid	Hypoglycemia, weight gain, allergy[a]
Nonsulfonylureas	Repaglinide	Prandin	2 mg tid	bid to qid	Hypoglycemia

[a]Indicates rare but serious side effects.
Bid, Twice a day; *tid,* three times a day.

determined that extremely tight glucose control in surgical and medical ICUs significantly increases the risk of hypoglycemia and is not associated with significantly reduced hospital mortality. However, tight control does seem to significantly reduce septicemia and improve wound healing. Current recommendations are to maintain serum glucose between 90 and 180 mg/dL.

8. **What are the complications of hyperglycemia in the perioperative setting?**
   - Impaired polymorphonuclear cellular phagocytic function, increased risk of infection, and increased length of hospitalization
   - Osmotic diuresis, dehydration, and hyperosmolarity
   - Ketogenesis and diabetic ketoacidosis
   - Proteolysis and decreased amino acid transport, resulting in retarded wound healing
   - Hyperviscosity, thrombogenesis, and cerebral edema (resulting in altered mental status)

9. **What considerations are important during the preoperative evaluation?**
   Important considerations include type of diabetes, duration of disease, oral hypoglycemic drugs or insulin therapy, and diabetic complications, including hypertension, renal disease, coronary artery disease (which may be silent or present atypically), and neuropathies (early satiety and reflux suggest gastroparesis). If patients have end-stage renal disease or require dialysis, fluid restrictions may be necessary.

10. **What is the significance of autonomic neuropathy? How can it be assessed?**
    Autonomic neuropathy may affect cardiovascular (silent ischemia), gastrointestinal (gastroparesis with increased risk of aspiration), thermoregulatory (decreased ability to alter blood vessel flow to conserve temperature), and neuroendocrine systems (decreased catecholamine production in response to stimulation). Autonomic neuropathy can be assessed by these tests:
    - An intact sympathetic nervous system can be assessed by the following: a normal response in diastolic pressure (from lying to standing) is a change of at least 16 mm Hg; an affected patient has a response of less than 10 mm Hg. Autonomic neuropathy is also evidenced by a large change in systolic blood pressure when changing from lying to standing posture. A normal decrease is less than 10 mm Hg; an affected patient has a decrease of at least 30 mm Hg
    - An intact parasympathetic nervous system can be assessed by observing heart rate response (i.e., rate variability) to breathing. Normal patients increase heart rate by at least 15 beats per minute. Affected patients have an increase of 10 or fewer beats per minute. Finally, concurrent with electrocardiogram (ECG) monitoring, the R-R ratio can be measured during a Valsalva maneuver. A normal ratio is greater than 1:2; an abnormal response is under 1

    Patients with autonomic neuropathy should be considered for preoperative aspiration prophylaxis, which may include an H_2-blocking agent, a gastric stimulant to decrease gastroparesis, and/or a nonparticulate antacid.

11. **What preoperative laboratory tests are appropriate for the patient with diabetes?**
    Evaluate electrolytes, phosphate, and magnesium, BUN and creatinine, blood glucose and ketones, urinalysis, and ECG. Proteinuria is an early manifestation of diabetic nephropathy. A cardiac stress test should be considered in sedentary patients with cardiac risk factors. Measuring hemoglobin A_1C will provide valuable information about the level of glucose control. Patients with hemoglobin A_1C greater than 9% are usually noncompliant and have an increased risk of dehydration.

12. **Are there any signs that oral intubation may be difficult?**
    Although the remainder of the airway examination may be normal, patients with diabetes may have decreased mobility in the atlantooccipital joint, which can complicate oral intubation. This can be evaluated radiographically. Patients may also have stiff joint syndrome with anterior fixation of the larynx. Stiff joint syndrome is suggested by the inability to approximate the palmar aspect of the metacarpal joints of the fingers (also known as the *prayer sign*, the patient cannot touch the palmar aspects of the fingers together when the palms are together). The palmar print is another way of assessing stiff joints.

13. **How should the patient with diabetes be prepared before surgery? Should all patients with diabetes receive insulin intraoperatively?**
    Patients receiving general anesthesia should be admitted to the hospital for overnight glucose testing. They should be scheduled as first case of the day. They require intravenous (IV) placement. Those patients having major surgery (>2 hours) require insulin infusion titrated to avoid ketoacidosis. Patients require testing hourly preoperatively and every 30 minutes during surgery to detect and prevent hypo- and hyperglycemia. If glucose rises to more than 250 between tests, check ketones.

14. **What else needs to be done for major surgery?**
    Patients planned for longer or more stressful surgeries have increased levels of counterregulatory hormones and are likely to benefit from tighter glucose control. Furthermore, insulin requirements are increased by infection, hepatic disease, obesity, steroids, and cardiovascular procedures and pain. An insulin infusion may be considered to establish tighter glucose control. Before surgery, hyperglycemia, fluid and electrolyte imbalances, and ketosis should be corrected. Ideally, in patients with renal failure, surgery should occur the day after hemodialysis.

Blood glucose levels under 200 mg/dL in the days preceding surgery are ideal and ensure adequate glycogen stores and insulin sufficiency. On the day before surgery, glucose should be monitored at bedside before each meal, at bedtime, and in the early morning. The goal is to have most glucose between 90 and 180 mg/dL. On the evening before surgery, give the usual evening long-acting insulin dose. Omit the usual morning insulin (short- and long-acting). Start an IV insulin infusion at least 2 hours before surgery. Dilute 50 units regular insulin in 50 mL of 0.9% saline so 1 unit = 1 mL. Also provide IV maintenance fluids consisting of 5% dextrose in normal saline. During surgery, aim to maintain blood glucose between 90 and 180 mg/dL by adjusting the IV insulin dose or the rate of the dextrose infusion. If glucose is under 70 mg/dL, give bolus of IV 10% dextrose 1 to 2 mL/kg and recheck in 15 minutes, repeating as necessary (2018 guidelines).

15. Describe the postoperative management of the patient with diabetes.

In significant procedures with prolonged recovery, it is easier to manage the patient by continuing the insulin and glucose infusion for up to 48 hours, matching increased or decreased insulin needs with changes in rate or concentration of the infusion. Continue bedside monitoring of glucose, electrolytes, and fluids. A blood glucose goal of 90 to 180 mg/dL is reasonable. If total parenteral nutrition is used, the insulin rate may need to increase and should be adjusted based on glucose monitoring.

With the resumption of oral feeding, insulin is given subcutaneously according to the patient's preoperative schedule. If pain or stress is still significant, it will be necessary to increase the dosage by as much as 20%. Monitor glucose at bedside before meals, at bedtime, and early in the morning, adjusting doses as necessary.

16. How do you manage patients using subcutaneous insulin pumps?

Insulin pumps are now commonly used and can ensure good glucose control. The pumps use one of the newer analog insulins (Humalog, NovoLog, and Apidra) and deliver both basal and bolus insulin doses. Because the basal rate is set to deliver necessary insulin for the fasting state, the pump can be used for insulin delivery during the perioperative and intraoperative periods, continuing the established basal rates. Check blood sugars at regular intervals, every hour pre-and postoperatively, and every 30 minutes intraoperatively, to ensure that the patient's blood sugar stays between 90 and 180 mg/dL. If the stress of a long surgery raises glucose levels, the basal infusion rate can be safely raised in increments of 0.1 unit per hour. If glucose levels fall, the rate can be safely reduced in increments of 0.1 unit per hour, or the pump can be suspended until glucose levels rise. When the patient is fully recovered, return to normal routines for pump use. For minor procedures under 2 hours, use the pump basal settings for the time of day. For longer or major procedures reduce the basal rates by 20%.

17. What insulins are preferred for pump use?

The rapid-acting analogs (NovoLog, Humalog, Apidra) are used in the insulin pumps. Interestingly, when insulin is given intravenously, there is no advantage to the analogs compared with regular human insulin. For that reason, the less expensive regular insulin is usually used for IV therapy.

18. How should I prepare patients for surgery who have type 2 diabetes and are only on oral medications?

Use of metformin has been associated with lactic acidosis, with a risk that is increased by renal insufficiency. For major surgery where there are additional risk factors (acute or chronic renal insufficiency, dehydration), discontinue metformin 24 hours before the surgery. For minor surgery, discontinue metformin on the day of the procedure. In all cases, metformin should be withheld for 48 hours after surgery and until normal renal function has been confirmed. For sulfonylureas, thiazolidinedione, dipeptidyl peptidase IV inhibitors, glucagon-like peptide-1 analogs, and sodium-glucose transport protein-2 inhibitors, stop the medication on the day of surgery (see Table 47.1).

19. Describe the management of patients with diabetes requiring urgent surgery.

If at all possible, electrolyte and glucose imbalance should be corrected before surgery. Sufficient rehydration, electrolyte replacement, and insulin treatment can be achieved in 4 to 6 hours, improving hyperglycemia, ketosis, and acidosis. Rehydration is initiated with 10 to 20 mL/kg of normal saline (NS). Infuse insulin at 0.1 unit/kg/h using 0.45 NS (or D_{10} in 0.45 NS if glucose is <150 mg/dL). Patients in ketoacidosis requiring emergency surgery may receive insulin therapy according to the guidelines in Table 47.2. Note that ketoacidosis may present with symptoms of an acute abdomen!

20. Are regional anesthetics helpful in patients with insulin-dependent diabetes? Can epinephrine be added to local anesthetic solutions?

Regional anesthetic techniques decrease the stress response and may help maintain a more stable blood glucose and decrease stress on the cardiovascular system. Epinephrine should not be used in peripheral nerve blocks (e.g., ankle blocks) because of the risk of decreasing blood flow to an area possibly already affected by impaired microcirculation. In blocks with high systemic absorption, such as brachial plexus or intercostal blocks, low-dose epinephrine may be used.

21. Is it possible to achieve continuous monitoring of glucose levels in the operating room and in the perioperative period?

The technology is commercially available to have continuous glucose monitoring before, during, and after a procedure. Currently, there are two continuous glucose-monitoring (CGM) systems that have US Food and Drug Administration

Table 47.2 Insulin Therapy Guidelines

	ONSET OF ACTION	PEAK	DURATION OF ACTION
Long Acting (Basal)			
Lantus (glargine)	2–3 hours	None	24 hours
Levemir (detemir)	2–3 hours	None	24 hours
Tresiba	Continuous	None	72 hours
Tujeo	Continuous	None	72 hours
Intermediate Acting			
Regular[a]	30–60 minutes	2–4 hours	6–9 hours
NPH (suspension)[a]	4 hours	4–8 hours	8–13 hours
Rapid Acting			
Humalog (lispro)	10–30 minutes	30–90 minutes	3–4 hours
NovoLog (aspart)	10–30 minutes	30–90 minutes	3–4 hours
Apidra (glulisine)	10–30 minutes	30–90 minutes	3–4 hours
Ultra-Rapid Acting			
Fiasp	15 minutes	60 minutes	2 hours

[a]No longer preferred or in common use.

approval. There is also one flash glucose monitoring system. CGM systems (Dexcom and Medtronic Guardian) sample interstitial fluid every few minutes and display the values. The Flash system uses an inserted sensor, but gives a glucose reading whenever a sensor wand is passed over the site. There is a risk that such systems might fail intraoperatively and the current recommendation is to use them only under research protocols and with additional blood glucose assessments.

KEY POINTS: DIABETES MELLITUS

1. Careful attention to glucose control before, during, and after surgery is important to reduce risk of infection, promote more rapid healing, avoid metabolic complications, and shorten hospital stay.
2. The goal for insulin management during surgery is to maintain glucose between 90 and 180 mg/dL.
3. Intraoperative glucose control in all but the shortest cases is best achieved by using a glucose-insulin IV infusion or a pump.
4. Patients with diabetes have a high incidence of coronary artery disease with an atypical or silent presentation. Maintaining perfusion pressure, controlling heart rate, continuous ECG observation, and a high index of suspicion during periods of refractory hypotension are key considerations.
5. The inability to touch the palmar aspects of index fingers when palms touch (the prayer sign) can indicate a difficult oral intubation in patients with diabetes.

Websites

American Diabetes Association: http://www.diabetes.org
Children's Diabetes Foundation: http://www.childrensdiabetesfoundation.org
Juvenile Diabetes Research Foundation: http://www.jdrf.org

Suggested Readings

Burant CF, Young LA, eds. Medical Management of Type 2 Diabetes, 7th ed. Alexandria: American Diabetes Association; 2012:101–103.
Davidson MB. Standards of medical care in diabetes. Diabetes Care. 2005;28(Suppl):S4–S36.
Dronge AS, Perkal MF, Kancir S, et al. Long-term glycemic control and postoperative infectious complications. Arch Surg. 2006;141(4):375–380.
Ferrari LR. New insulin analogues and insulin delivery devices for the perioperative management of diabetic patients. Curr Opin Anaesthesiol. 2008;21(3):401–405.
Jefferies C, Rhodes E, Rachmiel M, et al. ISPAD Clinical Practice Consensus Guidelines 2018: Management of children and adolescents with diabetes requiring surgery. Pediatr Diabetes. 2018;19(Suppl) 27:227–236.
Macrae D, Grieve R, Allen E, et al. A randomized trial of hyperglycemic control in pediatric intensive care. N Engl J Med. 2014;370(2):107–118.
Rhodes ET, et al. Perioperative management of pediatric surgical patients with diabetes mellitus. Anesth Analg. 2005;101(4):986–999.
Riddle MC. Standards of medical care in diabetes—2018. Diabetes Care. 2018;41(Suppl 1):S12–S155.
van den Berghe G, Wouters P, Weekers F, et al. Intensive insulin therapy in the critically ill patients. N Engl J Med. 2001;345:1359–1367.
Wiener RS, Wiener DC, Larson RJ. Benefits and risks of tight glucose control in critically ill adults: a meta-analysis. JAMA. 2008;300(8):933–944.

CHAPTER 48

NONDIABETIC ENDOCRINE DISEASE

Peiman Lahsaei, MD

1. Review the thyroid hormone laboratory tests.
   Thyroid hormone laboratory tests include:
   - Total thyroxine (T_4) level
   - Total triiodothyronine (T_3) level—formed from the peripheral conversion of T_4
   - Thyroid-stimulating hormone (TSH) level—formed in anterior pituitary
   - Resin T_3 uptake (T_3RU). T_3RU is useful in conditions that alter levels of thyroid-binding globulin, which would alter total T_4 results (Table 48.1)
   - Thyrotropin-releasing hormone (TRH)—produced by the hypothalamus

2. What are common signs and symptoms of hypothyroidism?
   - Symptoms include fatigue, cold intolerance, constipation, dry skin, hair loss, weight gain.
   - Signs include bradycardia, hypothermia, decreased tendon reflexes, hoarseness, periorbital edema.
   - Long-term, untreated hypothyroidism may progress to myxedema coma, which can be fatal. Myxedema is characterized by hypoventilation, hypothermia, hypotension, hyponatremia, and hypoglycemia (the "hypos"), as well as obtundation and adrenal insufficiency. Note, Addisonian crisis can have a similar presentation to hypothyroidism.

3. Review the causes of hypothyroidism.
   The most common causes of hypothyroidism include surgical or radioiodine ablation of thyroid tissue during the treatment of hyperthyroidism and, most commonly, Graves disease. Other causes of hypothyroidism include chronic thyroiditis (Hashimoto thyroiditis), drug effects, such as amiodarone and lithium, iodine deficiency, and pituitary or hypothalamic dysfunction. It can also be cause by infiltrative disorders, such as amyloidosis, sarcoidosis, hemochromatosis, and scleroderma.

4. Which manifestations of hypothyroidism have the greatest anesthetic consideration?
   Hypothyroidism causes depression of myocardial function. Cardiac output declines as a result of decreased heart rate and stroke volume. Decreased blood volume, baroreceptor reflex dysfunction, and pericardial effusion may also accompany hypothyroidism. Conduction delays, symptomatic bradycardia and prolonged QT interval, leading to polymorphic ventricular tachycardia are also possible in severe hypothyroidism. Subsequently, the hypothyroid patient will be more sensitive to the hypotensive effects of anesthetics.
   Hypoventilation may also be a feature of hypothyroidism. The ventilatory responses to both hypoxia and hypercarbia are impaired, making the hypothyroid patient sensitive to drugs that cause respiratory depression. Hypothyroidism also decreases the hepatic and renal clearance of drugs. Lastly, patients are prone to hypothermia because of lowered metabolic rate and consequently, lowered heat production.

5. How does hypothyroidism affect the minimum alveolar concentration of anesthetic agents?
   Animal studies show that minimum alveolar concentration (MAC) is not affected by hypothyroidism. But in clinical cases, it has been noted that hypothyroid patients have increased sensitivity to anesthetic agents. This is caused not by a decrease in MAC per se, but by the patient's metabolically depressed condition.

6. Should elective surgery be delayed in a hypothyroid patient?
   Patients with mild to moderate hypothyroidism are not at increased risk when undergoing elective surgical procedures. Some authorities suggest that elective surgery in patients who are symptomatic should be delayed until the patient is rendered euthyroid. In patients with severe hypothyroidism, elective surgery should be delayed until they have been rendered euthyroid. This may require 2 to 4 months of replacement therapy for complete reversal of the cardiopulmonary effects. Normalization of the patient's TSH level reflects reversal of hypothyroid-induced changes.
   In the event of emergency surgery and severe hypothyroidism, administration of intravenous (IV) T_3/T_4 is the appropriate measure. One should also consider administration of steroids, given high likelihood of adrenal insufficiency. While administering IV T_3/T_4, one must monitor for ST changes and myocardial ischemia.

7. What is the most common electrolyte deficiency in hypothyroidism?
   Hyponatremia is the most common electrolyte abnormality seen in hypothyroidism. It is caused by the impaired free water excretion that results from renal impairment and excess vasopressin excretion. Extreme hyponatremia can affect mental status and should be corrected cautiously, as it can lead to cerebral osmotic demyelination syndrome.

Table 48.1 Usefulness of Thyroid Function Tests in the Diagnosis of Hypothyroid or Hyperthyroid States

DISEASE	T_4	T_3	TSH	T_3RU
Primary hypothyroidism	−	−	+	−
Secondary hypothyroidism	−	−	−	−
Hyperthyroidism	+	+	0	+
Pregnancy	+	0	0	+

T_4, Thyroxine; T_3, tri-iodothyronine; *TSH*, thyroid-stimulating hormone; T_3RU, resin T_3 uptake; +, increased; −, decreased; *0*, no change.

8. List common signs and symptoms of hyperthyroidism.
   - Symptoms include anxiety, tremor, heat intolerance, and fatigue.
   - Signs include goiter, tachycardia, proptosis, atrial fibrillation, weight loss, and weakness.
   - Causes of hyperthyroidism include Graves disease, thyroiditis, toxic multinodular goiter, and excessive iodine intake.

9. How is hyperthyroidism treated?
   - Antithyroid drugs, such as propylthiouracil (PTU) inhibit iodination and coupling reactions in the thyroid gland, thus reducing production of T_3 and T_4. PTU also inhibits peripheral conversion of T_4 to T_3. Iodine in large doses not only blocks hormone production but also decreases the vascularity and size of the thyroid gland, making iodine useful in preparing hyperthyroid patients for thyroid surgery.
   - Radioactive iodine, ^{131}I, is actively concentrated by the thyroid gland, resulting in destruction of thyroid cells and a decrease in the production of hormone.
   - Surgical subtotal thyroidectomy

10. Review the concerns of hyperthyroidism on anesthetic management.
    In a hyperthyroid state, metabolic rate is increased, impacting the cardiovascular system, the magnitude of which is proportional to the severity of thyroid dysfunction. Because of increased global oxygen consumption, the cardiovascular system is hyperdynamic. Tachycardia and elevated cardiac output are present, and tachyarrhythmias, atrial fibrillation, left ventricular hypertrophy, and congestive heart failure may develop. Also of note, hyperthyroid patients with proptosis are more susceptible to ocular damage during surgery because of difficulty with taping their eyelids closed.

11. How is MAC affected by hyperthyroidism?
    As in hypothyroidism, MAC is not affected by hyperthyroidism, although clinically hyperthyroid patients appear to be resistant to the effects of anesthetic agents. Inhalation induction is slowed by the increased cardiac output. Also the rate of drug metabolism is increased, giving the appearance of resistance.

12. Review thyrotoxicosis and its treatment
    Also known as *thyroid storm*, this is an acute exacerbation of hyperthyroidism usually caused by some stress, such as surgery or infection. It is characterized by extreme tachycardia, hyperthermia, and possibly severe hypotension. Perioperatively, it usually occurs 6 to 18 hours after surgery, but can occur intraoperatively and be mistaken for malignant hyperthermia. In the OB (obstetrics) population, thyroid storms are possible with molar pregnancy.
    Treatment consists of judicious β-adrenergic blockade, infusion of IV fluids, and temperature control if hyperthermia is present. Corticosteroids should be considered for refractory hypotension because hyperthyroid patients may have a relative cortisol deficiency. Antithyroid drugs should be added after surgery.

13. What complications may occur after thyroidectomy?
    Adjacent to the thyroid gland are the trachea and larynx, and cervical hematoma may lead to airway obstruction. Chronic pressure on the trachea from, for example, a goiter, may lead to tracheomalacia, and postextubation tracheal collapse is also a consideration. Inadvertent resection of the parathyroid glands may lead to hypocalcemia and, subsequently, laryngospasm or seizure. Damage to the recurrent laryngeal nerves (RLNs) may impair vocal cord function and lead to hoarseness (if unilateral) or airway obstruction. Bilateral partial RLN injury can result in vocal cord adduction and airway obstruction. Total destruction of the bilateral RLNs results in the vocal cords being in midposition and rarely produces total airway obstruction.

14. Describe parathyroid hormone function.
    Parathyroid hormone (PTH), also known as *parathormone*, has a significant effect on serum calcium levels. Inadequate PTH levels are usually associated with hypocalcemia and commonly have observed tetanic effects. Hyperparathyroidism and hypoparathyroidism are associated with hypercalcemia and hypocalcemia, respectively.

15. Why are parathyroid glands commonly removed?

Parathyroid adenomas, a common source of hyperparathyroidism, are most commonly removed. Roughly speaking, unplanned total removal of all parathyroid glands during thyroidectomy occurs about 0.5% to 5% of the time. On occasion, one parathyroid gland is reinserted in an arm so that parathyroid function persists. One parathyroid gland is thought suitable to maintain serum PTH and calcium levels.

16. Describe complications posthyperparathyroidectomy.

Hypocalcemia may result in laryngospasm. Hematoma may obstruct the airway. RLNs may be transected, leading to vocal cord dysfunction and possible airway obstruction. Unlike other hormones, there is no replacement analog for parathormone.

17. Describe the anatomy and physiology of the adrenal gland.

The suprarenal adrenal gland is functionally divided into the adrenal cortex and the adrenal medulla. The adrenal cortex principally produces the steroid hormone cortisol (the main glucocorticoid) and aldosterone (the main mineralocorticoid). Aldosterone is secreted by the adrenal cortex and is regulated by the renin-angiotensin system (discussed in Chapter 30). Production of cortisol is regulated by adrenocorticotropic hormone (ACTH), which is produced by the anterior pituitary gland. The release of ACTH is promoted by corticotropin-releasing hormone (CRH), derived from the hypothalamus, thus completing the hypothalamic-pituitary-adrenal (HPA) axis. Cortisol inhibits release of both CRH and ACTH, establishing negative feedback control. Ectopic ACTH can be produced by various neoplasms, such as small-cell lung carcinomas.

The adrenal medulla secretes epinephrine and norepinephrine. Their release is governed by the sympathetic nervous system, discussed in Chapter 4.

18. How much cortisol is produced by the adrenal cortex?

Normally approximately 20 to 30 mg of cortisol per day is produced. This amount increases dramatically in response to a stress, such as infection or surgery. Under stressful conditions, 75 to 150 mg/day may be produced, with the increase in production being generally proportional to the severity of the stress.

19. How do exogenous steroids compare with cortisol?

See Table 48.2.

20. What are the most common causes of HPA axis disruption?

Causes of HPA axis disruption include central nervous system mass lesions (tumor or abscess), head injury or subarachnoid hemorrhage, tuberculosis, vascular injury, and adrenal causes (etomidate, ketoconazole, hemorrhage, infection, autoimmune adrenalitis, adrenal hemorrhage, bilateral adrenal metastases), septic shock, and other acute illness.

21. What is the impact of steroid administration on the HPA axis?

Exogenous steroids (glucocorticoids) result in HPA axis suppression. Short-term steroid administration—7 to 10 days—results in suppression of CRH and ACTH release, which usually returns to normal about 5 days after discontinuation of steroid therapy. Long-term administration of exogenous steroids results in adrenocortical atrophy secondary to a lack of ACTH. This results in prolonged adrenocortical insufficiency, which can last a year or more following steroid discontinuation. Therefore long-term steroid administration should not be terminated abruptly; rather it should be gradually tapered off over a period of 1 to 4 weeks.

22. What is an Addisonian crisis?

Also referred to as *acute adrenocortical insufficiency*, an Addisonian crisis is caused by a relative lack of cortisol or other glucocorticoid. It is a shock state characterized by refractory hypotension, hypovolemia, and electrolyte disturbances.

Table 48.2 Relative Potency of Cortisol and Exogenous Steroids

STEROID	GLUCOCORTICOID	MINERALOCORTICOID	HALF-LIFE (HOURS)
Cortisol	1	1	8–12
Cortisone	0.8	0.8	8–12
Prednisone	4	0.25	12–36
Methylprednisolone	5	0.25	12–36
Triamcinolone	5	0.25	12–36
Dexamethasone	20–30	—	26–54
Fludrocortisone	5	200	12–36

23. **Is perioperative stress steroid supplementation for patients on chronic steroid therapy necessary?**

Few documented cases of acute perioperative adrenal insufficiency (i.e., Addisonian crisis) exist. Studies have shown that patients who have been on long-term steroid therapy, undergoing even major surgery, rarely become hypotensive because of glucocorticoid deficiency. If observed, hypotension is usually the result of hypovolemia or cardiac dysfunction. Possible side effects of perioperative steroid supplementation include:

- Hyperglycemia
- Gastric ulceration
- Fluid retention
- Impaired wound healing
- Aggravation of hypertension
- Immunosuppression

One approach might be that no supplementation is required unless hypotension refractory to standard treatment occurs. Few data indicate any significant problems related to short-term perioperative steroid supplementation. Despite its rarity, acute adrenal insufficiency is associated with significant morbidity and mortality. Therefore because perioperative steroid supplementation is associated with few risks in itself and because acute adrenal insufficiency can potentially lead to death, supplemental steroids should be given. Currently, this seems to be the view of most authorities.

24. **What dosage of corticosteroids should be administered when considered perioperatively?**

Often debated, recent guidelines suggest lower doses and shorter durations than those recommended in the past. Patients ordinarily receiving 5 mg/day or less of prednisone should receive their normal daily replacement but do not require supplementation. For minor surgery, no supplementation or minimal supplementation may suffice. Hydrocortisone, 25 mg, may suffice. For moderate surgery, give 50 to 75 mg of hydrocortisone on the day of procedure and taper the dose quickly over 1 to 2 days. For major surgery, a variety of dosages have been suggested, with none being shown to be superior to the rest. A suggested regimen would be 100 to 150 mg of hydrocortisone, on the day of procedure, with a quick 1- to 2-day taper. The goal of these regimens is to give the lowest dose possible that provides sufficient supplementation, while avoiding potential side effects.

25. **Review the impact of steroids when patients are critically ill.**

On occasion, there is HPA axis suppression and decreased cortisol synthesis. Oftentimes, serum cortisol levels may be difficult to interpret. IV hydrocortisone, 50 mg every 6 hours, should be considered.

26. **Should anabolic steroid use be considered when planning an anesthetic?**

Yes. Anabolic steroids are ingested to enhance physical performance. Increased muscle mass increases oxygen requirements. Cardiomyopathies are common, as is atherosclerosis. Hypertension and diastolic cardiac dysfunction have been noted. Hepatic dysfunction is a risk, as is hypercoagulopathy. Resistance to nondepolarizing muscle relaxants has been reported. Athletes ingesting anabolic steroids may be hyperaggressive and have other behavioral disturbances. Prompt discontinuation of anabolic steroids before surgery may result in Addisonian effects.

27. **What is a pheochromocytoma?**

A pheochromocytoma is a catecholamine-producing tumor that is associated with multiple syndromes including multiple endocrine neoplasia-IIA/B and neurofibromatosis 1. Unrecognized, this can lead to significant perioperative morbidity and mortality. It should be ruled out in patients on multiple antihypertensive medications who present with uncontrolled hypertension. Additional signs/symptoms include paroxysmal sweating, headaches, and tachycardia. Elevated urine metanephrines is usually diagnostic. Such patients may have myocarditis from excessive endogenous catecholamines.

28. **What are the anesthetic considerations for pheochromocytoma?**

Patients should be started on an α blocking agent, such as phenoxybenzamine, for 10 to 14 days, until symptoms and blood pressure are controlled before elective surgery. Of note, patients should not be started on a β blocker before being on an α blocking agent first.

The anesthesia care team should be prepared for intraoperative hemodynamic shifts and should use short-acting agents for blood pressure control. Once the tumor is removed, patients my developed hypotension and require pressure support and volume. For these reasons, invasive monitors and central access is recommended for the perioperative management of this patient population.

KEY POINTS: NONDIABETIC ENDOCRINE DISEASE

1. Perioperatively mild to moderate hypothyroidism is of little concern even for elective surgery. Patients with severe, symptomatic hypothyroidism should be treated before surgery.
2. MAC of volatile anesthetics is unchanged in both hypothyroid and hyperthyroid states.
3. Thyrotoxicosis ("thyroid storm") may mimic malignant hyperthermia. It is detected by an increased serum T_4 level and treated initially with β blockade, followed by antithyroid therapy.
4. Perioperative glucocorticoid supplementation should be considered for patients receiving exogenous steroids.
5. Chronic exogenous glucocorticoid therapy should not be discontinued abruptly. Doing so may precipitate acute adrenocortical insufficiency.

Suggested Readings

Axelrod L. Perioperative management of patients treated with glucocorticoids. Endocrinol Metab Clin North Am. 2003;32:367–383.

Bouillon R. Acute adrenal insufficiency. Endocrinol Metab Clin North Am. 2006;35:767–775.

Connery LE, Coursin DB. Assessment and therapy of selected endocrine disorders. Anesthesiol Clin North Am. 2004;22:93–123.

Cooper MS, Stewart PM. Adrenal insufficiency in critical illness. J Intensive Care Med. 2007;22:348–362.

Jonklaas J, Bianco AC, Bauer AJ, et al. Guidelines for the treatment of hypothyroidism: prepared by the American thyroid association task force on thyroid hormone replacement. Thyroid. 2014;24:1670–1751.

Kam PC, Yarrow M. Anabolic steroids abuse: physiological and anaesthetic considerations. Anaesthesia. 2005;60:685–692.

Moskovitz JB, Bond MC. Molar pregnancy-induced thyroid storm. J Emerg Med. 2010;38(5):e-71–e-76.

Neuman HPH. Pheochromcytoma. In: Fauci AS, ed. Harrison's Principles of Internal Medicine. 17th ed. New York: McGraw-Hill; 2008:2269.

Shoback D. Hypoparathyroidism. N Engl J Med. 2008;359:391–403.

Wald DA. ECG manifestations of selected metabolic and endocrine disorders. Emerg Med Clin North Am. 2006;24:145–157.

Yasumasa I, Yutaka O, Kazuyuki Y, et al. Osmoregulation of plasma vasopressin in myxedema. J Clin Endocrinol Metabol. 1990;70(2):534–539.

CHAPTER 49

OBESITY AND OBSTRUCTIVE SLEEP APNEA

Brian M. Keech, MD

1. **Define obesity.**
   Obesity is defined using the body mass index (BMI) (Table 49.1).

$$BMI = \frac{Mass}{Height^2} \left(\frac{kg}{m^2}\right)$$

2. **Describe the implications of obesity as they pertain to anesthetic management.**
   - Anesthetic Plan—Procedures that are normally performed under sedation and/or monitored anesthetic care may not be safe or feasible to perform in obese patients.
   - Induction of Anesthesia—Decreased lung volumes (i.e., functional residual capacity [FRC]) and increased oxygen consumption because of body habitus, in conjunction with a short, fat neck, and decreased pulmonary compliance can make mask ventilation and intubation difficult.
   - Relaxation—Procedures that usually do not require neuromuscular blockade may not be feasible in obese patients without it.
   - Pulmonary—Decreased pulmonary compliance predisposes to hypoventilation and atelectasis, which increases the risk of hypercarbia and hypoxemia, respectively.
   - Airway—High incidence of obstructive sleep apnea (OSA) and pulmonary complications, all of which is exacerbated by the respiratory depressant effects of anesthesia and opioids.
   - Positioning—Procedures requiring Trendelenburg or lateral positioning can present challenges regarding patient safety and/or operating room equipment stability.
   - Monitoring—Noninvasive blood pressure monitoring may be inaccurate or ineffective in obese patients necessitating invasive arterial blood pressure monitoring.

3. **Discuss the cardiovascular considerations in patients who are obese.**
   Systemic and pulmonary hypertension, as well as left- and right-sided heart failure and coronary artery disease, can be found in obese patients. As body mass increases, so does oxygen consumption, causing a compensatory increase in circulating blood volume and cardiac output to meet increased demand. Chronic systemic hypertension, in the setting of compensatory increased cardiac output, can lead to left ventricular hypertrophy and left heart failure. Chronic hypercapnia and hypoxia, commonly associated with OSA, can increase pulmonary artery pressure (i.e., hypoxic pulmonary vasoconstriction), leading to right ventricular hypertrophy and right heart failure.

4. **What are the main pulmonary abnormalities associated with obesity?**
   - Decreased pulmonary compliance ($\Delta V/\Delta P$)
   - Decreased FRC
   - Increased oxygen consumption ($\dot{V}O_2$)

5. **Review pulmonary and respiratory considerations in caring for patients with obesity.**
   Considerations include the possibility of a difficult airway, increased incidence of asthma, OSA, obesity hypoventilation syndrome (OHS), and pulmonary hypertension. Obesity is a major risk factor for hypoxemia in the perioperative environment.

6. **How does obesity affect pulmonary mechanics and predispose a patient to hypoxemia?**
   - Decreased FRC—Obesity causes "restrictive lung disease" because of a decrease in compliance of both the chest wall and the lung itself. Recall, FRC is determined when the opposing forces of the expanding chest wall and the recoil forces of the lung are equal. Increased chest wall mass reduces chest wall compliance, which reduces the outward force of the chest. Increased abdominal mass displaces the diaphragm cephalad and reduces "chest wall" compliance. Together, this leads to a decrease in FRC. A decrease in FRC causes atelectasis, where atelectasis causes: (1) hypoxemia (i.e., shunt), and (2) decreased lung compliance (i.e., collapsed alveoli are less compliant than recruited alveoli).
   - Increased oxygen consumption ($\dot{V}O_2$)—Increasing body mass, increases total body oxygen consumption. Recall, FRC is the volume of lung that oxygenates the blood, particularly when a patient is apneic. Increased oxygen consumption in the setting of decreased FRC greatly increases the risk of hypoxemia.

Table 49.1 Classification of Body Mass Index

BODY MASS INDEX	CLASSIFICATION
$\leq$18.5	Underweight
18.5–25	Normal weight
25–30	Overweight
30–35	Class I obesity
35–40	Class II obesity
$\geq$40	Class III obesity

7. **What is the best method to improve pulmonary mechanics for patients with obesity?**
   Pulmonary mechanics for patients with obesity can significantly be improved with ramp positioning (Fig. 49.1). A ramp is made by stacking folded blankets, using a commercial foam wedge, or positioning the operating room table in reverse Trendelenburg. Ramp positioning has the following benefits: (1) increases FRC, and (2) increases chest wall compliance. Ramp positioning improves pulmonary mechanics by displacing the diaphragm in the caudal direction and reduces the gravitational effects of chest wall tissue from directly compressing the lungs. Ramp positioning before induction of anesthesia, increases chest wall compliance, which facilitates easier bag mask ventilation and yields a larger FRC, providing more time for laryngoscopy before hypoxemia ensues.

8. **What are some of the common comorbidities seen in patients with obesity?**
   - Metabolic syndrome
   - OSA
   - OHS
   - Systemic and pulmonary hypertension
   - Cardiovascular disease (i.e., coronary artery disease, congestive heart failure, and atrial fibrillation)
   - Dyslipidemia
   - Diabetes mellitus type 2
   - Renal disease

9. **What is metabolic syndrome?**
   Metabolic syndrome is a cluster of comorbidities associated with abdominal obesity. The core features are abdominal obesity, dyslipidemia, diabetes mellitus or insulin resistance, and hypertension. Increased visceral adipose tissue or increased waist circumference is a core tenant of metabolic syndrome and has a better correlation to the syndrome than BMI.

10. **What is OSA?**
    OSA is characterized by repetitive episodes of apnea or reduced inspiratory airflow during sleep and is caused primarily by airflow obstruction. Symptoms include snoring, daytime somnolence, poor concentration, and fatigue. Risk factors include advanced age, male gender, obesity, hypertension, nasal congestion, craniofacial dysmorphology, and upper airway soft tissue abnormalities.

11. **What is OHS?**
    OHS is the triad of obesity, daytime hypoventilation, and sleep-disordered breathing. Such patients often have OSA, restrictive lung disease, and pulmonary hypertension. Daytime hypercapnia is distinctly common and more prevalent compared with patients with OSA alone.

12. **How do we screen for OSA?**
    Laboratory polysomnography is the definitive diagnostic study when OSA is suspected; however, the specific criteria for making a formal diagnosis is beyond the scope of this text. Preoperatively, in the absence of a formal diagnosis, it is advantageous to screen for OSA. This process begins with the history and continues with the physical examination. Common physical examination findings in patients with OSA include:
    - Obesity—Even mild obesity is associated with OSA.
    - Narrow airway—Conditions associated with this include retrognathia, micrognathia, macroglossia, tonsillar hypertrophy, and a high Mallampati score.
    - Large neck—OSA is prominent among men with a shirt collar size greater than 17 inches (16 inches for women).
    - Elevated blood pressure—Almost half of all patients with OSA have hypertension.

    Common screening tools include the STOP-Bang, Berlin, and Sleep Apnea Clinical Score questionnaires. These tools generally have a high false positive rate, meaning that when the score is high, patients do not always have the condition. However, when the score is low, they are unlikely to have it. Thus these questionnaires are sensitive but not specific and are generally only helpful when they are negative.

A Supine with correct sniffing position

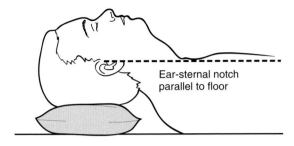

Ear-sternal notch
parallel to floor

B Ramp with incorrect sniffing position

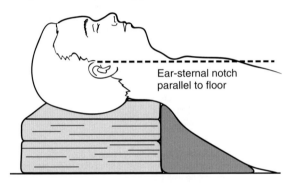

Ear-sternal notch
parallel to floor

C Ramp with correct sniffing position

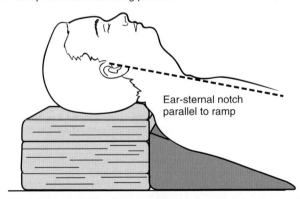

Ear-sternal notch
parallel to ramp

Fig. 49.1 Proper ramp positioning. (A) Proper sniffing position (alignment of airway axes by flexing the neck and extending the head to facilitate laryngoscopy and intubation success) is said to occur when an imaginary line, connecting the ear to sternal notch, is parallel to the floor in the supine patient. (B) Ramp positioning should avoid excessive neck extension, which can occur if the ear to sternal notch line is parallel to the floor in the ramp position. Excessive neck extension can make laryngoscopy and subsequent intubation more difficult. Although this position may improve pulmonary mechanics, it could make intubation more difficult. (C) Ideal ramp positioning should also include sniffing position (neck flexion and head extension), which would imply that the ear to sternal notch line is parallel to the ramp itself (or parallel to the floor if the ramp was removed). This position will improve pulmonary mechanics and facilitate alignment of the airway axes, which will improve the grade of view on laryngoscopy and intubation success.

13. **How do you manage induction of anesthesia for a morbidly obese patient? Are there any methods that can reduce problems with hypoxemia on induction?**

Induction of anesthesia for a morbidly obese patient can pose several challenges, such as difficult intubation, difficult mask ventilation, and reduced time to hypoxemia. The most important intervention is to perform a proper history and physical examination, such that patients deemed high risk undergo an awake fiberoptic intubation. For patients undergoing intubation, following induction of anesthesia (also known as asleep intubation), the most important intervention is proper patient positioning using a ramp. Other adjuncts to consider are the following:

- Rapid sequence induction to avoid mask ventilation and proceed directly to laryngoscopy. Patients may be a difficult mask but easier intubation.
- First, attempt with a video laryngoscope or at least have one immediately available.
- Preoxygenate with 5 to 10 cm H_2O continuous airway positive pressure using the adjustable pressure-limiting valve on the anesthesia machine.
- Use high flow nasal cannula at 60 liters per minute ([LPM]; ideally) or a regular nasal cannula at 10+ LPM to prolong time before hypoxemia during laryngoscopy (i.e., apneic oxygenation).

14. **What should the set tidal volume be for patients with morbidly obesity? What other ventilator strategies should be used to optimize oxygenation?**

All patients who are intubated should be managed using lung protection strategies using tidal volumes of 5 to 8 mL/kg of ideal body weight (IBW). In patients with obesity, it is crucial that IBW is used and not actual or total body weight (TBW) as the patient's lungs are not proportional to the patient's body habitus. Other strategies include using a higher positive end expiratory pressure (i.e., 8–10 cm H_2O) and frequent alveolar recruitment maneuvers every 30 minutes (10–20 seconds duration, holding a plateau pressure of 40 cm H_2O).

15. **What are the advantages and disadvantages with regional anesthesia in obese patients?**

Advantages
- Decreased cardiopulmonary depression
- Improved postoperative analgesia with decreased need for narcotics
- Less postoperative nausea and vomiting
- Decreased postanesthetic care unit stay

Disadvantages
- Technical difficulties arise in performing the blocks because of body habitus
- Failed peripheral nerve or neuraxial blocks may require intubation under suboptimal conditions
- Positioning is difficult and may not be well tolerated

16. **Describe bariatric surgery as treatment for obesity. What are the anesthetic concerns?**

Bariatric surgery broadly encompasses several surgical weight-loss procedures used in the treatment of obesity. Bariatric operations can be categorized as restrictive, malabsorptive, or a combination of both. Indications for bariatric surgery include a BMI greater than 40 kg/m^2 or a BMI between 30 and 40 kg/m^2 for patients with obesity-related comorbidities, who have failed nonsurgical management. The most common restrictive operation is sleeve gastrectomy, where the Roux-en-Y gastric bypass is the most common operation that has both restrictive and malabsorptive properties. Bariatric surgery is very effective with studies showing resolution of metabolic syndrome in more than 95% of cases and a 90% reduction in the relative risk of death after 5 years.

Bariatric surgical procedures are often performed laparoscopically. The increased intraabdominal pressure of obesity, combined with a pneumoperitoneum, results in venous stasis, reduced intraoperative portal venous blood flow, decreased urinary output, lower respiratory compliance, increased airway pressure, impairment of cardiac function, and hypercapnia. In addition, there is less efficient elimination of carbon dioxide and increased arterial partial pressure of carbon dioxide, when compared with nonobese patients. Postoperative complications include deep venous thrombosis, anastomotic leaks, wound infection, bleeding, herniation, and small bowel obstruction.

17. **How does obesity change the pharmacokinetics of medications? Redistribution? Clearance? What body weight should you use to dose medications?**

In general, the loading dose of a drug is based on the volume of distribution and the maintenance dose or time interval between doses on clearance. For example, a patient with hepatorenal disease will still generally require the same loading dose, but the dosing intervals are increased. Obesity complicates dosing of medications because the volume of distribution for lipophilic drugs is increased compared with hydrophilic drugs. Further, there is a spectrum of drugs that may be partially hydrophilic or partially lipophilic. In other words, some hydrophilic drugs are more hydrophilic than others and the corollary is true with lipophilic medications. In general, there are several dosing weights that can be used:

- TBW—A patient's total scale weight
- IBW—Weight based on gender and height. IBW is calculated as follows:
  Male: IBW = 50 kg + 2.3 kg/inch for every inch over 5 feet
  Female: IBW = 45 kg + 2.3 kg/inch for every inch over 5 feet

- Lean body weight (LBW)—Calculated by subtracting body fat weight from TBW. Although obesity is primarily because of an increase in body fat composition, approximately 20% to 30% of their TBW is because of an increase in LBW. LBW is likely the most accurate weight in obese patients to determine the proper loading dose for hydrophilic medications or for medications that have a rapid effect before redistribution (e.g., induction dose of propofol). It can be calculated as follows:

$$LBW \approx IBW + (20\% - 30\%)\,(IBW)$$

Most drugs can safely be dosed using LBW and titrated to effect, with the realization that a spectrum exists where some drugs are slightly more hydrophilic or lipophilic than others. Succinylcholine, however, is one medication that should be dosed using TBW.

KEY POINTS: OBESITY AND OBSTRUCTIVE SLEEP APNEA

1. Patients with obesity often have multiple comorbidities, such as OSA, hypertension, heart disease, diabetes, and renal disease.
2. Obesity decreases pulmonary compliance, causing decreased FRC and is associated with increased oxygen consumption because of a larger body habitus.
3. Hypoxemia (and hypercarbia) is a frequent problem in this patient population and many patients have other comorbidities, such as OSA, which increases the risk of hypoxemia because of opioid and anesthetic related upper airway obstruction.
4. Ramp positioning before the induction of anesthesia can improve pulmonary mechanics and reduce the incidence of hypoxemia on induction.
5. The loading dose for most medications in patients with obesity should be based on LBW.

SUGGESTED READINGS

American Society of Anesthesiologists Task Force on Perioperative Management of patients with obstructive sleep apnea: Practice guidelines for the perioperative management of patients with obstructive sleep apnea: an updated report by the American Society of Anesthesiologists Task Force on Perioperative Management of patients with obstructive sleep apnea, Anesthesiology. 2014;120:268–286.

Nightingale CE, Margarson MP, Shearer E, et al. Peri-operative management of the obese surgical patient 2015. Association of Anaesthetists of Great Britain and Ireland Society for Obesity and Bariatric Anaesthesia. Anaesthesia. 2015;70(7):859–876.

CHAPTER 50

ALCOHOL AND SUBSTANCE ABUSE

Dominique Schiffer, MD

1. **How is alcohol absorbed and metabolized?**

   Alcohol is absorbed across the gastrointestinal mucosa, more so in the small intestine than in the stomach. It enters into the portal vein and proceeds to the liver, where it is metabolized.

   Most consumed alcohol is converted to acetaldehyde by the enzyme alcohol dehydrogenase and secondarily by cytochrome P450 2E1, as alcohol blood levels rise. Alcohol metabolism follows Michaelis–Menten zero-order kinetics, meaning that once the enzyme is saturated with ethanol, the rate of metabolism is constant, even though blood alcohol concentration may continue to increase. Some 5% to 10% of consumed alcohol is excreted unchanged in the breath and urine. Alcohol easily crosses the blood-brain barrier. Blood levels of alcohol correlate well with the concentration in lung alveoli, thus the basis of the breathalyzer test used by law enforcement officers.

2. **What are the acute and chronic effects of alcohol on the nervous system?**

   Acutely, alcohol depresses the central nervous system by inhibiting polysynaptic function, which is characterized by a generalized blunting and eventual loss of higher motor, sensory, and cognitive function. Although the behavioral effects of alcohol consumption may seem excitatory or stimulating to observers and users, this effect is probably caused by a depressive effect on inhibitory pathways (disinhibition).

   Chronic alcohol use is associated with peripheral nerve and neuropsychiatric disorders, many of which (e.g., Wernicke encephalopathy and Korsakoff psychosis) may be linked to nutritional deficiencies (e.g., thiamine B-1). Alcohol-related neuropathy may be present in the lower extremities, often with concomitant weakness of the intrinsic muscles of the feet. It is a symmetrical, bilateral mixed sensory and motor peripheral neuropathy, often presenting as pain and numbness of the feet. Generalized weakness in the proximal limb musculature may also be noted in chronic alcoholic myopathy.

3. **What are the effects of alcohol on the cardiovascular system?**

   Although controversial, some evidence suggests that small amounts of alcohol may be cardioprotective. However, even modest ingestion over the long-term is associated with atrial fibrillation, hypertension, left ventricular hypertrophy, and cardiomyopathy. "Holiday Heart syndrome," following an alcohol binge, is well characterized by acute onset of atrial fibrillation. Acutely, moderate ingestion of alcohol produces no significant changes in blood pressure or myocardial contractility. Cutaneous vasodilation generally occurs, and heart rate increases. At high levels of acute ingestion, a decrease in central vasomotor activity causes respiratory and cardiac depression.

   The leading cause of death in chronic users of alcohol is cardiac dysfunction. Consumption of 60 oz of ethanol per month (8 pints of whiskey or 55 cans of beer) may lead to alcohol-induced hypertension. An intake over 90 oz per month over a 10-year period may result in cardiomyopathy, with associated pulmonary hypertension, right-sided heart failure, and dysrhythmias. Ventricular tachydysrhythmias, ventricular fibrillation, and sudden death are also risks.

4. **How does alcohol affect the respiratory system?**

   Acute alcohol intake may cause hyperventilation via disinhibition of central respiratory regulation centers and increases dead-space ventilation. Despite this, alcohol depresses the ventilatory response to carbon dioxide. Chronic alcohol users are susceptible to pulmonary infections because of greater airway colonization, often by staphylococci or gram-negative organisms, associated with frequent aspiration of gastric contents. There is also a generalized decrease in all lung capacities (vital, functional residual, and inspiratory capacity).

5. **How does alcohol affect the gastrointestinal and hepatobiliary systems?**

   Acutely, alcohol use may cause esophagitis, gastritis, and pancreatitis. Chronically, alcohol use leads to delayed gastric emptying and relaxation of the lower esophageal sphincter, increasing the risk of aspiration. Also acutely, the liver undergoes transient and reversible fatty infiltration. Although such changes resolve with abstinence, prolonged alcohol exposure leads to chronic infiltration of fat, which, over time, progresses to necrosis and fibrosis of liver tissue. The initial presentation of fatty liver is hepatomegaly. As necrosis, fibrosis, and cirrhosis progresses, the liver regresses in size. Chronic severe consumption of alcohol leads to irreversible cirrhosis and alcohol-induced hepatitis. Hepatic synthetic function is impaired. Production of albumin and coagulation Factors II, V, VII, X, and XIII are decreased. Reduction of albumin results in lower intravascular oncotic pressure and may lead to tissue edema. A reduction in circulating coagulation factors may predispose to bleeding, which is evidenced by a prolonged prothrombin time.

6. **Which nutritional deficiencies are seen in chronic alcohol users?**

   Chronic alcohol abuse can impair intestinal absorption of essential amino acids and vitamins, especially thiamine and folate. Deficiency of thiamine leads to Wernicke encephalopathy, polyneuropathy, and cardiac failure characterized by high cardiac output, low systemic vascular resistance, and loss of vasomotor tone. Folic acid deficiency causes bone-marrow depression and thrombocytopenia, leukopenia, and anemia.

7. **What are the effects of alcohol on inhalational anesthetics?**

   Acutely, in nonhabituated, intoxicated patients, the minimal alveolar concentration (MAC) of inhalational agents is reduced. For chronic users, the MAC for inhalational agents is increased. Acutely intoxicated patients are also more sensitive to the effects of barbiturates, benzodiazepines, and opioids. Cross-tolerance to intravenous anesthetic agents may also be present in patients who are chronically exposed to alcohol.

8. **How does alcohol affect the metabolism of neuromuscular blocking drugs?**

   Patients with liver disease may have decreased levels of circulating plasma cholinesterase, prolonging the effects of succinylcholine. Cirrhotic patients, with poor liver function, have a greater Volume of distribution V_D for injected drugs and thus require larger doses of nondepolarizing neuromuscular blocking drugs (NMBDs). Nondepolarizing relaxants that rely on hepatic clearance may have a prolonged duration of action. Muscle relaxants that are metabolized independently of organ function (e.g., cisatracurium) are good choices for patients with liver disease. Regardless of the NMBD chosen, close monitoring of neuromuscular blockade is recommended.

9. **Describe special considerations in the perioperative assessment of alcohol-abusing patients**

   Special consideration must be given to the cardiovascular system of chronic alcohol users. Tachycardia, dysrhythmias, or cardiomegaly may indicate alcohol-related cardiac dysfunction, and a 12-lead electrocardiogram (ECG) should be evaluated. Patients with alcohol-induced cardiac disease are less sensitive to endogenous or parenteral catecholamines. Also alcoholic patients are often volume depleted and may require fluid resuscitation. Hypokalemia and hypoglycemia are common. Anemia, thrombocytopenia, and altered coagulation are indicators of significant liver disease and may be present. Instrumentation of the esophagus should be undertaken carefully in patients with known liver disease, as the possibility of rupturing esophageal varices exists.

10. **What are the signs and symptoms of alcohol withdrawal?**

    Alcohol withdrawal presents as anorexia, insomnia, weakness, combativeness, tremors, dilated pupils, disorientation, auditory and visual hallucinations, and convulsions. Onset is usually 10 to 30 hours after abstinence has begun, and the symptoms may last for 40 to 50 hours. Prolonged abstinence may lead to delirium tremens or autonomic hyperactivity (tachycardia, diaphoresis, fever, anxiety, and confusion). Alcohol withdrawal syndrome may occur, while under anesthesia, and manifest as uncontrolled tachycardia, diaphoresis, and hyperthermia. The treatment is administration of benzodiazepines.

KEY POINTS: CONCERNS IN CHRONIC ALCOHOLICS

1. May present with cardiomyopathy and cardiac dysrhythmias.
2. Predisposed to aspiration and have diminished pulmonary function/reserve.
3. Portal hypertension and varices (avoid orogastric and nasogastric tubes).
4. Impaired synthetic liver function (important screening tests are albumin and prothrombin time).
5. Alcohol withdrawal may precipitate seizures.

11. **Review the differences between addiction, dependence, and tolerance according to the American Pain Society.**
    - Dependence implies "a state of adaptation that is manifested by a drug class–specific withdrawal syndrome that can be produced by abrupt cessation, rapid dose reduction, decreasing blood level of the drug, and/or administration of an antagonist."
    - Opioid tolerance is "a state of adaptation in which exposure to a drug induces changes that result in a diminution of one or more of the drug's effects over time."
    - Addiction "is a primary, chronic, neurobiological disease, with genetic, psychosocial, and environmental factors influencing its development and manifestations. It is characterized by behaviors that include one or more of the following: impaired control over drug use, compulsive use, continued use despite harm, and craving."

12. **List complications of chronic opioid use:**
    Oral intake (prescribed use or illicit use)
    - Tolerance
    - Opioid induced hyperalgesia
    - Immunosuppression
    - Increased risk of cardiovascular death
    - Testosterone depletion
    - Accidental overdose

- Sleep disordered breathing
- Atelectasis

Intravenous (IV)/intramuscular intake (usually illicit use, in addition to the aforementioned)

- Cellulitis
- Abscess formation
- Subacute bacterial endocarditis
- Thrombophlebitis
- Hepatitis, human immunodeficiency virus
- Pneumonia
- Acute pulmonary edema
- Sepsis
- Systemic and pulmonary emboli

13. **Discuss common perioperative concerns associated with the chronic opioid abuser**
It is necessary to know the patient's usual opioid requirements to avoid under medication. Associated behavioral and psychological problems may make general anesthesia a better option than regional or local anesthesia. These patients may be in acute withdrawal and be uncooperative. IV access may be difficult, and central venous catheterization may be necessary. A substantially increased dose of opioids to achieve the desired effect is not unusual. Consultation with a pain-management team may help with development of a realistic postoperative pain-management strategy. It is important to note that the perioperative period is an inappropriate time to attempt opioid withdrawal/weaning.

14. **Describe the time frame and stages of opioid withdrawal**
The onset and duration of withdrawal vary depending on the drug used. For example, heroin withdrawal symptoms usually peak within 36 to 72 hours and may last for 7 to 14 days. Symptoms of withdrawal include restlessness, sweating, nausea, rhinorrhea, nasal congestion, abdominal cramping, lacrimation, mydriasis, and drug craving. Overt withdrawal results in piloerection, emesis, diarrhea, muscle spasms (thus the term *kicking the habit*), fever, chills, tachycardia, and hypertension.

15. **What medications are used to stabilize and detoxify the withdrawing opioid patient?**
Long-acting medications (e.g., methadone and sustained-release morphine) are used because they have a slower onset of action and the high experienced is less prominent. Autonomic hyperactivity and other symptoms of acute opiate withdrawal are treated with β-adrenergic antagonists and α_2 agonists, such as clonidine.

16. **Which arrhythmias are patients being treated with methadone prone to?**
There are multiple reports of these patients having prolonged corrected QT intervals, torsades de pointes, and even sudden death. Other important characteristics of methadone are that it has no effect on seizure disorders, has no active metabolites, is relatively safe in renal failure, and has not been associated with hepatic toxicity.

17. **What is Suboxone and how should it be managed perioperatively?**
Suboxone is a combination of buprenorphine and naloxone and is an effective treatment for patients with opioid use disorder. Buprenorphine is used to treat chronic pain. It is a partial mu agonist with very high receptor affinity and a half-life of 24 to 60 hours. Because of its high affinity and long half-life, buprenorphine can block other opioids from binding to the mu receptor for several days. Naloxone cannot be absorbed orally and therefore functions as an antitampering agent.

In essence, Suboxone and buprenorphine block the effects of all standard mu-opioid receptor analgesics (e.g., fentanyl, morphine) and can therefore make the anesthetic management of these patients difficult. For major elective surgery, it is recommended that patients stop taking Suboxone (or buprenorphine) 3 days before surgery. During this period, they can begin replacing the Suboxone (buprenorphine) with full mu agonist therapy. For less painful operations or when pain can be controlled with regional anesthesia/analgesia and/or multimodal analgesia, discontinuation of Suboxone (buprenorphine) may not be necessary. Ideally, cessation of Suboxone/buprenorphine should be undertaken with the knowledge and assistance of the Suboxone/buprenorphine prescribing physician.

18. **What are the signs and symptoms of acute cannabis intoxication?**
In the acute setting, patients may exhibit increased heart rate and systolic blood pressure, conjunctival injection, dry mouth, orthostatic hypotension, and drowsiness. Anxiety and panic attacks are also possible, as well as short-term memory loss and hallucinations.

19. **Are cannabis smokers at increased risk for pulmonary complications?**
Though marijuana smoking is not associated with chronic pulmonary disease syndrome, chronic marijuana smokers do often experience chronic cough, increased sputum production, dyspnea and chest tightness, and frequent respiratory infections. However, ironically, recent long-term studies have shown that cannabis smoking is associated with an increased force vital capacity.

20. **Do cannabis users require more or less opioid medication in the perioperative period?**
There are limited studies in this regard and the full picture is complicated. There are data that indicate there are decreased rates of opioid prescriptions and opioid related deaths in states that have enacted medical cannabis laws.

21. What are the anesthetic considerations for the cannabis user?

Briefly, autonomic hyperactivity, slowed gastric emptying, increased airway reactivity, and concomitant use of other substances may all be present. With this in mind, regional anesthesia or a general anesthetic, with a rapid sequence induction, should be considered. Postoperative pain control may be an issue; therefore a multimodal pain management plan is recommended.

22. What are the various forms of cocaine and routes of administration?

A hydrochloride salt of cocaine is a powdery, white crystalline, water-soluble substance that can be sniffed or injected, or applied mucosally. A lipid-soluble form, called *crack or free-base cocaine*, is inexpensively manufactured by mixing the hydrochloride salt with an alkali. Crack is more stable on heating, vaporizes readily, and has high bioavailability when smoked.

23. How is cocaine metabolized and excreted?

Peak plasma concentrations occur 15 to 60 minutes after intranasal ingestion; its biological half-life is about 45 to 90 minutes. Plasma (pseudocholinesterase) and liver esterases hydrolyze cocaine to ecgonine methyl ester (EME) and benzoylecgonine. EME and benzoylecgonine constitute 80% of the metabolites of cocaine and are detected in urine for 14 to 60 hours after cocaine use. Only 1% to 5% is cleared unmetabolized in the urine.

24. What are the physiological effects of cocaine?

Cocaine causes inhibition of norepinephrine, dopamine, and serotonin transporter mechanisms. However, the physiological effects are caused principally by increases in norepinephrine levels. At adrenergic nerve endings, cocaine inhibits the reuptake of norepinephrine into the neuron. Increases in synaptic norepinephrine levels within the autonomic nervous system increase systolic, diastolic, and mean arterial pressure, heart rate, and body temperature.

25. List the common signs and symptoms of acute cocaine intoxication

- Nausea and vomiting
- Headache
- Rapid or irregular heartbeat
- High or low blood pressure
- Hallucinations
- Chest pain
- Convulsions and stroke
- Mydriasis

26. What is the most life-threatening toxic side effect of cocaine abuse and its treatment?

Cardiac ischemia and subsequent acute myocardial infarction are present in approximately 6% of all hospital admissions for chest pain secondary to cocaine use. Cocaine causes a myocardial oxygen supply/demand mismatch by increasing heart rate and blood pressure, through alpha adrenergic stimulation. At the same time, through coronary vasoconstriction, oxygen supply is decreased. Cocaine causes both systolic and diastolic dysfunction, arrhythmias and atherosclerosis. Cocaine also promotes thrombosis through a number of mechanisms. All told, the risk of myocardial infarction increases 24-fold within the first 60 minutes of cocaine use. Treatment of cocaine-induced chest pain includes the use of selective β_1-adrenergic blockade, nitrates, calcium channel blockers, and α-adrenergic blockers. Selective β_2 blockade should generally be avoided, because it may lead to unopposed α_1-mediated coronary and peripheral vasoconstriction.

27. List the signs and symptoms of cocaine withdrawal

- Anhedonia
- Anxiety and mild depressive symptoms
- Fatigue, difficulty maintaining concentration
- Increased appetite
- Increased sleep
- Tremors
- Myalgias

28. What are the anesthetic concerns in the acutely intoxicated cocaine user?

Cocaine may prolong the QT interval, making preoperative assessment of the ECG useful. Sedation and a deep level of general anesthesia inhibit adrenal release of catecholamines, potentially reducing the dysrhythmic effects of cocaine. The patient should be well anesthetized, before airway instrumentation is attempted, to avoid severe tachycardia and hypertension. It is important to note that cocaine sensitizes the cardiovascular system to the effects of endogenous catecholamines, making the maintenance of adequate anesthetic depth throughout the operation important. Ketamine can potentiate the cardiovascular toxicity of cocaine and should be avoided. The MAC of inhalational anesthetic agents is increased in the setting of acute cocaine intoxication. Should hypotension require pressor therapy, direct-acting agents, such as phenylephrine may be better because these patients may be catecholamine depleted.

KEY POINTS: CONCERNS IN PATIENTS TAKING COCAINE

1. The use of cocaine promotes vascular disease in general. Myocardial ischemia is not uncommon in cocaine-abusing patients, and selective β_2 blockade should be avoided because it may cause vasoconstriction and worsen the ischemia. Alpha adrenergic blockade should be used instead.
2. Severe hypertension and tachycardia are risks during airway management, unless the patient is deeply anesthetized.
3. Cocaine sensitizes the cardiovascular system to the effects of endogenous catecholamines. Ketamine can potentiate the cardiovascular toxicity of cocaine and should be avoided.

29. **What is crystal methamphetamine, and what are its properties?**
Crystal methamphetamine looks like glass fragments or shiny bluish white rocks, hence the name. It is a stimulant, similar to the drug amphetamine (trade names Vyvanse, Desoxyn) used to treat attention deficit hyperactivity disorder and narcolepsy. Methamphetamine use produces a rapid pleasurable rush followed by euphoria, heightened attention, and increased energy. These effects are caused by release of norepinephrine, dopamine, and serotonin. It is quite similar to cocaine in its manifestations, except longer lasting (4–8 hours).
    Recommendations for anesthetizing a methamphetamine-abusing patient are similar to those for cocaine. Avoid anesthetizing the acutely intoxicated patient for elective procedures. Anesthesia is probably safely started in patients who are chronic users but not acutely intoxicated. There may be an increased incidence of dental trauma because of the common finding of dental decay.

30. **What are the signs of symptoms of methamphetamine intoxication and withdrawal?**
Signs and symptoms of intoxication include anorexia, diaphoresis, hypertension, tachycardia, hyperthermia, agitation, and psychosis. Patients can also have myocardial infarctions, seizures, strokes, rhabdomyolysis, and renal failure. The withdrawing patient will experience fatigue, irritability, insomnia, anxiety, and psychotic reactions. An unusual sign seen in chronic methamphetamine users is dental decay, known as *meth mouth* (secondary to decreased salivary flow).

31. **What is ecstasy, and what are its mechanism of action and route of administration?**
Ecstasy, or 3,4-methylenedioxymethamphetamine, is a synthetic, psychoactive drug similar to the stimulant methamphetamine and the hallucinogen mescaline. It increases the activity of multiple neurotransmitters, including serotonin, dopamine, and norepinephrine. It is taken orally in capsule or tablet form. Its effects last 3 to 6 hours. Additional doses slow its enzymatic degradation, resulting in increased duration of action and increased risk of toxicity.

32. **What are the cognitive, physical, and psychological effects of ecstasy?**
Abusers experience a sense of well-being and decreased anxiety. Memory impairment may occur. Adverse reactions include nausea, chills, involuntary teeth clenching, muscle cramping, and blurred vision. More serious side effects, such as hypertension, loss of consciousness, and seizures are less common. Rarely, hyperthermia develops, which may precipitate cardiovascular collapse and multiorgan failure. Withdrawal may involve drug craving, depression, confusion, and severe anxiety. In nonhuman primates, as little as a 4-day exposure has been associated with damage to neurons involved in mood, thinking, and judgement.

33. **What is phencyclidine, and what is its mechanism of action?**
Phencyclidine (PCP) is a cyclohexylamine that was developed in the 1950s as a general anesthetic but was subsequently taken off the market because of its tendency to produce hallucinations. The precise mechanism of action of PCP is unknown, but it is thought to depress cortical and thalamic function, while stimulating the limbic system. PCP may block afferent impulses associated with the affective component of pain perception and suppress spinal cord activity. PCP can also inhibit pseudocholinesterase. Of note, the IV anesthetic, ketamine, is produced by chemical modification of PCP.

Websites
https://painmed.org/
World Health Organization: Management of substance abuse: http://www.who.int/substance_abuse

SUGGESTED READINGS

Bachi K, Mani V, Jeyachandran D, et al. Vascular disease in cocaine addiction. Atherosclerosis. 2017;262:154–162.
Beaulieu P. Anesthetic implications of recreational drug use. Can J Anesth. 2017;64(12):1236–1264.
Courtney KE, Ray LA. Methamphetamine: an update on epidemiology, pharmacology, clinical phenomenology, and treatment literature. Drug Alcohol Depend. 2014;143:11–21.
Hassan SF, Wearne TA, Cornish JL, et al. Effects of acute and chronic systemic methamphetamine on respiratory, cardiovascular and metabolic function, and cardiorespiratory reflexes. J Physiol. 2016;594(3):763–780.
Havakuk O, Rezkall SH, Kloner RA. The cardiovascular effects of cocaine. J Am Coll Cardiol. 2017;70(1):101–113.
Maguire DR, France CP. Impact of efficacy at the μ-opioid receptor on antinociceptive effects of combinations of μ-opioid receptor agonists and cannabinoid receptor agonists. J Pharmacol Exp Ther. 2014;351(2):383–389.

Mirijello A, Tarli C, Vassalo GA, et al. Alcoholic cardiomyopathy: what is known and what is not known. Eur J Intern Med. 2017;43:1–5.

Molina PE, Gardner JD, Souza-Smith FM, et al. Alcohol abuse: critical pathophysiological processes and contribution to disease burden. Physiology (Bethesda, Md.). 2014;29(3):203–215.

Ribeiro LI, Ind PW. Effect of cannabis smoking on lung function and respiratory symptoms: a structured literature review. NPJ Primary Care Respir Med. 2014;26(1):16071.

Singh A, Saluja S, Kumar A, et al. Cardiovascular complications of marijuana and related substances: a review. Cardiol Ther. 2018;7:45.

CHAPTER 51

NEONATAL ANESTHESIA

Lee D. Stein, MD

1. **Why are neonates and preterm infants at increased anesthetic risk?**
   - Pulmonary factors. Differences in the neonatal airway, including large tongue and occiput, floppy epiglottis, small mouth, and short neck predispose infants to upper airway obstruction. The more premature the infant, the higher the incidence of airway obstruction. The carbon dioxide response curve is shifted further to the right in neonates than in adults (i.e., infants have a comparatively decreased ventilatory response to hypercarbia). Newborn vital capacity is about one-half of an adult's vital capacity, respiratory rate is at least twice that of an adult (respiratory rate in the 30s would be normal for a term neonate and even higher values are acceptable for preterm neonates), and oxygen consumption is 2 to 3 times greater. Consequently, when neonates receive medications that decrease their respiratory drive they will desaturate much faster than adults. Neonates will also fatigue more easily because their diaphragms have less type 1 muscle fibers than adults
   - Cardiovascular factors. Newborn infants have noncompliant ventricles that function at close to maximal contractility. Cardiac output is dependent on heart rate. Neonates are highly sensitive to the myocardial depressant effects of many anesthetic agents, especially those that may produce bradycardia. Inhalational agents should be used cautiously
   - Temperature regulation. Infants have poor central thermoregulation, thin insulating fat, increased body surface area-to-mass ratio, and high minute ventilation. These factors make them susceptible to hypothermia in the operating room (OR). Shivering is an ineffective mechanism for heat production because infants have limited muscle mass. Nonshivering thermogenesis uses brown fat to produce heat, but it is not an efficient method to restore body temperature and increases oxygen consumption significantly. Cold-stressed infants may develop cardiovascular depression and hypoperfusion acidosis
   - Pharmacological factors. Neonates have a larger volume of distribution and less tissue and protein binding of drugs than older children and adults. They also have immature livers and kidneys, which are less efficiently able to eliminate medications. There is a larger distribution of their cardiac output to the vessel-rich tissues. The uptake and elimination of inhalational anesthetics is more rapid than in an adult.

2. **Do neonates have normal renal function?**
   Glomerular function of the kidneys is immature, and the concentrating ability is impaired. Renal clearance of drugs may be delayed. Extra salt and water are not handled well. Neonates will not compensate for hypovolemia, as efficiently as adults, but will still become tachycardic and have decreased urine output.

3. **Why is it important to provide infants with exogenous glucose?**
   Neonates have low stores of hepatic glucose, and mechanisms for gluconeogenesis are immature. Infants who have fasted may develop hypoglycemia. Symptoms of hypoglycemia include apnea, cyanosis, respiratory difficulties, seizures, high-pitched cry, lethargy, temperature instability, and sweating. Hypoglycemia may be associated with long-term neurological sequelae. For this reason, in neonates, it is typical to give glucose containing fluid (e.g., D10NS) during operative procedures.

4. **What are the differences in the gastrointestinal or hepatic function of neonates?**
   Gastric emptying is prolonged, the lower esophageal sphincter is incompetent, and neonates spend much of their time on their backs; thus the incidence of reflux may be increased. Elevated levels of bilirubin are common in neonates. Kernicterus, a complication of severely elevated levels of bilirubin, will lead to neurological dysfunction and even death in extreme cases. Commonly used medications, such as furosemide and sulfonamide, may displace bilirubin from albumin and increase the risk of kernicterus. Diazepam contains the preservative benzyl alcohol, which also may displace bilirubin. Hepatic metabolism is immature, and hepatic blood flow is less than that in older children or adults. Drug metabolism and effect may be prolonged.

5. **What is retinopathy of prematurity?**
   Retinopathy of prematurity is a disorder that occurs primarily in premature infants who have been exposed to high inspired concentrations of oxygen. Proliferation of the retinal vessels, retinal hemorrhage, fibroproliferation, scarring, and retinal detachment may occur, with decreased visual acuity and blindness. Premature infants should have limited exposure to high concentrations of inspired oxygen. Oxygen saturation should be maintained between 92% and 95%, except during times of greater risk for desaturation. Use of an oxygen blender to control the fraction of inspired oxygen is useful.

6. How is volume status assessed in neonates?

Findings in neonates that are hypovolemic are tachycardia, sunken fontanelles, decreased skin turgor, delayed capillary refill, weight loss, crying without tears, and decreased urine output. Hypotension is a late finding. Capillary refill after blanching of the big toe should be less than 3 seconds. The extremities should not be significantly cooler than the rest of the body. Finally, the skin should look pink and well perfused—not pale, mottled, or cyanotic.

7. What problems are common in premature infants?

See Table 51.1.

8. What special preparations are needed before anesthetizing a neonate?

The room should be warmed before the start of the procedure to minimize radiant heat loss. Use emergency warming of the OR, if available, and there is little time before emergently starting a procedure. A warming blanket, head cover, and infrared warming lights also help to decrease heat loss. Covering the infant with plastic decreases evaporative losses. Forced-air warming blankets have been shown to be effective at keeping infants warm. Temperature should be monitored carefully because it is easy to overheat a small infant.

- Routine monitors in a variety of appropriately small sizes should be available. At least two pulse oximeter probes are helpful in measuring preductal and postductal saturation.
- Calculate estimated blood volume, maintenance, and maximal acceptable blood loss.
- Placing 25 to 50 mL of balanced salt solution in a buretrol prevents inadvertent administration of large amounts of fluid. Glucose should be added to the solution.
- Ensure 5% albumin and blood is readily available.

9. Why might you measure pre- and postductal oxygen saturations?

Preductal oxygen saturations are measured in the right hand, whereas postductal saturations are measured in the foot. Measuring both would help detect a right to left cardiac shunt, because deoxygenated blood from the right side of the heart would lower the postductal saturation compared with the preductal saturation. This occurs when there is pulmonary hypertension along with a patent ductus arteriosus (PDA).

10. What intraoperative problems are common in small infants?

See Table 51.2.

11. What are common neonatal surgeries?

- Tracheoesophageal fistula (TEF)
- Gastroschisis
- Omphalocele
- Congenital diaphragmatic hernia
- PDA
- Intestinal obstruction
- Pyloric stenosis (presents in young infants more than neonates)

Table 51.1 Common Problems in Premature Infants

PROBLEM	SIGNIFICANCE
Respiratory distress syndrome	Surfactant, which is produced by alveolar epithelial cells, coats the inside of the alveolus and reduces surface tension. Surfactant deficiency causes alveolar collapse. BPD occurs in about 20% of cases.
Bronchopulmonary dysplasia (BPD)	Interstitial fibrosis, cysts, and collapsed lung, all impairing ventilatory mechanics and gas exchange, may accompany bronchopulmonary dysplasia.
Apnea and bradycardia (A and B)	This is the most common cause of morbidity in the postoperative period. Sensitivity of chemoreceptors to hypercarbia and hypoxia is decreased. Immaturity and poor coordination of upper airway musculature also contribute. If apnea persists >15 seconds, bradycardia may result and worsen hypoxia.
Patent ductus arteriosus (PDA)	Incidence of hemodynamically significant PDA varies with degree of prematurity, but is usually high. Left-to-right shunting through the PDA may lead to fluid overload, heart failure, and respiratory distress.
Intraventricular hemorrhage (IVH)	Hydrocephalus may result from IVH. Avoiding fluctuations in blood pressure and intracranial pressure may reduce the risk of IVH.
Retinopathy of prematurity	See Question 5.
Necrotizing enterocolitis	Infants develop distended abdomen, bloody stools, and vomiting. They may present in shock and require surgery to resect ischemic intestines.

Table 51.2 Common Intraoperative Problems in Infants

PROBLEM	POSSIBLE CAUSES	SOLUTION
Hypoxia	Short distance from cords to carina may cause hypoxia because ETT is easily dislodged or displaced into main stem bronchus. Pressure on abdomen or chest by surgeons may decrease FRC and vital capacity.	At intubation, place the ETT into right mainstem, carefully listen to breath sounds, pull the tube back so that breath sounds are bilateral. Tape ETT 1–2 cm above level of carina. Inform surgeons when they are interfering with ventilation. Hand ventilation helps to compensate for changes in peak pressure.
Bradycardia	Hypoxia Volatile anesthetics Succinylcholine	Preoxygenate before intubation or extubation. All airway manipulations should be performed expeditiously. Minimize amount of volatile agent administered. Give atropine before administering succinylcholine to blunt vagal effects and ensure oxygenation.
Hypothermia	See Question 1	Facilitate a warm operating room by having a warming blanket, warming lights, warm fluids, and humidifier, and keep the infant covered whenever possible.
Hypotension	Bradycardia Volume depletion	Treat bradycardia with anticholinergics and ensure oxygenation. Many neonatal surgeries are associated with major fluid loss. Volume status should be carefully assessed, with deficits replaced appropriately.

ETT, Endotracheal tube; *FRC,* functional residual capacity.

12. Discuss the incidence and anesthetic implications of congenital diaphragmatic hernia.
   - The incidence is 1 to 2 out of 5000 live births.
   - The diaphragm fails to close completely, allowing the peritoneal contents to herniate into the thoracic cavity. Abnormal lung development and hypoplasia usually occur on the side of the hernia but may be bilateral.
   - The majority of hernias occurs through the left-sided foramen of Bochdalek.
   - Associated cardiovascular abnormalities present in 23% of patients and associated central nervous system abnormalities present in 28%.
   - Patients present with symptoms of pulmonary hypoplasia. The severity of symptoms and prognosis depend on the severity of the underlying hypoplasia. Pulmonary hypertension is very common.
   - Mask ventilation may cause visceral distention and worsen oxygenation. The infant should be intubated while awake. Low pressures must be used for ventilation to prevent barotrauma. Pneumothorax of the contralateral (healthier) lung may occur when high pressures are needed. Some patients may require high-frequency ventilation or extracorporeal membrane oxygenation.
   - A nasogastric tube should be used to decompress the stomach.
   - A transabdominal approach is used for the repair.
   - Good intravenous (IV) access is mandatory. An arterial line may be necessary if the infant has significant lung or cardiac abnormalities.
   - Pulmonary hypertension may complicate management by impairing oxygenation and decreasing cardiac output. Most patients need to remain intubated in the postoperative period.
   - Opioids and muscle relaxants should be the primary agents used. Inhalational agents may be used to supplement the anesthetic if tolerated by the infant.

13. Which congenital anomalies are associated with TEF?
   TEFs may occur alone or as part of a syndrome. The two most common syndromes are the VATER and the VACTERL syndromes. Patients with VATER have vertebral anomalies, imperforate anus, tracheoesophageal fistula, and renal or radial abnormalities. Patients with VACTERL have all of the aforementioned plus cardiac and limb abnormalities.

14. How should patients with TEF be managed?
   - Patients usually present with excessive secretions, inability to pass a nasogastric tube, and regurgitation of feedings. Respiratory symptoms are uncommon.
   - Positive-pressure ventilation may cause distention of the stomach. In a spontaneously breathing patient, either an awake intubation or inhalational induction may be carried out.

- Preoperative echo will determine the laterality of the aortic arch and will determine which side surgeons will enter the chest. Surgeons will perform bronchoscopy before intubation to evaluate the location of the fistula.
- The endotracheal tube (ETT) should be placed into the right mainstem and gradually withdrawn, until bilateral breath sounds are heard. Alternatively, a fiberoptic bronchoscope can be used to ensure the ETT is advanced past the fistula. The stomach should be auscultated to ensure that it is not overinflated. If the infant has significant respiratory distress because of overinflation of the stomach, it may be necessary to perform a gastrostomy before anesthetizing the patient.
- An arterial line is sometimes not necessary if the infant is otherwise a healthy infant and has no other congenital anomalies. In selected patients, it may be helpful to monitor blood gas values.
- Pulse oximetry is invaluable. Probes should be placed at a preductal (right hand or finger) and postductal site (feet).
- Once the airway has been secured, the infant is typically placed in the left lateral decubitus position. Placing a precordial stethoscope on the left chest helps to detect displacement of the ETT.
- Surgical repair involves either thoracotomy or video-assisted thoracoscopic repair. The fistula is divided. If possible, the esophagus is reanastomosed; if not, a gastrostomy tube is placed. Maintenance of adequate ventilation and oxygenation can be extremely challenging.
- It is desirable to extubate the infant as soon as possible to prevent pressure on the suture line; however, this must be weighed against the potential need for reintubation, which could also disrupt the sensitive surgical site.

15. **What are the differences between omphalocele and gastroschisis?**
An omphalocele is a hernia within the umbilical cord caused by failure of the gut to migrate into the abdomen from the yolk sac. The bowel is completely covered with chorioamniotic membranes, but otherwise usually normal. Patients with omphalocele frequently have associated cardiac, urological, and metabolic anomalies.
In gastroschisis, the bowel is not covered with chorioamniotic membranes; often there is an inflammatory exudate, and the bowel anatomy may be abnormal. The exact cause of gastroschisis is unknown; it may be the result of occlusion of blood supply to the abdominal wall or fetal rupture of an omphalocele. It is not typically associated with other anomalies.

16. **How are patients with omphalocele or gastroschisis managed in the perioperative period?**
    - It is important to prevent evaporative and heat loss from exposed viscera. The exposed bowel should be covered with warm, moist saline packs, and plastic wrap, until the time of surgery. The OR should be warmed before the arrival of the infant. Warming lights and a warming blanket help to decrease conductive and radiation heat loss. Covering the head and extremities with plastic prevents evaporative loss. Placing the baby on a forced air blanket can substantially reduce heat loss.
    - Respiratory distress can occur when an omphalocele is associated with pulmonary hypertension; however, children will often present to the OR breathing spontaneously. Rapid-sequence induction quickly establishes airway control.
    - Ventilation is controlled with muscle relaxants to facilitate return of the bowel into the abdomen.
    - After intubation, a nasogastric tube should be placed if not already present.
    - Patients need good IV access to replace third-space and evaporative losses. An arterial line can be helpful.
    - Once the surgeons begin to put the viscera into the abdomen, the ventilatory requirements change, because of increased intraabdominal and intrathoracic pressure. Hand ventilation during this phase allows the anesthesiologist to feel peak airway pressures and changes in airway pressures.
    - If peak airway pressures are greater than 40 cm H_2O, the surgeons must be notified because primary closure will not be possible. The surgeons can choose either to do a fascial closure or to place a synthetic mesh silo over the defect. Both approaches necessitate return trips to the OR for the final corrective procedure.
    - The abdominal cavity may be too small for the viscera. Venous return from or blood flow to the lower extremity may be compromised. A pulse oximeter on the foot helps to detect such changes. Renal perfusion may decrease and manifest as oliguria.
    - Patients usually remain intubated after surgery.
    - Surgeons are increasingly performing placement of a silo device at the bedside in the neonatal intensive care unit and bringing patients to the OR for the final repair.

17. **How does pyloric stenosis present?**
Pyloric stenosis is a common surgical problem, occurring in 1 out of 500 to 1000 live births. First-born males are more commonly affected, and it usually presents between 3 and 5 weeks of age. Patients present with persistent projectile vomiting. Dehydration, hypochloremia, and metabolic alkalosis can develop. Continued severe vomiting and dehydration can lead to metabolic acidosis. An olive-like mass may be felt in the epigastrium, but is commonly not able to be palpated. Confirmation of the diagnosis by upper gastrointestinal study has largely been replaced by abdominal ultrasound. Surgeons may choose to repair the pylorus laparoscopically or by an open approach.

18. **Discuss the perioperative management of patients with pyloric stenosis.**
    - This is a medical emergency, but not a surgical emergency. Electrolyte and volume imbalances need to be corrected before surgery.

- A gastric tube should be placed and continuous suction applied. The patient may have a large gastric volume of oral x-ray film contrast.
- Patients are at risk for aspiration; therefore rapid-sequence intubation or modified rapid-sequence intubation should be performed. Awake intubation in this situation has been associated with greater desaturation and a longer time to intubate.
- Opioids are usually unnecessary and should be avoided intraoperatively. The procedure is only minimally painful, and these patients can have increased respiratory sensitivity.
- Patients need to be closely monitored for postoperative apnea.

19. Are there any benefits to specific ventilator strategies in neonates?

Evidence has emerged that strongly supports the use of lung protective ventilation (4–6 mL/kg) in the management of neonates with respiratory distress syndrome (RDS), meconium aspiration syndrome, or congenital diaphragmatic hernia. Injury that has resulted in heterogeneous lung mechanics may cause a particular susceptibility to overdistention because of small absolute lung volumes and a highly compliant chest wall. Regional overdistention from large tidal volumes and elevated airway pressures may be more significant in neonates because of the difference in chest wall compliance and abdominal compartment pressures. In addition to barotrauma caused by high airway pressure, atelectotrauma, related to repeated alveolar recruitment and derecruitment, has been identified as potentially injurious in patients at risk for RDS.

20. At what age should the former premature infant be allowed to go home after surgery?

Premature infants are at increased risk for the development of postoperative apnea, even after relatively minor surgery. Postoperative apnea has been reported in ex-premature infants up to 60 weeks' postconceptual age (PCA). Côté and associates showed that, in ex-premature infants born at a gestational age of 32 weeks, undergoing inguinal herniorrhaphy, the risk of postoperative apnea was not less than 1%, until 56 weeks' PCA. Other risk factors for postoperative apnea are history of apnea, mechanical ventilation after birth, intraventricular hemorrhage, chronic lung disease, PDA, necrotizing enterocolitis, and anemia. Full-term neonates are at low risk after 45 weeks' PCA.

KEY POINTS: NEONATAL ANESTHESIA

1. Neonates are at increased anesthetic risk because:
   - They desaturate quickly.
   - They are prone to airway obstruction.
   - Noncompliant ventricles depend on adequate heart rate to maintain cardiac output.
   - They become hypothermic quickly.
   - Immature kidney and liver function affects the pharmacology of administered medications.
2. Common neonatal surgeries include:
   - TEF
   - Gastroschisis
   - Omphalocele
   - Congenital diaphragmatic hernia
   - PDA
   - Intestinal obstruction
   - Pyloric stenosis
3. When anesthetizing neonates, the following procedures are followed:
   - Warm the room and have warming lights, blankets, head covers, and convection air warming blankets available to maintain body heat.
   - Have multiple endotracheal sizes available.
   - Estimate fluid maintenance, deficit, blood volume, and acceptable blood loss before the surgery.
   - Prevent accidental overhydration by limiting the amount of volume in the buretrol.

21. Does regional anesthesia protect the patient from developing postoperative apnea?

Spinal anesthesia without supplemental sedation has been associated with less early apnea (0–30 minutes postoperative) than general anesthesia, although there has been no difference found with late apnea (30 minutes to 12 hours postoperative). Caudal epidural blockade may also be used. The addition of sedation may increase the incidence of postoperative apnea.

SUGGESTED READINGS

Bachiller PR, Chou JH, Romanelli TM, et al. Neonatal emergencies. In: Côté CJ, Lerman J, Anderson BJ, eds. A Practice of Anesthesia for Infants and Children. 5th ed. Philadelphia: Saunders; 2013:746–765.

Côté CJ, Zaslavsky A, Downes JJ, et al. Postoperative apnea in former preterm infants after inguinal herniorrhaphy: a combined analysis. Anesthesiology. 1995;82:809–822.

Davidson AJ, Morton NS, Arnup SJ, et al. Apnea after awake regional and general anesthesia in infants: The General Anesthesia Compared to Spinal Anesthesia Study—Comparing Apnea and Neurodevelopmental Outcomes, a Randomized Controlled Trial. Anesthesiology. 2015;123:38–54.

Feldman JM, Davis PJ. Do new anesthesia ventilators deliver small tidal volumes accurately during volume-controlled ventilation? Anesth Analg. 2008;106:1392–1400.

Gregory G, Andropoulos DA. Pediatric Anesthesia. 5th ed. Oxford: Wiley-Blackwell; 2011.

Schultz MJ, Haitsma JJ, Slutsky AS, et al. What tidal volumes should be used in patients without acute lung injury? Anesthesiology. 2007;106:1226–1231.

Vitali SH, Arnold JH. Bench-to-bedside review: ventilator strategies to reduce lung injury—lessons from pediatric and neonatal intensive care. Crit Care. 2005;9:177–183.

CHAPTER 52

PEDIATRIC ANESTHESIA

Nicole Arboleda, MD, Brian M. Keech, MD

1. **Compare and contrast the adult and pediatric airways.**
   Compared with adults, children have larger heads, shorter necks, smaller nares, and larger tongues. Infants and neonates are obligate nose breathers. They have a large tongue, which can obstruct the airway and make laryngoscopy more difficult. Their large occiput places them in a flexed cervical position when supine, so a shoulder roll can be helpful for positioning for intubation. The glottis is located higher in the neck at C3–C4 compared with C5 in adults making the larynx appear more anterior. The narrowest part of the pediatric airway is subglottic, at the level of the cricoid cartilage, which may increase their risk of postextubation stridor. They should have an endotracheal tube (ETT) leak is less than 30 cm H_2O to prevent excessive pressure on this part of the tracheal mucosa. The vocal cords slant anteriorly, making visualization of the glottis and successful insertion of the ETT more difficult. Lastly, the epiglottis is elongated, omega shaped, and is situated at an acute angle to the long axis of the trachea, making control of the epiglottis during laryngoscopy more difficult.

2. **Highlight the differences between the adult and pediatric pulmonary systems.**
   Compared with adults, neonates, infants, and small children have:
   - Increased lung and chest wall compliance, leading to closure of noncartilaginous airways at tidal volume breathing.
   - Smaller and fewer alveoli, reaching adult levels in adolescence.
   - Increased airway resistance because of small diameter of airways, increasing work of breathing (WOB).
   - Inefficient chest wall mechanics secondary to more horizontal, more pliable ribs and cartilage.
   - Fewer type 1 high-oxidative muscle fibers, making infants fatigue more easily.
   - Quicker desaturation during apnea because of smaller functional residual capacity (FRC) and increased oxygen consumption.

3. **Highlight the differences between the adult and pediatric cardiovascular systems.**
   Compared with adults, neonates, infants, and small children have:
   - Less compliant ventricles and limited ability to increase cardiac output (CO) by increasing contractility; they increase CO only by increasing heart rate. They are also more dependent on extracellular calcium for maintaining cardiac contractility.
   - Infants have an immature baroreceptor reflex and limited ability to compensate for hypotension. As a result, they are more susceptible to the cardiac depressant effects of volatile anesthetics and most intravenous anesthetics.
   - Infants have increased vagal tone and are prone to bradycardia. The three major causes of bradycardia are hypoxia (most common), vagal stimulation (e.g., laryngoscopy), and volatile anesthetics.

4. **What are normal vital signs in children?**
   See Table 52.1.

5. **When should children be premedicated for surgery? Which drugs are most commonly used?**
   Children frequently experience fear and anxiety when they are separated from their parents for surgery. These children are at increased risk for emergence delirium and may later experience negative postoperative behavioral changes. In general, children who are 2 to 6 years old who have had previous surgery, no preoperative tour or education, or who fail to interact positively with healthcare providers are candidates for premedication.

   Premedication with midazolam may reduce the incidence of negative postoperative behavioral changes. Distraction techniques, involving pediatric recreational therapists using video games or active play, are increasingly used to reduce perioperative anxiety, and may obviate the need for premedication in some instances.

6. **Should parents be allowed to accompany their children to the operating room for anesthetic induction?**
   Allowing parents to accompany children to the operating room (OR) may facilitate anesthetic induction in some cases. Parents and children should be educated and prepared for what to expect, and parents should be prepared to leave when the anesthesiologist believes it appropriate. Anxious parents may interfere with the provision of care and create problems for the care team. Although parents often wish to be present during induction, premedication with midazolam and/or distraction techniques are associated with lower levels of anxiety in the child. The benefit of both premedication and parental presence during anesthesia does not appear to be additive.

7. **What medications are available for premedication?**
   See Table 52.2.

Table 52.1 Normal Vital Signs in Children

AGE (YEARS)	HR (beats/min)	RR (breaths/min)	SBP (mm Hg)	DPB (mm Hg)
<1	100–160	30–60	60–95	35–69
1–3	90–140	24–40	70–105	50–65
3–5	75–110	18–30	80–110	50–65
6–12	75–100	18–30	80–110	57–71
12–16	60–90	12–16	100–130	60–80

DBP, Diastolic blood pressure; *HR*, heart rate; *RR*, respiratory rate; *SBP*, systolic blood pressure. A good rule of thumb is normal SBP = 70 mm Hg + (2 × age in years).

Table 52.2 Drugs Used for Premedication in Children

DRUG	ROUTE	COMMENTS	DISADVANTAGES
Midazolam	PO, PR, IN, IV, SL	Quick onset, minimal side effects, short half-life	Tastes badly when given orally, intranasal administration burns
Ketamine	PO, PR, IN, IV, SL	Quick onset, good analgesia	May slow emergence, tastes bad, intranasal administration burns
Diazepam	PO, PR, IM	Cheap, minimal side effects	Long onset time (peak sedation within 1 hour), may prolong emergence
Dexmedetomidine	IN, IV, IM	Does not burn with intranasal administration	Long onset time, may prolong emergence, bradycardia

IM, Intramuscular; *IN*, intranasal; *IV*, intravenous; *OTFC*, oral transmucosal fentanyl citrate; *PO*, by mouth; *PR*, per rectum; *SL*, sublingual.

8. **Describe the common anesthetic induction techniques used in children.**
   Inhalational induction is the most common induction technique in children younger than 10 years of age who do not have intravenous (IV) access. The child is asked to breathe a mixture of 70% nitrous oxide (N_2O) and 30% oxygen for approximately 1 minute; sevoflurane is then added. The sevoflurane concentration can be increased slowly or rapidly.
   Rapid inhalational induction is used with uncooperative children. The child is held down, and a mask containing 70% N_2O, 30% oxygen, and 6% to 8% sevoflurane is placed on the child's face. This unpleasant technique should be avoided if possible.
   Steal induction may be used if the child is already sleeping. Inhalational induction is accomplished by holding the mask near the child's face, while gradually increasing the concentration of sevoflurane. The goal is to induce anesthesia without awakening the child.
   IV induction is used in children who already have an IV in place. Children older than 10 years are usually candidates for preoperative IV placement. Topical lidocaine or subcutaneous lidocaine injectors (J-Tip) can be used to make IV placement less traumatic. Typical medications used for IV induction are propofol, 2 to 3 mg/kg and ketamine, 2 to 5 mg/kg.
   Lastly, intramuscular (IM) induction with midazolam, ketamine, and atropine may be used as a reliable, but potentially painful induction.

9. **How does the presence of a left-to-right shunt affect inhalational and intravenous induction?**
   In a left-to-right shunt (e.g., atrial septal defects, patent foramen ovale, ventricular septal defects, patent ductus arteriosus), blood from the system arterial circulation mixes with systemic venous blood. This leads to volume overload of the right heart and pulmonary circulation, resulting in congestive heart failure and decreased lung compliance. Uptake and distribution of inhaled agents are minimally affected; onset time for IV agents is slightly prolonged.

10. **How does the presence of a right-to-left shunt affect inhalational and intravenous induction?**
    In a right-to-left shunt (truncus arteriosus, tetralogy of Fallot, tricuspid atresia, Eisenmenger syndrome), deoxygenated blood from the right heart bypasses the lungs and mixes directly with systemic arterial blood. This causes hypoxemia and left ventricular overload. Patients compensate by increasing blood volume and hematocrit. It is important to maintain a high systemic vascular resistance (SVR) to prevent increased shunting from right to left. Such shunts may slightly delay inhalation induction and shorten the onset time of IV induction agents.

11. **Briefly discuss the special precautions that need to be considered in a child with congenital heart disease.**
    - The anatomy of the lesion(s) and direction of blood flow should be determined and its physiological implications understood.
    - Pulmonary vascular resistance (PVR) needs to be maintained at normal values if possible. If the PVR increases, right-to-left shunting may increase and worsen oxygenation. A patient with a left-to-right shunt and elevated PVR may develop a reversal in the direction of blood flow (Eisenmenger syndrome). If a patient has a left-to-right shunt, decreasing the PVR may increase blood flow to the lungs and lead to pulmonary overcirculation and edema. Decreasing the PVR in patients with a right-to-left shunt may improve hemodynamics. Conditions that can increase shunting are listed in Table 52.3.
    - IV air bubbles must be meticulously avoided. Use of an IV line filter for the distal end of the IV is sometimes warranted. If there is communication between the right and left sides of the heart (ventricular septal defect, atrial septal defect, patent foramen ovale), air injected intravenously may travel across the communication and enter the arterial system. This may lead to cardiac and/or central nervous system symptoms if the air obstructs the blood supply to the heart, brain, or spinal cord (paradoxical air embolus).
    - Prophylactic antibiotics should be given to prevent infective endocarditis. Recommendations for medications and doses can be found in the American Heart Association guidelines from 2017.
    - Avoid bradycardia.
    - Understand how to recognize and treat a "tet spell." Children with tetralogy of Fallot have right ventricular outflow tract (RVOT) obstruction (pulmonary artery stenosis or atresia), an overriding aorta, ventricular septal defect, and right ventricular hypertrophy. They may or may not have cyanosis at rest. However, many are prone to hypercyanotic spells ("tet" spells) as they get older. Such episodes are characterized by worsening RVOT obstruction, possibly as a result of hypovolemia, increased contractility, or tachycardia during times of stimulation or stress. These patients are frequently treated with β blockers, which should be continued perioperatively. Hypovolemia, acidosis, excessive crying or anxiety, and increased airway pressures should be avoided, and SVR maintained. If a hypercyanotic spell occurs in the perioperative period, treatment includes maintaining the airway, volume infusion, increasing the depth of anesthesia, or decreasing the surgical stimulation. Phenylephrine is valuable in increasing SVR. Additional doses of β blockers may also be useful. Metabolic acidosis should be corrected.

12. **How does one choose the correct ETT size in pediatrics?**
    Before induction of anesthesia, an array ETT sizes should be available. They should range in size between a half size above and a half size below the estimated size in Table 52.4. In general, the appropriate ETT size can be estimated using the following equations:
    Appropriate ETT size, uncuffed = [Age in years/4] + 4
    Appropriate ETT size, cuffed = [Age in years/4] + 3.5

Table 52.3 Conditions That Can Increase Shunting

LEFT-TO-RIGHT SHUNT	RIGHT-TO-LEFT SHUNT
Low hematocrit	Decreased SVR
Increased SVR	Increased PVR
Decreased PVR	Hypoxia
Hyperventilation	Hypercarbia
Hypothermia	Acidosis

PVR, Pulmonary vascular resistance; *SVR,* systemic vascular resistance.

Table 52.4 Guidelines for Endotracheal Tube Size

AGE	SIZE—INTERNAL DIAMETER (mm)
Preterm (<1250 g)	2.5–3.0 uncuffed
Newborns	3.0 cuffed–3.5 uncuffed
Newborn–12 months	3.5–4.0 cuffed
12–18 months	4.0 cuffed
2 years	4.0–4.5 cuffed
>2 years	ETT size = (16 + age)/4

ETT, Endotracheal tube.

The leak around the ETT should be less than 30 cm H_2O, and it should be inserted to 1 cm depth of approximately 3 times its internal diameter when measured at the alveolar ridge, for example, a 4.0 mm uncuffed ETT should be inserted to a depth of 12 cm at the gums/teeth.

See Table 52.4.

13. Discuss the use of cuffed ETTs in children.

Teaching has traditionally been that cuffed ETTs should not be used in children younger than 8 years old. The reasons are as follows:

i. Uncuffed ETTs avoid the potential of trauma and subsequent mucosal inflammation to what was traditionally held to be the narrowest part of the pediatric airway—the cricoid. Early studies were done in cadavers; in cadaveric models, the airway is cone shaped, with the cricoid at its apex. More recent magnetic resonance imaging studies to assess laryngeal and tracheal dimensions in anesthetized, nonparalyzed spontaneously breathing children found that, although the airway was cone shaped, the apex and narrowest portions were at the level of the vocal cords. Although tracheal mucosal inflammation and injury are related to a number of factors, including duration of intubation and number of intubation attempts, several recent studies have found that cuffed ETTs decrease the number of intubation attempts and are associated with decreased air leak (resulting in less OR pollution and greater ability to use low fresh gas flows). In addition, they provide better protection against aspiration.

ii. Uncuffed ETTs allow for the use of a larger ETT to be passed, thereby decreasing resistance to air flow. Many patients who are intubated (in either the OR or intensive care unit) are mechanically ventilated; thus the WOB is not as much of an issue as it used to be. Newer circuits and anesthesia machines have also helped decrease the problem of WOB.

In summary, cuffed ETTs can be used safely in children and neonates. Of course, the cuff takes up space, thus limiting the size of the ETT that can be used, but the major advantages of using cuffed ETTs are that they avoid the need for repeat laryngoscopy and may allow use of lower fresh gas flows.

Microcuff ETTs are a newer iteration of the cuffed ETT formulated to seal the airway with half the pressure of conventional cuffed ETTs. Their cuff is short and cylindrical and placed near the tube tip. This positions the cuff lower in the airway and less likely to causes pressure at the level of the cricoid cartilage.

14. Discuss the use of laryngeal mask airways in children.

Laryngeal mask airways (LMAs) are also useful in pediatrics. They can help secure a difficult airway, either as the primary airway device or as a conduit for endotracheal intubation. In addition, their use may be helpful during difficult mask ventilation situations. The LMA is used frequently for routine airway management in minor procedures and is now included in the Neonatal Resuscitation Program protocol for airway management.

See Table 52.5.

15. How does the pharmacology of commonly used anesthetic drugs differ in children?

- The minimal alveolar concentration (MAC) of the volatile agents is higher in children than adults. The highest MAC is in infants 1 to 6 months old. Premature babies and neonates have a lower MAC.
- Children have a higher tolerance to the dysrhythmic effects of epinephrine during general anesthesia with volatile agents.
- In general, children have higher drug requirements (mg/kg) because they have a greater volume of distribution (more fat, more body water).
- Opioids should be used judiciously in children younger than 1 year old because they are more sensitive to the respiratory depressant effects than are older children and adults.

Table 52.5 Laryngeal Mask Airways for Children	
SIZE OF CHILD	LMA SIZE
Neonates up to 5 kg	0.5–1
Infants 5–10 kg	$1^1/_2$
Children 10–20 kg	2
Children 20–30 kg	$2^1/_2$
Children/small adults >30 kg	3
Children/adults >70 kg	4
Children/adults >80 kg	5

LMA, Laryngeal mask airway.

16. **How is perioperative fluid managed in children who are nothing by mouth?**
    - Maintenance fluids are calculated as follows:
      - Under 10 kg: 4 mL/kg/h
      - 10 to 20 kg: 40 mL/h plus 2 mL/kg/h for every kg over 10 kg
      - Child over 20 kg: 60 mL/h plus 1 mL/kg/h for every kg over 20 kg
    - Estimated fluid deficit (EFD) should be calculated and replaced as follows:
      - EFD = maintenance fluid requirements × hours since last oral intake
      - ½ EFD + maintenance given over the first hour
      - ¼ EFD + maintenance given over the second hour
      - ¼ EFD + maintenance given over the third hour
    - EFD should be replaced for major cases. For minor cases, 10 to 20 mL/kg of a balanced salt solution (BSS), with or without glucose, is usually adequate

17. **What is the most common replacement fluid used for children and why?**
    In infants and small children, lactated Ringers or normal saline, with or without added glucose, is recommended. Hypoglycemia is rare in healthy, older children undergoing minimally invasive procedures, and administration of 5% glucose-containing solutions often results in hyperglycemia. Regardless of whether or not glucose-containing solutions are used for maintenance IVFs (intravenous fluids), nonglucose containing, isotonic fluids should always be used to replace third space and/or blood losses. In major pediatric surgical operations, it is prudent to check serial glucose levels periodically.

18. **How does one calculate estimated blood volume in children?**
    See Table 52.6.

19. **How is maximum allowable surgical blood loss calculated?**
    Maximum allowable blood loss (MABL) is calculated by the following equation:

    $$MABL = EBV \times (Starting\ Hct - Target\ Hct)$$

    Starting Hct
    EBV, estimated blood volume; Hct, hematocrit
    The lowest acceptable hematocrit varies with circumstances. Blood transfusion is usually considered when the hematocrit is less than 21% to 25%, depending on the circumstances.
    As an example of how this calculation can be useful, consider the following case:
    A 6 kg, 4-month-old infant is scheduled for craniofacial reconstruction. He is otherwise healthy, and his last oral intake was 6 hours before arrival to the OR. Preoperative Hct = 33%, lowest acceptable Hct = 25%.
    - Maintenance fluid requirement = kg weight × 4 mL/h = 24 mL/h
    - EFD = Maintenance fluid requirement × 6 h = 144 mL
    - EBV = kg weight × 80 mL/kg = 480 mL
    - MABL = (EBV × [Starting Hct − lowest acceptable Hct])/average Hct = (480 × [33 − 25])/29 = 132 mL
      So, assuming that the child's fluid deficit and ongoing losses have been kept up with, a 132-mL blood loss during surgery would drop the Hct from 33% to 25%.

20. **How do the manifestations of hypovolemia differ in children as compared with adults?**
    Healthy children have the ability to compensate for an acute volume loss of 30% to 40% before manifesting blood pressure changes. The most reliable early indicators of compensated hypovolemic shock (i.e., acute volume loss <30%–40%) in a child are persistent tachycardia, cutaneous vasoconstriction, and diminution of pulse pressure.

21. **Discuss the physiological responses to blood loss in children.**
    See Table 52.7.

Table 52.6 Guidelines for Estimated Blood Volume in Children	
AGE	**EBV (mL/kg)**
Preterm	100
Neonate	90
Infant up to 1-year-old	80
Older than 1 year	70

EBV, Estimated blood volume.

Table 52.7 Physiologic Response to Blood Loss in Children

ORGAN SYSTEM	<25% BLOOD LOSS	25%–40% BLOOD LOSS	>40% BLOOD LOSS
Cardiac	Weak, rapid, pulse; thready pulse	Tachycardia	Hypotension, tachycardia; bradycardia indicates severe blood loss and impending circulatory collapse
Central nervous system	Lethargic and confused	Obtunded, dulled response to pain	Comatose
Skin	Cool, clammy	Cyanotic, decreased capillary refill, cold extremities	Pale, cold
Kidneys	Oliguria	Minimal UOP	Minimal if any UOP

UOP, Urine output.

22. **What is the most common type of regional anesthesia performed in children? Which local anesthetic is used, and what dose is appropriate?**
Caudal epidural block is the most common regional technique. It is usually performed in an anesthetized child and provides intraoperative and postoperative analgesia. It is used for surgery of the lower extremities, perineum, and lower abdomen.
   Bupivacaine (0.125%–0.25%) or ropivacaine 0.2% are most commonly used. Bupivacaine 0.25% produces intraoperative analgesia and decreases the required volatile anesthetic; however, motor blockade may occur. The toxic dose of bupivacaine in children is 2.5 mg/kg; in neonates, 1.5 mg/kg. Commonly used doses are listed in Table 52.8.

23. **What are the common pediatric postoperative complications?**
   • Postoperative nausea and vomiting (PONV) is the most common cause of delayed discharge or unplanned admission. Factors associated with PONV in children include age over 6 years, length of surgery longer than 20 minutes, previous history of PONV, eye surgery, inner ear procedures, history of motion sickness, tonsillectomy/adenoidectomy, preoperative nausea or anxiety, hypoglycemia, use of opioids, and N_2O.
      The best treatment for PONV is prevention. Prophylactic administration of an antiemetic medication should be considered for all patients at high risk for PONV. Avoiding opioids decreases the incidence of PONV, as long as pain relief is adequate (e.g., patient has a caudal block), as does administering adequate amounts of IV fluid, dexamethasone, ondansetron, and using propofol maintenance anesthetic (in lieu of volatile anesthetic).
   • **Laryngospasm** and **stridor** are more common in children than in adults. Management for laryngospasm includes oxygen, positive pressure ventilation, jaw thrust, succinylcholine, propofol, and reintubation if necessary. Stridor is usually treated with humidified oxygen, steroids, and racemic epinephrine.
   • **Emergence agitation** (EA) has increased in incidence with the development of short-acting volatile agents (sevoflurane and desflurane). EA occurs postoperatively and can cause patient harm and lead to parental dissatisfaction. Risk factors include early school age, preoperative anxiety, pain, baseline behavioral abnormalities, and method of anesthesia. EA can be prevented and/or managed with opioids (if pain is present), dexmedetomidine, midazolam, and propofol.

24. **What is the significance of masseter muscle rigidity during anesthetic induction?**
Rigidity of the masseter muscles occurs in 1% of children receiving succinylcholine (and, historically, halothane). Masseter muscle rigidity (MMR) may be an early symptom of malignant hyperthermia (MH), but it may also occur in patients who are not MH susceptible.
   When MMR develops, the major consideration is whether or not to proceed with surgery, versus postponing and waking the child up. Unless other signs of MH develop, or the severity of MMR is such that it impedes intubation, a prudent course of action is to convert to a nontriggering anesthetic technique and proceed with surgery.

Table 52.8 Commonly Used Doses of Local Anesthetic for Caudal Block

DOSE (mL/kg)	LEVEL OF BLOCK	SITE OF OPERATION
0.5	Sacral/lumbar	Penile, lower extremity
1	Lumbar/thoracic	Lower abdominal
1.2	Upper thoracic	Upper abdominal

Doses are typical for bupivacaine 0.25% or ropivacaine 0.2%

After the completion of surgery, patients should be admitted and observed for signs of MH (tachycardia, hypercarbia, acidosis, blood pressure lability, muscle rigidity, hyperthermia, and myoglobinuria). The development of hyperthermia is considered a late sign. If creatine phosphokinase (CPK) is greater than 20,000, the patient likely has MH. If the CPK is less than 20,000 but still significantly elevated, an MH workup should be undertaken, including muscle biopsy. If CPK is normal or minimally elevated, the patient is probably not at increased risk for MH.

25. Should children with upper respiratory infections receive general anesthesia?

The risk of perioperative adverse respiratory events is much greater after an upper respiratory infection (URI). This risk persists for up to 6 weeks and occurs secondary to heightened airway irritability. The underlying pulmonary derangements associated with URI include decreased diffusion capacity for oxygen, decreased lung compliance, increased airway resistance, increased ventilation-perfusion mismatch, hypoxemia, and increased airway reactivity. Adverse perioperative events include laryngospasm, bronchospasm, postextubation croup, atelectasis, mucous plugging and impaired oxygenation. Factors associated with an increased likelihood of perioperative complications include airway instrumentation, fever, productive cough, lower respiratory tract involvement, prior history of asthma and/or snoring, passive smoking, copious secretions, and nasal congestion.

Recommendations for a child presenting for surgery with a mild URI include the following:

- Discuss the increased risk of adverse perioperative events with parents and the surgical team.
- Try to avoid intubation if possible (LMA or mask use has a lower risk).
- Preoperative albuterol treatment can be used to prophylax against perioperative bronchospasm.
- Humidification of inspired gases is thought to decrease airway dryness and maintain ciliary clearance.
- The febrile child presenting for an elective procedure with wheezing, rhonchi that do not clear with coughing, an abnormal chest x-ray film, elevated white count, or decreased activity level should be rescheduled.
- The well-appearing, afebrile child with a recent, uncomplicated URI and clear secretions may be able to safely undergo anesthesia.

26. Discuss the implications of sleep-disordered breathing in children.

Sleep-disordered breathing (SDB) is part of a continuum that ranges from normal breathing and oxygenation to chronic intermittent desaturation and obstructive sleep apnea (OSA). OSA is known to be associated with a decreased ventilatory response to CO_2 and a higher incidence of perioperative respiratory problems, including desaturation, obstruction, apnea, and heightened opioid sensitivity. It is important to ascertain the severity of SDB, as well as the presence of other comorbidities, before inducing anesthesia.

SDB can be caused by upper airway obstruction secondary to adenotonsillar hypertrophy, obesity, neuromuscular problems, or craniofacial abnormalities. Children with SDB may also exhibit significant behavioral and school performance issues. Tonsillectomy and adenoidectomy have been shown to eliminate airway obstruction in 85% to 95% of healthy patients with OSA and results in significant clinical improvement.

Of note, children with SDB and/or OSA can demonstrate clinically significant increased sensitivity to the respiratory depressant effect of opioids. These medications should always be dosed conservatively in this patient population, and consideration should be given to admitting children with severe OSA after undergoing anesthesia.

KEY POINTS: PEDIATRIC ANESTHESIA

1. Neonates, infants, and small children may be difficult to intubate because they have a more anterior larynx, relatively large tongues, and a long, floppy epiglottis. The narrowest part of the larynx has been found to be below the vocal cords at the cricoid cartilage.
2. Neonates, infants, and small children desaturate more rapidly than adults because of increased oxygen consumption and decreased FRC.
3. Premedication with midazolam and/or distraction techniques are arguably superior in decreasing anxiety when compared with placebo or parental presence at the time of induction.
4. The decision to proceed with elective surgery in the presence of a URI requires careful consideration of the child's medical history, comorbidities, surgery type, and anesthetic indicated.
5. Children with SDB/OSA require postoperative monitoring and judicious opioid dosing.

SUGGESTED READINGS

Francis A, Eltaki K, Bash T, et al. The safety of preoperative sedation in children with sleep-disordered breathing. Int J Pediatr Otorhinolaryngol. 2006;70:1517–1521.
Gregory GA, Andropoulos DA. Pediatric Anesthesia. 5th ed. Oxford: Wiley-Blackwell; 2011.
Miller RD, Cohen NH, Eriksson LI, et al. Miller's Anesthesia. 8th ed. Philadelphia: Elsevier; 2015:2757–2798.

CHAPTER 53

CONGENITAL HEART DISEASE

Lawrence I. Schwartz, MD, Megan L. Albertz, MD

1. **What is the incidence of congenital heart disease?**
   Congenital heart disease (CHD) is the most common type of birth defect. Although a variable range can be found in the literature, a reasonable estimate of the incidence is one in 250 live births. Ventricular septal defect is the most common type of CHD, comprising 25% of all congenital heart defects.

2. **What are some of the unique features of the neonatal heart?**
   The newborn myocardium is not fully mature at birth. The following features of the neonatal heart can make caring for these patients very challenging:
   - The newborn myocardium is poorly organized and has fewer myofibrils with fewer contractile elements, leading to decreased tension development.
   - Underdeveloped calcium cycling and excitation-contraction coupling, leading to cytosolic calcium dependence.
   - Incomplete sympathetic innervation combined with intact parasympathetic system provides the "heightened" vagal tone that can cause bradycardia.
   - Beta-adrenergic receptors are less sensitive, and may be downregulated in children with congenital heart disease.
   These cellular differences result in a newborn heart that is less compliant, develops less contractile force, and is less responsive to inotropic support than mature hearts. This can contribute to cardiac dysfunction in newborns with CHD pre- and postsurgical repair. Myocardial maturation is generally complete by 6 to 12 months of age.

3. **What are the three shunts of the fetal circulation?**
   The fetal circulation is a parallel circulation containing three shunts that function to provide the most highly oxygenated fetal blood from the placenta to the developing heart and brain. The ductus venosus shunts well-oxygenated, nutrient-rich blood in the umbilical vein from the liver to the right atrium. This blood is then shunted through the foramen ovale to the left side of the heart, ultimately exiting through the aorta. In the presence of atelectatic, amniotic fluid filled lungs and high pulmonary vascular resistance (PVR), deoxygenated blood returning to the right ventricle is shunted from the main pulmonary artery through the ductus arteriosus to the descending aorta. It can then flow by a lower systemic vascular resistance (SVR) pathway back to the placenta for reoxygenation, via the umbilical artery.

4. **How are different types of congenital heart disease classified?**
   CHD can be classified in multiple ways, including segmentally, anatomically, and physiologically. Anesthesiologists most commonly use the physiological classification. Physiologically, specific CHDs can be classified as acyanotic or cyanotic. Acyanotic heart defects can further be divided into acyanotic disease, with left-to-right shunt, and acyanotic disease, without left-to-right shunt. Cyanotic heart disease can be classified as having "ductal-dependent" pulmonary blood flow, "ductal-dependent" systemic blood flow, and mixing lesions, without "ductal-dependent" blood flow. See Table 53.1.

Table 53.1

CLASSIFICATION OF CONGENITAL HEART DISEASE	EXAMPLES
Acyanotic CHD with left-to-right shunt	Atrial septal defect, ventricular septal defect, partial anomalous pulmonary venous return
Acyanotic CHD without left-to-right shunt	Coarctation of the aorta, aortic valvar disease, cardiomyopathies
Cyanotic CHD with ductal-dependent pulmonary blood flow	Ebstein's anomaly, tetralogy of Fallot + pulmonary atresia, tricuspid atresia
Cyanotic CHD with ductal-dependent systemic blood flow	Hypoplastic left heart syndrome, interrupted aortic arch, critical aortic stenosis
Mixing lesions without ductal-dependent blood flow	Atrioventricular septal defect, transposition of the great arteries, double outlet right ventricle

5. **What is meant by "ductal-dependence" when describing cardiac lesions?**
In some forms of CHD, there is complete obstruction of either pulmonary or systemic blood flow. The ductus arteriosus is a fetal blood vessel that shunts deoxygenated blood from the right ventricle to the descending aorta to return blood to the placenta for reoxygenation. In lesions, such as pulmonary atresia or hypoplastic left heart syndrome, a patent ductus arteriosus is the only means of supplying pulmonary or systemic blood flow. However, the ductus arteriosus normally closes in the presence of higher arterial partial pressure of oxygen (PaO_2), seen following birth. Therefore an infusion of prostaglandin E_1 is vital to maintaining ductal patency and supporting life, until a palliative or corrective surgery can be performed.

6. **What are the common genetic disorders associated with CHD?**
Some 15% of CHD is associated with a genetic disorder. It is recommended that children diagnosed with one of these genetic disorders have a transthoracic echocardiogram before undergoing anesthesia. See Table 53.2.

7. **How are shunt fractions calculated?**
Using cardiac catheterization data, relative flows in the pulmonary, and systemic circulations can be calculated using the Fick principle (flow is inversely related to oxygen extraction):

$$Qp/Qs = (SaO_2 - SvO_2)/(SpvO_2 - SpaO_2)$$

where Qp = pulmonary blood flow; Qs = systemic blood flow; SaO_2 = systemic arterial oxygen saturation; SvO_2 = systemic mixed venous oxygen saturation; $SpvO_2$ = pulmonary venous oxygen saturation; and $SpaO_2$ = pulmonary arterial oxygen saturation.

8. **What are the anesthetic considerations for children with left-to-right shunts?**
A left-to-right shunt will ultimately lead to volume overloading of both ventricles, and may result in congestive heart failure (CHF). In the pediatric patient, CHF may present as feeding difficulties, failure to thrive, tachycardia, and poor perfusion. Excess blood flow through the shunt (atrial septal or ventricular septal defect) and through the developing pulmonary vascular bed can lead to increased PVR and pulmonary hypertension (referred to as *arterialization*). The anesthetic management of these patients may include:
- Judicious use of oxygen, so as not to increase the left-to-right shunt and decrease cardiac output in the face of CHF.
- Treatment of CHF with inotropic agents, such as milrinone, dopamine, or epinephrine.
- Management of pulmonary hypertension with pulmonary vasodilators, such as inhaled nitric oxide.
- Management of arrhythmias that commonly arise during surgical repair: complete atrioventricular block, junctional ectopic tachycardia.
Note that in children with left-to-right shunts, there will be little to no effect on the speed of either inhalational or intravenous induction.

9. **What are the anesthetic considerations for children with right-to-left shunts?**
Right-to-left shunts occur when there is an atrial septal defect, ventricular septal defect, or patent ductus arteriosus, and right-sided heart pressures exceed those on the left. These can be caused by elevated pulmonary pressures from pulmonary hypertension (most commonly idiopathic in children) or long-standing left-to-right shunts, resulting in Eisenmenger syndrome. Right-to-left shunt physiology can also occur in CHD, with obstruction or restriction to pulmonary blood flow. Anesthetic consideration for these patients may include:
- Management of pulmonary hypertension.
- Careful inspection of intravenous fluids, so as to avoid injecting any air bubbles. Air bubbles inadvertently injected into a vein can cross to the left side of the heart, enter the systemic arterial circulation and can cause stroke or myocardial ischemia.

Table 53.2 Genetic Disorders and Their Associated Phenotypes

GENETIC DISORDER	COMMON NONCARDIAC FINDINGS	COMMON CARDIAC LESIONS
Down syndrome (Trisomy 21)	Macroglossia, atlantooccipital instability, developmental delay, hypotonia, obstructive sleep apnea	Atrial septal defect, ventricular septal defect, atrioventricular septal defect, tetralogy of Fallot
DiGeorge syndrome	Thymic hypoplasia, hypocalcemia, low-set ears, speech, and learning disorders	Interrupted aortic arch, truncus arteriosus, tetralogy of Fallot
Turner syndrome	Short webbed neck, short stature, lymphedema of hands and feet	Coarctation of the aorta, bicuspid aortic valve, hypoplastic left heart syndrome
Williams syndrome	Infantile hypercalcemia, elfin facies, social personalities	Supravalvular aortic stenosis, supravalvular pulmonary stenosis, coronary artery stenosis

Note that in children with right-to-left shunts, speed of inhalational induction will be slower and more affected by insoluble anesthetics. Intravenous induction may actually be faster, as anesthetics will bypass the lungs and go to the brain more quickly.

10. **What is a pulmonary hypertensive crisis? How is it treated?**
In patients with pulmonary hypertension, the pulmonary vasculature is often hyperreactive to various stimuli that cause pulmonary vasoconstriction. These stimuli include hypoxia, acidosis, hypercarbia, hypothermia, and pain. When PVR increases to a point at which right ventricular pressure equals or exceeds left ventricular pressure, a pulmonary hypertensive crisis may result. This is a potentially lethal situation in which right ventricular failure may ensue, diminishing pulmonary blood flow and subsequent cardiac output, and decreasing coronary perfusion. The subsequent table outlines the treatment of pulmonary hypertension. See Table 53.3.

11. **What is tetralogy of Fallot?**
The tetrad of anatomic findings described by Fallot for this congenital heart lesion is ventricular septal defect, overriding aorta, right ventricular outflow tract (RVOT) obstruction, and right ventricular hypertrophy. Depending on the degree of pulmonary obstruction, these patients can present with normal blood oxygen saturation or hypoxemia. When patients present for surgical repair, one of the primary concerns for the anesthesiologist is an acute hypercyanotic episode, or "tet spell."

12. **What is a "tet spell," and how is it treated?**
The RVOT obstruction in tetralogy of Fallot can have a dynamic component. The subvalvular RVOT is muscular and contracts in response to inotropic stimuli, such as catecholamine release. When such contraction occurs—or if SVR decreases significantly—less blood will flow through the pulmonary artery, and the desaturated blood will be shunted right-to-left across the ventricular septal defect into the left ventricle and into the systemic circulation. The subsequent hypoxemia and acidosis increases PVR further and worsens the right-to-left shunt. This acute hypercyanotic episode can create a downward spiral, ultimately leading to cardiopulmonary collapse.
Treatment of a "tet spell" includes increasing SVR, lowering PVR, relaxing the hyperdynamic RVOT, and increasing right ventricular stroke volume. See Table 53.4.

Table 53.3 Treatment of Pulmonary Hypertension

GOAL	METHOD
Increase oxygen partial pressure	Increase fraction of inspired oxygen (FiO_2) Treat atelectasis Control ventilation
Alkalosis	Hyperventilation Treat metabolic acidosis
Control stress response	Adequate analgesia
Pulmonary vasodilation	Inhaled nitric oxide Intravenous prostacyclin (PGI_2)
Maintain coronary perfusion pressure	Maintain systemic vascular resistance with intravenous vasopressin, phenylephrine, or epinephrine

Table 53.4 Treatment of Hypercyanotic Spells

GOALS	METHODS
Relax the RVOT	Beta blockers Deepening anesthesia (too deep can decrease SVR further)
Increase SVR	Phenylephrine 5 to 10 mcg/kg (or more)
Decrease PVR	Increase FiO_2 Hyperventilation Sodium bicarbonate
Increase stroke volume	Intravenous fluid balance

13. **What is single ventricle physiology?**
    Patients born with single ventricle physiology have only one functioning ventricle to provide both pulmonary and systemic cardiac output. Single ventricle physiology is a parallel circulation that, if not repaired, will lead to chronic cyanosis and volume overload CHF. By definition, single ventricle physiology exists in any CHD that requires Fontan palliation surgery.

14. **How is a single ventricle congenital heart defect repaired?**
    The ultimate goal of single ventricle repair is to provide a series circulation without intracardiac shunt or obstruction. This is done in a stepwise fashion over the patient's first 2 to 3 years of life, and there are classically three successive surgeries performed to achieve this goal.
    1. Stage I palliation is performed in the newborn period, and involves securing pulmonary blood flow. This is often done with a modified Blalock-Taussig shunt. A small gortex graft is sewn from the subclavian artery to the right pulmonary artery. In the case of hypoplastic left heart syndrome, a neoaorta is also created to stabilize systemic blood flow. This is known as the *Norwood operation*.
    2. Stage II palliation occurs at a few months of life. A cavopulmonary anastomosis is created by taking the superior vena cava off the right atrium and connecting it to the branch pulmonary artery. This surgery, commonly called a *modified bidirectional Glenn operation*, begins the process of reducing the volume overload on the single ventricle. From this point onward, the patient's pulmonary blood flow is dependent on direct venous flow into the lungs.
    3. Stage III palliation in performed at approximately 2 years of life. This is the Fontan completion and involves creating an inferior cavopulmonary artery anastomosis. This establishes the series circulation; the single ventricle is now only responsible for directly to the lungs.
       The anesthetic management of these surgeries is very complex and requires close attention to balancing PVR and SVR blood flow. In addition, these patients often require intraoperative treatment for myocardial dysfunction and arrhythmias.

15. **What is the prognosis for children with congenital heart disease following surgery?**
    As surgical, anesthetic, and postoperative care have improved over the last 50 years, survival, following surgical intervention, has improved to well over 90% at major CHD centers. However, long-term outcomes are still associated with significant morbidity and mortality. Of note, up to 50% of mortality associated with birth defects in infants and children results from CHD.

16. **Are there adults with congenital heart disease?**
    With advances in the care of patients with CHD, many children now survive into adulthood. Currently in the United States, there are more adults with CHD than children, with adults accounting for about two-thirds of the CHD patients in the general population. Although these patients are living longer lives, they are at risk for multiple long-term sequelae and often require lifelong medical surveillance and therapy.

17. **What are the long-term cardiac complications associated with congenital heart disease?**
    Numerous complications can occur in patients with repaired or palliated CHD. Residual shunts, obstructions, heart valve abnormalities, surgical trauma, inflammation, foreign material implants, and myocardial injury can lead to many long-term consequences, including ventricular failure, cardiac arrhythmia, heart block, requiring a pacemaker, pulmonary hypertension, subacute bacterial endocarditis, and chronic cyanosis.

18. **What are the long-term noncardiac complications associated with congenital heart disease?**
    As patients with CHD live longer, they are at risk of developing chronic multiorgan diseases that can contribute to morbidity and mortality. Adult patients with CHD may be more susceptible to organ injury from ventricular failure and impaired neurohumeral control. See Table 53.5.

Table 53.5 Noncardiac Complications Associated with Congenital Heart Disease

Renal	Chronic kidney disease
Lung	Restrictive lung disease, pulmonary hypertension, plastic bronchitis (specifically in Fontan patients)
Gastrointestinal/Liver	Congestive hepatopathy, cirrhosis, enteropathy
Neurological	Cerebrovascular disease, depression, anxiety
Hematological	Anemia, polycythemia, thrombosis

19. Describe the clinical problems associated with cyanotic congenital heart disease

In response to chronic hypoxemia, these patients can develop polycythemia. When hematocrit exceeds about 65%, increased blood viscosity is associated with a greater risk of thrombosis, stroke, coagulopathy, and poor blood flow in the microcirculation. The combination of hypoxemia and impaired blood flow can lead to tissue ischemia and organ dysfunction. In the heart, ventricular dysfunction occurs as the myocardium is subjected to chronic ischemia and is exacerbated by the hypertrophy, associated with ventricular outflow obstruction, as in pulmonary stenosis.

KEY POINTS: PATHOPHYSIOLOGICAL EFFECTS OF CYANOTIC HEART DISEASE

1. Polycythemia
2. Increased blood viscosity
3. Coagulopathy
4. Decreased tissue perfusion
5. End-organ ischemia

20. What neuromonitoring and neuroprotective strategies are used to improve outcomes following cardiac surgery in children?

Children with CHD undergoing cardiopulmonary bypass (CPB) surgery are at risk for neurological injury because of the risk of thrombosis, low cardiac output, and hemodynamic instability. Near infrared spectroscopy monitoring is commonly used in pediatric cardiac surgery. Sensors are placed on the patient's forehead to assess regional oxygenation to the brain, and this is used as a marker for oxygen delivery. Electroencephalogram and transcranial Doppler are other modalities available to monitor neurological function and perfusion but are often impractical to use in the operating room.

Beyond the risk of stroke, major emphasis has been placed on understanding neurodevelopmental outcomes, such as behavior and learning. During CPB, neuroprotection is attempted by maintaining adequate mean arterial blood pressure and cooling the patient to minimize metabolic demands. Many anesthetics necessary to provide analgesia and immobility, during cardiac surgery, have been shown to cause apoptosis and brain injury in animal models. A relatively new anesthetic, dexmedetomidine may provide neuroprotection when given in combination with other anesthetics and has been associated with improved morbidity and mortality in patients undergoing cardiac surgery.

21. What is subacute bacterial endocarditis and how can it be prevented?

Turbulent or high-velocity blood flow in the heart, associated with congenital heart defects, can cause damage to the endocardium of the heart or valves. Damaged endocardium can be a nidus for infection in the presence of bacteremia or septicemia. Bacteremia can occur during dental or surgical procedures and can lead to bacterial endocarditis. Prophylactic administration of antibiotics during these procedures can prevent the development of endocarditis. However, the overall risk from surgery is still low, and the latest recommendations from the American Heart Association restrict the use of prophylactic antibiotics to the highest risk populations only. Dental and oral surgical procedures carry the greatest risk of infection. Box 53.1 "Cardiac conditions with the highest risk of endocarditis" outlines the current recommendations for treatment with antibiotic prophylaxis. Except for the conditions listed, antibiotic prophylaxis is no longer recommended for any form of CHD.

Patients at risk can be treated with amoxicillin, ampicillin, cefazolin, or clindamycin if they have a penicillin allergy. Surgical patients should continue to receive prophylactic antibiotic treatment, as indicated for their surgical procedure. In these cases, it is reasonable to choose a medication that will also provide prophylaxis for subacute bacterial endocarditis.

Box 53.1 Cardiac Conditions Associated With the Highest Risk of Endocarditis for Which Prophylaxis With Dental Procedures is Reasonable

Prosthetic cardiac valve or prosthetic material used for cardiac valve repair

Previous infective endocarditis

Congenital heart disease (CHD)

Unrepaired cyanotic CHD, including palliative shunts and conduits

Completely repaired CHD with prosthetic material or device, whether placed by surgery or catheter intervention, during the first 6 months after procedure

Repaired CHD with residual defects at the site or adjacent to the site of a prosthetic patch or device

Cardiac transplantation recipients who develop cardiac valvulopathy

Suggested Readings

Andropoulos DB. Anesthesia for Congenital Heart Disease. 3rd Edition. John Wiley & Sons, Inc: New Jersey; 2015.

Marelli AJ, Mackie AS, Ionescu-Ittu R, Rahme E, Pilote L. Congenital heart disease in the general population: changing prevalence and age distribution. Circulation. 2007;115:163–172.

Fischer LG, Van Aken H, Burkle H. Management of pulmonary hypertension: Physiological and pharmacological considerations for anesthesiologists. Anesth Analg. 2003;96:1603–1616.

Garson A Jr, Bricker JT, Fisher DJ, Neish SR (eds). The Science and Practice of Pediatric Cardiology. 2nd ed. Baltimore, Lippincott, Williams & Wilkins, 1998.

Gilboa SM, Salemi JL, Nembhard WN, Fixler DE, Correa A. Mortality resulting from congenital heart disease among children and adults in the United States, 1999 to 2006. Circulation. 2010;122:2254–2263.

Laird TH, Stayer SA, Rivenes SM, et al. Pulmonary-to-systemic blood flow ratio effects of sevoflurane, isoflurane, halothane, and fentanyl/midazolarn with 100% oxygen in children with congenital heart disease. Anesth Analg. 2002;95:1200–1206.

Lui GK, Saidi A, Bhatt AB, et al. Diagnosis and management of noncardiac complications in adults with congenital heart disease: a scientific statement from the American Heart Association. Circulation. 2017;136:.

Perez-Zoghbi JF, Zhu W, Grafe MR, et al. Dexmedetomidine-mediated neuroprotection against sevoflurane-induced neurotoxicity extends to several brain regions in neonatal rates. Br J Anaesth. 2017;119:506–516.

Rivenes SM, Lewin MB, Stayer SA, et al. Cardiovascular effects of sevoflurane, isoflurane, halothane, and fentanyl-midazolam in children with congenital heart disease: An echocardiographic study of myocardial contractility and hemodynamics. Anesth Analg. 2001;94:223–229.

Schwartz LI, Twite M, Gulack B, et al. The perioperative use of dexmedetomidine in pediatric patients with congenital heart disease: an analysis from the congenital cardiac anesthesia society-society of thoracic surgeons congenital heart disease database. Anesth Analg. 2016;123:715–721.

Tabbutt S, Ramamoorthy C, Montenegro LM, et al. Impact of inspired gas mixtures on preoperative infants with hypoplastic left heart syndrome during controlled ventilation. Circulation. 2001;104(Suppl 11):1159–1164.

Williams W. Surgical outcomes in congenital heart disease: expectations and realities. Eur J of Cardiothoracic Surg. 2005;27:937–944.

Williams GD, Ramamoorthy C. Brain monitoring and protection during pediatric cardiac surgery. Semin Cardiothorac Vasc Anesth. 2007; 11(1):23–33.

Wilson W. Prevention of infective endocarditis: guidelines from the American Heart Association: a guideline from the American Heart Association Rheumatic Fever, Endocarditis, and Kawasaki Disease Committee, Council on Cardiovascular Disease in the Young, and the Council on Clinical Cardiology, Council on Cardiovascular Surgery and Anesthesia, and the Quality of Care and Outcomes Research Interdisciplinary Working Group. Circulation. 2007;116(15):1736–1754.

CHAPTER 54

FUNDAMENTALS OF OBSTETRIC ANESTHESIA

Thomas R. Gruffi, MD, Mahesh Vaidyanathan, MD, MBA

1. **What are the cardiovascular adaptations to pregnancy?**

   Increased progesterone levels associated with pregnancy are presumed to increase the production of nitric oxide and prostacyclin. This is coupled with a decreased response to catecholamines and angiotensin, resulting in vasodilation. The subsequent decrease in systemic vascular resistance (SVR) is demonstrated by a decrease in blood pressure. Increased levels of relaxin, responsible for increased tissue elasticity, may lead to aortic dilation, especially in patients with connective tissue disorders. A parturient's plasma volume increases partly, as a response to increased water and sodium retention, from increased renin levels. Table 54.1 summarizes the major cardiovascular changes.

2. **When is the greatest increase in cardiac output (CO) experienced by parturients?**

   The most notable increase in CO (see Table 54.1) is achieved immediately postpartum, as a result of autotransfusion during uterine contractions. This physiological change is one of the most important changes and can potentially be life threatening in patients with pulmonary hypertension or stenotic valvular lesions. Anatomically, the increase in blood volume results in ventricular hypertrophy, as demonstrated by an enlarged cardiac silhouette on chest x-ray. A new grade I–II systolic murmur can often be heard on physical examination. By the second half of pregnancy, the third heart sound can frequently be detected on auscultation, with a fourth heart sound heard in up to 16% of patients.

3. **What hematological changes accompany pregnancy?**

   Table 54.2 summarizes the hematological changes during pregnancy. Relative to the nonpregnant state, plasma volume increases by 55% and total blood volume increases by 45% (1000–1500 mL). Red cell volume increases by 30%, which is offset by the increase in plasma volume, resulting in a dilutional anemia. The average hemoglobin and hematocrit is 11.6 g/dL and 35.5%, respectively. Maternal anemia occurs as a result of iron deficiency, particularly when the hemoglobin and hematocrit levels fall below 10 g/dL and less than 30%, respectively. Parturients may also experience a noninfectious leukocytosis with a concomitant decrease in cell-mediated immunity. Parturients are known to have an increased risk of developing viral infections, presumably from altered immunity from pregnancy.

4. **What hematological complications are parturients at increased risk for developing?**

   Pregnancy is associated with a hypercoagulable state as a result of increased activity of coagulation factors, particularly I, VII, VIII, IX, X, and XII, with a concomitant decrease in activity of anticoagulant factors, such as protein S and acquired activated protein C resistance. Accordingly, parturients are at increased risk for thrombotic events (e.g., deep venous thrombosis and pulmonary embolism). This is counterbalanced by increased fibrinolysis as a consequence of decreased levels of factors XI and XIII, which normally act as antifibrinolytics. There is increased platelet consumption, which is counterbalanced by increased platelet production. As a result, the platelet count is usually normal, although thrombocytopenia (platelet count $<150,000/mm^3$) can occur in 7.6% of women, and 0.9% of patients can have a platelet count less than $100,000/mm^3$. Thrombocytopenia in pregnancy can also occur in pathological conditions, specifically with preeclampsia or with hemolysis, elevated liver enzymes, and low platelet count (HELLP) syndrome.

5. **What pulmonary and respiratory changes occur with pregnancy?**

   Parturients experience a cephalad displacement of the diaphragm, in addition to an increase in the anteroposterior diameter of the chest wall during pregnancy. These anatomic changes cause a decrease in functional residual capacity (FRC). Minute ventilation significantly increases in pregnant women because of increased oxygen consumption (Table 54.3). The upper airway becomes more edematous with significant capillary engorgement, secondary to increased intravascular volume. The airway mucosa is often friable and prone to bleeding with manipulation or trauma.

   The decrease in FRC, coupled with an increase in oxygen consumption, significantly increases the risk of rapid desaturation with apnea. Airway edema associated with pregnancy further complicates managing the airway, where the risk of difficult/failed intubation is increased eight-fold. Therefore because of the combined risk of difficult intubation and the risk of rapid desaturation with apnea, it is extremely important to ensure adequate and effective preoxygenation, proper ramp positioning (see Chapter 49, "Obesity and Sleep Apnea"), and the availability of other equipment (e.g., flexible scope).

Table 54.1 Cardiovascular Changes During Pregnancy

CARDIAC OUTPUT	INCREASE 50% (PLATEAUS BY 28 WEEKS)
During labor	Additional 30%–40% increase
Immediately postpartum	75% increase above prelabor value
48 hours postpartum	At or below prelabor value
2 weeks postpartum	10% above prepregnant value (returns to normal by 12–24 weeks postpartum)
Stroke volume	Increase 25% (between 5 and 8 weeks)
Heart rate	Increase 25% (increases 15% by end of first trimester)
Mean arterial pressure	Decrease 15 mm Hg (normal by second trimester)
Systemic vascular resistance	Decreases 21%
Pulmonary vascular resistance	Decreases 34%
Central venous pressure	No change
Uterine blood flow	10% maternal cardiac output (600–700 mL/min at term)

Table 54.2 Hematological Changes During Pregnancy

Plasma volume	Increases 55% by term (15% by end of first trimester)
Red blood cell volume	Increases 30%
Blood volume	Increases 45%
Hemoglobin	Decrease 15% by midgestation ($\approx$11.6 g/dL)
Platelet count	No change or decrease
PT and PTT	Decreased
Fibrinogen	Increased
Fibrinolysis	Increased
Factors I, VII, VIII, IX, X XII	Increased

PT, Prothrombin time; *PTT*, partial thromboplastin time.

Table 54.3 Respiratory Changes at Term in Pregnancy

Minute ventilation	50% increase (can go up to 140% of prepregnancy values in the first stage of unmedicated labor and up to 200% in the second stage)
Alveolar ventilation	70% increase
Tidal volume	40% increase
Oxygen consumption	20% increase
Respiratory rate	15% increase
Dead space	No change
Lung compliance	No change
Residual volume	29% decrease
Vital capacity	No change
Total lung capacity	5% decrease
Functional residual capacity	15%–20% decrease
FEV1	No change

FEV$_1$, Forced expiratory volume in 1 second.

6. **What is a normal arterial blood gas in a pregnant patient?**
   Given the rise in minute ventilation, pregnant women develop a respiratory alkalosis (Table 54.4). Hyperventilation during active labor further contributes to the preexisting metabolic disturbance and is the second most important physiological change during labor, as it can result in uterine vasoconstriction and decreased placental perfusion, hypoxemia, and fetal distress.

7. **What gastrointestinal changes occur during pregnancy?**
   The expanding uterus displaces the stomach cephalad, resulting in incompetence of the lower gastroesophageal sphincter (GES) and increased intragastric pressure. Increased progesterone levels also decrease the tone of the lower GES. These changes place parturients at higher risk for reflux, regurgitation, and aspiration on both induction and emergence from anesthesia. Therefore all pregnant laboring patients are considered to have a full stomach and are managed accordingly (e.g., rapid sequence induction and intubation, cricoid pressure).

8. **What renal changes are associated with pregnancy?**
   Renal plasma flow, glomerular filtration rate (GFR), and creatinine clearance increase by the fourth month of gestation. Blood urea nitrogen (BUN) and creatinine are decreased; normal values in pregnancy are 6 to 9 and 0.4 to 0.6 mg/dL, respectively. Glycosuria up to 10 g/dL and proteinuria up to 300 mg/dL is not abnormal. Urinary stasis contributes to the frequency of urinary tract infections seen in pregnancy.

9. **What changes occur in the central nervous system of pregnant patients?**
   Progesterone in both the plasma and cerebrospinal fluid increases 10- to 20-fold in late pregnancy. Progesterone is sedating and potentiates the effects of volatile anesthetics. Pregnant patients are also more sensitive to local anesthetics and may need dose reductions by as much as 30%. Minimal alveolar concentration for inhaled agents is decreased with studies showing a 28% reduction, starting with the first trimester of pregnancy. An enlarged uterus compresses the inferior vena cava (IVC), in conjunction with increased vasodilation from pregnancy, causing distention of the epidural venous plexus and increased epidural blood volume. This must be taken into consideration when providing neuraxial analgesia, as the potential epidural space is smaller, increasing the risk for dura puncture or intravascular catheter placement.

10. **What hepatic alterations occur with pregnancy?**
    Liver size, blood flow, and morphology do not change during pregnancy. Lactate dehydrogenase, serum bilirubin, alanine aminotransferase, aspartate aminotransferase, and alkaline phosphatase (of placental origin) increase with pregnancy. Elevated progesterone levels inhibit the release of cholecystokinin, thus resulting in incomplete emptying of the gallbladder. When coupled with altered bile acid formation, pregnant women are at increased risk of gallstone formation. Because of the elevated plasma volume, the total protein, albumin concentration, and oncotic pressure all decrease during pregnancy. As a result, the serum free fraction of protein-bound drugs increases because of decreased albumin levels. Plasma cholinesterase concentrations may decrease up to 75%, causing a mild pseudocholinesterase deficiency and a mildly prolonged duration of action of succinylcholine. However, this is often not clinically significant.

11. **What is the uterine blood flow at term?**
    Uterine blood flow is approximately 50 to 190 mL/min before pregnancy and reaches approximately 10% of maternal CO (600–700 mL/min) at term. Accordingly, this increases the pregnant patient of peripartum hemorrhage because of uterine rupture, uterine atony, placenta previa, or placental abruption.

12. **How quickly do the physiological alterations of pregnancy return to normal after delivery?**
    - Cardiovascular: CO returns to slightly above prepregnancy values at about 2 to 4 weeks after delivery.
    - Respiratory: FRC and residual volume rapidly return to normal. Alveolar ventilation returns to baseline by 4 weeks after delivery with a gradual rise in maternal partial pressure of carbon dioxide in arterial blood.
    - Hematological: Dilutional anemia and hematocrit values return to normal within 4 weeks secondary to postpartum diuresis.
    - Renal: Serum creatinine, GFR, and BUN return to normal levels in less than 3 weeks
    - Gastrointestinal: The effects of the gravid uterus on the gastrointestinal system resolve in about 2 to 3 days following delivery.

Table 54.4 Normal Arterial Blood Gas Values in Pregnant and Nonpregnant Women

	pH	PaO_2	$PaCO_2$	HCO_3
Pregnant	7.41–7.44	85–109 mm Hg	27–33 mm Hg	21–27 mmol/L
Nonpregnant	7.35–7.45	60–100 mm Hg	35–45 mm Hg	24 mmol/L

HCO_3, Bicarbonate; $PaCO_2$, partial pressure of carbon dioxide in arterial blood; PaO_2, partial pressure of oxygen in arterial blood.

13. What are the three stages of labor?
    - Stage 1: Cervical dilation and effacement begin with the onset of regular, painful contractions and end when dilation of the cervix is complete ($\sim$10 cm). The latent phase is characterized by slow cervical dilation and effacement. The active phase is defined as the period of progressive cervical dilation, which usually begins around 4 to 5 cm.
    - Stage 2: The second stage ends with delivery of the neonate.
    - Stage 3: The third stage ends with delivery of the placenta.

14. Where does labor pain derive from? Which levels of the spinal cord are involved in transmitting labor pain during stages 1 and 2?
    Pain during the first stage of labor is caused by uterine contractions and cervical dilation, as transmitted by the sympathetic fibers entering the dorsal horn of the spinal cord at T10–L1. As labor progresses, the fetal head descends into the pelvis (i.e., stage 2) and pain is transmitted from the pelvic floor, lower vagina, and perineum via the pudendal nerve, entering the spinal cord at S2–S4.

15. What is aortocaval or caval compression syndrome? How is it treated?
    Historically, it was thought aortocaval compression syndrome was because of the gravid uterus compressing both the IVC and aorta, causing hypotension and tachycardia. Subsequently, this caused a decrease in uterine and placental blood flow manifesting as nonreassuring fetal heart rate (FHR) changes. However, a recent magnetic resonance imaging study found that vena cava compression is much more profound than aorta compression. *Caval compression decreases the mother's venous return, causing a decrease in CO and perfusion to the fetus. Accordingly, left uterine displacement (lateral position or a wedge under the right hip) is a helpful maneuver to prevent caval compression and to increase venous return. Symptomatic patients should be placed in the left uterine displacement position and may be treated with intravenous fluid administration, supplemental oxygen, and sometimes the use of a vasopressor.

16. Describe the anatomy of the placenta and umbilical cord.
    The maternal side of the placenta consists of a basal plate. Within the basal plate are spiral arteries, which are divisions from the uterine arteries and veins. The fetal side is the chorionic plate, made up of villi surrounded by chorion. The space where these two surfaces meet is the intervillous space. The villi contain divisions from two umbilical arteries, which carry blood to the placenta, and divisions from the single umbilical vein, which carries the nutrient-rich blood back to the fetal circulation.

17. What factors influence uteroplacental perfusion?
    Caval compression by the gravid uterus can decrease uteroplacental perfusion. Uterine blood flow may also decrease with maternal hypotension. In addition, uterine contractions, conditions, such as preeclampsia and placental abruption, and administration of some medications, such as ketamine and oxytocin, can all result in significant increases in uterine vascular resistance, which can decrease uterine blood flow. Finally, increased maternal catecholamines levels (i.e., pain during labor), maternal hypoxia, hypercarbia, and hypocarbia have all been associated with decreased uteroplacental perfusion.

18. How should hypotension associated with spinal anesthesia be treated in a cesarean section or laboring patient?
    Historically, treatment of hypotension under spinal anesthesia was guided by the goal to maintain uteroplacental blood flow. Ephedrine was the preferred vasopressor of choice because other agents (i.e., phenylephrine) decreased uteroplacental blood flow, but ephedrine did not. However, more recent studies suggest that large doses of ephedrine may be detrimental to the fetus (dose-dependent fetal metabolic acidosis, tachycardia, and abnormal FHR variability), whereas infusions or large doses of phenylephrine did not result in depression of fetal pH. Although α-adrenergic agonists (i.e., phenylephrine) produces peripheral vasoconstriction, with uterine vascular resistance greater than SVR, it has not been clinically shown to decrease uteroplacental blood flow. Problems observed with ephedrine are likely related to the direct β-agonist activity on fetal metabolism and is less likely secondary to decreased uteroplacental perfusion. However, it is important to note that all of these studies were done in healthy parturients at term, undergoing cesarean section. Some clinicians advocate for the routine use of prophylactic ephedrine to prevent any adverse effects of maternal hypotension following spinal anesthesia. Although this practice may prevent hypotension, evidence does not support improved neonatal outcomes.

19. What is the role of intravenous fluid preloading before regional anesthesia for cesarean delivery?
    Intravenous fluid preloading before regional anesthesia to prevent hypotension remained controversial for years, until recently. A metanalysis from 2017 showed that women who received crystalloid coload (fluid given after intrathecal injection) compared with preload (fluid given before intrathecal injection) had less incidence of hypotension, need for vasopressors, and nausea and vomiting. However, similar to prophylactic ephedrine administration, there was no difference in neonatal outcomes. Studies have also shown no difference in outcomes with crystalloid versus colloid administration.

20. How are drugs and other substances transported across the placenta? Which drugs cross the placenta?

    Placental transfer of drugs occurs by simple diffusion, active transport, bulk flow, facilitated diffusion, and breaks in the chorionic membrane. Anesthetic compounds cross the placenta mostly by simple diffusion. Compounds that are low in molecular weight, small in spatial configuration, poorly ionized, and lipid soluble have high rates of placental transfer. Most anesthetic agents are highly lipid soluble, have low molecular weights, and easily transfer across the placenta. Some anesthetic agents known to cross the placenta include atropine, scopolamine, β-adrenergic antagonists, nitroglycerin, diazepam, propofol, isoflurane, nitrous oxide, local anesthetics, opioids, neostigmine, and ephedrine. The basic principle is that small, nonionized molecules will more easily cross the placenta compared with large, ionized molecules. However, it is important to note that a change in pH can change the degree of ionization for a given molecule thus "ion trapping" the molecule in the fetal circulation. Specifically, in the presence of fetal acidosis, nonionized local anesthetics delivered via neuraxial technique can cross the placenta, bind to a proton, and become "ion trapped" in the fetal circulation.

    A helpful acronym for drugs that do not cross the placenta is HIGNS: *H*eparin, *I*nsulin, *G*lycopyrrolate, *N*ondepolarizing muscle relaxants, and *S*uccinylcholine.

21. What methods are used to evaluate fetal wellbeing during labor?

    FHR values and trends are recorded routinely in conjunction with external or internal monitoring of uterine activity. The baseline FHR is measured between contractions and is normally 110 to 160 beats per minute. Fetal tachycardia (>160) may indicate fever, hypoxia, use of β-sympathomimetic agents, maternal hyperthyroidism, or fetal hypovolemia. Fetal bradycardia (<110) may be because of hypoxia, complete heart block, β-blockers, local anesthetics, or hypothermia. The beat-to-beat variability is thought to represent an intact neurological pathway in the fetus. Increased variability is seen with uterine contractions and maternal activity. Decreased variability can be seen with central nervous system depression, hypoxia, acidosis, sleep, narcotic use, vagal blockade, and magnesium therapy for preeclampsia. Absence of beat-to-beat variability, especially in the presence of FHR decelerations or bradycardia, is a particular concern for fetal acidosis (Table 54.5).

22. What is the significance of FHR decelerations?
    - Early decelerations: caused by head compression (vagal stimulation). Typically, they are uniform in shape, begin near the onset of a uterine contraction, with its nadir at the same time as the peak of the contraction, and are benign (Fig. 54.1).
    - Variable decelerations: caused by umbilical cord compression. They are nonuniform in shape and are abrupt in onset and duration (lasting >15 seconds but <2 minutes). Although they usually do not reflect fetal acidosis, repetitive variable decelerations can lead to fetal hypoxia and acidosis.
    - Late decelerations: caused by uteroplacental insufficiency. They are uniform in shape, with a gradual onset (just after onset of contraction) and return to baseline, with their nadir and recovery after the peak and recovery of the contraction. These are associated with maternal hypotension, hypertension, diabetes, preeclampsia, or intrauterine growth restriction, and are an ominous indicator that the fetus is unable to maintain normal oxygenation and pH in the face of decreased blood flow.

    The treatment for nonreassuring FHR changes involves maintaining maternal blood pressure and placing the parturient in the left uterine displacement position.

Table 54.5 Fetal Heart Rate Pattern Classification

CATEGORY	CHARACTERISTICS
1—Normal	Baseline rate 110–160 beats per minute Baseline variability: moderate Late or variable decelerations: absent Early decelerations: present/absent
2—Indeterminate	All tracings not categorized as 1 or 3, which include examples such as: Baseline variability: minimal or marked Absent variability without recurrent decelerations Prolonged deceleration Absence of induced accelerations after fetal stimulation
3—Abnormal	Baseline variability: absent and recurrent late or variable decelerations Bradycardia

Modified from Macones GA, Hankins GD, Spong CY, et al. The 2008 National Institute of Child Health and Human Development workshop report on electronic fetal monitoring: update on definitions, interpretation and research guidelines. Obstet Gynecol. 2008;112:661–666.

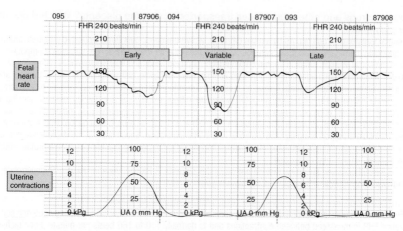

Fig. 54.1 Early, variable, and late fetal heart rate (FHR) deceleration during labor.

Table 54.6 Apgar Score

SCORE	HEART RATE	RESPIRATORY EFFORT	MUSCLE TONE	REFLEX IRRITABILITY	COLOR
0	Absent	Apneic	Flaccid	No response	Pale or blue
1	<100	Irregular, shallow, or weak cry	Some flexion of extremities	Grimace or weak cry	Acrocyanosis
2	>100	Good and crying	Active motion	Sneeze, cough, or cry	Pink

23. **What is the Apgar score?**
    Dr. Virginia Apgar, an anesthesiologist and first female full professor at Columbia University College of Physicians and Surgeons, developed a simple and repeatable method to assess newborn wellbeing 1 and 5 minutes after birth. It is the most widely accepted and used system to evaluate neonates, determine which neonates need resuscitation, and measure the success of resuscitation (Table 54.6). The score is comprised of separate scores (from 0 to 2) assigned to variables, including heart rate, respiratory effort, muscle tone, reflex irritability, and color to provide a total score of 10. The Apgar score can be measured again at 10 and 20 minutes, as resuscitative efforts are continued. A score of 0 to 3 indicates a severely depressed neonate, whereas a score of 7 to 10 is considered normal.

24. **Describe the management of the pregnant patient undergoing nonobstetric surgery.**
    Organogenesis occurs as early as the fifth week of gestation; because this is the most crucial time for fetal development, it is best to avoid all nonemergent surgery during this time. The safest period is during the second trimester because organogenesis is complete and preterm contractions and spontaneous abortions are less likely. The most common surgical conditions include appendicitis, cholecystitis, pancreatitis, bowel obstruction, ovarian torsion, ovarian cyst rupture, or hemorrhage and trauma. In emergent situations, surgery is obviously unavoidable, and the primary goal is maternal safety.
    There is no evidence that any drug or technique is preferred over another, as long as maternal oxygenation and perfusion are maintained. Furthermore, there is no evidence that any anesthetic agent currently in use is associated with teratogenic effects, particularly at standard recommended doses. However, the use of nitrous oxide is controversial, as it can impair DNA synthesis and should be avoided if possible. Although the type of anesthesia (regional, general, sedation) does not affect outcome, it is recommended to provide regional anesthesia whenever possible. If surgery is performed after the fetus is deemed viable (~24 weeks), fetal monitors should be placed (assuming they do not interfere with surgical exposure) to assess fetal wellbeing intraoperatively, and to assist in deciding whether delivery is prudent or necessary. If intraoperative fetal monitoring cannot be done, the FHR should be assessed both preoperatively and postoperatively. Obstetric personnel and pediatricians should be involved and informed.

If general anesthesia is needed, the patient should receive aspiration prophylaxis with sodium citrate and rapid-sequence intubation. It is critical to avoid maternal hypotension and uteroplacental hypoperfusion, using fluids and vasoactive agents, as appropriate. Patients should be positioned in left uterine displacement to avoid caval compression.

KEY POINTS: FUNDAMENTALS OF OBSTETRIC ANESTHESIA

1. Physiological alterations in pregnancy include an increase in CO, heart rate, plasma volume, minute ventilation, and oxygen consumption; decreases in SVR and FRC; dilutional anemia; and a hypercoagulable state.
2. Pregnant patients can pose airway management problems because of airway edema, large breasts that make laryngoscopy difficult, full stomachs that render them prone to aspiration, and rapid oxygen desaturation because of decreased FRC and increased oxygen consumption.
3. Pregnant patients are sensitive to both volatile and local anesthetics.
4. Nonemergent surgical procedures should be avoided if possible during pregnancy. If necessary, they should ideally be scheduled for the second trimester and with appropriate FHR monitoring.

SUGGESTED READINGS

American College of Obstetricians and Gynecologists. Obstetric analgesia and anesthesia. ACOG Practice Bulletin No. 177. Obstet Gynecol. 2017;129(4):e73–e89.

American Society of Anesthesiologists Task Force on Obstetric Anesthesia. Practice guidelines for obstetric anesthesia an updated report by the American Society of Anesthesiologists Task Force on Obstetric Anesthesia and the Society for Obstetric Anesthesia and Perinatology. Anesthesiology. 2016;124(2):270–300.

Conklin KA, Chang AB. Physiologic changes in pregnancy. In: Chestnut DH, Wong CA, Tsen LC, et al., eds. Obstetric Anesthesia: Principles and Practice. 5th ed. Philadelphia: Saunders; 2014.

Eisenach JC, Weiner CP. Uteroplacental blood flow. In: Chestnut DH, Wong CA, Tsen LC, et al., eds. Obstetric Anesthesia: Principles and Practice. 5th ed. Philadelphia: Saunders; 2014.

Lee JE, George RB, Habib AS. Spinal-induced hypotension: incidence, mechanisms, prophylaxis, and management: summarizing 20 years of research. Best Pract Res Clin Anaesthesiol. 2017;31(1):57–68.

Ni HF, Liu HY, Zhang J, et al. Crystalloid coload reduced the incidence of hypotension in spinal anesthesia for cesarean delivery, when compared to crystalloid preload: a meta-analysis. Biomed Res Int. 2017;2017:3462529.

CHAPTER 55

OBSTETRIC ANALGESIA AND ANESTHESIA

Thomas R. Gruffi, MD, Mahesh Vaidyanathan, MD, MBA

1. **What modes of analgesia are available to the parturient?**
   Parenteral opioids, inhaled nitrous oxide, epidural, spinal, and combined spinal-epidural (CSE) are all acceptable modes of analgesia, depending on the patient's comorbidities, time of presentation, clinical condition, and personal preference.

2. **What are the most commonly used parenteral opioids for labor analgesia? Which side effects are of special concern?**
   Although intravenous medications may decrease the intensity of labor pain, they do not provide complete analgesia and may cause maternal sedation, itching, and nausea. Parenteral opioids readily cross the placenta and may cause a decrease in fetal heart rate variability. If opioids are administered in close proximity to newborn delivery, neonatal respiratory depression may occur. Table 55.1 summarizes commonly used parenteral opioids and their side effects.
   Remifentanil, because of its rapid onset and ultra-short half-life ($\sim$3–4 minutes), is gaining popularity, and has proven efficacy, as shown by several trials. It is often administered by patient-controlled analgesia (PCA). Despite its ultra-short half-life, remifentanil may cause significant maternal respiratory depression, including apnea, so parturients need to be in a closely monitored setting.

3. **What advantages does PCA offer over conventional intermittent bolus dosing?**
   PCA is associated with greater patient satisfaction, less risk of maternal respiratory depression, less antiemetic requirements, and better pain relief despite lower drug doses. PCA is an intravenous form of opioid delivery and is especially useful if epidural anesthesia is contraindicated or not available. Currently, fentanyl and remifentanil are the most commonly used PCA medications for labor pain.

4. **Discuss the benefits of epidural analgesia for labor and delivery.**
   Uterine contractions and labor pain increase catecholamine levels. High levels of catecholamines (i.e., epinephrine and norepinephrine) may prolong labor by decreasing uterine contractility through β_2-agonism. Note, this is the same mechanism of action for some tocolytics (e.g., terbutaline). Increased catecholamine levels may result in decreased placental perfusion, fetal acidosis, and prolonged labor. Respiratory alkalosis because of hyperventilation from pain, may shift the oxyhemoglobin dissociation curve to the left, decreasing oxygen delivery to the fetus, causing fetal acidosis. Epidural analgesia provides the most effective pain relief in most laboring women, reduces maternal catecholamine levels, facilitates uterine contraction, and may potentially improve uteroplacental perfusion. Finally, epidural *analgesia* can be used for epidural *anesthesia*, if emergent cesarean section becomes necessary (e.g., poor fetal heart tracing), thus avoiding the need for general anesthesia with endotracheal intubation.

5. **What are the indications and contraindications for epidural analgesia during labor and delivery?**
   Patient request is the main indication and *analgesia* can readily be converted to *anesthesia* by increasing local anesthetic concentration. Absolute contraindications to epidural anesthesia include:
   - Patient refusal
   - Coagulopathy
   - Uncontrolled hemorrhage
   - Elevated intracranial pressure
   - True allergy to local anesthetics
   - Infection at the site of needle introduction
     Relative contraindications include:
   - Severe stenotic valvular disease
   - Maternal bacteremia
   - Certain neurologic diseases
   - Prior spinal instrumentation with hardware is not a contraindication, but can make placement more difficult

6. **Discuss the importance of a test dose and suggest an epidural test dose regimen. When and why is this regimen used?**
   The test dose is performed to diagnose subarachnoid or intravenous placement of the epidural catheter, thereby preventing total spinal anesthesia or systemic toxicity from local anesthetics. A common test dose is 3 mL of 1.5% lidocaine (45 mg) with 1:200,000 epinephrine (15 mcg). If the test dose of local anesthetic is administered

Table 55.1 Intravenous Analgesics for Labor

DRUG	USUAL DOSE	ONSET	DURATION	PCA DOSING
Fentanyl	0.5–1 mcg/kg IV	3–4 minutes	45 minutes	10–25 mcg q5–12 min
Comments: Short acting, no active metabolites, potent respiratory depressant for mother, minimal sedation and nausea. Context-sensitive half-life increases with infusion duration.				
Remifentanil	0.5–1 mcg/kg IV	1 minute	5–10 minutes	0.25–0.5 mcg/kg q2–3 min
Comments: Equipotent to fentanyl, quick onset, short acting, and constant context-sensitive half-life (3–4 min), does not depend upon hepatorenal elimination, requires maternal monitoring for respiratory depression.				
Butorphanol	1–2 mg IV	5 minutes	2–3 hours	N/A
Comments: Sedating for mother, ceiling effect for both analgesia and respiratory depression, dysphoric reactions or withdrawal symptoms in opioid-dependent patients can occur.				
Nalbuphine	10 mg IV	5 minutes	2–3 hours	N/A
Comments: Similar profile as butorphanol.				

IV, Intravenous; *N/A,* not applicable; *PCA,* patient-controlled analgesia.

Table 55.2 Common Local Anesthetics for Obstetric Anesthesia and Analgesia

DRUG	CLASS	ADVANTAGES	DISADVANTAGES
Bupivacaine (0.125%–0.5%)	Amide	Limited placental transfer (highly protein bound) Intermediate onset of action (15–20 minutes to peak effect) Analgesia lasts ≈2 hours	Intermediate motor blockade Cardiovascular toxicity (slower dissociation channels)
Ropivacaine (0.1%–0.2%)	Amide	Onset, duration, and sensory block similar to bupivacaine Less motor block Less cardiotoxic	Less potent than bupivacaine More expensive
Lidocaine (0.75%–2%)	Amide	Quick onset (10 minutes)	Crosses placenta readily Greater motor blockade Short duration of analgesia (45–90 minutes)
2-Chloroprocaine (3%)	Ester	Rapid onset (6–12 minutes) Allergic actions because of the metabolite PABA	Short half-life because of rapid metabolism (30–60 minutes)

*PABA, p-*Aminobenzoic acid.

intrathecally, motor and sensory block will rapidly appear along with hypotension. If the test dose is injected intravenously, tachycardia results within 45 seconds because of the epinephrine additive. If there is any doubt in the practitioner's mind about the exact location of the epidural catheter, the catheter should be removed and replaced.

7. What are the characteristics of the ideal local anesthetic to treat labor pain? How does epinephrine affect the action of local anesthetics?
The ideal local anesthetic for labor would have rapid onset of action, minimal risk of toxicity, minimal motor blockade with effective sensory blockade, minimal effect on blood pressure and placental perfusion, and would not impair the ability of the parturient to "push" during contractions. Bupivacaine and ropivacaine are the most commonly used epidural agents for labor analgesia. Lidocaine and chloroprocaine are the most commonly used epidural agents for obstetric surgical anesthesia. The addition of epinephrine (1:200,000) speeds the onset and prolongs the duration of action by decreasing vascular absorption of local anesthetic, but it also increases the intensity of motor blockade (not desirable in laboring patients). The addition of epinephrine to a local anesthetic does not appear to affect uterine blood flow adversely, and it decreases the risk of maternal toxicity.

8. What are the most commonly used local anesthetics for obstetric anesthesia? What are their advantages and disadvantages?
See Table 55.2.

9. **What are common complications of neuraxial anesthesia? What are their treatments?**
The most common complication of epidural analgesia/anesthesia is hypotension, defined as a decrease in systolic blood pressure of 20% to 30% from baseline. This may result in decreased uteroplacental perfusion and fetal hypoxia and acidosis, so avoidance is paramount to decrease risk of fetal distress. Hypotension results from sympathetic blockade, peripheral venodilation, and decreased venous return to the heart. Treatment includes fluid administration, left uterine displacement, and vasoactive agents (e.g., phenylephrine).

The incidence of accidental dural puncture is approximately 1.5%. This complication can cause a severe headache known as *postdural-puncture headache* (PDPH) in approximately 50% of patients. If cerebrospinal fluid (CSF) is found when placing an epidural, there are two options: (1) the needle can be removed, and the epidural placed at an alternate interspace; or (2) the catheter may be left in situ within the subarachnoid space. Placing an epidural catheter at a different interspace has the theoretical risk for local anesthetic to migrate and pass into the subarachnoid space, through the large dural puncture conduit created by the Touhy needle, resulting in a block that is unexpectedly high or dense. Alternatively, threading the catheter into the subarachnoid space effectively "plugs the hole" and can reduce the incidence of PDPH, but has the risk of a provider inadvertently dosing drugs through the spinal catheter, thinking the catheter is an epidural causing a high spinal.

Other common complications or known side effects include pruritus, nausea/vomiting, and shivering. Shivering may be treated with opioid agents (e.g., meperidine) and antiemetic medications (e.g., ondansetron). Pruritis often occurs with intrathecal or epidural opioid agents and various treatment options exist, such as serotonin 5-HT$_3$ antagonists (e.g., ondansetron) and mixed agonist–antagonist opioids (e.g., nalbuphine, butorphanol). The best method to prevent pruritis is to limit the dose of intrathecal/epidural opioid (i.e., 100 mcg morphine intrathecal or 3 mg morphine epidural), as higher doses cause more side effects than analgesia benefit. Note, that diphenhydramine is not effective in treating opioid-induced pruritis.

10. **What is local anesthetic systemic toxicity? How do you treat it?**
Intravenous local anesthetic injection may produce dizziness, restlessness, tinnitus, seizures, and loss of consciousness. Cardiovascular toxicity often follows neurologic toxicity. Cardiovascular toxicity can range from dysrhythmias to cardiac arrest and bupivacaine, specifically, is associated with the highest incidence of cardiac toxicity compared to other local anesthetic agents. Anesthetic systemic toxicity (LAST) is often thought to occur immediately after injection of local anesthetic, intravenous injection, and that neurologic symptoms should precede cardiac symptoms. However, up to half of all cases are found to occur 30 minutes after local anesthetic administration, may occur despite no apparent intravenous injection, and may present with no apparent neurologic symptoms. The treatment of LAST includes the following:
- Supportive care (e.g., intubation, vasoactive agents, benzodiazepines for seizures) and advanced cardiac life support for cardiac arrest. Note, that epinephrine doses should be reduced (<1 mcg/kg) and vasopressin should be avoided, based on empiric data from animal studies showing worse outcomes with high dose epinephrine and vasopressin. Amiodarone is the first-line agent for dysrhythmias and local anesthetics should, for obvious reasons, not be given for this indication.
- Immediately give intralipid for severe symptoms of LAST. You do not have to wait until the patient is in cardiac arrest. Intralipid acts as a lipid "sink" and binds local anesthetics, removing them from maternal circulation. Intralipid can be lifesaving with its main side effect being pancreatitis, although data firmly establishing other side effects are is limited. Note that intralipid may be used in other clinical settings to reverse toxicity from lipid soluble agents in general (e.g., serotonin syndrome).
- Early delivery (<5 minutes) of the fetus, if return of spontaneous circulation is not quickly restored such that delivery can occur soon after cardiac arrest. Note that delivery of the fetus helps facilitate more effective cardiopulmonary resuscitation (e.g., better venous return).

11. **What is a "high spinal"? How do you treat it?**
A high spinal occurs when local anesthetics migrate cephalad, causing a large sympathectomy similar to neurogenic shock from spinal cord trauma. The incidence of an unexpected high block or total spinal block is approximately 1 in 4500 lumbar epidurals for labor analgesia. The signs and symptoms of a total spinal block include hypotension, bradycardia, dyspnea, inability to speak, loss of consciousness, and cardiac arrest. Risk is minimized by aspirating the epidural catheter every time a local anesthetic is administered, giving a single test dose immediately after placement, and avoiding multiple intrathecal injections after a failed spinal anesthetic. Treatment includes intubation, oxygen administration, ventilation, and support of maternal circulation with vasoactive medications. Note that *direct* vasoactive agents (epinephrine, norepinephrine, etc.) are much more effective in treating a high spinal compared to *indirect* agents (i.e., ephedrine).

12. **Explain the mechanism of action of intrathecal and epidural opioids. What effect do they have on pain perception, sympathetic tone, sensation, and movement?**
Opioids administered intrathecally or epidurally provide excellent analgesia, without appreciably affecting sympathetic tone, sensation, or voluntary motor function. Opioids given via these routes bind to presynaptic and postsynaptic receptor sites in the dorsal horn of the spinal cord (Rexed laminae I, II, and V), altering nociceptive transmission. Some of the effects of lipid-soluble opioids (i.e., fentanyl) may be caused by their systemic absorption.

13. **Which opioids are most commonly used as a neuraxial analgesia adjuvant? Name their most common side effects.**

    The most commonly used neuraxial opioids are fentanyl (12.5–25 mcg intrathecal/100–200 mcg epidural) and morphine (100–150 mcg intrathecal/3–4 mg epidural). Pruritus, nausea, and vomiting are the most common side effects. Neuraxial morphine can cause delayed respiratory depression, although it is very uncommon in this population. Intrathecal or epidural opioids alone may provide adequate relief for the early stages of labor, but they are unreliable in producing adequate analgesia for the active phase of labor. Concurrent administration of local anesthetic is necessary for late cervical dilation and delivery of the infant. Finally, the nonopioid central α_2 agonist, clonidine, can be used as an intrathecal (15–30 mcg) and epidural (75 mcg) analgesic/anesthetic adjunct. It has also been shown to extend the duration of analgesia and strengthen the degree of sensory and motor blockade.

14. **Does epidural analgesia cause prolongation of labor or increase the risk of assisted vaginal delivery?**

    No. This issue *was* highly controversial. It was thought that epidural analgesia was *associated* with prolonged labor and increased assisted vaginal delivery, but recent studies do not support this assertion. The association is likely because anesthesiologists and obstetricians may be more likely to strongly recommend that the patient receive neuraxial analgesia if she is more at risk for assisted vaginal delivery (i.e., morbidly obese, significant labor pain in early first stage of labor) and that patients with the longest duration of labor (nulliparous women) are more likely to receive an epidural. Although epidural labor analgesia may slightly prolong the second stage by about 30 minutes, there appears to be no harm to mother or fetus, and the American College of Obstetricians and Gynecologists (ACOG) recommends allowing an extra hour of pushing for mothers with an epidural block in place. ACOG has stated: "Neuraxial analgesia techniques are the most effective and least depressant treatments for labor pain … more recent studies have shown that epidural analgesia does not increase the risk of cesarean delivery." As a matter of fact, one study compared cesarean section rates before and after institution of regional anesthesia as the primary mode of anesthesia delivery and found no change in the incidence of cesarean deliveries.

15. **What are the advantages and disadvantages of spinal anesthesia for cesarean section? Which drugs are frequently used in this technique?**

    Spinal anesthesia produces a reliable and dense, neuraxial block, is relatively easy to perform, is rapid in onset, and carries no risk of local anesthetic systemic toxicity. The development of small-gauge, noncutting needles has significantly reduced the incidence of PDPH to 1% or less. Hypotension can be significant and can occur rapidly, requiring rapid intravenous fluid administration, left uterine displacement positioning to avoid caval compression, and administration of phenylephrine (100–200 mcg) or ephedrine (5–10 mg intravenous). Commonly used drugs are summarized in Table 55.3.

16. **What are the advantages and disadvantages of cesarean section with epidural anesthesia versus spinal anesthesia?**

    If an epidural is used for labor analgesia, high concentrations of local anesthetics can easily be administered through the catheter to provide surgical anesthesia, if cesarean section later becomes necessary. The local anesthetic should be given in increments, titrating to the desired sensory level of T4. Titration of local anesthetic results in more controlled sympathetic blockade; thus the risk of hypotension and reduced uteroplacental flow may be avoided. Typically, epidural anesthesia produces less intense motor and sensory blockade than spinal anesthesia.

    Disadvantages of epidural anesthesia include slower onset, larger local anesthetic dose requirement, occasional patchy block unsuitable for surgery, and the risk of total spinal anesthesia or systemic toxicity, if the epidural catheter migrates subarachnoid or intravascular. Accidental dural puncture may occur when placing an epidural (~1.5%) and approximately 50% to 85% of such patients experience PDHP.

17. **How is a CSE performed? What are its advantages?**

    A CSE is a technique often performed using a needle-through-needle approach. The needle-through-needle approach involves identification of the epidural space by loss-of-resistance technique with a Tuohy needle, followed by insertion

Table 55.3 Drugs Used for Spinal Anesthesia for Cesarean Section

DRUG	DOSE	DURATION (MINUTES)
Bupivacaine	10–12 mg	60–120
Lidocaine	75 mg	45–75
Adjuvant Drugs		
Epinephrine	100–200 mcg	
Morphine	100–150 mcg	
Fentanyl	10–25 mcg	

of a long (120-mm), small-gauge (24- to 27-G), noncutting spinal needle, until the dura is punctured and clear CSF is noted. Subsequently, a spinal dose of local anesthetic and/or an opioid is injected into the subarachnoid space, and the spinal needle subsequently removed. Finally, an epidural catheter is threaded into the epidural space. The advantage of a CSE technique is rapid and reliable analgesia (because of the spinal anesthetic component) and confirmation of the epidural space before threading the catheter reducing the risk of a failed epidural.

A novel technique called the *dural puncture epidural* has recently been introduced. It is essentially a CSE without administering intrathecal medication through the spinal needle. It is thought that this allows local anesthetic delivered by the epidural catheter to transverse through a conduit created by the dural puncture into the CSF at a slower, sustained rate. It has been shown to combine (to a lesser extent) the benefits of both epidural and CSE techniques regarding speed of onset, block density, and confirmation of epidural space with less side effects of hypotension, pruritus, and uterine hypertonus.

18. List the indications for general anesthesia for cesarean section.
    • Extreme fetal distress (in the absence of a functioning epidural catheter)
    • Significant coagulopathy
    • Inadequate regional anesthesia (without time to replace catheter)
    • Acute maternal hypovolemia/hemorrhage
    • Patient refusal of regional anesthesia

19. What concerns the practitioner when administering general anesthesia for cesarean section? How is it performed?
    The obstetric population is at greater risk for difficult intubation, rapid oxygen desaturation, and aspiration of gastric contents. The goal is to minimize maternal risk and neonatal depression. This goal is accomplished by following guidelines and managing all obstetric patients as high aspiration risk. After monitors are placed, while the patient is being preoxygenated, the abdomen is prepared and draped. When the obstetricians are scrubbed and ready to make skin incision, a rapid-sequence induction with cricoid pressure is performed, and incision occurs after correct placement of the endotracheal tube is verified. Propofol is generally used on induction, but if the patient is hemodynamically unstable, ketamine or etomidate may be administered. Succinylcholine is the muscle relaxant of choice for most patients because of its fast onset and offset duration. To prevent maternal awareness, approximately 1 minimum alveolar concentration (MAC) of an inhaled volatile agent is administered between tracheal intubation and delivery of the neonate. After delivery, the MAC of the inhaled volatile agent is reduced from 0.5 to 0.75, while simultaneously starting nitrous oxide (50%), to reduce the risk of uterine atony and hemorrhage. Following delivery, opioids are administered in addition to oxytocin to facilitate uterine contraction.

KEY POINTS: OBSTETRIC ANALGESIA AND ANESTHESIA

1. Opioids administered intravenously to the mother readily cross the placenta and may cause a decrease in fetal heart rate variability.
2. Intravenous PCA is associated with greater patient satisfaction, less respiratory depression, less antiemetic requirements, and better pain relief along with lower drug doses.
3. Epidural analgesia is effective, safe, and reduces maternal catecholamine levels, which may improve uteroplacental perfusion and facilitate uterine contractions.
4. The contraindications to epidural anesthesia include patient refusal, coagulopathy, uncontrolled hemorrhage, increased intracranial pressure, and infection at the site of needle insertion. Relative contraindications include systemic maternal infection, back surgery with hardware placement, severe aortic stenosis, and certain neurologic diseases.
5. Bupivacaine, ropivacaine, lidocaine, and chloroprocaine are the most commonly used local anesthetics in obstetric anesthesia.
6. Spinal anesthesia for cesarean delivery produces reliable and dense sensory and motor block, is relatively easy to perform, has a rapid onset, and carries no risk of local anesthetic toxicity.

SUGGESTED READINGS

American College of Obstetricians and Gynecologists. Obstetric analgesia and anesthesia. ACOG Pract Bull. 2017;177.
American Society of Anesthesiologists Task Force on Obstetric Anesthesia: Practice guidelines for obstetric anesthesia: an updated report by the American Society of Anesthesiologists Task Force on Obstetric Anesthesia and the Society for Obstetric Anesthesia and Perinatology. Anesthesiology. 2016;124(2):270-300.
Tsen, LC. Anesthesia for cesarean delivery. In: Chestnut DH, Wong CA, Tsen LC, et al, eds. Obstetric Anesthesia: Principles and Practice. 5th ed. Philadelphia: Saunders; 2014.

CHAPTER 56

HIGH-RISK OBSTETRICS

Thomas R. Gruffi, MD, Mahesh Vaidyanathan, MD, MBA

1. **Define high-risk pregnancy.**
   High-risk pregnancies are those that involve either a maternal or fetal condition that increases the likelihood of maternal or fetal morbidity and/or mortality. They comprise approximately 6% to 18% of total pregnancies (Table 56.1); however, the true incidence and particular comorbidity is highly dependent up on the demographic, socioeconomic status, and geographic region. Specifically, high-risk pregnancy is associated with age (<15 or >35 years old), lower socioeconomic status, rural areas, and lower educational achievement.

2. **How many women die per day from pregnancy? What are the most common causes of death because of pregnancy?**
   The World Health Organization reports (2017 data) that approximately 810 women die every day (~300,000 per year) from preventable causes related to pregnancy, of which 94% of maternal deaths occur in low income countries (i.e., sub-Saharan Africa and Southern Asia). Common causes of pregnancy-related death include hemorrhage, infection, stroke, thrombotic pulmonary embolism, and cardiac disease. The most common cause of death in low-income countries is hemorrhage, whereas cardiac disease is the most common cause of death in high-income countries. The risk of pregnancy-related death is 1:45 in low-income countries compared with 1:5400 in high-income countries.

3. **What are the hypertensive disorders of pregnancy?**
   Hypertensive disorders complicate up to 10% of pregnancies and are one of the leading causes of maternal morbidity and mortality worldwide. Chronic hypertension (HTN) is often diagnosed prepregnancy, but may go undiagnosed until the first prenatal visit. Chronic HTN is defined as HTN (i.e., >140/90 mm Hg) before 20 weeks' gestation and does not resolve postpartum. Alternatively, gestational HTN is defined as HTN occurring after 20 weeks' gestation and does resolve postpartum. Neither presents with proteinuria. Preeclampsia is defined as new onset HTN after 20 weeks' gestation presenting with either proteinuria (≥300 mg/24 h, protein-creatinine ratio ≥0.3, or 2+ on urine dipstick) or other evidence of severe features, such as the following:
   a. Thrombocytopenia
   b. New-onset headache or visual disturbances
   c. Impaired liver function
   d. Serum creatinine >1.1 mg/dL or >2 times baseline
   e. Pulmonary edema
      Preeclampsia may initially present as gestational HTN and up to 50% of women with gestational HTN later develop proteinuria or other severe features consistent with the diagnosis of preeclampsia. If preeclampsia is left untreated, it can progress to eclampsia (defined by seizures). Table 56.2 summarizes the types of hypertensive disorders found in pregnant patients.

4. **Describe the characteristics of preeclampsia and review associated risk factors.**
   Preeclampsia is a hypertensive disorder of pregnancy distinguished by proteinuria and/or other associated features (e.g., thrombocytopenia, acute kidney insufficiency, impaired liver function). Although parturients with preeclampsia may have peripheral edema, suggesting hypervolemia, clinically they are intravascularly hypovolemic because of the loss of oncotic pressure from proteinuria and systemic inflammation causing increased vascular permeability. Box 56.1 lists known risk factors for preeclampsia. Interestingly, maternal smoking history has shown to reduce the risk of developing preeclampsia. Patients with a history of preeclampsia and/or who have several risk factors may be given prophylactic low-dose aspirin to reduce its occurrence and/or severity when started early in pregnancy (≤16 weeks' gestation).

5. **What is HELLP syndrome?**
   HELLP (*h*emolysis, *e*levated *l*iver enzymes, and *l*ow *p*latelet count) syndrome occurs in approximately 20% of patients with preeclampsia. HELLP syndrome is a microangiopathic hemolytic anemia associated with thrombocytopenia and elevated liver enzymes. The pathophysiology is complex, but is likely caused by activation of the clotting cascade, leading to a consumptive coagulopathy (thrombocytopenia), hemolysis, and liver ischemia. Symptoms may include headache, nausea/vomiting, and right upper quadrant pain secondary to liver ischemia or hepatic hemorrhage. Interestingly, around 12% of patients with HELLP syndrome may present as normotensive. Parturients who develop HELLP syndrome after 34 weeks, especially when associated with laboratory evidence of disseminated intravascular coagulation (DIC), require immediate delivery, regardless of gestational age.

Table 56.1 High-Risk Conditions in Pregnancy

HIGH-RISK CONDITION	PREVALENCE
Obesity	6%–38%
Preterm birth	5%–10%
Mental disorders	10%
Hypertension (chronic, gestational, preeclampsia, eclampsia)	10%
Diabetes (including gestational DM)	6%–8%
Asthma	3%–8%
Substance abuse	4%–5%
Hypothyroidism	2%–3%
Chorioamnionitis	1%
Cardiac disease	1%
Renal disease	1%
Hyperthyroidism	0.2%–0.4%

DM, Diabetes mellitus.
Above data are approximate, and significant variation exists between patient populations.

Table 56.2 Hypertensive Disorders of Pregnancy

TYPE	BLOOD PRESSURE	ONSET	PROTEINURIA
Chronic	≥140/90 mm Hg	Before 20 wk EGA	Absent, does not resolve PP
Gestational	≥140/90 mm Hg	After 20 wk EGA	Absent, resolves PP
Preeclampsia	≥140/90 mm Hg	After 20 wk EGA	≥300 mg/24 h, protein/Cr ≥0.3, or 2+ on urine dipstick
Preeclampsia with Severe Features	≥160/110 mm Hg	After 20 wk EGA	Same as earlier or other end-organ damage

EGA, Estimated gestational age; PP, postpartum.
Modified from the ACOG Practice Bulletin No. 202. Gestational hypertension and preeclampsia. Obstet Gynecol. 2019;133(1):e1–e25.

Box 56.1 Risk Factors of Preeclampsia

Nulliparity
Black race
Extremes of age
Personal history or family history of preeclampsia
Multiple gestation
Maternal obesity

Chronic hypertension
Diabetes mellitus
Thrombotic vascular disease
Assisted reproductive technology
Limited exposure to paternal sperm

However, some women with HELLP syndrome are managed expectantly and may receive systemic corticosteroids for fetal lung maturity.

6. How do you differentiate HELLP syndrome from thrombocytopenic purpura (TTP) and hemolytic uremic syndrome (HUS)?
The pathophysiology and presentation of HELLP syndrome overlaps TTP and HUS in that they are all associated with hemolysis, transaminitis, renal injury, and thrombocytopenia. However, the primary difference is that the

predominant clinical presentation of the latter two are neurological abnormalities and renal failure, respectively, whereas HELLP syndrome predominantly affects the liver and is associated with a more severe transaminitis. It is important to differentiate HELLP syndrome from other thrombotic microangiopathies, as the thrombocytopenia is usually less severe with HELLP syndrome and the mainstay of treatment is different: delivery of the fetus for HELLP syndrome and plasma exchange for TTP/HUS.

7. **What is the most common cause of death in patients with preeclampsia?**
Hemorrhagic stroke, followed by cardiac disease, is the leading cause of mortality in preeclampsia. The risk for stroke in preeclampsia is likely related to a combination of systemic inflammation, coagulopathy (e.g., HELLP syndrome), and uncontrolled HTN. Therefore control of blood pressure (BP) with antihypertensive agents (i.e., systolic BP <160 mm Hg), in addition to initiating magnesium therapy (reduces cerebral edema and is neuroprotective), is of the utmost importance to minimize patient mortality. Other cause of mortality in preeclampsia are the following (in order of frequency): cardiovascular, disseminated intravascular coagulopathy, acute respiratory distress syndrome, renal failure, sepsis, and hepatic hemorrhage.

8. **What is the etiology of preeclampsia?**
Although the etiology of preeclampsia is unknown, abnormal placentation likely plays a significant role. Abnormal placentation occurs as a result of failure of trophoblastic invasion of the spiral arteries. The abnormal spiral arteries result in a high resistance placental circulation. Placental perfusion is reduced with subsequent release of vasoactive substances, ultimately resulting in fetal growth restriction, thus increasing the risk for preterm delivery and associated complications (e.g., respiratory distress syndrome and intraventricular hemorrhage). This is the asymptomatic first stage. The second stage is characterized by systemic endothelial dysfunction and inflammation, resulting in vasoconstriction and possible development of thromboemboli.

9. **How is preeclampsia managed?**
The mainstay of management is magnesium therapy and BP control. Magnesium sulfate is given for seizure prophylaxis, although the mechanism by which it prevents seizures is unknown. Magnesium is both a natural calcium and NMDA receptor antagonist. The side effects of magnesium are in part related to its calcium receptor antagonism. Magnesium also has analgesic properties because of its *N*-methyl-D-aspartate (NMDA) receptor antagonism similar to ketamine and nitrous oxide. Proposed mechanisms include reduced cerebral edema because of its calcium channel blocking properties and antiepileptic properties because of NMDA antagonism. Moreover, magnesium is a vasodilator and attenuates the vascular response to endogenous and exogenous vasopressors, again, similar to calcium channel blockers. Magnesium sulfate is also advantageous for fetal neuroprotection as it has been shown to decrease the incidence of neurological insult in preterm neonates, likely because of its NMDA antagonism.
　　First-line intravenous antihypertensive medications are labetalol and hydralazine. Because cerebral autoregulation is disrupted in preeclampsia, cerebral blood flow is not constant and is a function of BP, even within normal BP limits. Therefore antihypertensives are administered to *control* BP (i.e., goal systolic BP <160 mm Hg), not to normalize BP because overcorrection could lead to cerebral hypoperfusion, particularly if the autoregulation curve has shifted to the right because of chronically uncontrolled HTN.

10. **What are the side effects of magnesium sulfate administration?**
The therapeutic range of magnesium sulfate is 4 to 8 mEq/L. As plasma concentrations increase, patients develop electrocardiogram changes, such as widening of the QRS complex and QT interval prolongation. Deep tendon reflexes are absent at 10 mEq/L, atrioventricular block and respiratory paralysis occur at 15 mEq/L, and cardiac arrest occurs at 25 mEq/L. In therapeutic doses, magnesium sulfate increases the sensitivity to muscle relaxants, especially nondepolarizing muscle relaxants. Because magnesium sulfate also crosses the placenta, newborns may demonstrate decreased muscle tone, respiratory depression, and apnea.

11. **How do you treat magnesium toxicity?**
The mainstay of treatment is intravenous calcium. Diuretics with intravenous fluids should also be considered.

12. **What are the anesthetic considerations for patients with preeclampsia?**
A thorough preoperative evaluation should be completed, including review of past medical history, airway examination, and evaluation of coagulation status. Preeclampsia will cause even more oropharyngeal edema than is normally apparent with pregnancy, thus airway evaluation is crucial and should be rechecked because the edema (and Mallampati score) can worsen throughout labor. These patients may be at increased risk for difficult mask ventilation and intubation.
　　Because up to 20% of patients with preeclampsia will develop HELLP syndrome, an evaluation of the patient's platelet count and coagulation status (prothrombin time and partial thromboplastin time) is recommended before performing neuraxial techniques. The main concern is the risk of causing an epidural hematoma when performing a spinal or epidural in the setting of coagulopathy attributed to thrombocytopenia. Recent studies show that the incidence of epidural hematoma is extremely low, when the platelet count is greater than 70,000 mm^{-3}. However, it is important to consider the trend of the platelet decrease, medications, and other comorbidities that may impair platelet function itself or cause coagulopathy.

Care must be taken to avoid acute hypotension because of sympathetic blockade from neuraxial anesthesia, as patients with preeclampsia are frequently intravascularly hypovolemic. Although spinal anesthesia is more likely to produce sudden hypotension, recent studies have confirmed its safety for cesarean delivery. Neuraxial anesthesia is preferable to general anesthesia, as the latter increases the risk for difficult intubation, aspiration, and HTN from laryngoscopy, increasing the risk of hemorrhagic stroke. Further, judicious use of intravenous fluids is important as these patients are prone to developing noncardiogenic pulmonary edema (i.e., acute respiratory distress syndrome [ARDS]) because of the increased vascular permeability from systemic inflammation.

13. What is eclampsia?

Eclampsia is the development of peripartum seizures and/or coma that is not caused by an underlying neurological disease. Patients may experience headache, visual disturbances, and epigastric pain before the onset of seizure activity. Parturients may have evidence of cerebral edema and multifocal hemorrhage. Other complications include hemorrhagic stroke, ARDS, and other complications of HELLP syndrome, such as liver infarction, liver failure, acute kidney injury, DIC, and coagulation disturbances.

14. How are eclamptic seizures treated?

Most eclamptic seizures are self-limited; however, maternal airway management and intrauterine resuscitation are the main concerns. If the seizure does not resolve or if there are concerns that the patient is not protecting their airway, then the patient may need to be intubated. Magnesium sulfate is the first-line antiepileptic drug (AED) for eclamptic seizures and should be given as a bolus (4–6 grams intravenous [IV]) for a loading dose and started on an infusion (2–4 g/h IV). Other AEDs that may be considered to treat seizures because of eclampsia include propofol, lorazepam, midazolam, and levetiracetam. Immediate delivery may also be indicated.

15. Discuss preterm labor. How is it managed?

Preterm labor is the onset of frequent uterine contractions associated with progressive cervical dilation or effacement occurring before 37 weeks' gestation and often results in preterm delivery. Preterm labor is associated with placental abruption, uterine abnormalities, cervical insufficiency, multiple gestations, premature rupture of the membranes, and urinary tract, systemic, or gynecological infection (Box 56.2). Although preterm delivery occurs in only 5% to 10% of pregnancies, it accounts for the majority of neonatal morbidity secondary to pulmonary immaturity and neonatal deaths. Survival is around 50% at 25 weeks or less but significantly increases to around 90% at 28 weeks' (or more) gestation.

Premature labor can be suppressed with tocolytics, such as calcium channel blockers, magnesium sulfate, cyclooxygenase inhibitors, and β-agonists (Table 56.3). Nonsteroidal antiinflammatory drugs (NSAIDs) should be

---

Box 56.2 Risk Factors for Preterm Delivery

African descent	Polyhydramnios (uterine distention)
History of preterm delivery	Trauma
History of tobacco/substance abuse	Abdominal surgery during pregnancy
Acute or chronic systemic disease	Multiple gestation
Low prepregnancy body mass index	Low socioeconomic status

Table 56.3 List of Common Tocolytics and Side Effects

CLASS	DRUG	MATERNAL SIDE EFFECTS	FETAL SIDE EFFECTS
Cyclo-oxygenase inhibitors (NSAIDs)	Indomethacin	Nausea Heartburn	Closure of PDA Pulmonary HTN Renal dysfunction (reversible) Oligohydramnios IVH
Magnesium sulfate	Magnesium sulfate	Flushing Lethargy Muscle weakness Hypocalcemia/demineralization Hypocalcemia Pulmonary edema Cardiac arrest	Hypotonia Respiratory depression

Table 56.3 List of Common Tocolytics and Side Effects (*Continued*)

CLASS	DRUG	MATERNAL SIDE EFFECTS	FETAL SIDE EFFECTS
β-Adrenergic agonists	Terbutaline Ritodrine	Dysrhythmias Pulmonary edema Hypotension Hyperglycemia Hypokalemia N/V, fever	Tachycardia Hyperglycemia Hypertrophy (Neonatal—hypoglycemia hypocalcemia, hypotension)
Calcium channel blockers	Nifedipine Nicardipine	Transient hypotension Flushing Headache Dizziness	None

HTN, Hypertension; *IVH*, intraventricular hemorrhage; *NSAIDs,* nonsteroidal antiinflammatory drugs; *N/V*, nausea/vomiting; *PDA*, patent ductus arteriosus.

selectively used if patients have NSAID-sensitive asthma, active peptic ulcer disease, or coagulation abnormalities. Magnesium sulfate is a weak tocolytic and is not clinically effective in suppressing premature labor, but it improves fetal neurological outcomes in premature newborns.

16. What are the causes of antepartum hemorrhage?

Placenta previa, placental abruption, and uterine rupture, are all causes of antepartum hemorrhage that concern the anesthesiologist.

Placenta previa is caused by abnormal placentation either near or completely covering the internal cervical os. The classic presentation is painless vaginal bleeding. Risk factors include prior uterine surgery, prior cesarean delivery, recurrent abortions, and advanced maternal age.

Placental abruption is caused by premature separation of the placenta before delivery of the fetus. Acute placental abruption classically presents with vaginal bleeding, uterine tenderness, and increased uterine activity; however, chronic placental abruption can also occur with a more insidious presentation. Risk factors include a previous abruption, trauma, HTN, smoking, and cocaine use.

Uterine rupture is caused by a tear of the uterine wall, which results in fetal distress and maternal hemorrhage. The presentation is variable and can range from mild uterine tenderness with nonreassuring fetal heart patterns to severe abdominal pain and hemorrhagic shock. Risk factors include trauma, prior uterine surgery, prior cesarean delivery, uterotonic drugs, dystocia, and abnormal placentation.

17. What is the most common cause of postpartum hemorrhage? How is it managed?

The most common cause of postpartum hemorrhage is uterine atony because of failure of the uterus to contract following delivery. Conditions which cause uterus overdistention will increase the risk of uterine atony, such as multiple gestation, fetal macrosomia, and polyhydramnios. Other risk factors for uterine atony include high parity, prolonged labor, chorioamnionitis, precipitous labor, augmented labor, and tocolytic agents.

Obstetric management includes bimanual compression, uterine massage, and uterotonics. Oxytocin (Pitocin®), the first-line treatment, is a synthetic hormone structurally similar to vasopressin and is administered as an infusion (20–50 units/1000 mL crystalloid). Its main side effect is hypotension. Methylergonovine (Methergine®) is an ergot alkaloid derivative and is administered (0.2 mg) intramuscularly and is known to cause HTN. It is contraindicated in hypertensive disorders, peripheral vascular disease, and ischemic heart disease. Methyl prostaglandin $F_{2\alpha}$ (Hemabate®) is administered into the uterine myometrium or skeletal muscle (250 mcg) for the treatment of refractory uterine atony. Its main side effect is bronchospasm and is contraindicated in patients with asthma. Other options include intrauterine balloon tamponade (e.g., Bakri® Postpartum Balloon), which is a balloon placed within the uterus that serves as a tamponade to stop bleeding. Medically refractory uterine atony may require uterine artery ligation or embolization, or hysterectomy.

18. What are the anesthetic concerns for diabetes mellitus (DM) and obesity?

Obesity and DM increases the risk for spontaneous abortions, stillbirth, preeclampsia, polyhydramnios, fetal macrosomia, fetal malformations, and cesarean delivery. Pregestational diabetes is associated with preterm labor and delivery. Obesity causes reduced lung volumes (i.e., reduced functional residual capacity) and increases baseline oxygen consumption, where both are already adversely affected by pregnancy. Further, obesity decreases chest wall compliance making mask ventilation difficult. Therefore obese patients are at a much higher risk of airway complications (i.e., hypoxemia and difficult mask ventilation) on induction of anesthesia. Therefore neuraxial analgesia/anesthesia is strongly preferred in this patient population whenever possible.

19. **What are the causes of DIC in obstetric patients?**
DIC is a consumptive coagulopathy, resulting from abnormal activation of the coagulation cascade with the formation of large amounts of thrombin, depletion of coagulation factors, activation of the fibrinolytic system, and hemorrhage. In obstetrics, the most frequent causes are preeclampsia, HELLP syndrome, sepsis, fetal demise, placental abruption, and amniotic fluid embolism.

20. **What is the most common cardiac disease that complicates pregnancy?**
Congenital heart disease is the most common cardiac disease in pregnant women in the United States. It accounts for approximately 60% to 80% of cardiac disease during pregnancy.

21. **How is congenital heart disease managed during pregnancy?**
Pulmonary artery catheterization is rarely required for most patients with congenital heart disease. Intrathecal opioid is a good option for labor analgesia when patients will not tolerate a decrease in systemic vascular resistance and venous return. Epidural anesthesia, as opposed to a spinal, may be considered in patients with significant valvular heart disease provided that the induction of anesthesia through the epidural is slow, and hemodynamic changes are promptly treated. Single-injection spinals for cesarean delivery are contraindicated in many patients with congenital heart disease. However, neuraxial anesthesia/analgesia may be advantageous for these patients as it can blunt the sympathetic response to labor pain and the hemodynamic changes that accompany labor and delivery.

KEY POINTS: HIGH-RISK OBSTETRICS

1. Maternal morbidity and/or mortality from hypertensive disorders often results from cerebrovascular and cardiovascular complications.
2. The risk of epidural hematoma as a complication of neuraxial techniques is extremely low when the platelet count is greater than 70,000 mm^{-3}. However, it is also important to consider the trend of the platelet decrease, medications, and other comorbidities that may impair platelet function itself or cause coagulopathy.
3. Magnesium toxicity progressively cause the following: sedation, nausea, vomiting, flushing, urinary retention, ileus, hyporeflexia, skeletal muscle weakness, vasodilation, bradycardia, myocardial depression, coma, and cardiopulmonary arrest.
4. Magnesium toxicity can be treated with calcium and diuretics.
5. Common causes of antepartum hemorrhage include the following: placenta previa (painless vaginal bleeding), placental abruption (painful vaginal bleeding), uterine rupture (variable presentation ranging from mild symptoms to painful, life-threating vaginal bleeding).
6. Uterine atony is the most common cause of postpartum hemorrhage and often results in substantial blood loss.
7. Obesity and diabetes mellitus increases the risk of preeclampsia, preterm labor and delivery, painful labor, fetal macrosomia, and operative delivery. A preference towards neuraxial techniques should strongly be considered in this patient population because of the concerns with airway management on induction of general anesthesia.

SUGGESTED READINGS

American Society of Anesthesiologists Task Force on Obstetric Anesthesia. Practice guidelines for obstetric anesthesia: an updated report by the American Society of Anesthesiologists Task Force on Obstetric Anesthesia and the Society for Obstetric Anesthesia and Perinatology. Anesthesiology. 2016;124(2):270–300.

American Society of Anesthesiologists Task Force on Pulmonary Artery Catheterization. Practice guidelines for pulmonary artery catheterization: an updated report. Anesthesiology. 2003;99:988–1014.

Bateman BT, Polley LS. Hypertensive disorders. In: Chestnut DH, Wong CA, Tsen LC, et al., eds. Obstetric Anesthesia: Principles and Practice. 5th ed. Philadelphia: Saunders; 2014.

Mayer DC, Spielman FJ, Bell EA, et al. Antepartum and postpartum hemorrhage. In: Chestnut DH, Wong CA, Tsen LC, et al., eds. Obstetric Anesthesia: Principles and Practice. 5th ed. Philadelphia: Saunders; 2014.

Reid RW, Chestnut DH. Renal disease. In: Chestnut DH, Wong CA, Tsen LC, et al., eds. Obstetric Anesthesia: Principles and Practice. 5th ed. Philadelphia: Saunders; 2014.

Sibai BM. Preeclampsia and hypertensive disorders. In: Gabbe SG, Niebyl JR, Simpson JL, et al., eds. Obstetrics: Normal and Problem Pregnancies. 7th ed. Philadelphia: Elsevier; 2017:661–705.

Thornhill ML, Camann WR, Harnett M, et al. Cardiovascular disease. In: Chestnut DH, Wong CA, Tsen LC, et al., eds. Obstetric Anesthesia: Principles and Practice. 5th ed. Philadelphia: Saunders; 2014.

CHAPTER 57

TRAUMA ANESTHESIA

Bethany Benish, MD

1. Outline and prioritize the initial assessment and management of a trauma patient.

   The American College of Surgeons Committee on Trauma has developed a systematic and concise guideline for management of trauma patients and is taught as Advanced Trauma Life Support (ATLS). Initial assessment includes:
   - Primary survey (ABCDEs)
   - Resuscitation
   - Secondary survey
   - Continued postresuscitation monitoring and reevaluation
   - Definitive care

   The goal of the primary survey is to identify and manage immediately life-threatening conditions. The primary survey is carried out in the following sequence:

   Airway—establish and maintain a patent airway using advanced airway management if needed (such as endotracheal intubation, cricothyrotomy, or tracheostomy)
   Breathing—ensure adequate gas exchange and assist with ventilation if needed
   Circulation—control external hemorrhage and replace intravascular volume
   Disability—perform a rapid neurological evaluation
   Exposure/**E**nvironmental control—undress to evaluate for other injuries, then cover to avoid hypothermia

   The secondary survey begins once the ABCs are stabilized and includes a head to toe evaluation of the trauma patient, as well as indicated diagnostic studies (radiographs, focused sonography, laboratory tests, and invasive diagnostic procedures).

2. Using the aforementioned guideline, describe the specific assessment and management of an unconscious, hemodynamically unstable trauma patient arriving in the operating room.

   First priorities are always the ABCs (airway, breathing, and circulation). An unconscious trauma patient requires prompt securement of the airway, best accomplished with rapid-sequence induction (RSI) and tracheal intubation. RSI means minimizing the time between loss of consciousness and establishment of a secure endotracheal airway. RSI is performed to minimize risk of pulmonary aspiration of gastric contents. Succinylcholine is the preferred paralytic agent because of its rapid onset. The Sellick maneuver (firm pressure applied to cricoid ring) may prevent regurgitation of gastric contents during induction of anesthesia.

   The next priority should be establishing appropriate intravenous access, using short, large bore (14 or 16 gauge) peripheral catheters, rapid infusion catheters (RICs) or central access, using 9F introducers (internal jugular, subclavian, or femoral veins). Arterial cannulation is then obtained for continuous blood pressure monitoring and for frequent blood analysis (arterial blood gases, hematocrit, platelet count, coagulation studies, and blood chemistry).

3. Describe the specific concerns during airway management of trauma patient with known or suspected cervical spine injury.

   The incidence of cervical spine injury in a trauma patient is 2% to 5%, and this increases to 10% in the presence of a severe head injury. In these situations, airway management must be performed without excessive movement of the cervical spine. There are, unfortunately, no airway management techniques that result in complete cervical immobility, but attempts are made to minimize neck movement. A jaw-thrust maneuver is used to establish a patent airway, while avoiding neck hyperextension. Manual in-line stabilization (MILS) should be used to stabilize the neck during laryngoscopy. MILS is performed by an assistant placing his/her hands on each side of the patient's head and neck to immobilize the cervical spine. Use of video laryngoscopy or fiberoptic bronchoscopy can improve success of intubation in these patients.

   In the setting of a known cervical spinal cord injury, awake fiberoptic intubation using topicalization and carefully titrated sedation may be the safest way to secure the airway and may allow for postintubation assessment of neurological status before induction of anesthesia. A bloody airway and/or an uncooperative patient, however, may reduce the utility of this technique during initial airway management.

4. How is the American Society of Anesthesiologists difficult airway algorithm altered in trauma?
   See Figure 57.1.

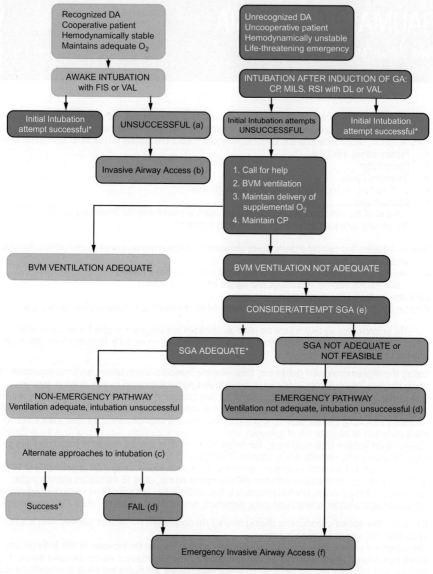

Fig. 57.1 Difficult airway algorithm (modified for trauma patients). *DA,* Difficult airway.

5. When is emergency invasive airway access indicated? How is it performed?

When ventilation is inadequate and intubation attempts are unsuccessful, invasive airway management is indicated. In the setting of trauma, oropharyngeal hemorrhage, neck hematoma, glottic edema, or laryngeal injury, conventional methods of achieving tracheal intubation may not work and emergency invasive airway access is indicated.

Options for invasive airway access include needle cricothyroidotomy and open surgical cricothyroidotomy. Cricothyroidotomy is preferable to tracheostomy because it is faster to perform and does not require neck extension.

Needle cricothyroidotomy is performed by inserting a large gauge (14-G) plastic cannula through the cricothyroid membrane beyond the level of obstruction. Oxygen is then delivered via jet insufflation, until a definitive airway can be established.

Surgical cricothyroidotomy is performed with either a percutaneous or open technique.

Percutaneous cricothyroidotomy is performed using commercially available kits, in which the Seldinger technique is used to convert a needle cricothyroidotomy over a wire and dilator to a 6.0 cuffed airway catheter.

Open cricothyroidotomy is performed by making a midline 4-cm vertical skin incision starting just below the thyroid cartilage prominence, followed by palpation, identification, and a horizontal cut through the cricothyroid membrane. A curved hemostat can be inserted to dilate the opening and a small endotracheal or tracheostomy tube (5–7 mm) can be inserted into the airway.

This open technique may be faster and more successful than percutaneous, but is dependent on the skills and training of the proceduralist.

6. Which anesthetic induction agents are best for trauma patients?

In the setting of hypovolemia, choosing an induction agent that has the lowest cardiovascular depressant effect is vital. More important than the specific drug chosen, is reduction of dose to minimize hypotension through loss of sympathetic tone.

Ketamine is the preferred induction agent in a hypovolemic patient because it usually maintains blood pressure via direct stimulation of the sympathetic nervous system. It is the only agent that increases peripheral vascular resistance. Ketamine can, however, have direct myocardial depressant effects that may result in hypotension, in the setting of severely ill patients with depleted adrenal reserves.

Etomidate is another induction agent commonly used in trauma patients because of its minimal effects on hemodynamics. The dose should be reduced by 25% to 50% in hypovolemic patients and caution should be used in patients relying on sympathetic tone to maintain cardiac output. In addition, etomidate inhibits cortisol synthesis by the adrenal gland, resulting in adrenal suppression, even after a single induction dose. The clinical significance of this short-term adrenal suppression is unclear.

7. Review the ATLS classifications of hemorrhagic shock (class 1–IV)

See Figure 57.2.

8. In addition to vital signs listed in Figure 57.2, are there other clinical indicators of the severity of hemorrhagic shock?

Markers of organ perfusion, such as serum lactate and base deficit indicate severity of shock and can be used during early management to demonstrate adequacy of resuscitation. Base deficit on arterial blood gas indicates changes in oxygen delivery in the setting of hypoperfusion. Base deficit is superior to the ATLS classification of hemodynamic shock in predicting transfusion need and mortality. A base deficit greater than 6 mmol/L on admission indicates moderate shock and predicts increased mortality. Base deficit greater than 6 mmol/L also predicts the likely presence of trauma-induced coagulopathy (TIC) and hypofibrinogenemia, both of which contribute to ongoing blood loss.

Serum lactate is a less specific marker of organ hypoperfusion and tissue hypoxia compared with base deficit. Elevation may be seen in several clinical scenarios, in addition to trauma, including alcohol intoxication. Nevertheless, failure to clear elevated lactate in setting of trauma is another predictor of increased mortality.

9. What is damage control surgery? What is damage control resuscitation?

Damage control surgery refers to providing only interventions that are immediately necessary to control hemorrhage, contamination, and protect from further injury, leaving definitive repairs for a later time.

Class of haemorrhagic shock				
	I	II	III	IV
Blood loss (mL)	Up to 750	750–1500	1500–2000	> 2000
Blood loss (% blood volume)	Up to 15	15–30	30–40	> 40
Pulse rate (per minute)	< 100	100–120	120–140	> 140
Blood pressure	Normal	Normal	Decreased	Decreased
Pulse pressure (mm Hg)	Normal or increased	Decreased	Decreased	Decreased
Respiratory rate (per minute)	14–20	20–30	30–40	> 35
Urine output (mL/hour)	> 30	20–30	5–15	Negligible
Central nervous system/mental status	Slightly anxious	Mildly anxious	Anxious, confused	Confused, lethargic

Fig. 57.2 Advanced Trauma Life Support (ATLS) classification of hemorrhagic shock.

Damage control resuscitation combines the principles of hypotensive resuscitation, immediate control of bleeding, replacement of blood loss with transfused blood instead of intravenous fluids, and early correction of coagulopathy with component therapy.

10. What is the "bloody vicious cycle" of trauma?

The "bloody vicious cycle" also known as the *lethal triad* of the hemorrhaging trauma patient consists of acidosis, hypothermia, and coagulopathy. Acidosis and hypothermia significantly worsen coagulopathy by interfering with platelet and clotting factor function. Resuscitation efforts with only packed red blood cells (PRBCs) and crystalloids further dilute platelets and coagulation factors. Uncontrolled bleeding further consumes factors and platelets, thereby worsening the coagulopathy, leading to more bleeding. In addition, hypothermia, common in the trauma patient because of factors, such as the need for exposure and large volume resuscitation, worsens coagulopathy by impairing clotting factor function.

11. Discuss the initial management of hypovolemic shock.

Historically, initial replacement of blood loss was with balanced crystalloid solutions, usually in a ratio of 3 to 4 times the estimated blood loss. Administering large volumes of crystalloid, however, results in a dilutional coagulopathy, and contributes to the often lethal coagulopathy of trauma. Instead, modern hemostatic resuscitation protocols in trauma restrict the use of crystalloid, while encouraging early plasma and platelet transfusion. In the setting of severe trauma, early resuscitation using fixed ratios of 1:1:1 of PRBCs, fresh frozen plasma, and platelets is recommended. In addition to fixed ratios, viscoelastic hemostatic assays (thromboelastography [TEG] or rotational thromboelastometry [ROTEM]) provide rapid, comprehensive, in vivo evaluation of clot formation, strength, and breakdown, and can be used for specific, goal-directed clotting factor replacement.

12. What is TIC?

TIC is characterized by varying degrees of dysfibrinogenemia, hyperfibrinolysis, endothelial dysfunction, and impaired platelet function. It develops rapidly following tissue trauma and hemorrhagic shock.

One-third of trauma patients are coagulopathic upon arrival to the Emergency Department and this is an independent predictor of transfusion, multiorgan failure, and mortality. In patients with the similar Injury Severity Scores (ISS), the presence of coagulopathy nearly doubles mortality.

Correction of this coagulopathy is one of the primary goals of trauma management.

13. How can TIC be assessed?

As discussed earlier, viscoelastic hemostatic assays (TEG or ROTEM), as well as traditional coagulation studies (prothrombin time [PT]/partial thromboplastin time [PTT], international normalized ratio [INR], fibrinogen) are used to diagnose and manage TIC (Fig. 57.3).

14. What are the limitations of traditional coagulation studies?

Traditional coagulation studies, such as PT/PTT/INR, often take too much time to process to be of use during trauma resuscitation. In addition, PTT and PT/INR are performed on plasma (platelet poor) to evaluate clotting factor deficiency in isolation, which excludes the cellular component of coagulation. Finally, PTT and PT/INR tests are terminated once the first fibrin strands are formed, which is when only 5% of the total amount of thrombin has been generated.

15. What is the significance of hyperfibrinolysis in trauma? How is it diagnosed?

Fibrinolysis is an important component of the normal balance of clot formation and breakdown. Pathological fibrinolysis, termed *hyperfibrinolysis*, results in nonsurgical bleeding because of the premature breakdown of formed clot.

The incidence of hyperfibrinolysis varies widely in the trauma literature, ranging from 2% to 15% of trauma patients on arrival to the Emergency Department and one-third of trauma patients requiring massive transfusion. Hyperfibrinolysis independently predicts mortality.

Hyperfibrinolysis is diagnosed using viscoelastic hemostatic assays (TEG or ROTEM). On rapid TEG, it is defined by LY30 (lysis at 30 min) greater than 7.5% or EPL (estimated percent lysis) over 15%.

Fibrinolysis in trauma is complex, as severely injured patients have both promotors and inhibitor of fibrinolysis.

16. What is tranexamic acid? What is its role in trauma?

Tranexamic acid (TXA) is a synthetic lysine derivative that irreversibly inhibits the proteolytic action of plasmin on fibrin clots and platelet receptors, thereby inhibiting fibrinolysis. TXA has been shown to decrease RBC transfusion in a variety of elective surgeries.

In 2011 the Clinical Randomisation of an Antifibrinolytic in Significant Haemorrhage 2 (CRASH-2) trial, a large randomized placebo-controlled trial, evaluating the effect of early TXA in over 20,000 trauma patients, showed a significant reduction in all-cause mortality when TXA was given within 3 hours of injury. Other military (Military Application of Tranexamic Acid in Trauma Emergency Resuscitation [MATTERs] trial) and smaller civilian studies initially confirmed this early mortality reduction. More recently, however, studies at US major trauma centers have shown increased mortality in the highest injury acuity patients when given TXA. In addition, there have been many criticisms of the CRASH-2 trial and whether it should be applied to US trauma patients.

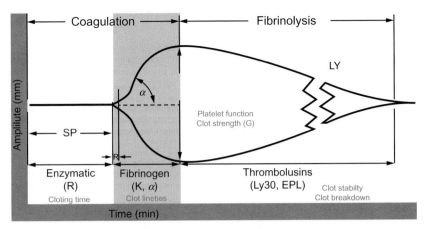

Fig. 57.3 Thromboelastography.

At present, the use of TXA in trauma is still controversial. If available, viscoelastic hemostatic assays (TEG or ROTEM) should be used to guide its administration, but more studies are needed to predict which patients will benefit from TXA in trauma.

17. **Are there other agents used for hemostatic resuscitation?**

Prothrombin complex concentrate (PCC) is a concentrate of donor pooled plasma containing Factors II, VII, IX, and X, as well as Protein C and S. It allows for rapid reversal of warfarin and some Factor Xa inhibitors, with minimal risk of transfusion-related acute lung injury or volume overload. The role of PCC in coagulopathic trauma patients is still being evaluated.

Fibrinogen concentrate is another plasma-derived hemostatic concentrate with future potential use in trauma. Initial studies demonstrate safety, with no increase in thromboembolic events but again, larger quality trials are needed.

18. **Why do trauma patients become hypothermic? How does hypothermia affect outcome?**

Hypothermia is common in all surgical patients because of loss of hypothalamic regulation, peripheral vasodilation, and exposure to a cold operating room environment. Trauma patients are often hypothermic on arrival because of prehospital environmental exposure, and infusion of unwarmed fluids and blood.

Hypothermia directly contributes to coagulopathy by interfering with factor and platelet function. Measures should be taken to reduce the potential for hypothermia in trauma patients by warming the room, warming all fluids and blood products (except platelets), and using forced air warming devices.

19. **How does cardiac tamponade present? What is Beck's triad? How should anesthesia be managed in a patient with tamponade?**

Cardiac tamponade is compression of the heart through the accumulation of fluid (often blood) in the pericardial sac. It can arise in the setting of both blunt and penetrating chest trauma. Beck's triad consists of hypotension, distant heart sounds, and distended neck veins, all the classic signs of cardiac tamponade. Because the heart floats freely in the accumulating fluid/blood within the pericardial sac, electrical alternans, that is, a constantly changing axis, can be seen on electrocardiogram.

A patient with cardiac tamponade is preload dependent and can have cardiovascular collapse during induction of anesthesia. To avoid this, it may be necessary to drain the pericardium under local anesthesia, via a subxiphoid pericardial window, before induction. If induction must occur before drainage, ketamine is the induction agent of choice and maintaining spontaneous ventilation is key, as positive pressure ventilation will decrease venous return and greatly reduce cardiac output.

20. **Describe the clinical presentation and treatment of tension pneumothorax.**

Tension pneumothorax is a progressive accumulation of air in the pleural space often caused by lung injury (e.g., rib fracture, penetrating wound, or central venous line placement). If the pleural cavity does not communicate with the ambient environment, this air space will expand quickly with positive-pressure ventilation. Signs of tension pneumothorax include unexplained tachycardia, hypotension, and increased airway pressures, as well as possible tracheal and neck vein distention (if euvolemic).

Treatment includes emergent needle decompressive thoracostomy, in which a large-bore needle is placed through the chest wall in the second intercostal space, at the midclavicular line. A rush of air confirms the diagnosis. Tension pneumothorax is a clinical diagnosis and is life-threatening; treatment should not be delayed for radiographic confirmation. Of note, nitrous oxide is avoided in trauma patients because it can cause expansion of a pneumothorax by rapidly diffusing into air-filled cavities.

21. Describe the presentation of blunt cardiac injury in the setting of trauma.

Blunt cardiac injury includes a spectrum of injuries, ranging from myocardial contusion to cardiac wall rupture. Blunt cardiac injury can present as dysrhythmia or conduction block, as well as injury to the valves or papillary muscles and thrombosis/dissection of coronary arteries (most commonly right coronary). Because of its anterior position, the right heart is most commonly injured.

Echocardiography should be performed if blunt cardiac injury is suspected, to evaluate for segmental wall motion defects, as well as valvular or septal injuries. Transesophageal echocardiography is much more sensitive than transthoracic echocardiography in identifying injuries that may require intervention.

22. How is an air embolism diagnosed and managed?

Chest trauma, specifically penetrating lung injuries, can result in a systemic air embolism, secondary to communication between the pulmonary vasculature and the airways (bronchovenous or alveolocapillary fistulae). Pulmonary vascular air embolism often presents as cardiovascular collapse following intubation and positive pressure ventilation in patients at risk.

This is a rare and often unrecognized complication that requires a high index of suspicion in the context of chest trauma. To minimize risk, use small tidal volumes with low inspiratory airway pressure and avoid the use of excessive positive end-expiratory pressure. Lung isolation may be required and can facilitate surgical evaluation and repair. Emergency thoracotomy and cross-clamping of pulmonary hilum, on the side of injury, may be life saving.

23. Discuss the anesthetic considerations for acute spinal cord injury.

Airway management, discussed briefly earlier, focuses on cervical spine immobilization and use of direct or indirect laryngoscopy (video-assisted), while maintaining MILS. Depending on urgency and cooperation of the patient, awake fiberoptic intubation may be considered, although it has not been shown to be superior to asleep techniques.

Succinylcholine remains the preferred paralytic for emergent intubation in acute spinal cord injured patients but should be avoided between 48 hours and 12 months postinjury to avoid the risk of life-threatening hyperkalemia caused by denervation hypersensitivity.

Traumatic spinal cord injuries, especially those above the mid-thoracic level, are associated with some degree of neurogenic shock. As for all trauma patients, other causes for systemic hypotension must be evaluated and managed, including hemorrhage, tension pneumothorax, pericardial tamponade, myocardial injury, and sepsis. Hypotension in the setting of spinal cord injury must be managed promptly, as this reduction in spinal cord perfusion pressure (SCPP) can contribute to a secondary neurological injury. General recommendations regarding hemodynamic goals in spinal cord trauma include maintaining mean arterial pressure (MAP) over 90 mm Hg. It is thought that aggressive hemodynamic management may provide an improvement of axonal function and may improve neurological outcome. Adequate fluid resuscitation is an important first step in managing hypotension but often infusion of vasopressors, such as phenylephrine, are required for sufficient hemodynamic improvement. Spinal cord injuries above T6 can interrupt sympathetic cardioaccelerator fibers, resulting in bradycardia. These injuries often require chronotropic support in addition to vasoconstriction. Medications, such as norepinephrine or epinephrine, can accomplish this. Anesthetic agents should be carefully titrated as these patients are unable to compensate for blood pressure drops by increasing sympathetic tone. In addition to managing neurogenic shock, large volume blood loss may occur during spinal cord surgery. Transfusion of RBCs, as well as coagulation factors, and platelets are often required. Viscoelastic hemostatic assays (TEG or ROTEM) provide a comprehensive evaluation of in vivo coagulation and can assist with goal-directed transfusion in this setting.

24. What are the anesthetic considerations for adult traumatic brain injury? What is the significance of a Glasgow Coma Scale score of 8 or less?

Patients with moderate to severe traumatic brain injury (TBI) often require emergent surgical intervention. As with all trauma patients, initial management should focus on airway, breathing, and circulation. In addition, the patient's neurological assessment is performed using the Glasgow Coma Scale (GCS) (see Table 57.1).

If GCS score is 8 or less, the TBI is classified as severe and endotracheal intubation is indicated. A secure airway and adequate ventilation is key to prevention of secondary neurological injury from hypoxia and hypercarbia in the setting of TBI. Intraoperative anesthetic management involves maintaining a cerebral perfusion pressure (CPP) of 60 to 70 mm Hg (CPP = intracranial pressure [ICP] – MAP), correction of anemia/coagulopathy, and interventions to decrease intracranial pressure, including:

- Elevating head of bed more than 15 degrees
- Avoiding neck vein congestion through neutral positioning
- Maintaining arterial partial pressure of carbon dioxide 35 to 40 mm Hg, unless transtentorial herniation is suspected
- Administering intravenous mannitol (0.25–1 g/kg) to acutely lower ICP
- Considering hypertonic saline as an additional agent for hyperosmolar therapy

Tight glucose control and avoidance of hyperthermia are also important considerations in the anesthetic management of TBI patients.

Table 57.1 Glasgow Coma Scale

SCORE	MOTOR	VERBAL	EYE OPENING
6	Obeys commands	N/A	N/A
5	Localizes stimulus	Oriented	N/A
4	Withdraws from stimulus	Confused	Spontaneously
3	Flexes arm	Words/phrases	To voice
2	Extends arm	Makes sounds	To pain
1	No response	No response	Remain closed

Scores from 3 to 15.

25. Describe the management of the pregnant trauma patient.

Trauma in a pregnant woman offers unique challenges related the anatomical and physiological changes of pregnancy, as well as consideration for fetal wellbeing. Initial management, as always, focuses on the ABCs of resuscitation. Airway management is complicated by glottic and supraglottic edema, decreased apneic reserve, and higher risk of pulmonary aspiration. For these reasons, rapid sequence intubation, after adequate preoxygenation, should be performed with availability of smaller endotracheal tubes (size 6.0 or 6.5) and preparation for emergent surgical airway if necessary.

Hemodynamic stabilization and aggressive fluid and blood resuscitation are important for both maternal and fetal outcome. Significant blood loss (1.5–2 L) may occur with minimal alteration in maternal vital signs. Fetal distress can be an early and often the only sign of inadequate resuscitation in a healthy mother. Compression of the inferior vena cava by the gravid uterus (>20 weeks) may cause hypotension. Positioning the patient with left uterine displacement should minimize this effect.

An obstetrician should be notified for fetal monitoring if more than 20 weeks' gestation and must be immediately available should emergent caesarian section be required

In the event of maternal cardiac arrest, advanced cardiovascular life support should be performed. If the patient does not respond to initial cardiopulmonary resuscitation efforts, emergency caesarian section should be performed because delivery of the child improves resuscitative efforts.

26. Review anesthetic concerns for the geriatric trauma patient.

With an aging population, the elderly represent a growing segment of trauma patients. Geriatric patients can have significant life-threatening injury from often low impact mechanisms, making triage challenging. With age-related decline in physiological reserve, coexisting organ dysfunction and comorbid chronic diseases, geriatric patients may not be able to compensate for the stress of trauma. In addition to comorbidities, elderly patients are often on numerous medications that may affect resuscitative efforts (beta-blockers and vasodilators) or increase bleeding risk (antiplatelet medications and anticoagulants). Overall, geriatric trauma patients have increased mortality when compared with younger cohorts.

KEY POINTS: TRAUMA ANESTHESIA

1. Initial management of trauma patients focuses on the ABCs: airway, breathing, and circulation. Once the airway is secure, placement of multiple large bore intravenous catheters for hypovolemic resuscitation is a priority.
2. TIC is an independent predictor of transfusion, multiorgan failure, and mortality. Correction of coagulopathy is one of the primary goals of acute trauma management. Early ratio-driven transfusion of 1:1:1 RBC: plasma: platelet should be used until viscoelastic hemostatic assays (TEG/ROTEM) are available for goal directed hemostatic resuscitation.
3. Acute cardiovascular collapse, following initiation of positive pressure ventilation in the setting of blunt or penetrating chest trauma, may be caused by cardiac tamponade, tension pneumothorax, or venous air embolism.
4. In the setting of TBI and spinal cord injury, anesthetic goals focus on maintaining adequate perfusion of the brain and spinal cord to minimize secondary ischemic insult and improve neurological outcome.

SUGGESTED READINGS

Hagberg CA, Kaslow O. Difficult airway management algorithm in trauma updated by COTEP. ASA Monitor. 2014;78:56–60.
Tobin JM, Varon AJ. Update in trauma anesthesiology: perioperative resuscitation management. Anesth Analg. 2012;11(6):1326–1333.
Varon A, Smith C, eds. Essentials of Trauma Anesthesia. Cambridge: Cambridge University Press; 2017.

CHAPTER 58

THE BURNED PATIENT

Thomas Phillips, MD, Marshall Lee, MD

1. **Who gets burned?**

   In the United States, there are over 450,000 burn injuries each year responsible for 40,000 hospitalizations and approximately 3400 deaths. The majority of burns are thermal injuries. Electrical burns usually cause tissue destruction by thermal and associated injuries. In chemical burns, the degree of injury depends on the particular chemical, its concentration, and duration of exposure. The majority of burn patients are men, with 70% occurring in a residential home.

2. **What are the consequences of skin damage?**

   The skin is the largest organ of the human body. It has three principal functions, all of which are disrupted by burn injury:
   - Sensory organ—Burn patients may have absent pain sensation particularly with deeper burns.
   - Thermoregulation—Burn patients have extensive evaporative heat and water loss, leading to hypothermia.
   - Infection—The skin serves as a barrier to protect the body against the entrance of microorganisms in the environment. Burn patients are at profound risk for infection and sepsis.

3. **How are burns classified?**
   - Superficial (first-degree)
     - Damage is limited to the epidermis. The burn site is red and painful but often resolves without sequelae. No surgical interventions are typically required.
   - Superficial partial thickness (superficial second-degree)
     - Papillary dermis is damaged. This is often severely painful and appears swollen with blistering. Such injuries generally require cleaning and sterile dressing for appropriate healing.
   - Deep partial thickness (deep second-degree)
     - Reticular dermis is damaged with decreased pain sensation to touch. This will require cleaning and sterile dressing, in addition to possible excision and skin grafting.
   - Full thickness (third-degree)
     - Damage extends into the epidermis, dermis, and subcutaneous tissue. Burn site appears white or charred. No pain sensation to superficial touch. Treatment is as previously discussed, with early skin grafting.
   - Fourth-degree
     - Damage includes deep tissues including bones, muscles, and tendons. This often requires surgical intervention for adequate healing.

4. **What systems are affected by burns?**

   Large burns cause massive tissue destruction and activation of a cytokine-mediated inflammatory response affecting virtually all organ systems. This includes the cardiovascular and respiratory systems; hepatic, renal, and endocrine system; the gastrointestinal tract; hematopoiesis; coagulation; and the immune system. The pathophysiology of major burn injuries has two characteristic phases: the early phase ($<$48 hours after injury), followed by the hypermetabolic phase ($>$48 hours after injury). A notable characteristic of the first phase is intravascular hypovolemia because of increased vascular permeability and that of the second phase is intravascular hypervolemia because of fluid reabsorption. Edema, particularly laryngeal edema, is a major concern in both phases.

5. **How is the cardiovascular system affected?**

   The early phase ($<$48 hours) of a burn injury is characterized by an increase in vascular permeability, resulting in "third spacing" of intravascular fluid, causing tissue edema and intravascular hypovolemia. This causes the cardiac output to decrease and the systemic vascular resistance (SVR) to increase. This is in contrast to the second phase of burn injury (i.e., hypermetabolic phase), which is characterized by an increase in oxygen consumption, CO_2 production, and cardiac output and a decrease in SVR. Fluid shifts during the second phase is opposite to that of the first phase, where fluid from the interstitial space reaccumulates into the intravascular space, causing problems, such as pulmonary edema. This is exacerbated by the fact that many patients received aggressive fluid resuscitation during the early phase. Complicating the second phase is the development of sepsis, which also increases cardiac output and decreases SVR.

6. **How is the respiratory system affected?**

   Pulmonary complications of burn injuries and smoke inhalation can often go unrecognized. Chest x-rays are often normal, until multiple days after the initial insult. Smoke or carbonaceous material around the mouth or nose can clue providers to the presence of damage to the pulmonary system. Pulmonary complications can be divided into three distinct syndromes, based on clinical features and temporal relationship to the injury. Early complications, occurring the first 24 hours postburn, include carbon monoxide (CO), cyanide poisoning, and direct inhalation injury to the airway and lungs. This may lead to upper airway obstruction and pulmonary edema. Delayed injury, occurring 2 to 5 days after injury, includes adult respiratory distress syndrome (ARDS) and pneumonia. Damage to the mucociliary transport system increases the risk of developing pulmonary infections. Late pulmonary complications, which occurs days to weeks after injury include pneumonia, atelectasis, and pulmonary embolism (PE).

It is important to appreciate that patients with burn injuries often require aggressive volume resuscitation. Aggressive volume resuscitation during the initial, "early phase" of burn injury and/or fluid reabsorption during the latter phase of burn injury (i.e., hypermetabolism phase) can exacerbate these pulmonary complications: (1) pulmonary edema, and (2) upper airway obstruction because of edema.

7. What is inhalation injury?

Inhalation injury occurs when hot gases, toxic substances, and reactive smoke particles reach the tracheobronchial tree and damage tissues. These substances result in wheezing, bronchospasm, corrosion, and airway edema. Inhalation injury can cause damage to the upper airway (i.e., airway compromise, nasal obstruction, and acute laryngitis with varying degrees of laryngeal edema), damage to the conducting airway (i.e., tracheitis and bronchitis), and injury to the lower respiratory tract (i.e., pneumonitis, pulmonary edema, and ARDS). Bronchoscopy can be useful in the diagnosis of inhalation injury, as radiographic imaging often underestimates the extent of injury.

8. What is the best way to treat inhalation injury?

Management is generally supportive. Oxygen should be provided as necessary to ensure adequate oxygenation. Bronchospasm should be treated with beta-agonists. Pulmonary hygiene is important in these patients, as there can be excessive carbonaceous material in the lungs and some patients may require intubation because of laryngeal edema or respiratory failure.

9. How should the airway of a burn patient be managed?

Providers should have a low threshold to intubate patients with burns or injuries to the face and oropharynx. Patients with heat and smoke injury, plus extensive face and neck burns, usually all require intubation. Subsequent edema to the airway can rapidly develop, causing upper airway obstruction and potential loss of the airway. Careful examination of the airway during laryngoscopy should be performed, if possible, to examine the extent of injury to the airway. Patients with oral burns but no smoke injury should be considered for early intubation, as well because airway edema may ensue making intubation especially difficult.

10. What are the features of carbon monoxide poisoning?

CO poisoning is one of the leading causes of death in fires. CO is produced by incomplete combustion associated with fires, exhaust from internal combustion engines, cooking stoves, and charcoal stoves. Its affinity for hemoglobin is 200 times that of oxygen. CO combines with hemoglobin to form carboxyhemoglobin (COHb) and a standard pulse oximeter cannot differentiate between COHb and oxyhemoglobin, causing overestimation of the measured oxygen saturation. COHb causes tissue hypoxia because of decreased oxygen carrying capacity (CO preferentially binds to hemoglobin) and the oxygen-hemoglobin dissociation curve shifts to the left impairing oxygen delivery to tissue.

11. How do you treat carbon monoxide poisoning?

The mainstay for treatment of CO toxicity is 100% oxygen, which decreases the serum half-life of COHb from 4 to 5 hours to 80 to 100 minutes. Hyperbaric oxygen (2–3 ATM) produces a more rapid displacement of CO with a COHb half-life of 20 minutes. The drawback of hyperbaric oxygen pertains to the logistics in transporting an unstable burn patient to a center that has such capabilities, in a timely fashion, such that the patient may derive benefit without compromising their safety. The vast majority of cases can successfully be managed with 100% oxygen, as the benefit it affords (20 minutes COHb half-life) versus 100% oxygen (80–100 minutes COHb half-life) may be lost in the time spent transporting the patient.

12. What are the features of cyanide poisoning?

Cyanide poisoning should be on the differential diagnosis for any patient with a history of smoke inhalation who has a persistent anion gap metabolic acidosis, despite adequate oxygen delivery. Cyanide is a gas produced from burning nitrogenous materials. It binds to cytochrome oxidase, preventing the production of adenosine triphosphate from aerobic metabolism, resulting in "histotoxic hypoxia" and lactic acidosis. It can also stimulate neurotransmitter release, resulting in neurotoxicity and seizures. The mixed venous oxygen saturation in patients suffering from cyanide poisoning is often greatly increased. If suspected, treatment is initially supportive. Antidotes include hydroxocobalamin, sodium thiosulfate, and amyl/sodium nitrate.

13. How is renal function affected in burn patients?

Renal blood flow and glomerular filtration diminish rapidly during the early phase, activating the renin angiotensin aldosterone system and the release of antidiuretic hormone. Electrolyte abnormalities are common, including low potassium, calcium, and magnesium. The incidence of acute renal failure in burn patients varies from 0.5% to 38%, depending primarily on the severity of the burn. The associated mortality rate is very high (77%–100%). Hemoglobinuria caused by hemolysis and myoglobinuria, secondary to muscle necrosis, can lead to acute tubular necrosis and acute renal failure. In general, early acute kidney disease (AKI) is the result of poor renal perfusion because of hypovolemia and cardiac suppression. Late AKI is usually secondary to sepsis, multiorgan failure, and nephrotoxic drugs.

14. **How is myoglobinuria treated?**
Myoglobinuria is treated by vigorous fluid resuscitation with isotonic crystalloid targeting an endpoint of urine output greater than 2 mL/kg/h. Evidence does not support the use of bicarbonate and/or mannitol adjuncts.

15. **What is the endocrine response to a burn?**
The endocrine response to a thermal burn involves massive release of catecholamines, glucagon, adrenocorticotropic hormone, antidiuretic hormone, renin, angiotensin, and aldosterone. Glucose levels may be elevated, and patients are susceptible to nonketotic hyperosmolar coma. Patients with larger burns are at higher risk for the development of adrenal insufficiency.

16. **What are the hematological complications that occur with burn patients?**
Patients are often initially hemoconcentrated because of the loss of fluid from the intravascular to the interstitial space. However, red cell production is often decreased because of decreased erythropoiesis (i.e., anemia of critical illness). In addition, ongoing infection can result in subacute activation of the coagulation cascade, causing a consumptive coagulopathy. Platelet function is both qualitatively and quantitatively depressed.

17. **What are the immunological complications that occur with burns?**
Infection in the burn patient is a leading cause of morbidity and mortality and remains one of the most demanding concerns for the burn team. Initially, wounds are often colonized by gram-positive and gram-negative organisms. Fungal colonization is commonly caused by *Candida albicans* and occurs typically in the subsequent weeks, following the initial injury. Risk factors for infection include the size of the initial burn wound and wound manipulation (e.g., dressing changes), which may cause bacteremia. Systemic antimicrobials are only indicated to treat documented infections, such as pneumonia, bacteremia, wound infection, and urinary tract infection. Prophylactic antimicrobial therapy is only recommended if the burn wound must be excised or grafted in the operating room and should only be continued in the immediate postoperative period.

18. **How are patients with burns resuscitated?**
The goal of fluid resuscitation is to correct hypovolemia and optimize organ perfusion. Adequate fluid administration is critical to prevent "burn shock" and other complications of thermal injury. Burns cause a generalized increase in capillary permeability, with loss of fluid and protein into the interstitial space. This loss is greatest in the first 48 hours (i.e., early phase). It should be appreciated that the edema is primarily caused by systemic inflammation and that up to 50% of this edema may occur at sites distant from the burn injury site. The most common formula used today for fluid replacement is the Parkland formula. The Parkland formula involves giving 4 mL of lactated Ringer's (LR) solution per kilogram of body weight per percent of total body surface area (TBSA) burned (4 mL/kg/% TBSA). Half of the calculated amount is given during the first 8 hours, and the remainder is given over the next 16 hours, in addition to daily maintenance fluid. Most burn centers use crystalloid (i.e., LR) as the primary fluid for resuscitation; however, early use of colloids (i.e., albumin) may be considered.

19. **How do you calculate the percent of TBSA burned?**
The severity of a burn injury is based on the surface area covered in deep partial-thickness, full-thickness, and subdermal burns. The rule of nines method allows reasonable estimation (Table 58.1). Because of the difference in body habitus (particularly head and neck), the rule of nines must be altered in children (Table 58.2).

20. **What is important in the preoperative history for burn patients?**
It is important to know at what time the burn occurred to accurately assess if the patient is in the early phase (i.e., intravascular hypovolemia) or the hypermetabolic phase (i.e., intravascular hypervolemia). The type of burn is also important in assessing airway damage, associated injuries, and the possibility of more extensive tissue damage than initially appreciated (e.g., electrical burns).

Table 58.1 Rule of Nines for Adults	
Head and neck	9%
Upper extremities	9% each
Chest (anterior and posterior)	9% each
Abdomen	9%
Lower back	9%
Lower extremities	18% each
Perineum	1%

Table 58.2 Rule of Nines for Children: Percent Body Surface According to Age

BODY PART	NEWBORN	3 YEARS	6 YEARS
Head	18	15	12
Trunk	40	40	40
Arms	16	16	16
Legs	26	29	32

21. **What should the anesthesiologist look for on the preoperative physical examination?**
In addition to the conventional concerns of any patient about to undergo surgery, the status of the patient's airway should be the number one priority. A complete airway examination is a must. Excessive sputum, wheezing, and diminished breath sounds may suggest inhalation injury to the lungs. The cardiovascular system should also be evaluated, noting pulse rate and rhythm, blood pressure, cardiac filling pressures (if available), and urine output. Special attention should be given to the neurological examination, to assess their level of consciousness and orientation.

22. **What preoperative tests are required before induction?**
Special emphasis should be placed on correcting the acid-base and electrolyte imbalance during the early phase of injury. Therefore an arterial blood gas (ABG) analysis and a chemistry panel is recommended. In the presence of CO poisoning, the pulse oximeter will overestimate the saturation of hemoglobin. It is important to know that many ABG analyzers cannot measure the COHb, which can only be done if the ABG analyzer includes a cooximeter. Coagulation tests are also helpful, because these patients are at risk of coagulopathy. A urine myoglobin should be done in patients with a history of electrical injury or pigmented urine.

23. **What monitors are needed to give a safe anesthetic?**
Access for monitoring may be difficult. Needle electrodes or electrocardiogram (ECG) pads stapled to the patient may be required for the ECG monitor and nerve stimulator. A blood pressure cuff may be placed on a burned area, but this is often avoided in favor of an arterial catheter and great care must be taken to avoid any burn injury site. Alternate sites of pulse oximetry may be necessary, such as the ears, nose, or forehead because of burn injury to the fingers or toes. Accurate temperature monitoring is a must because of the exaggerated decrease in body temperature in this patient population.

24. **Is succinylcholine safe to administer to a burn patient? How are other neuromuscular blocking agents affected in this patient population?**
Succinylcholine is safe to administer in the first 24 hours after a burn; however, 24 to 48 hours following the initial injury, succinylcholine should be avoided. This is because of the proliferation of extrajunctional neuromuscular receptors, leading to hyperkalemia and cardiac arrest. Patients are thought to be at risk of this complication up to a year past the initial burn injury. Conversely, burn patients tend to be resistant to the effects of nondepolarizing muscle relaxants (e.g., rocuronium) and may need 2 to 5 times the normal dose.

25. **How should temperature be managed for burn patients in the perioperative setting?**
Burn patients are at high risk for intraoperative hypothermia because of faster than normal heat loss. Methods to combat this include increasing the room temperature, forced-air warming systems, warmed intravenous fluids, and minimizing exposed body surface area. Intraoperative hypothermia should be avoided and is associated with increased mortality, surgical site infections, and coagulopathy.

26. **How should the nutritional needs of a burn patient be managed?**
Nutrition is extremely important in burn patients, secondary to the significant metabolic derangements that these injuries cause. Burns cause a persistent hypermetabolic state, which can last almost a year past the initial injury. Early enteral nutrition is proven to be beneficial, balancing the need for maintaining caloric goals, while avoiding overfeeding. Among carbohydrates, lipids, and proteins, priority is given to achieving carbohydrate goals because this has shown to have a positive effect on wound healing and spares muscle degradation.

27. **Describe specific features of electrical burns.**
Care of electrical burns is similar to that of thermal burns, except that the extent of injury may be misleading. Because bone is highly resistant to electrical current, tissue near bone (i.e., muscle) is highly susceptible to thermal injury and necrosis. This may cause large areas of necrotic tissue to form that is disproportionate to what is grossly observed because the tissue injury is under intact skin. This may lead to underfluid resuscitation when using the Parkland formula. Myoglobinuria is common, and urine output must be kept high to avoid renal injury. The development of neurological complications after electrical burns is common, including peripheral neuropathies or spinal cord deficits. Apnea may also result at the time of injury from titanic contraction of respiratory muscles or cerebral medullary injury. Cardiac dysrhythmias, including cardiac arrest, may occur up to 48 hours after injury.

KEY POINTS: THE BURNED PATIENT

1. The initial goal of resuscitation in burn patients is to correct hypovolemia. Burns cause a generalized increase in capillary permeability, with loss of significant fluid and protein into the interstitial space.
2. The Parkland formula involves giving (4 mL/kg/% TBSA) of crystalloid fluid and is a common method used to guide initial fluid resuscitation. Half of the calculated amount is given during the first 8 hours, and the remainder is given over the next 16 hours.
3. The persistence of metabolic acidosis in a patient with adequate volume resuscitation and cardiac output suggests a problem with either oxygen delivery (i.e., carboxyhemoglobin) and/or oxygen utilization by the mitochondria (i.e., cyanide toxicity).
4. There should be a low threshold for elective intubation in patients presenting with burns, as diffuse edema is common, including laryngeal edema.
5. Succinylcholine may cause hyperkalemia and cardiac arrest if given 24 to 48 hours after the initial injury. This is because of the proliferation of extrajunctional neuromuscular receptors.
6. Burned patients tend to be resistant to the effects of nondepolarizing muscle relaxants and may need 2 to 5 times the normal dose.
7. Electrical burns may cause tissue injury that is much larger than what appears on examination, as the injury is primarily because of tissue near bones under intact skin.
8. Early enteral nutrition is important for burn patients in the second phase of injury (i.e., hypermetabolism).
9. Infections are a common cause of morbidity and mortality.

SUGGESTED READINGS

Bittner EA, Shank E, Woodson L, et al. Acute and perioperative care of the burn-injured patient. Anesthesiology. 2015;122(2):448–464.
Clark A, Imran J, Madni T, et al. Nutrition and metabolism in burn patients. Burns Trauma. 2017 Apr 17;5:11.

CHAPTER 59

GERIATRIC ANESTHESIA

Paul Garcia, MD, Sona S. Arora, MD, Andrew Bowman, MD, Brian M. Keech, MD

1. **From an anesthetic perspective, what makes a patient elderly?**
   There is no universal age that defines a patient as aged/geriatric/elderly, although 65 years is used most commonly. Many debate whether considering physiological age may be more appropriate than using chronological age. Overall, elderly patients have decreased functional reserve and are at higher risk for surgical and anesthetic complications.

2. **What constitutes frailty?**
   Frailty represents a decline in multiple bodily systems and is typically associated with other geriatric syndromes, including falls and fractures, delirium and dementia, and the increased likelihood of perioperative complications. Factors associated with frailty include advanced age, lower educational level, depression, smoking, intellectual disability, poor family support, and lower socioeconomic status. Markers of frailty include weight loss, muscle weakness, decreased activity level, and the subjective experience of exhaustion from routine daily activities.

3. **Which types of procedures do geriatric patients undergo most frequently?**
   Relative to younger patients, the geriatric population has a higher rate of procedures involving the cardiovascular and urological systems, and incurs a higher number of orthopedic injuries (i.e., from falls and/or chronic degenerative arthritis). Geriatric patients also undergo emergent procedures more often than younger patients and are at greater risk for complications associated with emergent surgery.

4. **What are the overriding characteristics and principles governing age-related physiological changes as they relate to anesthesia in geriatrics?**
   Basal function of most organ systems is relatively unchanged by the aging process per se, but functional reserve and the ability to compensate for physiological stresses are reduced. However, because of the diversity of this population, the extent of age-related physiological changes for any particular individual is difficult to predict.

5. **What age-related changes occur to the cardiovascular systems of geriatric patients?**
   - Age-related wall thickening and stiffening of large elastic arteries leads to decreased arterial compliance, increased afterload and compensatory left ventricular hypertrophy (LVH).These vascular changes can occur in the absence of atherosclerosis or hypertension and are independent predictors of mortality.
   - LVH can result in diastolic dysfunction and impaired ventricular filling. Commonly in these patients, atrial contraction is necessary to maintain adequate preload and problems with atrial conduction (e.g., atrial flutter/fibrillation, junctional rhythms) can lead to profound changes in cardiac output.
   - LVH leads to elevated left ventricular end diastolic pressure and a subsequent decline in coronary blood flow, irrespective of the degree of coronary atherosclerosis present. Note the ischemic risk to the thickened left ventricular myocardium that this scenario presents.
   - Decreased venous compliance results in an impaired ability to buffer changes in intravascular volume, presenting a challenge to the maintenance of consistent preload during changing perioperative conditions. Too much intravenous fluid given too quickly may result in volume overload and flash pulmonary edema, whereas not enough can lead to hypotension and myocardial ischemia.
   - Geriatric patients have decreased adrenergic receptor mass, limiting the sympathetic nervous system's ability to respond to stress and/or hypotension. Coupled with beta blocker therapy (common in this patient population), cardiac output now becomes more dependent on stroke volume, resulting in a potentially significant decrease in cardiac output, with alterations in preload and/or afterload.
   - Baroreceptor function declines with age, resulting in labile blood pressure and orthostatic hypotension.

6. **What age-related changes occur to the pulmonary systems of geriatric patients?**
   - Decreased thoracic compliance requires increased work of breathing to maintain minute ventilation.
   - With age, closing capacity surpasses functional residual capacity, increasing the risk of atelectasis and hypoxemia, and the need for supplemental oxygen.
   - Both anatomic and physiological dead space increase with age.
   - The incidence of obstructive sleep apnea (OSA) increase with age.
   - Carotid body function declines with age, resulting in decreased compensatory responses to both hypoxemia and hypercarbia, especially with sedation.
   - Impaired swallowing mechanisms (dysphagia) and decreased pulmonary ciliary clearance increase the risk of aspiration. Couple this with a decline in muscle strength (cough) and the risk for development of perioperative pneumonia increases.

7. **What age-related changes occur to the renal systems of geriatric patients?**
   - With age, renal blood flow decreases. This leads to a decline in glomerular filtration rate (GFR), even though serum creatinine may not correspondingly increase (secondary to decreased overall muscle mass.)
   - Renal tubular function declines, resulting in impaired ability to concentrate and dilute urine when necessary. This may lead to dehydration or volume overload, respectively.
   - The ability to excrete electrolytes and medications may be affected. There is also reduced ability to renally metabolize medications.
   - Decreased renal blood flow and impaired renal autoregulation may predispose these patients to perioperative acute renal failure. Special attention needs to be paid toward the careful administration of intraoperative fluids.

8. **What age-related changes occur to the endocrine systems of geriatric patients?**
   - Geriatric patients have both decreased insulin production and decreased end organ responsiveness to insulin, predisposing them to perioperative hyperglycemia, even in the absence of diabetes. High glucose levels can lead to increased perioperative infection risk, impaired wound healing, altered mental status, and volume/electrolyte abnormalities.
   - The sympathetic response to stress is diminished because of receptor downregulation and the possible presence of antiadrenergic medications.

9. **What age-related changes occur to the gastrointestinal systems of geriatric patients?**
   - Delayed gastric emptying and dysphagia are common and probably underdiagnosed in this population. Couple these with concurrent dysfunction of the autonomic nervous system commonly seen in diabetes, and the risk for aspiration pneumonia increases.
   - There is decreased hepatic mass, blood flow, conjugating ability, and hematological protein production, resulting in several physiological changes that can impact a patient's perioperative course. Among them are altered drug metabolism and protein binding, and blood coagulation.

10. **What age-related changes occur to the nervous systems of geriatric patients?**
    - Elderly patients have increased sensitivity to the sedating effects of all anesthetic agents, decreasing minimum alveolar concentration (MAC) and MAC-awake, and possibly prolonging emergence.
    - They have decreased cerebral mass, decreased neurotransmitter synthesis, and decreased gamma-aminobutyric acid, opioid, serotonin, acetylcholine, and dopamine receptors.
    - Geriatric patients are at increased risk for the development of multiple perioperative neurocognitive disorders, including postoperative delirium (POD) and/or cognitive decline. Cognitive decline may be diagnosed up to 30 days after surgery (delayed neurocognitive recovery) or for up to 12 months (postoperative neurocognitive disorder).

11. **What is POD?**
    POD is a state of altered mental status presenting in the perioperative period and is characterized by inattention, disorganized thinking, and fluctuations in level of consciousness (either hyper or hypoactive). Common causes of delirium (perioperative or otherwise) include pain, hypoxia or hypercarbia, medications (especially polypharmacy), metabolic derangements, electrolyte and/or glucose dysregulation, urinary retention, ethanol withdrawal, and infection.

12. **Is all delirium the same?**
    No. The features of delirium can be diverse, including changes in perception, memory, language, reasoning, and visuospatial processing. From a motor perspective, patients can present as hyperactive, hypoactive, or both. Conducting a standardized cognitive assessment, preoperatively (e.g., mini-mental state examination), can assist with the postoperative evaluation of patients who are at risk by providing a baseline.

13. **Is a patient who is hyperactive upon emergence from anesthesia considered delirious?**
    No. POD is commonly confused with emergence delirium, which is also referred to as *emergence agitation*. Emergence agitation/delirium occurs upon emergence from anesthesia and typically lasts less than 30 minutes. Agitation after emergence is most common in children and young adults but may be associated with increased surgical pain in patients of any age. The association of POD with the onset of any detrimental long-term cognitive effects is questionable.

14. **How is postoperative cognitive function described outside of the perioperative period?**
    Previously, the term *postoperative cognitive decline* was used to describe abnormal cognition associated with surgery and general anesthesia. However, it has been recommended that any cognitive decline occurring up to 30 days after surgery be referred to as *delayed neurocognitive recovery*. The term *postoperative neurocognitive disorder* is used to describe cognitive declines occurring up to 12 months postoperatively. Regardless of nomenclature, risk factors for postoperative cognitive dysfunction are the same and include increased age, lower educational level and socioeconomic status, prolonged operative time (> 2 hours), major or emergency surgery, the presence of surgical complications, and previous stroke. It is difficult to determine for any single individual if the patient was destined for this dysfunction before surgery or if events occurring perioperatively were contributory.

15. **What are some strategies to help prevent the development of a perioperative neurocognitive disorder?**
    - Avoid hyperglycemia because it correlates with the occurrence of delayed neurocognitive recovery and persistent postoperative neurocognitive disorder.
    - Avoid burst suppression (and deep anesthesia), as it has been linked to POD and, in some studies, persistent perioperative neurocognitive disorders.
    - Avoid certain medications associated with PNDs perioperative neurocognitive disorders, including benzodiazepines, long-acting narcotics, anticholinergics that cross the blood-brain barrier, and certain antinausea agents, such as scopolamine, promethazine, metoclopramide, droperidol, and prochlorperazine.
    - Return assistive devices, such as glasses, hearing aids, and dentures, as soon as possible.
    - Geriatric patients are often prescribed multiple daily medications (polypharmacy), and there is a high risk for drug interactions, which may lead to PND.
    - Preventing other known causes of delirium, such as medication or alcohol withdrawal in the perioperative period should be considered.
    - No pharmacological intervention has been proven to be effective in either the prevention or treatment of perioperative neurocognitive disorders. However, risk awareness, brain monitoring for titration of anesthetic medications, and postprocedural assessments may decrease the incidence and severity.

16. **Does regional anesthesia reduce the incidence of postoperative mental status changes?**
    When used as a primary anesthetic or adjunct, regional techniques may reduce the geriatric patient's overall exposure to potentially harmful medications. The specific benefits remain controversial, but data appear to point toward reduced morbidity with the use of regional techniques in geriatric patients. It is especially helpful in the setting of skeletal fractures or elective orthopedic procedures, both of which occur at a higher rate in the geriatric population, and has been found to reduce 30-day mortality in hip fracture repair. The use of regional anesthesia may also reduce the risk of perioperative venous thromboembolism (VTE).

17. **How should perioperative drug dosing be managed for elderly patients?**
    - In general, drug dosages should be reduced for elderly patients.
    - Total body water is decreased, leading to increased serum drug concentrations with lower initial doses. In addition, reduced renal and/or hepatic clearance leads to prolonged drug half-life.
    - Circulation time may be slower in elderly patients, leading to a delayed onset of drug effect. One exception to this rests with volatile anesthetics. Alveolar concentration of a volatile anesthetic will increase more rapidly in the face of this age-related decline in circulation time, hastening the onset of induction.
    - Total body fat is increased relative to lean tissue, allowing adipose tissue to act as a medication reservoir, thereby prolonging drug elimination time for highly soluble medications.
    - Despite having a smaller muscle mass, elderly patients are not more sensitive to muscle relaxants, probably because there are fewer receptors at the neuromuscular junction.
    - Over the age of 40 years, MAC decreases by 6% per decade.
    - Analgesia can be difficult to control in the elderly because both pain and heightened sensitivity to the sedating effects of opioids can lead to delirium and respiratory depression. Despite this, pain medicine should not be withheld in elderly patients. Multimodal management of pain may be helpful. If given the choice between decreasing hypnotic agents and decreasing centrally acting opioids in an elderly patient—the hypnotic agents should be the first considered for decrease (or elimination).

18. **How are the pharmacokinetics and quality of spinal anesthesia affected by age?**
    Elderly patients have decreased blood flow to the subarachnoid space, resulting in slower absorption of spinal anesthetic solutions. They also have a smaller volume of cerebrospinal fluid (CSF), the specific gravity of which tends to be higher than that of younger patients. In addition, elderly patients may have accentuated degrees of lumbar lordosis and thoracic kyphosis, increasing both cephalad spread and pooling in the thoracic segments. Together, these lead to a higher final CSF concentration for a given drug dose and altered spread of local anesthetic. Clinically, one might see higher levels of spinal anesthesia accompanied by faster onset of action and prolonged duration. Also of note, older patients have a lower incidence of postdural puncture headaches compared with younger patients.

19. **How does epidural anesthesia change with age?**
    Neuraxial techniques are often more difficult from a technical standpoint in older patients because of calcification of the spinal ligaments and the presence of osteoarthritis and spondylosis. In addition, attaining optimal positioning can be challenging. Pharmacologically, smaller local anesthetic doses are required to achieve the same level of block when compared with younger patients, likely because of the narrowing of the vertebral canal that occurs with age.

20. **Is airway management more difficult in elderly patients?**
    Yes. It is more common for geriatric patients to be obese, edentulous, and have OSA, all increasing the likelihood for difficult mask ventilation. In addition, decreased atlantooccipital mobility, and the possibility of prior cervical spine procedures limit neck mobility.

21. **What are some other practical considerations for the perioperative care of elderly patients?**
    - Obtaining vascular access can be challenging. Neoplastic disease, frequent blood draws, and/or other chronic health conditions can make vascular access challenging. Connective tissue changes can make existing veins more susceptible to infiltration, and arterial cannulation can be more difficult secondary to arterial calcification.
    - Fragile skin calls for the judicious use of surgical tape.
    - Neuraxial techniques may be more difficult because of narrowed spinal foramina and calcified ligaments.
    - Obtaining surgical and anesthesia consent may become difficult in the setting of hearing difficulty, delirium and/or dementia.

22. **Why are elderly patients prone to hypothermia?**
    Elderly patients have a reduced basal metabolic rate, produce less body heat, and have diminished reflex cutaneous vasoconstriction to prevent heat loss. As mentioned, aging is also associated with a decrease in β-adrenergic receptors, which are integral to temperature homeostasis.

23. **Are geriatric patients at higher risk for VTE?**
    Geriatric patients can have multiple risk factors, which predispose them to VTE, including the presence of hypercoagulable states, smoking, and prior history of VTE. They also have risk factors for venous stasis, including immobility, congestive heart failure, obesity, varicose veins, and venous compression.

24. **Do all geriatric patients need higher level monitoring, that is, arterial and/or central lines?**
    Age alone is not an indication for invasive monitoring. Each patient should be assessed individually with respect for their individual comorbidities and the surgical procedure being performed. Because of the increased susceptibility to POD and/or PND, it may be prudent to use electroencephalogram monitoring to reduce exposure to anesthetic agents.

KEY POINTS:

1. There is no universal age that defines a patient as aged/geriatric/elderly, although 65 years is used most commonly.
2. Age-related physiological changes include LVH, increased reliance on preload for cardiac output, decreased venous compliance, increased closing capacity, decreased GFR, decreased hepatic function, and increased risk for the development of perioperative neurocognitive disorders.
3. Geriatric patients are more sensitive to the sedating effects of anesthetic agents.
4. In general, drug dosages should be reduced for elderly patients.

SUGGESTED READINGS

Chow WB, Rosenthal RA, Merkow RP, et al. Optimal preoperative assessment of the geriatric surgical patient: a best practices guideline from the American College of Surgeons National Surgical Quality Improvement Program and the American Geriatrics Society. J Am Coll Surg. 2012;215:453–466.

Deiner S, Silverstein JH. Postoperative delirium and cognitive dysfunction. Br J Anaesth. 2009;103(suppl 1):i41–i46.

Evered L, Silbert B, Knopman DS, et al. Recommendations for the nomenclature of cognitive change associated with anaesthesia and surgery—2018. J Alzheimer Dis. 2018;66(1):1–10.

Fried LP, Tangen CM, Walston J, et al. Frailty in older adults: evidence for a phenotype. J Gerontol A. 2001;56(3):M146–M157.

Inouye SK, Studenski S, Tinetti ME, et al. Geriatric syndromes: clinical, research, and policy implications of a core geriatric concept (editorial comments by Dr. William Hazzard on pp 794–796). J Am Geriatr Soc. 2007;55(5):780–791.

Monk TG, Weldon BC, Garvan CW, et al. Predictors of cognitive dysfunction after major noncardiac surgery. Anesthesiology. 2008;108:18–30.

LAPAROSCOPIC SURGERY

Katelyn O'Connor, MD, Raj Parekh, MD

CHAPTER 60

1. **What are the benefits of minimally invasive procedures?**
   Improvements in scope technology have allowed many procedures to be performed without large surgical incisions, affording the patient rapid recovery of function, less postoperative pain and analgesic requirements, improved postoperative pulmonary function, smaller incisions, fewer wound infections, decreased postoperative ileus, decreased length of hospitalization, and a more rapid resumption of normal daily activities.

2. **What are some currently practiced minimally invasive procedures?**
   - **General surgery:** Gastrectomy, colectomy, cholecystectomy, appendectomy, pancreatectomy, splenectomy, hepatectomy, adrenalectomy, hernia repairs, diagnostic laparoscopy, gastric bypass, gastric banding, Nissen fundoplication, feeding tube placement.
   - **Gynecological procedures:** Hysterectomy, tubal ligation, pelvic lymph node dissection, hysteroscopy, myomectomy, oophorectomy, and laser ablation of endometriosis.
   - **Thoracoscopic procedure/video-assisted thoracic surgery:** Lobectomy, pneumonectomy, wedge resection, drainage of pleural effusions and pleurodesis, evaluation of pulmonary trauma, resection of solitary pulmonary nodules, tumor staging, repair of esophageal perforations, pleural biopsy, excision of mediastinal masses, transthoracic sympathectomy, pericardiocentesis, and pericardiectomy.
   - **Cardiac surgery:** Coronary artery bypass and valve repair.
   - **Orthopedics:** Various joint procedures.
   - **Urological procedures:** Laparoscopic nephrectomy, pyeloplasty, orchiopexy, cystoscopy/ureteroscopy, and prostatectomy.
   - **Neurosurgery:** Ventriculoscopy, microendoscopic discectomy, spinal fusion, and image-guided techniques to approach masses/tumors easily.

   The focus of this chapter will be the physiological concerns associated with abdominal laparoscopy because they are common operations with profound effects on physiology.

3. **Are there any contraindications for laparoscopic procedures?**
   Relative contraindications for laparoscopy include increased intracranial pressure, patients with ventriculoperitoneal or peritoneal-jugular shunts, hypovolemia, congestive heart failure, severe cardiopulmonary disease or coagulopathy.

4. **Why has carbon dioxide become the insufflation gas of choice during laparoscopy?**
   The ideal gas would be physiologically inert, colorless, inflammable, and capable of undergoing pulmonary excretion (Table 60.1). The choice of an insufflating gas for the creation of pneumoperitoneum, pneumothorax, etc., is influenced by the blood solubility of the gas, tissue permeability, combustibility, expense, and potential to cause side effects. Carbon dioxide (CO_2) has become the gas of choice because it offers the best compromise between its advantages and disadvantages.

5. **How does CO_2 insufflation affect the partial pressure of carbon dioxide?**
   CO_2 insufflation increases the partial pressure of carbon dioxide ($PaCO_2$). The degree of increase in $PaCO_2$ depends on the intraabdominal pressure (IAP), the patient's age, underlying medical conditions, patient positioning, and mode of ventilation. In healthy patients, the primary mechanism of increased $PaCO_2$ is absorption via the peritoneum. $PaCO_2$ rises approximately 5 to 10 minutes after CO_2 insufflation and reaches plateau in 20 to 25 minutes.

6. **What is considered a safe IAP?**
   An IAP under 15 mm Hg is generally safe for surgical operations. Intraabdominal hypertension is defined as an IAP over 12 mm Hg, which can impair abdominal perfusion to vital organs, decrease pulmonary compliance, and decrease cardiac output. Because laparoscopic procedures are often performed with an IAP in the 12 to 15 mm Hg range, these operations can share the same pathophysiology, albeit to a lesser degree, as abdominal compartment syndrome (ACS). ACS is caused by edema from excess fluid administration, such as after a liver transplant or in sepsis and requires a sustained IAP over 20 mm Hg, with evidence of organ failure (e.g., renal failure) for diagnosis. To minimize the harm of iatrogenic intraabdominal hypertension, insufflation machines are often set to alarm at 15 mm Hg.

7. **How does intraabdominal hypertension affect cardiopulmonary physiology?**
   CO_2 insufflation increases IAP, causing cephalad displacement of the diaphragm, reducing functional residual capacity (FRC) and pulmonary compliance, while increasing peak airway pressures. This decrease in FRC causes atelectasis, which increases intrapulmonary shunting and promotes hypoxemia (Table 60.2). Trendelenburg position further

Table 60.1 Comparison of Gases for Insufflation

	ADVANTAGES	DISADVANTAGES
Carbon dioxide (CO_2)	Colorless Odorless Inexpensive Decreased risk of air emboli compared with other gases because of its high blood solubility	Hypercarbia Respiratory acidosis Cardiac dysrhythmias, in rare cases resulting in sudden death More postoperative neck and shoulder pain, resulting from diaphragmatic irritation (compared with other gases)
Nitrous oxide (N_2O)	Decreased peritoneal irritation Decreased cardiac dysrhythmias (compared with CO_2)	Supports combustion and may lead to intraabdominal explosions when hydrogen or methane is present Greater decline in blood pressure and cardiac index (compared with CO_2)
Air		Supports combustion Higher risk of gas emboli (compared with CO_2)
Oxygen (O_2)		Highly combustible
Helium	Inert Not absorbed from abdomen	Greatest risk of embolization

Table 60.2 Pulmonary Changes Associated With Laparoscopy

INCREASED	DECREASED
Peak inspiratory pressure	Functional residual capacity
Intrathoracic pressure	Respiratory compliance
$PaCO_2$	pH
Atelectasis and Shunt	PaO_2/FiO_2

FiO_2, Fraction of inspired oxygen; $PaCO_2$, partial pressure of carbon dioxide; PaO_2, partial pressure of oxygen.

aggravates these changes. Vascular compression from intraabdominal hypertension can increase systemic vascular resistance (increased afterload) and decrease venous return (decreased preload), which together can decrease cardiac output, which may only be clinically apparent in patients with a history of heart failure or situations with severely elevated IAP.

8. How do you calculate abdominal perfusion pressure? How does a decreased abdominal perfusion pressure affect visceral organs?

$$APP = MAP - IAP$$

APP, abdominal perfusion pressure; MAP, mean arterial pressure; IAP, intrabdominal pressure
   Decreased abdominal perfusion pressure (APP) is caused by an elevated IAP, which may be exacerbated by a low cardiac output, causing decreased mean arterial pressure. One of the most sensitive end organs to low perfusion is the kidney, which initially manifests as low urine output and in severe situations as acute kidney injury. Together, these hemodynamic effects result in catecholamine release and activation of the renin-angiotensin system. Hepatoportal arterial and venous blood flow may also decrease and elevated liver enzymes have been noted after prolonged laparoscopic cases. Splanchnic microcirculation is also decreased.

9. What hemodynamic effects may occur upon entering the peritoneal cavity?
   Insertion of the trocar (portal used to introduce instruments into the peritoneal cavity) or Veress needle (spring-loaded needle used to create pneumoperitoneum) can cause vagal stimulation, such as bradycardia, atrioventricular dissociation, nodal rhythm, and even asystole. Peritoneal stretch from gas insufflation can also result in vagal stimulation.

10. Describe anesthetic techniques used for minimally invasive surgery.
   Minimally invasive surgery can be performed under local anesthesia with intravenous sedation (i.e., monitored anesthesia care), regional anesthesia (e.g., spinal), and general anesthesia (GA), the most common technique. In the case of laparoscopic surgery, unexpected conversion from a laparoscopic to an open procedure must be

considered when choosing an anesthetic technique. Advantages of GA include optimal muscle relaxation, ability to position the patient as needed, ability to control ventilation, protection from gastric aspiration, and a quiet surgical field. Urinary bladder and gastric decompression are often done to decrease the risk of visceral puncture and improve the surgical field in laparoscopic operations.

11. **Should inhaled nitrous oxide be used as an anesthetic adjuvant during laparoscopy?**
Nitrous oxide (N_2O) is often avoided because of concerns of bowel distention and increased postoperative nausea and vomiting.

12. **Can laparoscopy be performed on children or pregnant women?**
Laparoscopic surgery is commonly performed in pediatric populations. Children undergo similar physiological changes and experience similar benefits of laparoscopic procedures as adults. CO_2 absorption in infants may be faster and more profound than in adults because of a greater peritoneal surface area to body weight ratio.

Pregnancy was initially considered to be a contraindication to laparoscopic surgery because of concerns regarding decreased uterine blood flow, increased intrauterine pressure, and resultant fetal hypoxia and acidosis. Multiple reports have since determined that laparoscopic surgery is safe in pregnancy and does not result in increased rates of fetal morbidity or mortality. Procedures should be performed in the second trimester if possible. Body positioning should avoid inferior vena cava compression (i.e., left uterine displacement). Abdominal insufflation pressure should be kept as low as possible in pregnant patients to minimize its physiologic effects on perfusion and venous return.

13. **What complications are associated with laparoscopic surgery and CO_2 pneumoperitoneum?**
Complications are most likely to occur during placement of the trocar/Veress needle through the abdominal wall and CO_2 insufflation.
   - **Intraoperative complications:** Major vessel injury, hemorrhage, organ perforation, bladder and ureter injury, burns, cardiac arrhythmias (atrioventricular dissociation, nodal rhythms, bradycardia, and asystole), hypercapnia, hypoxemia, CO_2 subcutaneous emphysema, pneumothorax, gas embolism, endobronchial intubation, increased intracranial pressure, and aspiration. Other complications are also possible depending on the specific procedure performed.
   - **Postoperative complications:** Postoperative nausea and vomiting, pain, shoulder and neck pain secondary to diaphragmatic irritation, deep venous thrombosis, delayed hemorrhage, peritonitis, wound infection, pulmonary dysfunction, and incisional hernia have all been noted.

14. **What is robotic laparoscopic surgery?**
The use of robotic operations, such as the Da Vinci system, has recently exploded in the field of surgery. Although very similar to laparoscopic surgery in terms of insufflation, extra care must be taken in terms of space in the operating room and positioning of the patient because of the size of the robot. Access to the patient in general, and most importantly to the airway, is extremely limited, and careful planning should be implemented before the start of the procedure.

SUGGESTED READINGS

Hayden P, Cowman P. Anaesthesia for laparoscopic surgery. Cont Educ Anaesth Crit Care Pain. 2011;11(5):177–180.
Antoniou SA, Antoniou GA, Antoniou AI, et al. Past, present, and future of minimally invasive abdominal surgery. J Soc Laparoendosc Surg. 2015 Jul-Sep;19(3).
Galaal K, Donkers H, Bryant A, et al. Laparoscopy versus laparotomy for the management of early stage endometrial cancer. Cochrane Database Syst Rev. 2018 Oct 31;10:CD006655.
Miller RD. Miller's Anesthesia. 8th ed. Philadelphia, PA: Elsevier Saunders; 2015.
Barash PG, Cahalan MK, Cullen BF, et al. Clinical Anesthesia. 8th ed. Philadelphia, PA: Wolters Kluwer/Lippincott Williams & Wilkins; 2017.

CHAPTER 61

MAJOR VASCULAR SURGERY

Sama Ansari, MD, Raj Parekh, MD

1. **What are some examples of major vascular surgery?**
   - Endovascular aneurysm repair (EVAR): stents passed through an artery (usually femoral) and guided to the aorta via fluoroscopy without operating directly on the aorta.
   - Open aortic surgery: direct repair of the aorta via abdominal or retroperitoneal incision.
   - Carotid endarterectomy: removing an atherosclerotic plaque in the carotid artery to correct stenosis and reduce risk of stroke.
   - Vascular bypass: procedure that redirects blood flow by reconnecting blood vessels to bypass a diseased artery (e.g., fem-fem, fem-tib, aortoiliac).
   - Arteriovenous fistula creation: surgical connection between artery and vein to provide vascular access for hemodialysis.
   - Vein stripping: surgical removal of varicose veins.
   - Angioplasty: endovascular procedure to widen stenosed arteries and veins.

2. **Define aortoiliac occlusive disease.**
   Aortoiliac occlusive disease is a type of peripheral arterial disease (PAD) that is characterized by atherosclerotic changes within the aorta (usually abdominal) that extend into the iliac and femoral arteries, which results in hypoperfusion of vital organs and the lower extremities. Involvement at the iliac bifurcation and renal arteries is common; aneurysmal changes may be found as well.

3. **Define abdominal aortic aneurysm.**
   An abdominal aortic aneurysm (AAA) is a focal dilation that is 1.5 times the artery's normal diameter and is a relatively common cause of sudden death in the elderly (approximately 5% of sudden deaths). A normal aortic diameter is approximately 2.0 cm; therefore an AAA is 1.5 times this diameter or 3 cm. The majority of AAAs are asymptomatic, but some patients may present with abdominal pain and other complications (e.g., thrombus). Approximately 50% of patients with a ruptured AAA reach the hospital alive and half of those patients do not survive. Aneurysm size is the greatest predictor of potential rupture and the risk of rupture increases substantially with diameters greater than 5.5 cm. Elderly male patients (i.e., 65–75 years) that have a significant smoking history should be screened for AAA by ultrasound. An AAA found to be greater than 5.5 cm in diameter or increasing at a rate greater than 0.5 cm in diameter over the past 6 months, regardless of size, warrant surgical repair.

4. **What risk factors and coexisting diseases are common in patients with aortoiliac occlusive disease or AAA?**
   Risk factors include smoking, family history, obesity, atherosclerotic disease elsewhere, advanced age, and male gender. Common diseases include hypertension, ischemic heart disease, heart failure, chronic obstructive pulmonary disease (COPD), diabetes mellitus, chronic kidney disease, and carotid artery disease. Patients with AAA have a similar risk profile but smoking appears to be the strongest risk factor above all else.

5. **Describe the presence of coexisting cardiovascular disease in patients presenting for vascular surgery and how these patients may be optimized for surgery.**
   Coronary artery disease is the major cause of perioperative mortality and morbidity. Myocardial infarction occurs in 4% to 15% of patients and heart failure is noted in 30% of postoperative aneurysm repairs. Per American College of Cardiology (ACC)/American Heart association (AHA) guidelines, patients should generally undergo preoperative cardiac testing (e.g., stress echo) before undergoing large vascular operations if they have a history of cerebrovascular disease, diabetes mellitus, heart failure, and/or limited cardiopulmonary reserve, such as metabolic equivalents (METS) less than 4.

6. **List the appropriate intraoperative monitors for large vascular operations.**
   - Standard ASA monitors including electrocardiogram lead V5 to increase sensitivity to detect ischemia.
   - Intraarterial monitoring rapidly detects swings in blood pressure and facilitates laboratory analysis.
   - Foley catheter to monitor urine output.
   - Use of central venous pressures, pulmonary artery catheters, and/or transesophageal echocardiography is appropriate when severe heart failure, valvular disease, or pulmonary hypertension is present.
   - Somatosensory and motor-evoked potential can be considered if spinal cord ischemia is a significant risk.

7. Discuss the physiological implications of aortic clamping and unclamping.

Aortic cross-clamping increases systemic vascular resistance and left ventricular afterload, which is an enormous stress on the heart, particularly in a patient population that has significant risk factors for coronary artery disease and ischemic cardiomyopathy. Methods to minimize the physiological effects from cross-clamp include increasing the depth of anesthesia, vasodilator therapy, with nitroglycerin or sodium nitroprusside, and possible administration of α-blockers or calcium channel blockers. Suprarenal cross-clamp significantly increases the risk of postoperative acute kidney injury (AKI). The potential for a clinically profound decrease in anterior spinal artery blood flow is more likely in thoracic aortic operations and may necessitate a lumbar drain to remove cerebrospinal fluid to optimize spinal cord perfusion.

Hypotension and a decrease in systemic vascular resistance often occurs after unclamping because of venous return of acidotic blood containing ischemic metabolites, lactic acid, and potassium.

8. Review the anesthetic goals for large vascular operations.
- Maintain cardiac output and coronary perfusion, while limiting myocardial workload by controlling heart rate and afterload, especially during aortic cross-clamping.
- Aggressively replace blood loss with crystalloids, colloids, and blood products when necessary. This patient population may do better with a more liberal transfusion threshold.
- Maintain oxygenation and ventilation guided by blood gas analysis. Excessive ventilatory pressures may compromise preload.
- The best way to preserve renal function is to maintain normal intravascular volume, cardiac output, and oxygenation.
- Blood glucose should be monitored and controlled, regardless if they have a formal diagnosis of diabetes, as many patients are either at risk or have undiagnosed diabetes. Uncontrolled hyperglycemia can cause hypovolemia, electrolyte abnormalities, increased surgical site infections, and ketoacidosis in severe cases.
- Hypoperfusion of the anterior spinal artery during aortic cross-clamping or extended hypoperfusion places the patient at risk for paraplegia, especially during thoracic aortic surgery.
- Before unclamping, an intravenous bolus of fluid is wise. It may be necessary to reclamp the aorta or provide some minor degree of occlusion to allow the patient time to equilibrate and stabilize.

9. What can be done intraoperatively to preserve renal function?

Major factors that affect postoperative renal function include preoperative renal function, the degree of aortic disease, the duration of cross-clamp, and the amount of contrast agent given during an operation. Therefore optimizing renal function before surgery, maintaining euvolemia and renal perfusion, and minimizing cross-clamp time are paramount. Nephrotoxic medications (e.g., gentamicin, vancomycin) or medications that decrease renal blood flow (nonsteroidal antiinflammatory drugs) should be avoided. Urine output during the procedure does not necessarily correlate with kidney function (e.g., antidiuretic hormone is a stress hormone) and administering diuretics (e.g., furosemide and mannitol) to increase urine output does not reduce the incidence of postoperative AKI. Diuretics may lead to electrolyte abnormalities, such as hypokalemia, which increases the risk of dysrhythmias. Evidence does not support dopamine to prevent AKI.

10. What are the potential advantages to postoperative epidural analgesia?

Epidural anesthesia may suppress sympathetic tone and the stress response, while providing excellent analgesia. This limits myocardial work by attenuating tachycardia and hypertensive swings in patients predisposed to cardiac ischemia. It also provides titratable postoperative pain relief without excessive sedation. However, a concern with neuraxial procedures, such as an epidural, is hematoma formation causing acute cauda equina in the setting of anticoagulation with heparin, which is often given for vascular operations. In general, neuraxial techniques are considered safe practice, provided heparin is given at least 1 hour following spinal or epidural placement.

11. Describe endovascular repair of the aorta and its advantages over open repair.

EVAR uses stents passed through an artery (usually femoral) and guided to the aorta via fluoroscopy without operating directly on the aorta. It is most commonly used for AAA repair but may be used to treat thoracic aortic disease (i.e., TEVAR). An EVAR can be done under general, neuraxial, or local anesthesia. Compared with open repair, the endovascular approach involves reduced time under anesthesia, less fluid and hemodynamic support, reduced blood loss, less pain and trauma associated with major abdominal surgery, and reduced length of stay in the hospital. The risk of cardiac, pulmonary, and renal complications is reduced as well. Overall, the main benefit with EVAR over open surgical repair is lower perioperative mortality (0.5%–2% vs. 3%–5%). The open repair is considered more definitive and long-term outcomes appear to be similar between both approaches; however, this may change with improvements in stent technology.

12. What are the different types of aortic dissections?

An aortic dissection occurs when the innermost layer of the aorta is injured. Blood then flows into this tear causing the inner and middle layers to separate. There are two major types of aortic dissections (Stanford type A and type B) defined by the location of the tear. Type A dissections originate in the ascending aorta and may extend as far down to arteries in the lower extremities. Type A dissections may involve the aortic valve leading to aortic insufficiency. Conversely, a type B dissection involves a tear that originates distal to the left subclavian artery. Risk factors include, trauma, connective tissue disease, bicuspid aortic valve, hypertension, and illicit drugs, such as methamphetamine or cocaine.

13. **Discuss the medical management of aortic dissections.**
Management of aortic dissections depends on the type of dissection. Type A dissections are usually considered a surgical emergency because these patients are at a high risk for rupture, aortic valve involvement, stroke, myocardial infarction, and cardiac tamponade. They require immediate surgical treatment. Medical management is preferred for uncomplicated type B dissections, with surgery reserved for more complex cases. The primary goal of medical management is strict blood pressure control with a goal mean arterial pressure of 60 to 70 mm Hg and to minimize shearing forces on the aortic wall with beta blockers as first-line treatment (e.g., esmolol infusion). Vasodilating agents (e.g., nicardipine, sodium nitroprusside) are reserved for refractory cases.

14. **How do you manage a patient presenting with a ruptured AAA?**
Most patients should be taken immediately to the operating room, while being resuscitated, because rapid surgical intervention is necessary to prevent death. Multiple large-bore intravenous lines are necessary to facilitate volume resuscitation, along with intraarterial monitoring. The patient should have 10 units of blood available, universal donor blood if necessary, and the laboratory should be made aware that this case will probably require massive transfusion. Coagulopathy is ideally assessed with thromboelastography. A lower systolic blood pressure (i.e., <100 mm Hg) is ideal to minimize bleeding, although communication about hemodynamic goals should involve the surgical team.

KEY POINTS: MAJOR VASCULAR SURGERY

1. Comorbidities for patients undergoing vascular surgery include coronary artery disease, hypertension, COPD, chronic kidney disease, and diabetes mellitus.
2. Preoperative assessment, testing, and evaluation should be considered for patients with multiple comorbidities and/ or poor cardiopulmonary reserve (i.e., METS < 4) as per ACC/AHA guidelines.
3. The most common cause of perioperative mortality is cardiac disease. Postoperative renal failure is also an important independent predictor of mortality.
4. Cross-clamping increases systemic vascular resistance, blood pressure, and afterload, whereas unclamping causes vasodilation because of the return of acidotic blood containing ischemic metabolites, lactic acid, and potassium.
5. Stanford type A dissections involve the ascending aorta and are a surgical emergency, whereas type B dissections are distal to the left subclavian and can be medically managed.
6. Patients presenting with a ruptured AAA have a high mortality and should be taken emergently to the operating room for surgical intervention and volume resuscitated with blood products.

SUGGESTED READINGS

Barash PG, Cahalan MK, Cullen BF, et al. Clinical anesthesia. 8th Ed. Philadelphia, PA: Wolters Kluwer/Lippincott Williams & Wilkins; 2017.
Fann JI, Mitchell RS, Kaiser C, et al. Vascular surgery. In: Jaffe RA, Golianu B, Schmiesing CA, editors: Anesthesiologist's Manual of Surgical Procedures, 5th ed. Philadelphia: Lippincott Williams & Wilkins; 2014:405–458.
Fleisher LA, Fleischmann KE, Auerbach AD, et al. DN: 2014 ACC/AHA guideline on perioperative cardiovascular evaluation and management of patients undergoing noncardiac surgery: a report of the American College of Cardiology/American Heart Association Task Force on practice guidelines. J Am Coll Cardiol. 2014 Dec 9;64(22):e77–e137.
Mackey DC, Wasnick JD, Butterworth J. Morgan & Mikhail's Clinical Anesthesiology. 5th ed. New York: McGraw-Hill Education LLC; 2013.
Toshihiro F. Management of acute aortic dissection and thoracic aortic rupture. J Intensive Care. 2018;6:15.

CHAPTER 62

CARDIAC SURGERY: CARDIOPULMONARY BYPASS

Barbara Wilkey, MD, Nathaen Weitzel, MD

1. **What are the main functions of the cardiopulmonary bypass (CPB) circuit?**
   The CPB circuit functions as the temporary equivalent of the native cardiopulmonary system. The CPB circuit allows for perfusion of the patient's vital organs, while oxygenating the blood and removing carbon dioxide (CO_2). Isolation of the cardiopulmonary system allows for surgical exposure of the heart and great vessels along with cardiac electrical silence and a bloodless field.

2. **What are the basic components of the CPB circuit?**
   The CPB circuit has a venous line that siphons central venous blood from the patient into a reservoir. Blood reaches the venous reservoir via gravity or vacuum assist. Blood is then passed through an oxygenator, CO_2 removed, and then returned to the patient's arterial circulation. The pressure needed to perfuse the arterial circulation is generated by either a roller head or a centrifugal pump. The flow is usually nonpulsatile although some roller pumps can deliver pulsatile flow. The machine also has roller head pumps for cardioplegia administration, a ventricular vent to drain the heart during surgery, and a pump sucker to remove blood from the surgical field. In addition, the circuit contains filters for air and blood microemboli, because both can cause devastating central nervous system injury if delivered to the arterial circulation. A heat exchanger is present to produce hypothermia on bypass and warm the patient before separating from CPB. The venous reservoir must never be allowed to empty while on CPB because a life-threatening air embolism could result.

3. **Define the different levels of hypothermia. What are typical CPB temperatures?**
   - Mild: 32°C to 35°C
   - Moderate: 26°C to 31°C
   - Deep: 20°C to 25°C
   - Profound: 14°C to 19°C
     Typical CPB temperatures range from 28°C to 34°C Profound levels of hypothermia (14°C–19°C) is used for total circulator arrest, although this level of hypothermia is not necessary for all circulatory arrest cases.

4. **What are the adverse effects of hypothermia?**
   Adverse effects of hypothermia include coagulopathy because of platelet dysfunction and decreased synthesis and kinetics of clotting enzymes, hypocalcemia because of decreased metabolism of citrate, dysrhythmias, increased risk of infection, decreased oxygen unloading from hemoglobin, potentiation of neuromuscular blockade, and impaired cardiac contractility.

5. **Why is hypothermia used for patients on CPB?**
   Systemic oxygen demand decreases 9% for every degree of temperature drop. Hypothermia, therefore, allows for a lower CPB pump flow, while providing adequate oxygen delivery to vital organs. The main concern with CPB is the prevention of myocardial and central nervous system injury, along with renal and hepatic protection.

6. **What are the risk factors for acute kidney injury (AKI) in the peribypass period?**
   AKI is a common complication following CPB with an incidence of 20% to 30%. Risk factors include advanced age, female gender, preoperative renal insufficiency, ejection fraction less than 40%, diabetes mellitus, hemodilution on CPB, use of an intraaortic balloon pump, CPB duration, and complex cardiothoracic surgeries. Of these risk factors, preexisting renal dysfunction has the highest risk for postoperative AKI.

7. **What interventions reduce the risk of postoperative AKI?**
   There is no full-proof method for preventing AKI after CPB. Recommended methods include identifying high-risk patients, optimizing renal perfusion (e.g., goal-directed perfusion), avoiding a long CPB duration, and avoiding nephrotoxic medications.

8. **What is goal-directed perfusion (GDP)?**
   GDP is based on the theory that maintaining an adequate mean arterial pressure (MAP) does not guarantee adequate oxygen delivery to end organs. GDP evaluates multiple metabolic parameters, but in its simplest form, GDP

assesses oxygen delivery (DO_2) and carbon dioxide production (VCO_2). DO_2 can be altered by changing pump flow (i.e., cardiac output) and hemoglobin concentration. In the setting of tissue hypoxemia, acidosis develops and as a result VCO_2 increases. A DO_2 less than 270 mL/min/m^2 and a DO_2/VCO_2 ratio of less than 5 is associated with AKI after CPB.

9. **Discuss the traditional cannulation sites for CPB**
   Venous blood is typically obtained through cannulation of the right atrium, using a dual-stage cannula that drains both the superior and the inferior vena cava. Alternatively, for open-heart procedures, bicaval cannulation is used with direct, separate cannulation of the superior and inferior vena cavae. Arterial blood is returned to the patient via the ascending aorta proximal to the innominate artery. The femoral artery and vein can also be used as alternative cannulation sites. The drawbacks to femoral bypass include ischemia of the leg distal to the arterial cannula, inadequate venous drainage, possible inadequate systemic perfusion secondary to a small inflow cannula, and difficulty in cannula placement owing to atherosclerotic plaques. Axillary artery cannulation can be used for repeat sternotomies and is often carried out before the sternotomy to allow for arterial fluid or blood administration from the CPB machine during the sternal dissection if necessary. Cannulation of the brachiocephalic or axillary artery may be used if circulatory arrest is planned.

10. **How do the cannulation sites for minimally invasive valve operations compare to traditional cannulation sites for CPB?**
    Venous drainage is generally achieved by placing a single-stage catheter in the right atrium or superior vena cava via the femoral vein (Fig. 62.1). The drainage holes in the catheter should always sit in the right atrium. Venous drainage can be augmented using a vacuum assist system on the bypass machine. If needed, additional drainage may be achieved by placing a venous cannula via the internal jugular vein. In lieu of an internal jugular cannula, an endopulmonary vent catheter may be placed for additional drainage if the surgical approach is through the left atrium. Arterial cannulation can be peripheral (generally femoral) or direct (through thoracotomy). There are three general systems for antegrade cardioplegia administration: (1) either placement of a balloon in the aortic root that occludes and delivers cardioplegia, (2) cross-clamping through the sternotomy with direct placement of an aortic root vent, or (3) if the surgery is an aortic valve replacement, the surgeon can directly apply cardioplegia to the coronaries after the root is opened. Retrograde cardioplegia can be delivered by direct cannulation of the coronary sinus, through the thoracotomy incision or via a percutaneous technique (Fig. 62.2).

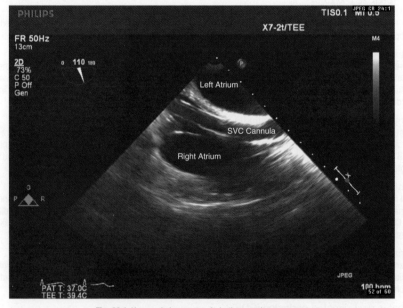

Fig. 62.1 Venous drainage cannula in the superior vena cava.

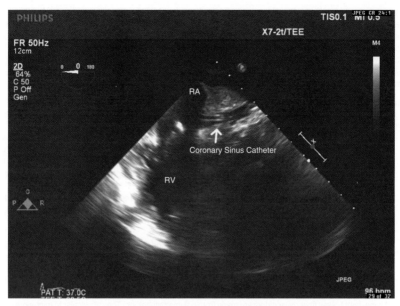

Fig. 62.2 Coronary sinus catheter for delivery of retrograde cardioplegia. *RA*, Right atrium; *RV*, right ventricle.

11. **What are the basic anesthetic strategies used for cardiac surgical operations that involve CPB?**
    Anesthetic strategies take into consideration the degree of systolic dysfunction, the extent of coronary disease, the magnitude of valvular disease, and the overall exercise tolerance. Patients undergoing CPB are considered high-risk for intraoperative awareness; however, this is likely from the previously popular high-dose opioid technique. The conduct of cardiac anesthesia has moved away from such techniques of the past, which involved high-dose opioid and long-acting neuromuscular blocking agents, as they were associated with prolonged time to extubation in the intensive care unit and delayed ambulation. Techniques that mitigate these problems and facilitate quick extubation (i.e., < 4 hours postoperatively) and early ambulation are known as *fast-tracking*. This involves administering short-acting and more carefully dosed neuromuscular blocking agents and opioids. In addition, medications, such as acetaminophen, ketorolac, dexmedetomidine, and ketamine along with regional techniques, such as parasternal blocks placed by the surgeons may be used for opioid sparing analgesia.

12. **What steps does an anesthesiologist need to take during conventional cannulation?**
    For a primary sternotomy, ventilation should be held. During aortic cannulation, hypertension should be avoided to minimize the risk of aortic dissection with a target systolic blood pressure of 120 mm Hg or less. During venous cannulation, the use of low tidal volume ventilation may improve surgical access, as the lungs will not encroach on the surgical field. Transesophageal echocardiography (TEE) is routinely used to guide coronary sinus catheter placement (e.g., to administer retrograde cardioplegia). In general, the anesthesiologist should visually follow progress on the field from sternotomy through cannulation, as this can be a time of significant blood loss and hemodynamic shifts.

13. **When and how is circulatory arrest used?**
    The technique of circulatory arrest is *most often* used when conditions (either anatomy or planned surgical procedure) are not amendable for flow through a bypass circuit. A common example is surgery on the aortic arch. In general, in aortic arch surgery, the patient is placed on CPB until: (1) he or she is cooled to the desired temperature, and (2) the surgeon is ready to place the aortic graft. At that point, flow is stopped through the bypass circuit. Hypothermia is used to decrease metabolic demand, but the degree of hypothermia targeted varies by each surgeon's clinical practice. Circulatory arrest can be accompanied by isolated cerebral perfusion or no cerebral perfusion. Isolated cerebral perfusion may be antegrade or retrograde, unilateral or bilateral. Antegrade cerebral perfusion is often delivered via a catheter in the axillary artery or innominate artery that directs blood up the carotid artery, as opposed to retrograde cerebral perfusion delivered via a catheter in the superior vena cava.

14. **What are additional anesthetic considerations associated with circulatory arrest?**
Patients who undergo hypothermic circulatory arrest are at increased risk for coagulopathy, neurologic sequelae, renal failure, and pulmonary dysfunction. In addition to standard monitoring during CPB, neurologic monitoring should be used, such as an electroencephalogram (EEG) or bispectral index. In theory, obtaining an isoelectric EEG before circulatory arrest will decrease cerebral oxygen demand during this low to no-flow state; however, strong data showing benefit is lacking. Packing the head in ice and administering lidocaine and steroids may also be neuroprotective.

15. **What are the different oxygenators used in CPB?**
Oxygenators are designed to allow gas exchange in a manner similar to the human lung. There are multiple types of oxygenators available for use, such as the following:
1. Direct contact oxygenators: Examples of direct contact oxygenators include bubble, screen, rotating disc, and drum oxygenators. All direct contact oxygenators work by: (1) creating oxygen bubbles that serve as the surface for gas exchange, and (2) placing the blood in direct contact with these bubbles. Although the device is simple, conceptually there are functional limitations with this design. Common problems are the buildup of foam on the oxygenators and damage to blood cells from direct contact
2. Membrane oxygenators use a semipermeable silicone membrane that allows for diffusion of O_2 and CO_2. Advantages of membrane oxygenators over direct contact oxygenators include the ability to control O_2 and CO_2 independently, and less cellular damage. However, they require a large surface area, and therefore a larger priming volume, which can absorb some medications
3. Microporous oxygenators are made of polypropylene fibers or sheets that use a countercurrent blood flow system. This design allows for a low surface area and a small priming volume compared with membrane oxygenators. Although plasma leak can occur over time, this is often not problematic within the time frame for most cardiac operations. If this type of oxygenator is used for long-term support (i.e., intensive care unit [ICU]) plasma leak may become problematic
4. Plasma-tight hollow fiber oxygenators are made from polymethylpentene. They are similar to micropore oxygenators in that they require low priming volumes, but they are not associated with problems because of plasma leakage. This feature makes this type of oxygenator ideal for long-term mechanical support in the ICU setting.

16. **What is meant by "pump prime"? What is the usual hemodynamic response to initiating bypass?**
"Pump prime" involves priming solutions (i.e., crystalloid, colloid, or blood) that are used to fill the CPB circuit. When bypass is initiated, the circuit must contain fluid to perfuse the arterial circulation until the patient's blood can circulate through the pump. Priming volumes historically were 1.5 to 2 L, but newer CPB circuits can achieve priming volumes as low as 650 to 800 mL for an open circuit, and even less with a so-called closed or mini-bypass circuit. Reductions in priming volume have resulted in decreased inflammatory response and a reduction in transfusion requirements. The acute hemodilution from the patient's circulating blood volume mixing with the prime volume can cause an acute reduction in MAP and hemoglobin concentration.

17. **Why is systemic anticoagulation necessary?**
Contact activation of the coagulation system occurs when nonheparinized blood contacts the synthetic surfaces of the CPB circuit, resulting in widespread thrombosis, oxygenator failure, and death. In a dire emergency, a minimum standard dose of 300 units/kg of heparin must be given through a central line before the initiation of bypass. If there is inadequate anticoagulation before the initiation of CPB, a clot will form within the CPB circuit. This is often a catastrophic event. Following separation from the CBP machine, protamine is used to bind heparin and reverse the anticoagulant effect.

18. **How is the adequacy of anticoagulation measured before and during bypass?**
An activated clotting time (ACT) is measured about 3 to 4 minutes after heparin administration and every 30 minutes on CPB. An ACT of 400 seconds or longer is considered acceptable. Heparin levels are frequently measured, but only the ACT is a measure of anticoagulant activity. This is particularly important in patients with heparin resistance (seen with preoperative heparin infusions) and antithrombin III deficiency.

19. **What must be ascertained before placing a patient on CPB?**
- Adequate arterial inflow of oxygenated blood with acceptable line pressures
- Sufficient venous return to the bypass pump
- Adequate anticoagulation (i.e., ACT > 400 seconds)
- If used, proper placement of retrograde cardioplegia cannula
- Arterial line to monitor real time blood pressure
- Core temperature monitoring
- Adequate depth of anesthesia

20. **Why is a left ventricular vent used?**
A left ventricular vent is used to prevent left ventricular distention during CPB, such as from aortic insufficiency or normally physiologic blood flow through the bronchial and thebesian veins. Left ventricular distention is problematic

as it can increase intraventricular pressure (i.e., myocardial wall tension), causing myocardial ischemia by precluding adequate subendocardial cardioplegia distribution and elevating myocardial oxygen demands. A left ventricular vent placed through the right superior pulmonary vein, decompresses the left side of the heart and returns blood to the CPB pump.

21. **What are the characteristics of cardioplegia?**
Cardioplegia can be crystalloid based or blood based. It can be dosed intermittently or continuously. Cardioplegia perfuses through the coronary vasculature and keeps the transmembrane potential in a resting state, thereby reducing myocardial oxygen and energy requirements to those of cellular maintenance. The mechanisms of various cardioplegia solutions include (but are not limited to) hyperkalemic arrest, hypocalcemia, high-dose adenosine/lidocaine/magnesium, and potassium adenosine triphosphate channel opening. Cardioplegia can be perfused either anterograde via the aortic root/coronary ostia or retrograde through a catheter in the right atrial coronary sinus.

22. **Discuss myocardial protection during CPB. What elements should be in place to optimize myocardial protection?**
Cellular integrity must be maintained during CPB to ensure cardiac performance after CPB. A critical factor to prevent cellular damage is intraoperative myocardial protection. Preservation of the balance between myocardial oxygen consumption and delivery can be optimized by the following:
- Adequate cardioplegia
- Hypothermia, specifically myocardial hypothermia with myocardial temperature goals below 12°C to 15°C
- Topical cooling of the heart with icy saline slush
- Left ventricular venting to prevent distention
- Insulating pad on the posterior cardiac surface to prevent warming from mediastinal blood flow
- Minimizing bronchial vessel collateral flow (which also rewarms the arrested heart)
  Inadequate preservation during CPB manifests as impaired cardiac output, ischemic electrocardiogram (ECG) changes, wall motion abnormalities on TEE, dysrhythmias, and the requirement for inotropic support.

23. **What is the function of an aortic cross-clamp?**
Clamping across the proximal aorta isolates the heart and coronary circulation. The arterial bypass inflow enters the aorta distal to the clamp. Antegrade cardioplegia is infused between the clamp and aortic valve, thus entering the coronary circulation. This isolation of the heart from the systemic circulation allows for prolonged cardioplegia activity, diastolic arrest of the heart, and profound myocardial cooling.

24. **Review the physiologic responses to CPB**
- Stress hormones, including catecholamines, cortisol, angiotensin, and vasopressin increase in part because of decreased metabolism
- Exposure of blood to the CPB circuit results in complement activation, initiation of the coagulation cascade, and platelet activation. A systemic inflammatory response is also initiated
- Platelet dysfunction associated with CPB may contribute to post-CPB bleeding
- Hemodilution associated with onset of CPB decreases the serum concentrations of most drugs but decreased hepatic and renal perfusion during CPB will eventually increase the serum concentration of drugs administered by continuous infusion

25. **What are the differences between pH-stat and α-stat methods of atrial blood gas measurement?**
There are differing opinions as to whether blood gases should be corrected for the temperature during CPB because the solubility of gases decreases with hypothermia. All blood gases are analyzed at 37°C. In pH-stat measurements, the obtained value is corrected on a nomogram, and the reported values refer to the partial pressure at the hypothermic temperatures. CO_2 is then added to the system to correct the acid-base status. More commonly, blood gases are reported uncorrected for patient temperature, a method referred to as α-stat blood gas management. Studies comparing the two methods show conflicting results, with the main concern related to the alteration in cerebral vascular tone because of the CO_2 management. In adults, α-stat management tends to show better neurologic outcomes and is the method most commonly used. Neonatal data, however, tend to show better neurologic outcomes with pH-stat management and is the most common method used for this population.

26. **Develop an appropriate checklist for discontinuing bypass**
- Check arterial blood gases and other laboratory results to assess acid-base balance, ensuring neutral pH, base deficit, and $PaCO_2$. Assess hemoglobin and electrolytes
- Ascertain adequate systemic rewarming, typically 37°C
- Recalibrate (i.e., "zero") all pressure transducers
- Ensure adequate cardiac rate and rhythm (patients may require pacing)
- Reexamine the ECG for rhythm and ischemia
- Evaluate TEE looking for signs of ischemia (regional wall motion abnormalities), along with evaluation of valves, specifically in operations of valve replacement or repair

- Remove intracardiac or intraaortic air if the aorta or cardiac chambers were opened. Note, TEE is an invaluable modality to assess for air
- Initiate ventilation of lungs

27. **How is the heparin effect reversed? What are the potential complications?**
Protamine, a positively charged protein molecule, binds the negatively charged heparin molecule and this complex is removed from the circulation by the reticuloendothelial system. Although there are different regimens to determine how much protamine should be administered, the simplest and most common method is to dose protamine based on the heparin administered (approximately 1 mg protamine per 100 units heparin). The efficacy of heparin reversal is most often assessed by ACT. Protamine administration is associated with systemic hypotension because of anaphylactoid or true anaphylactic reactions, along with catastrophic pulmonary hypertension because of anaphylactoid thromboxane release. Risk factors for such reactions include preexisting pulmonary hypertension, patients with diabetes mellitus treated with NPH insulin, and rapid bolus protamine administration.

28. **Why is cardiac pacing frequently needed after bypass?**
Between the ischemic insult of bypass, the residual effect of cardioplegia, and effects from hypothermia, cardiac conduction may be impaired and myocardial wall motion suboptimal. Sequential cardiac pacing at a rate of 80 to 100 beats per minute can significantly improve cardiac output. Remember, cardiac output equal heart rate times stroke volume!

29. **What are some of the things to consider if a patient has difficulty weaning from CPB?**
From a surgical standpoint, the adequacy of the surgical procedure (whether it be coronary artery bypass, valve replacement, or otherwise) should be reconsidered. TEE can evaluate regional wall motion abnormalities and valvular competency. The right and left ventricular filling pressure should be assessed by both TEE and invasive monitors. Other hemodynamic variables, such as cardiac index, mixed venous oxygen concentration, pulmonary artery pressure, pulmonary artery occlusion pressure, and systemic vascular resistance should be assessed.

30. **What are some therapies for the patient with impaired cardiac performance or difficulty weaning from CPB?**
Problems that might be encountered with weaning from CPB include reduced systemic vascular resistance (i.e., vasoplegia) and decreased cardiac contractility. Vasopressor agents and, in refractory cases, methylene blue is used to treat vasoplegia, whereas decreased contractility is treated with inotropic agents and, in refractory cases, an intraaortic balloon pump may be needed. Right heart dysfunction and/or pulmonary hypertension may also complicate weaning from bypass. Agents, such as nitric oxide or vasodilator therapy targeted toward the pulmonary system can be useful in this situation. TEE is invaluable in guiding these decisions along with the interpretation of the pulmonary artery catheter. If separation from CPB is not possible or sustainable with the methods noted earlier, extracorporeal membranous oxygenation (ECMO) should be considered.

31. **What is ECMO?**
ECMO is a mechanical method of providing oxygenation (venovenous ECMO) and or circulatory support (venous-arterial [V-A] ECMO) outside of the operating room. A full discussion of ECMO is beyond the scope of this chapter, but we will review basics here. When used to facilitate separation from CPB, V-A ECMO is almost always required. As with CPB, a venous cannula drains blood to an oxygenator, and a pump then moves the oxygenated blood through an arterial cannula to the body. Cannulation for ECMO can either be central or peripheral. Peripheral ECMO is often accomplished by cannulating the femoral artery and vein. If peripheral ECMO is used, an arterial line should be placed in the right radial artery to monitor for potential oxygenation mismatch between the upper and lower body. A problem that can occur with peripheral ECMO is a mismatch in oxygen delivery between the upper and lower body called *North-South (Harlequin) syndrome*. This is caused by an adequately functioning heart but poorly functioning lungs. Poorly oxygenated blood returns to the left heart and is subsequently ejected into the aorta. This preferentially delivers poorly oxygenated blood to the upper body, while the lower body receives well oxygenated blood from the peripheral ECMO circuit.

32. **Review the central nervous system complications of CPB**
There is about a 1% to 3% incidence of new neurologic events, defined as stroke (including vision loss), transient ischemic attack, or coma. There is also about a 3% incidence of deterioration in intellectual function, memory defects, or seizures, although sensitive neurocognitive testing reveals a much higher incidence (20%–60%) of cognitive dysfunction at 1-month and 6-month intervals. However, much of the cognitive dysfunction will resolve over a number of months. Cerebral microemboli, in particular platelet microemboli, are believed to be a contributing factor.

33. **What can decrease the incidence of such complications?**
- Reversible factors should be identified before surgery involving CPB. For instance, patients with significant carotid artery stenosis may require correction of this problem before undergoing CPB (perhaps during the same surgery). Because significant aortic atherosclerosis is an independent risk factor for stroke, avoiding aortic

cross-clamping by using an off-pump surgical strategy may benefit some of these patients. Alternatively, an anepiaortic probe may be used to find an atheroma-free area for cross-clamping
- Initially, it was thought that off-pump coronary artery bypass graft (CABG) would result in improved neurologic outcomes compared with patients undergoing CABG with CPB. Although study results vary, the majority of data do not support improved neurocognitive outcomes in patients who have undergone off-pump CABG
- Decrease cerebral oxygen consumption using hypothermia. Maintenance of adequate cerebral perfusion pressure (i.e., MAP > 60 mm Hg, assuming normal intracranial pressure/central venous pressure) and mixed venous oxygen saturation is important to optimize cerebral supply and demand
- TEE may identify a patent foramen ovale, significant atheromatous disease at the site of aortic cannulation, left atrial thrombi, and intracardiac air, all of which may contribute to a change in subsequent management
- Avoiding hypoglycemia and hyperglycemia is likely beneficial

KEY POINTS: CARDIOPULMONARY BYPASS

1. Patients must be completely anticoagulated before CPB is initiated; otherwise, a dire thrombotic complication may occur.
2. The CPB reservoir should never become empty while on CPB; otherwise, a dire complication from air embolism may occur.
3. Factors involved in myocardial preservation include cardioplegia, myocardial hypothermia, and ventricular venting. Consequences of inadequate myocardial preservation include decreased cardiac output, ischemia, dysrhythmias, and failure to wean from CPB.
4. Always consider imperfect surgical technique (e.g., kinking of graft, valve failure) when a patient is failing to wean from CPB.
5. Neurologic complications, in particular neurocognitive deficits, are common after CPB.

SUGGESTED READINGS

Gravlee G. Cardiopulmonary Bypass and Mechanical Support: Principles and Practice. 4th ed. Philadelphia: Wolters and Kluwer; 2016.
Kumar A, Suneja M. Cardiopulmonary bypass-associated acute kidney injury. Anesthesiology. 2011;114:964–970.
Ranucci M. Anaesthesia and cardiopulmonary bypass aspects of fast track. Eur Heart J Suppl. 2017;19:A15–A17.
Rupprecht L, Kunz D, Phillip A, et al. Pitfalls in percutaneous ECMO cannulation. Heart Lung Vessel. 2015;7(4):320–326.
Uyasl S, Reich D. Neurocognitive outcomes of cardiac surgery. J Cardiothorac Vasc Anesth. 2013;27:958–971.
Vernick W, Woo J. Anesthetic considerations during noninvasive mitral valve surgery. Semin Cardiothorac Vasc Anesth. 2012;16(1):11–24.
Wilkey BJ, Weitzel NS. Anesthetic considerations for surgery on the aortic arch. Semin Cardiothorac Vasc Anesth. 2016;20(4):266–272.
Welsby IJ, Um J, Milano CA, et al. Plasmapheresis and heparin reexposure as a management strategy in cardiac surgical patients with heparin-induced thrombocytopenia. Anesth Analg. 2010;110:30–35.

CHAPTER 63

THORACIC SURGERY: LUNG ISOLATION TECHNIQUES

Lawrence I. Schwartz, MD, Mark D. Twite, MB, BChir, FRCP, Monica Hoagland, MD

1. **What are the indications for lung isolation?**
   The absolute indications for lung isolation include:
   1. Protection of a healthy lung from contamination by a diseased lung (i.e., hemorrhage, pulmonary infection, or bronchopulmonary lavage)
   2. Provision of differential lung ventilation in the setting of unilateral lung disease (i.e., bronchopulmonary fistula or large pulmonary cysts or bullae)

   Lung isolation is relatively indicated to improve surgical exposure for procedures performed in the thoracic cavity. In the setting of difficult airway or severe patient comorbidities, the safety and need for lung isolation should be discussed with the surgeon before proceeding. For small children, surgical exposure is often achieved with CO_2 pneumothorax or manual retraction of the operative lung, rather than lung isolation.

2. **What types of surgical procedures usually require lung isolation?**
   Thoracic surgical procedures that may require lung isolation include:
   1. Surgery on the lung, bronchus, or pleura
   2. Surgery on the heart, great vessels, or pericardium
   3. Esophageal surgery
   4. Thoracic spine procedures from an anterior approach

3. **What are the techniques for achieving lung isolation?**
   There are three basic techniques for lung isolation:
   1. Left or right double-lumen endotracheal tube (DLT)
   2. Single-lumen endotracheal tube (ETT) with a bronchial blocker (BB)
   3. Single-lumen ETT placed in a mainstem bronchus (MSB)

4. **Describe DLTs.**
   A DLT consists of two ETTs of unequal lengths molded together with high-volume, low-pressure cuffs located proximal to each luminal opening (endotracheal and endobronchial). Each lumen can be used to isolate, selectively ventilate, or deflate the right or left lung independently, and is color-coded (white for tracheal and blue for bronchial) at the luminal cuff and at their respective pilot balloon. The tracheal cuff is proximal to the tip of the endotracheal lumen and is positioned above the carina; the smaller, blue bronchial cuff is proximal to the endobronchial lumen and is positioned within the MSB. Left and right DLTs are designed to have their respective bronchial lumen placed into the corresponding side MSB. The distal end of a DLT is bifurcated, with a color coded airway tube for each lumen, each attaching to a 15 mm circuit connector adapter.

5. **How does the right main stem bronchus differ from the left? How does this affect right-sided DLT design?**
   The right MSB has a wider lumen and leaves the trachea at a straighter trajectory than the left MSB. The right bronchus has three branches (upper, middle, and lower lobes), whereas the left has only two (upper and lower lobes). The left MSB is longer than the right, with the left upper and lower lobe bronchi diverging from the MSB about 5 cm from the carina. On the right, the upper lobe bronchus leaves the MSB about 1.5 to 2 cm from the carina. The right bronchus intermedius continues and divides into the middle and lower lobe bronchi more distally. Of note, the origin of the right upper lobe bronchus is variable and can sometimes arise from the carina or even the trachea (tracheal or porcine bronchus).

   Left- and right-sided DLTs differ in the angulation of the endobronchial lumen and in the location of the endobronchial cuff. Right DLTs have a less angulated bronchial lumen to accommodate the trajectory of the right MSB. Also they have a side port and bronchial cuff that is configured to allow ventilation of the right upper lobe bronchus (when properly positioned). The short length of the right MSB and potential anatomic variation can make proper placement of a right DLT difficult.

6. **Describe the placement and positioning of DLTs.**

   Under direct laryngoscopy, the lubricated DLT is passed through the vocal cords with the distal curvature (bronchial tip) concave anteriorly. The stylet is then removed and, as the tip passes the larynx, the tube is rotated 90 degrees toward the side of the bronchus to be intubated. Final positioning can be achieved either by auscultation or with fiberoptic bronchoscopy (FOB).

   Using auscultation, the DLT is advanced gently, until resistance is felt when the endobronchial lumen enters the bronchus. In turn, the endobronchial and tracheal cuffs are then inflated and their lumens clamped while the chest is auscultated bilaterally. A properly positioned left DLT will produce breath sounds on the left side exclusively when the endotracheal lumen is clamped and on the right side exclusively when the endobronchial lumen is clamped. The reverse is true for a right DLT. Note that auscultation alone is often unreliable for proper DLT placement, necessitating bronchoscopy.

   Using FOB, the bronchoscope is advanced through the endobronchial lumen of the DLT into the trachea and the appropriate side bronchus. Then, using the bronchoscope as a stylet, the DLT is advanced over the scope into the bronchus. Finally, the bronchoscope is withdrawn from the endobronchial lumen and passed through the tracheal lumen to confirm subcarinal position of the bronchial cuff and ensure patency of the opposite side MSB. It is important to note that the DLT can become dislodged during changes in patient position (e.g., turning to lateral decubitus or head movement), and positioning should be reconfirmed after any of these events. Lastly, when using a right-sided DLT, it must be ensured that the endobronchial cuff does not block the right upper lobe bronchial orifice. Because this often presents a challenge, many clinicians use left sided DLTs almost exclusively, even when isolation of the right lung is indicated. See Figure 63.1.

7. **What are the indications for a right DLT?**

   Right DLTs are indicated when there is left bronchial pathology (i.e., endoluminal tumors, endobronchial compression, trauma, or tracheobronchial disruption), or when the surgical procedure involves the left MSB (i.e., sleeve resection, lung transplantation, or bronchopleural fistula repair). The only contraindication to a right DLT is a porcine bronchus, in which the right upper lobe bronchus arises at or above the carina.

8. **How do you select the appropriate size DLT?**

   The optimal DLT size is the largest one that will pass atraumatically through the glottis and trachea into the bronchus, with only a small air leak detectable when the cuff is deflated. Using the largest possible DLT allows for better ventilation and clearance of secretions, lower ventilating pressures, faster operative lung collapse and less work of breathing during spontaneous ventilation at the end of the procedure. However, larger DLTs may be more difficult to place and/or cause airway trauma. Smaller DLTs may be easier to place, but the endobronchial cuff will require more volume to create an adequate seal, thereby increasing the potential for bronchial injury or cuff herniation across the carina. They are also more likely to become displaced during the procedure.

   Unfortunately, there is no reliable guideline for choosing the correct size DLT. MSB diameters do not reliably correlate with gender, height, or weight. The best estimate (when feasible) comes from measuring the airway diameter with radiological imaging. Many anesthesiologists will select 39 to 41 French ([Fr]; 1 Fr = 0.33 mm) DLTs for adult men (using height of 5′10″ as a cut-off) and 35 to 39 Fr DLTs for adult women (using heights of 5′5″ and 5′10″). The smallest DLT is a 26 Fr, which can be used in children as young as 8 years old.

9. **Describe bronchial blockers.**

   BBs are passed through (or alongside) a regular ETT and guided into either MSB using FOB to achieve lung separation (as opposed to lung isolation). They may also be used for selective lobar blockade. BBs have a balloon at the tip to occlude the ipsilateral bronchus and may possess a hollow center channel that can be used to provide continuous positive airway pressure (CPAP) or assist with suctioning of the operative lung.

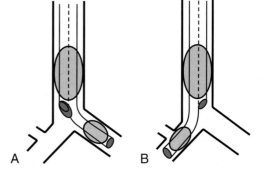

Fig. 63.1 (A) Double-lumen endotracheal tube correctly positioned in the left mainstem bronchus (MSB). (B) Double-lumen endotracheal tube correctly positioned in the right MSB. However, notice the position of the bronchial cuff on the endotracheal tube and the right upper lobe bronchus take off.

The surgeon must be notified when a BB is being used, as it may need to be repositioned to avoid inclusion into the staple line for procedures involving the MSB.

10. **Describe the placement of BBs.**

BBs are usually used in conjunction with standard oral ETTs, but they may also be used with nasotracheal tubes, tracheostomy tubes, or even laryngeal masks airway (LMAs). The BB and bronchoscope are ideally passed through the tracheal tube together, but this requires a tube with a minimum internal diameter of 4.5 mm. When smaller ETTs are used, the blocker is passed alongside the tracheal tube. Each type of BB has a unique mechanism for placement, but all require FOB guidance.

1. Arndt endobronchial blocker™ (Cook Medical): This BB has a nylon wire loop at its distal tip. The bronchoscope is threaded through the wire loop and then used to guide the blocker into position. Once positioned, the wire can be removed to allow suctioning and CPAP to the operative lung. Note that the nylon wire cannot be reinserted, making repositioning difficult if the BB becomes dislodged. The Arndt endobronchial blocker is the most commonly used BB for pediatric patients and the smallest available size is 5 Fr.

2. Cohen endobronchial blocker™ (Cook Medical): The proximal end of this blocker contains a wheel, which controls the distal tip. The wheel is used to guide the blocker into the correct bronchus under FOB visualization.

3. Univent tube™ (Fuji Systems Corporation): This is a single-lumen ETT with an external channel that houses a built-in bronchial blocker. The BB is composed of malleable material that allows the preshaped tip to be positioned into either MSB, under FOB guidance. The blocker of the Univent tube is also available separately as the Uniblocker. The Univent tube offers the advantage of greater stability (dislodgement is less likely as the blocker is secured to the ETT). However, the presence of the blocker channel decreases the cross-sectional area available for the ventilating lumen, causing a disproportionately high resistance to airflow, especially in smaller sized tubes. In larger tubes, CPAP and suctioning can be applied through the lumen of the BB.

4. Rüsch EZ-Blocker™ (Teleflex): Has a unique, "Y"-shape, with the bifurcation sitting just distal to the carina and one distal tip extending into each MSB. These BBs are easy to place and allow for right or left lung separation without any repositioning needed.

5. Vascular balloon catheters: Vascular catheters, such as the Fogarty arterial embolectomy catheter (Edwards Lifesciences), have been used successfully as off-label BBs. These are available in small sizes (2–3 Fr) and are used mainly in pediatric patients. The balloon cuff, unfortunately, possesses a low-volume, high-pressure cuff, which may increase the risk of a bronchial mucosal injury. Also, these lack a central channel for CPAP or suctioning.

Deflation of the operative lung for most BBs occurs by absorption atelectasis, which may increase the time required to achieve adequate surgical visualization.

11. **Can a single-lumen endotracheal tube be used to achieve lung isolation?**

Yes. A standard single-lumen ETT can be selectively advanced into the MSB of the nonoperative lung. The operative lung will then gradually become atelectatic and collapse. This is a simple and fast technique that can be useful in emergent situations, and for children who are too small for DLTs or BBs.

Placement of an ETT into the right MSB is easier because it diverges from the long axis of the trachea at a less acute angle than the left MSB does. Turning the patient's head to the right may better align the trachea and left MSB, improving the likelihood of success when attempting placement on the left side.

When using a cuffed ETT, the distance from the proximal cuff to the distal tip must be shorter than the length of the MSB to allow ventilation of all lung lobes. Pediatric microcuffed ETTs may not be as useful for right MSB intubation, as they lack a "Murphy eye" and, as a result, may compromise right upper lobe ventilation. Using an ETT with a Murphy eye avoids this potential problem.

12. **Discuss the relative advantages and disadvantages of each technique for lung isolation and/or lung separation?**

DLTs and bronchial blockers are the most commonly used techniques for achieving one-lung ventilation (OLV) in adults. DLTs can be placed without a bronchoscope and are more likely to remain positioned correctly than BBs. Once in place, they provide true lung isolation, as opposed to merely lung separation. Another important advantage is the ability to provide CPAP to the nonoperative lung during periods of hypoxemia. Disadvantages include an increased likelihood in such complications as sore throat, hoarseness, and airway injury. Initial tracheal cannulation can be more difficult than placing a single lumen ETT, and postoperative ventilation with a DLT is not recommended.

Bronchial blockers are more difficult to position and always require FOB guidance. However, they are advantageous in patients with a difficult airway or in those who may require postoperative ventilation. There is no significant difference between the two techniques in the time t, or quality of, lung collapse.

Mainstem placement of a single lumen ETT is an easy technique, but is generally reserved for emergency situations and pediatric patients (Table 63.1).

13. **What are the complications of OLV?**

1. Malposition: A correctly positioned device should allow ventilation of all lobes on the nonoperative side, while completely excluding all lobes on the operative side. Because of the anatomy of the tracheobronchial tree, devices placed into the right MSB may occlude the right upper lobe bronchus and impede ventilation or collapse of that lobe. In addition, a correctly placed device can migrate intraoperatively because of surgical manipulation

Table 63.1 Advantages and Disadvantages of Techniques Used for One-Lung Ventilation/Lung Isolation

TECHNIQUE	ADVANTAGES	DISADVANTAGES
Single-lumen tube in the nonoperative bronchus	Simple, fast placement No special equipment needed Useful technique for emergencies and small children	Cannot provide CPAP, suction or perform bronchoscopy to the operative lung Long time to operative lung collapse (absorption atelectasis) Difficult to obtain adequate seal (especially with uncuffed ETTs) Right mainstem placement may obstruct right upper lobe Left mainstem placement can be difficult
Balloon-tipped bronchial blocker in the operative bronchus	Can use with multiple different airways (oral or nasal ETT, tracheostomy, LMA) Can provide continuous ventilation during placement Can provide CPAP (marginally) to the operative lung Allows selective lobar isolation Easy return to two-lung ventilation if needed postoperatively Best device for patients with difficult airways	Requires FOB for placement Long time for placement Repositioning often required (frequent dislodgement and loss of seal) Small channel for suctioning and CPAP for the operative lung Cannot perform bronchoscopy in the operative lung
DLT	Rapid, more reliable placement Can place without FOB (but this is not recommended) Can ventilate, suction and perform bronchoscopy for either lung Can provide CPAP to the operative lung Easy conversion between one- and two-lung ventilation Best device for absolute lung isolation	Difficult to select appropriate size (not available for small children) Right-sided DLT may be difficult to position properly Difficult to place in patients with difficult laryngoscopy Risk of airway injury Not suitable for postoperative ventilation

CPAP, Continuous positive airway pressure; *DLT,* Double-lumen endotracheal tube; *ETT,* endotracheal tube; *FOB,* fiberoptic bronchoscopy; *LMA,* laryngeal mask airway.

or changes in patient position. Bronchial blockers may be particularly difficult to reposition once dislodged. This can lead to inadequate surgical exposure, contamination of the healthy lung or, in the case of proximal migration of the bronchial cuff into the trachea, complete obstruction of ventilation and acute hypoxemia.

2. Airway trauma: DLTs have a higher incidence of airway injury than BBs. These injuries include sore throat, hoarseness, and potentially catastrophic tracheal injuries. Bronchial injuries can be seen with both DLTs and BBs when the bronchial cuff is overinflated. This is more common when an inappropriately-sized, small DLT is used. To prevent overinflation, direct FOB visualization should be used to ensure that the cuff is inflated just enough to seal the bronchus (rarely >2 mL of air). The cuff should be deflated promptly when OLV is no longer required.

3. Hypoxemia and respiratory acidosis: Discussed later.

4. Surgical complications: A BB or the endobronchial lumen of a DLT can be accidentally incorporated into a surgical staple line across the MSB. Communication with the surgeon is imperative to prevent this complication.

14. Describe OLV techniques for patients with a difficult airway.
In patients who present with a difficult airway and require OLV, the safest approach is to first establish an airway with a single-lumen ETT. OLV may then be achieved by using a BB or by placement of a DLT, using an airway catheter exchange technique. Bronchial blockers are particularly useful in this patient population, as they can be used with oral or nasal ETTs, tracheostomy tubes, or even LMAs.

15. Describe OLV techniques for pediatric patients.
Lung isolation techniques are limited in pediatric patients because of the small size of the pediatric airway. OLV is not often required in children under 2 years old, as adequate surgical exposure can be achieved by CO_2 pneumothorax or manual retraction of the operative lung. In cases where OLV is required, mainstem placement of an ETT is the preferred technique for infants and small children. BBs can be used in children as young as 6 months of age. The smallest available DLT (26 Fr) can be used in children as young as 8 years of age (Table 63.2).

Table 63.2 Airway Devices for Pediatric Lung Isolation

AGE (YEARS)	MAINSTEM ETT (ID)	BRONCHIAL BLOCKER (FR)	UNIVENT TUBE (ID)	DLT (FR)
0–0.5	3.5			
0.5–2	4.0	5		
2–4	4.5	5		
4–6	5.0	5		
6–8	5.5	5	3.5	
8–10	6.0 (cuffed)	5–7	3.5	26
10–12	6.5 (cuffed)	5–7	4.5	26–28
12–14	6.5–7.0 (cuffed)	5–7	4.5–6.0	32
14–16	7.0 (cuffed)	7–9	6.0–7.0	35–37
16–18	7.0–7.5 (cuffed)	7–9	7.0–7.5	35–39

DLT, Double-lumen endotracheal tube; *ETT*, endotracheal tube.

16. **Describe the physiology of OLV.**
    Under normal physiological conditions, ventilation and perfusion are well matched because dependent portions of the lungs receive both greater perfusion and greater ventilation. This is because of gravitational effects on blood flow and lung compliance. The initiation of OLV stops all ventilation to one lung, which would theoretically create a 50% right-to-left shunt and relative hypoxemia if pulmonary perfusion remained unchanged. However, the actual shunt fraction is usually only around 25% because of the following:
    1. Atelectasis and surgical manipulation of the nonventilated lung obstruct vascular flow to that lung.
    2. Hypoxic pulmonary vasoconstriction (HPV) decreases blood flow to the nonventilated lung, redirecting it toward the ventilated lung. Of note, both anesthetic medication choice and ventilation strategy can impair compensatory HPV, resulting in hypoxemia.
    3. Lateral positioning of the patient increases perfusion to the dependent (ventilated) lung.

17. **Describe how patient positioning affects OLV physiology? How is this different for children?**
    For adults and older children undergoing OLV, ventilation/perfusion ($\dot{V}/\dot{Q}$) matching is best in the lateral decubitus position with the operative (or diseased) lung in the nondependent position, as is required for surgery. However, this is not the case for infants and small children. Positioning infants and young children with the ventilated lung in a dependent position worsens $\dot{V}/\dot{Q}$ matching for the following reasons:
    1. Infants have an easily compressible rib cage, which cannot fully support the dependent lung. The ventilated lung is therefore prone to atelectasis when in the dependent position.
    2. In adults, gravitational force increases perfusion to the dependent lung relative to the nondependent lung. This improves $\dot{V}/\dot{Q}$ matching during OLV. However, because of their small size, infants have a reduced hydrostatic pressure gradient and do not benefit from these gravitational effects in the lateral decubitus position.
    3. In adults, the elevated abdominal hydrostatic pressure on the dependent-side results in diaphragmatic loading on that side, and hence, a mechanical advantage during spontaneous ventilation. This gradient is also decreased in infants, reducing any functional advantage to lateral decubitus position for them.
    4. Infants and small children have a reduced functional residual capacity, resulting in airway and alveolar closure at tidal volume breathing.
    These factors, combined with the increased rate of oxygen consumption in small children leads to a greater incidence of hypoxemia when positioned in the lateral decubitus position.

18. **Discuss HPV.**
    HPV is a reflex constriction of vascular smooth muscle in the pulmonary circulation in response to low regional oxygen tension. It diverts blood from poorly ventilated to better-ventilated lung segments, thereby improving $\dot{V}/\dot{Q}$ matching and decreasing hypoxemia. During OLV, the maximal HPV response decreases blood flow to the nonventilated lung by approximately 40% to 50%. This response is biphasic, consisting of a rapid initial reduction (minutes) in perfusion, followed by a delayed, more robust reduction (hours) that has a slow offset. This pattern results in an arterial oxygen level that usually nadirs at around 20 to 30 minutes, after initiating OLV, then gradually increases over the next 1 to 2 hours.
    The slow offset has important clinical implications. Repeated cycling of OLV on an ipsilateral lung during a procedure will result in lesser degrees of hypoxemia because the HPV response is already active at the start of subsequent cycles. However, when patients undergo bilateral thoracic procedures, they will become more hypoxemic with OLV of the contralateral lung because the HPV reflex is still working to shift perfusion away from the previously deflated lung that is now being ventilated.

Table 63.3 Factors Affecting Hypoxic Pulmonary Vasoconstriction

HPV IS POTENTIATED (DECREASED SHUNT, IMPROVED OXYGENATION)	HPV IS ATTENUATED (INCREASED SHUNT, WORSENED OXYGENATION)
Acidosis (metabolic or respiratory)	Alkalosis (metabolic or respiratory)
Hyperthermia	Hypothermia
Decreased mixed venous oxygen saturation (decreased cardiac output)	Vasodilators
Vasoconstrictors	Volatile anesthetic agents (minimal clinical effect)

HPV, Hypoxic pulmonary vasoconstriction.

19. **What factors affect HPV?**
    HPV can be potentiated (causing decreased shunt/improved oxygenation) or attenuated (causing increased shunt/worsening oxygenation) by a variety of drugs and physiological factors (including acid-base status, temperature, and hemodynamic status.) The goals of anesthetic management during OLV include managing these variables as well as possible, so as to minimize their effects on HPV (Table 63.3).

20. **What anesthetic agents should be used during OLV?**
    All volatile anesthetic agents inhibit HPV in a dose-dependent fashion in vivo, theoretically worsening hypoxemia. However, this effect is often not clinically significant. One review found no evidence that the choice of inhalational or intravenous anesthetic agents affects patient outcomes, while another found that volatile agents are associated with a decrease in inflammatory mediators, pulmonary complications, and length of stay compared with intravenous agents. Based on these data, the classic recommendation for using total intravenous anesthesia during OLV may no longer be valid. Also of note, commonly used concentrations of epidural local anesthetics do not affect oxygenation during OLV.

21. **What ventilation strategies are appropriate during OLV?**
    OLV can result in hypoxemia attributed to V/Q mismatch, as well as lung injury because of the use of nonphysiological tidal volumes, loss of normal functional residual capacity, and hyperperfusion of the ventilated lung. These changes increase the risk of postoperative pulmonary complications, which are among the main causes of morbidity/mortality after lung surgery.
    - Lung protective ventilation strategies, including low tidal volumes (4–6 mL/kg), use of positive end-expiratory pressure (PEEP) of 5 cm H_2O or higher, permissive hypercapnia and recruitment maneuvers, are associated with decreased postoperative pulmonary complications and preserved gas exchange. The use of PEEP and alveolar recruitment maneuvers in the ventilated lung are particularly important when low tidal volume ventilation is used to prevent atelectasis and hypoxemia.
    - The inspired concentration of oxygen should be decreased to the lowest level required to maintain adequate oxygenation. Sustained exposure to 100% oxygen can cause resorption atelectasis and decrease the effectiveness of recruitment maneuvers.
    - An increased inspiratory:expiratory ratio is helpful to avoid auto-PEEP and lung overdistention.
    - Although pressure controlled ventilation provides theoretical benefits over volume controlled ventilation, including lower airway pressures and fewer hemodynamic effects, studies have not found a consistent benefit for pressure controlled ventilation during OLV.

22. **What are the causes of hypoxemia during OLV?**
    Hypoxemia (oxygen saturation <85%–90% or arterial partial pressure of oxygen [PaO_2] <60 mm Hg) occurs in approximately 5% of OLV cases. Reasons include:
    1. Patient factors: of note, patients who present preoperatively with obesity, low baseline PaO_2, and/or normal perfusion to the operative lung (diseased lungs often have reduced perfusion), have a higher incidence of hypoxemia during OLV. Pediatric patients are prone to atelectasis and V/Q mismatch, with subsequent hypoxemia during OLV in the lateral position.
    2. Surgical factors: right-sided surgery (i.e., requiring left-sided OLV) and procedures performed in the supine position are associated with higher rates of hypoxemia.
    3. Inappropriate ventilation strategies: atelectasis in the ventilated lung (low tidal volumes without PEEP or recruitment maneuvers) results in hypoxemia. In addition, high airway pressures in the ventilated lung can divert blood flow to the nonventilated lung, thereby increasing shunt and hypoxemia.
    4. Inadequate lung isolation: improperly positioned lung isolation devices can result in impaired ventilation and subsequent hypoxemia.

23. **How should hypoxemia be managed during OLV?**
    1. Increase the inspired oxygen concentration to 100%. Remember to bring it back to its previous levels (if possible) after resolution of the hypoxemic event.
    2. Check the position of the lung isolation device with FOB to rule out device malposition.
    3. Suction any blood or secretions present.

4. Optimize ventilation of the dependent lung, using recruitment maneuvers and PEEP to prevent atelectasis, and limiting inspiratory pressures to prevent diversion of blood flow to the nonventilated lung.
5. Provide oxygen to the operative lung via apneic oxygenation or CPAP. This will oxygenate the residual pulmonary blood that is not being shunted away from the operative lung by HPV.
6. Notify the surgeon. Returning to two-lung ventilation and/or placement of a clamp on the operative-side pulmonary artery may be required to treat hypoxemia.

24. **How do you resume intraoperative two-lung ventilation for the different lung separation devices?**

For patients with a MSB ETT, two-lung ventilation is easily resumed by withdrawing the tube to a tracheal position. BBs are simply removed and ventilation is continued through the in situ airway device (ETT, tracheostomy, or LMA). With a DLT, the bronchial cuff is deflated, and ventilation is resumed through both lumens of the DLT.

If postoperative ventilation is required, ideally, the DLT should be changed to a single lumen ETT to decrease the likelihood of ongoing airway trauma. It is important to note that this may be very difficult to do after a prolonged thoracic surgery in the presence of bleeding, increased secretions, and airway edema. If a DLT has to be left in place postoperatively, it is essential that receiving staff be familiar with its design and function.

KEY POINTS

1. OLV can be achieved with DLTs, BB, and standard single-lumen ETT, each of which has advantages and disadvantages.
2. Selection of an appropriate OLV device depends on surgical requirements, patient characteristics, and operator comfort. DLTs are more reliable, BBs may be advantageous for patients with a difficult airway.
3. Device malposition is a common complication during OLV. Positioning should be reassessed with FOB whenever circuit pressurization changes and/or a patient becomes hypoxemic.
4. Choice of anesthetic (inhalational vs. intravenous agents, with or without epidural placement) does not have a significant clinical effect on oxygenation during OLV.
5. Protective ventilation strategies during OLV include low tidal volume ventilation (4–6 mL/kg), PEEP (5 cm H_2O), limited peak airway pressures, and permissive hypercapnia.
6. Methods to improve oxygenation during OLV include increasing inspired oxygen, confirming placement of lung isolation device, clearing secretions from the airway, applying PEEP to the ventilated lung/CPAP to the nonventilated lung, asking the surgeon to manually restrict pulmonary blood flow to the nonventilated lung and, as a last resort, returning to two-lung ventilation.

Website

Thoracic Anesthesia: www.thoracic-anesthesia.com. Excellent site with many articles and an online bronchoscopy simulator.

SUGGESTED READINGS

Brodsky JB. Lung separation and the difficult airway. Br J Anaesth. 2009;103:i66–i75.
Campos JH. Hypoxia during one-lung ventilation: a review and update. J Cardiothorac Vasc Anesth. 2018;32(5):2330–2338.
Clayton-Smith A. A comparison of the efficacy and adverse effects of double-lumen endobronchial tubes and bronchial blockers in thoracic surgery: a systematic review and meta-analysis of randomized controlled trials. J Cardiothorac Vasc Anesth. 2015;29:955–966.
El Tahan MR. Impact of low tidal volumes during one-lung ventilation. A meta-analysis of randomized controlled trials. J Cardiothorac Vasc Anesth. 2017;31:1767–1773.
Fitzgerald J. Techniques for single lung ventilation in infants and children. Anesthesia Tutorial of the Week. Oct 23, 2015. www.wfsahq.org/resources/anaesthesia-tutorial-of-the-week
Letal M. Paediatric lung isolation. BJA Educ. 2017;17:57–62.
Lumb AB. Hypoxic pulmonary vasoconstriction. Anesthesiology. 2015;122:932–946.
Pedoto A. How to choose the double-lumen tube size and side: the eternal debate. Anesthesiol Clin. 2012;30:671–681.
Senturk M. Intraoperative mechanical ventilation strategies for one-lung ventilation. Best Pract Res Clin Anesthesiol. 2015;29:357–369.

CHAPTER 64

SPINE SURGERY

Anthony M. Oliva, MD, PhD

1. **What are the common indications for spine surgery?**

   By-and-large, spinal deformity is the most common reason a patient requires surgery. Causes of the deformity are usually developmental, such as scoliosis, or degenerative processes. Other reasons for spine surgery include injury from trauma, mass resection, osteomyelitis, and neurological decompensation. These procedures are usually elective but can be urgent or emergent in certain situations.

2. **What are the anesthetic considerations for spine surgery?**

   The site of surgery (i.e., lumbar, cervical, thoracic) and the planned surgery (fusion, microdiscectomy, number of levels, etc.) are the primary determinants of developing an anesthetic plan. Surgeons can approach the spine anteriorly, laterally, or posteriorly depending on the patient's pathology.

   - **Airway:** Surgery on the cervical spine may be associated with challenges in airway management because of significant limitations in neck range of motion. Moreover, with an anterior approach to the cervical spine, a specialized endotracheal tube that monitors vocal cord activity is typically used to provide information about possible recurrent laryngeal nerve injury. In the setting of cervical spine injury, great care is required to secure the airway in a safe manner. Direct laryngoscopy is rarely used for endotracheal tube placement. Instead, video laryngoscopy and fiberoptic bronchoscopy are commonplace, as they require less neck motion during laryngoscopy. In certain circumstances, an awake fiberoptic intubation is necessary. Postoperatively, airway swelling must be considered and the anesthesiologist needs to proceed with extubation cautiously. Airway edema is more likely to be encountered in cervical spine procedures, long procedures, and procedures with large volume of fluid administration.

   - **Positioning:** The surgical approach dictates patient positioning and the anesthesiologist is instrumental in ensuring the patient is properly positioned. Most often a posterior approach is used; thus the patient is positioned prone. In this instance, great care must be taken to ensure that pressure points are padded, that joints are in neutral positions, and that the face is protected from excessive pressure. Vision loss is a rare but devastating complication of spine surgery and proper prone positioning is an essential part of prevention. Anterior approaches to the spine require the patient to be supine and positioning is usually straightforward. In cervical spine surgery, anterior approaches may require coordinated positioning of the head and neck between the anesthesiologist and surgeon. Lateral approaches to the spine require the patient to be in a lateral decubitus position. In this position, an axillary roll on the dependent side is needed to prevent brachial plexus injury and the neck and arms need careful attention to be in neutral positions.

   - **Blood loss:** The amount of blood loss can be extremely variable, which requires the anesthesiologist to maintain vigilance and to frequently assess the extent of blood loss. A preoperative blood type and screen should be performed, when transfusion risk is low, and a blood type and cross, when transfusion risk is moderate or high. In most instances, at least two peripheral intravenous catheters are needed. When high-volume blood loss is expected, central venous catheters (i.e., an introducer sheath) should be considered. Placement of an arterial line should be considered when access to the arms during surgery is limited (cervical and thoracic spine surgery), when the volume of blood loss is anticipated to be high, when the duration of surgery is long, or when patient comorbidities warrant. On one end of the spectrum, spine surgery can be limited to one or two levels with a goal to relieve compression of the spinal cord or spinal nerve roots. These cases typically have less than 250 mL of blood loss. On the other end of the spectrum, surgery can span the entirety of the spine from the head to the pelvis. These procedures often require osteotomies, or cuts in the bone, to accomplish repair of extensive spinal deformities. Osteotomies can result in significant bleeding and a large surgery, such as the one described can have several liters of blood loss.

   - **Anesthetic agents:** Surgery on the spine requires general anesthesia. Anesthetic agents chosen for surgery often depend on whether the surgeon requests intraoperative neuromonitoring (IONM) for the procedure. If IONM is not used, then volatile anesthetic maintenance with muscle relaxation is often sufficient. However, when IONM is used, total intravenous anesthesia is commonly used, and patients often cannot be paralyzed.

   - **Special considerations:** Surgery on the thoracic spine, particularly with a lateral approach, requires one-lung ventilation. A double-lumen endotracheal tube or bronchial blocker is needed to facilitate surgical exposure.

3. **What adverse event is more common after spine surgery compared with other surgical procedures?**

   Postoperative visual loss (POVL) can occur following spine surgery and may appear with or without obvious signs of ocular trauma. Visual deficits range from blurring to complete blindness. The four types of visual loss encountered are central retinal artery occlusion, central retinal vein occlusion, cortical blindness, and ischemic optic neuropathy (ION). ION is the most common form of POVL after spine surgery.

4. What are the causes of POVL?

Occlusions of the central retinal artery or vein are most commonly associated with direct trauma to the globe of the eye (direct pressure on the globe) and less commonly with embolic events. Proper positioning of the patient with careful attention to protection of the eyes is important to prevent this injury. Cortical blindness is rare and is caused by ischemia of the visual cortex of the brain or the optic tracts within the cranium. The precise causes of ION are unknown, but the optic nerve and its blood supply are at risk within the orbit and at the lamina cribrosa where it penetrates the thick sclera. The blood supply is variable among individuals, and a watershed area exists along the midsection of the nerve, between the zones of perfusion from the more posterior hypophyseal branches of the carotid artery and the short posterior ciliary artery anteriorly. The nerve is damaged when there is a decrease in perfusion pressure to the optic nerve below the threshold of autoregulation, and severity and duration of the ischemia will influence the resulting injury. Although ION has occurred following other surgical procedures, most commonly it follows prone spine surgery. The estimated incidence of ION after spine surgery ranges from 0.01% to 0.2%.

5. What are the risk factors for POVL?

In an analysis of 80 patients from the American Society of Anesthesiologists POVL registry, patients undergoing prone spine surgery were studied with the goal to identify independent risk factors. Those factors are increasing duration of surgery, male sex, use of the Wilson frame for patient positioning, obesity, and lower percentage of colloid to crystalloid fluid replacement. Anemia, intraoperative blood pressure, and the presence of chronic hypertension, atherosclerosis, smoking, or diabetes were not found to affect risk. There is no known treatment for POVL.

6. What are the indications for use of IONM in spine surgery?

IONM is indicated in any setting with the potential for mechanical or vascular compromise of the sensory and/or motor pathways along the peripheral nerve, within the spinal canal, or within the brainstem or cerebral cortex. In general, the majority of spine surgeries will have some component of IONM. Procedures that may not use IONM are typically lumbosacral interventions where extensive decompression or hardware placement is not planned.

7. What is IONM and what modalities are used in spine surgery?

IONM allows ongoing assessment of neurological function, or dysfunction, in a patient undergoing a procedure. Information obtained from IONM can guide a surgeon's decisions about the surgical plan in real time and influence decisions of the anesthesiologist about anesthetic agents and blood pressure control. Surgery on the spine typically uses three IONM modalities: somatosensory-evoked potentials (SSEPs), motor-evoked potentials (MEPs), and electromyography (EMG).

   SSEPs provide information about ascending sensory pathways from the periphery to the cortex. An electric stimulus is given at a peripheral nerve and the signal propagates up the spinal cord, through the brainstem, ending in the somatosensory cortex. Electrodes in the scalp then measure this electrical signal, which reflect the ability of a specific sensory neural pathway to conduct an electrical signal from the periphery to the cerebral cortex. In most instances, the median nerves in the upper extremities and the posterior tibial nerves in the lower extremities are stimulated.

   MEPs provide information about descending motor pathways from the cortex to the periphery. An electric stimulus is applied at the cortex, specifically the precentral gyrus, and the signal descends through the brainstem and spinal cord to muscles in the periphery. Electrodes in muscles then measure this electrical signal, which reflect the ability of a specific motor neural pathway to conduct an electrical signal from the cerebral cortex to the periphery. Many different muscles can be monitored simultaneously. In the upper extremity, the adductor pollicis brevis muscle in the hand is most commonly monitored. In the lower extremity, the tibialis anterior muscle in the lower leg and the adductor hallucis muscle in the foot are most commonly monitored. MEPs may not be performed when the surgery is planned for spine levels lower than L2 because this level corresponds with where the spinal cord ends (the conus medullaris) in most individuals.

   There are two types of EMG tests and both provide information about the spinal cord or specific nerves and their associated muscles. The first type, called *spontaneous EMG*, is a continuous recording and no activity should be present at baseline. When activity is observed in a particular muscle, the corresponding nerve is subject to injury and the surgeon is notified. Activity is usually elicited from the surgeon working in close proximity to a nerve root or the spinal cord and from errant hardware placement. The second type, called *triggered EMG*, is a recording that enables surgeons to stimulate the spinal cord or specific nerves in the surgical field to elicit an EMG response. This allows for identification of functional tissue and to verify normal nerve function. It is important to monitor muscles that correspond to the surgical area. For example, in cervical spine surgery it is important to monitor the upper extremity muscles: deltoid, biceps, triceps, and adductor pollicis brevis.

8. What is the sensory pathway from a peripheral nerve to the cerebral cortex?

The axons of the peripheral sensory nerves enter the spinal cord via the dorsal spinal roots. These first-order neurons continue rostrally in the ipsilateral posterior column of the spinal cord until they synapse with nuclei at the cervicomedullary junction in the brainstem. Second-order neurons from these nuclei immediately decussate to the contralateral side of the brainstem, where they continue their ascent via the medial lemniscus through the midbrain, synapsing in the thalamus. Third-order neurons then travel via the internal capsule to synapse in the postcentral gyrus, known as the *primary somatosensory cortex.*

9. **What is the motor pathway from the cerebral cortex to a muscle?**
   The motor impulse originates in precentral gyrus upper motor neurons and their axons traverse through the brainstem where the vast majority decussate. The axons continue down the corticospinal tract in the spinal cord to synapse with lower motor neurons in the ventral horn of the spinal cord. The signal then propagates through the lower motor neurons to the motor end plate on muscles, resulting in muscle contraction.

10. **Describe the characteristics of the evoked potential waveforms.**
    Both SSEP and MEP waveforms are plotted as voltage versus time and are characterized by:
    - Amplitude: this is measured in microvolts from the waveform peak to valley.
    - Latency: this is measured in milliseconds from the onset of the stimulus to the occurrence of the first peak.
    - Morphology: this describes the overall shape of the waveform. SSEP waveforms in the cortex mimic the shape of a sine wave. MEP waveforms, on the other hand, are complex with multiple peaks and valleys.

11. **What constitutes a concerning change in evoked potential waveforms?**
    After the induction of anesthesia and before the start of surgery, baseline measurements of evoked potentials are collected. These baseline waveforms are used for comparison of future evoked potentials throughout the surgery to test for the presence of neurological injury or dysfunction. Any decrease in amplitude greater than 50% or increase in latency greater than 10% in SSEP waveforms satisfy alert criteria and may indicate a disruption of the sensory nerve pathways. Alert criteria are controversial for MEP waveforms because of variability from one trial to another; however, greater than 90% amplitude decrement is commonly used as the threshold for an alert.

12. **How do anesthetic agents affect evoked potential waveforms?**
    Generally speaking, the vast majority of anesthetic agents worsen evoked potential waveforms in a dose and time dependent fashion. These agents can prolong latency and decrease amplitude to levels that meet alert criteria. Volatile anesthetics impact waveforms to a greater degree compared with continuous intravenous anesthetics. Thus volatile agents are often avoided entirely or used at much lower concentrations (0.5 minimum alveolar concentration [MAC]) in combination with continuous intravenous agents when IONM is used. Ketamine is a notable exception because it can augment evoked potential waveforms and its administration during surgery is common for this reason, as well as for its analgesic properties.

13. **What other nonanesthetic variables can alter evoked potential waveforms?**
    - **Surgical:** mechanisms of injury during spine surgery include direct cord trauma (hooks, wires, and pedicle screws), epidural hematoma, distraction or compression of the spinal cord from correction by instrumentation, and excessive tension on blood vessels, leading to ischemia.
    - **Temperature:** hypothermia is a common culprit in the operating room. As temperature decreases below 36°C, increases in latency are seen, whereas amplitude is either decreased or unchanged. Hyperthermia ($>40°C$) is rarely encountered but if present can result in decreased amplitudes.
    - **Hypotension:** with a decrease of the mean arterial blood pressure, progressive decreases in amplitude are seen. MEP waveforms are more sensitive to hypotension and ischemia can be detected immediately. However, changes in SSEP waveforms may be delayed 10 to 20 minutes after the onset of ischemia.

14. **If evoked potentials change significantly, what can the anesthesiologist and surgeon do to decrease the insult to the monitored nerves or nerve pathways?**
    The anesthesiologist can:
    - Increase the mean arterial pressure (MAP), especially if induced hypotension is used. The extent of increase depends on numerous factors; however, a MAP greater than 85 mm Hg is a typical goal.
    - Administer intravenous steroids after discussion with the surgeon. Dexamethasone is a typical agent used in this scenario.
    - Correct anemia, if present.
    - Correct hypovolemia, if present.
    - Improve oxygen tension.
    - Correct hypothermia, if present.
    The surgeon can:
    - Reduce excessive retractor pressure.
    - Reduce surgical dissection in the affected area.
    - Decrease Harrington rod distraction, if indicated.
    - Check positioning of associated instrumentation (e.g., screws, hooks).
    If changes in the evoked potentials persist, despite corrective measures, then a wake-up test may be performed. However, this is rarely done. Instead, surgeons weigh the risks and benefits of the continuation of surgery in the light of possible neurological injury.

15. **Despite normal evoked potentials, can a patient awaken with neurological deficits after surgery?**
    Although IONM is a useful tool in preventing neurological damage during spinal surgery, it is by no means foolproof. The reported incidence of false-negative monitoring in a large (>50,000) series of cases is 0.06% (1 in 1500). The use of multiple IONM modalities provides a more complete assessment of neural pathway integrity.

KEY POINTS: SPINE SURGERY

1. Airway management for cervical spine surgery may be difficult, particularly in the setting of injury. Video laryngoscopy and fiberoptic bronchoscopy are preferred methods of securing the airway.
2. Patient positioning for surgery is dictated by how the surgeon wishes to approach the spine. The patient will be supine for an anterior approach, prone for a posterior approach, and lateral decubitus for a lateral approach.
3. Blood loss during spine surgery is highly variable. When the volume of blood loss is expected to be moderate or high, it is necessary to have adequate venous access and an arterial line for continuous hemodynamic monitoring.
4. Postoperative vision loss can follow spine surgery in rare instances and is most commonly caused by ischemic optic neuropathy, which is thought to be secondary to decreased blood flow to the optic nerve at select vulnerable locations.
5. Independent risk factors for ischemic optic neuropathy include male sex, prolonged surgery, use of the Wilson frame, obesity, and low percentage of colloid compared with crystalloid for fluid replacement. When positioning the patient prone, avoid direct pressure on the eye and place the head above the level of the heart.
6. When intraoperative neuromonitoring is used during spine surgery, an anesthetic technique that minimizes volatile anesthetic exposure is best to preserve evoked potential waveforms. Total intravenous anesthesia may be necessary.
7. Intraoperative neuromonitoring modalities used in spine surgery include SSEPs, MEPs, and EMG. These modalities are meant to test for neurological insult or injury during surgery.
8. When a worrisome neuromonitoring change occurs during surgery, the anesthesiologist and surgeon work together to determine the cause of the change and decide whether to implement any specific interventions.

SUGGESTED READINGS

Drummond JC, Patel PM, Lemkuil BP. Anesthesia for neurologic surgery. In: Miller RD, ed. Miller's Anesthesia. 8th ed. Philadelphia, PA: Elsevier Saunders; 2015:2158–2199.
Epstein NE. Perioperative visual loss following prone spinal surgery: a review. Surg Neurol Int. 2016;7(Suppl 13):S347–S360.
Jameson LC, Sloan TB. Neurophysiologic monitoring in neurosurgery. Anesthesiol Clin. 2012;30:311–331.
Pasternak JJ, Lanier WL. Neuroanesthesiology update. J Neurosurg Anesth. 2018;30:106–145.
Roth S. Postoperative visual loss. In: Miller RD, ed. Miller's Anesthesia. 8th ed. Philadelphia, PA: Elsevier Saunders; 2015:3011–3032.
Seubert CN, Mahla ME. Neurologic monitoring. In: Miller RD, ed. Miller's Anesthesia. 8th ed. Philadelphia, PA: Elsevier Saunders; 2015:1487–1523.
Sloan TB, Burger E, Klech CJ, et al. Neurophysiologic monitoring in thoracic spine surgery. In: Koht A, Sloan T, Toleikis R, eds. Monitoring the Nervous System for Anesthesiologists and other Health Care Professionals. 2nd ed. New York: Springer; 2017.
Urban MK. Anesthesia for orthopedic surgery. In: Miller RD, ed. Miller's Anesthesia. 8th ed. Philadelphia, PA: Elsevier Saunders; 2015:2386–2406.

CHAPTER 65

CRANIOTOMY

Anthony M. Oliva, MD, PhD

1. **How do anesthetic requirements differ during various time points in a craniotomy?**

   A craniotomy is unique in that the level of nociceptive stimulus varies greatly and the portions of the procedure that require deep anesthesia are mostly at the beginning. Deep anesthesia is essential during laryngoscopy (and intubation) to block any harmful increases in heart rate, blood pressure, and brain metabolic activity, which may increase intracranial pressure (ICP). Soon after intubation, placement of pins in the skull for head positioning is common and often necessitates deep anesthesia. Once these events conclude, considerable time may pass with little to no noxious stimuli. Patient positioning and operative preparation often takes considerable time, and maintenance of deep anesthesia may require vasoactive agents for hemodynamic support. If the plane of anesthesia is "light" during this period, careful anticipation that the depth of anesthesia will need to be increased immediately before incision of the scalp, opening of the skull, and reflection of the dura because these events provide increased surgical stimuli. Once the surgeon begins dissection of the brain or pathological tissue, noxious stimuli are minimal because these structures are essentially void of nociceptive nerve fibers.

2. **Discuss the various monitors used for a craniotomy.**

   Aside from the standard American Society of Anesthesiology monitors, patients may require invasive monitoring, central venous access, and neuromonitoring. Invasive monitoring typically includes an arterial line to assess hemodynamic changes and intravascular volume status. A central venous catheter should be considered if there is an elevated risk of venous air embolism, a high likelihood of using vasoactive infusions perioperatively, or to administer hypertonic saline to treat intracranial hypertension. Neuromonitoring, such as continuous electroencephalogram (EEG); somatosensory, motor, and brainstem auditory evoked potentials; and ICP monitoring may be helpful, depending upon the nature of the surgery and surgeon preference. Jugular bulb venous oxygen saturation and transcranial oximetry have been described as monitors of oxygen delivery and metabolic integrity of the brain globally, but are not used regularly in the intraoperative setting.

3. **What are the implications with fluid administration during a craniotomy?**

   The patient's intravascular volume status can significantly affect the surgeon's ability to visualize, dissect, and/or resect tissue. Sudden increases in intravascular volume, before opening the dura, may cause an exponential increase in ICP, especially in the setting of intracranial hypertension or when the ICP is already borderline elevated. However, hypotension because of hypovolemia may require volume resuscitation to restore normal cerebral perfusion. Therefore fluids should be administered judiciously to avoid both hypo- and hypervolemia.

4. **Which fluids are safe to administer? Which should be avoided?**

   Only isotonic or hypertonic intravenous fluids should be administered. Hypotonic fluids should be avoided, which can exacerbate cerebral edema. Recall, the tonicity of fluids refers to normal patient serum osmolarity where hypertonic (hyperosmolar) fluids will have a higher osmolarity compared with normal serum osmolarity (275–295 mOsm/L). Unless hypoglycemia is documented, glucose-containing solutions should also be avoided, because hyperglycemia can negatively affect neurological outcomes. Normal saline (0.9%) and balanced salt solutions are categorized as isotonic fluids and are safe to give; although, technically, normal saline (0.9%) has a slightly higher osmolarity compared with balanced salt solutions (i.e., PlasmaLyte, Ringer's lactate). Colloid solutions, such as isotonic 5% albumin or hypertonic 3% saline, are equivalent solutions for acute volume replacement. Hypertonic 25% albumin may be considered in situations where the patient is overall hypervolemic but intravascularly "dry," which often occurs with hypoalbuminemia (e.g., cirrhosis, malnutrition, nephrotic syndrome). There is a concern that albumin administration is associated with worse clinical outcomes in the setting of traumatic brain injury (TBI). However, the oft-cited study (Saline vs. Albumin Fluid Evaluation trial) found this association with *hypotonic* 4% albumin, so it is uncertain if this finding can also be extrapolated for isotonic (5%) or hypertonic (25%) albumin.

5. **What are the goals to "protect" the brain?**

   Brain protection refers to strategies to support the balance between brain metabolism and substrate delivery, while also preventing secondary injury to regions of the brain, following an episode of ischemia. The need for brain protection should be anticipated in the setting of TBI, stroke, and in various neurosurgical operations. Of primary importance is the adequate delivery of oxygen and energy substrates to brain tissue by maintaining optimal blood oxygen content and cerebral blood flow (CBF).

6. How can the brain be "protected"?

Long-acting barbiturates can be administered for cerebral metabolic suppression in the setting of refractory intracranial hypertension. However, this is often used in the intensive care unit, with little clinical evidence supporting improved neurological outcomes. Barbiturate coma therapy often requires the use of continuous EEG monitoring to titrate the agent to "burst-suppression" on EEG. The burst suppression pattern is characterized by predominant isoelectric activity with periodic "bursts" of electrical activity (e.g., 1 "burst" every 10 seconds). Although propofol may also achieve this goal, concerns surrounding propofol infusion syndrome limit its use in this setting.

In the intraoperative setting, cerebral metabolic suppression is needed when a major artery is temporarily clipped to facilitate access to an aneurysm. The EEG correlate, as previously discussed, is "burst suppression." This can be achieved by a rapid infusion or bolus of thiopental, propofol, or etomidate. Hypothermia reduces cerebral metabolism, CBF, cerebral edema, and ICP. Unfortunately, clinical studies show that mild to moderate hypothermia (32°C–34°C) does not improve neurological outcomes. However, control of temperature to avoid hyperthermia is shown to be beneficial in the intensive care setting and likely remains true in the intraoperative setting.

Other goals of cerebral protection include limiting secondary injury because of ischemia, cerebral edema, hematoma expansion, and brain herniation. Methods to prevent these complications include glucose control (140–180 mg/dL), maintain a normal cerebral perfusion pressure (50–70 mm Hg), avoid hypertension (e.g., goal systolic BP <140 mm Hg), avoidance of hypotonic fluids, and appropriate use of other modalities for treating ICP (See Chapter #44, "Intracranial Hypertension and Traumatic Brain Injury").

7. Is there an ideal anesthetic agent in patients undergoing a craniotomy?

The anesthetic agents administered for anesthesia is based on the understanding of the pharmacological properties of hypnotic agents, inhalation agents, opioids, muscle relaxants, and on a balancing their beneficial and adverse effects. Importantly, the intraoperative goal is to provide a motionless patient, hemodynamic stability, and an awake, neurologically assessable patient postoperatively. Regardless of the selected agent, it is important to use short-acting agents to facilitate rapid emergence from anesthesia and neurological examination after extubation. An overly sedated patient postoperatively may confound the clinical picture, leading to unnecessary imaging or procedures.

- Hypnotic agents: Thiopental effectively blocks conscious awareness and reduces ICP, CBF, and brain metabolism. Propofol has similar effects but is eliminated more rapidly with small doses; however, because of its context-sensitive half-life, its duration of action can significantly be prolonged when infused for an extended period. Etomidate and midazolam are only slightly less effective for metabolic suppression and are also useful.
- Inhalation agents: The differences between isoflurane, desflurane, and sevoflurane concerning metabolic suppression, CBF, and ICP are slight. All cause suppression of brain activity, while preserving or enhancing CBF. Costs and speed of elimination are major concerns in selecting an agent. Nitrous oxide increases ICP and CBF, although this effect may be modified by the coadministration of other hypnotic, analgesic, and anesthetic agents.
- Opioids: All opioids have negligible effects on CBF and small effects on cerebral metabolism. These agents block the adrenergic stimulation that increases brain activity. Morphine and hydromorphone are eliminated slowly and may cause respiratory depression after the procedure is completed. Hypercarbia caused by opioid-induced hypoventilation causes cerebral vasodilation, which increases CBF, cerebral blood volume, and ICP. All of which must be avoided after a craniotomy. Strong preference should be given to short-acting synthetic agents (i.e., remifentanil and sufentanil) to expedite emergence from anesthesia, facilitate neurological examination, following extubation, and minimize problems related to hypercapnia-induced elevation of ICP postoperatively.
- Muscle relaxants: Depolarizing neuromuscular blocking agents (i.e., succinylcholine) are generally not used in the setting of intracranial pathology, unless emergent control of the airway is necessary because of concerns of this agent causing a transient elevation in ICP. The main concern with nondepolarizing agents is masking neurological examination because of their longer half-life.

8. Is it better to use total intravenous anesthesia or inhalation agents? Does one affect CBF or ICP more than the other?

The ideal anesthetic agent would decrease cerebral metabolic rate of oxygen consumption, cerebral blood volume, and ICP. CBF is often used as a surrogate for cerebral blood volume, which often parallel each other; however, they are technically not the same and it is the cerebral blood volume that affects ICP, not CBF. Further, the majority of the cerebral blood volume is contained with the venous vasculature not the arterial vasculature, hence, agents that cause venodilation (e.g., nitroglycerin) affect ICP the most.

Propofol preserves cerebral autoregulation of CBF, whereas volatile agents, particularly when used at higher doses (i.e., >1 minimum alveolar concentration [MAC]), blunt cerebral autoregulation. However, when volatile agents are administered within usual clinical doses (~1 MAC), particularly with modern inhalation agents (i.e., sevoflurane), the effects on cerebral autoregulation are minimized. Studies show that total intravenous anesthesia (TIVA) with propofol is associated with a lower ICP and a higher cerebral perfusion pressure compared with inhaled volatile agents. However, evidence thus far show no difference in meaningful neurological outcomes between either strategy, despite the theoretical benefits of TIVA with propofol.

9. **Are there particular anesthetic problems associated with intracranial surgery?**

Space-occupying intracranial lesions are associated with disturbed autoregulation in adjacent tissue. Vascular malformations and aneurysms are accompanied by altered vasoreactivity (particularly if preceded by subarachnoid hemorrhage). Trauma patients in hemorrhagic shock with TBI may require conflicting goals with volume resuscitation. For example, a polytrauma patient in hemorrhage shock with a TBI will require volume resuscitation to treat hypotension (and to restore adequate cerebral perfusion); however, overzealous volume resuscitation may cause cerebral edema, leading to an increase in ICP and impairing cerebral perfusion. Intraoperative concerns include control of CBF and volume status, anticipation of the physiological effects of surgery, management of ICP, and maintenance of adequate cerebral perfusion pressure.

10. **What are the concerns for patient positioning during a craniotomy?**

Because of the long duration of these operations, protecting vulnerable peripheral nerves and pressure-prone areas from injury is essential. Provisions should be made to prevent antiseptic agents, such as chlorhexidine, from entering the eyes, which can lead to eye injury and blindness. Often, the head is in a fixed position with pins clamped against the outer skull. Because the head is in a fixed position, any patient movement will stress the cervical spine. Muscle paralysis should be maintained when the head is secured in a holding device, unless contraindicated with neuromonitoring modalities. Specific neuromonitoring where paralysis is contraindicated include motor evoked potentials and electromyography neuromonitoring.

In every craniotomy, the risk of air entrainment into the venous system should be assessed. Whenever the surgical site is positioned above the right atrium, a potential "negative" pressure exists between the surgical site and the central venous system. Air entrained in the central venous system may collect into the right heart, causing right heart strain by impairing preload and/or significantly increasing right heart afterload. Note, the pathophysiology resembles pulmonary embolism. Significant air entrainment can result in profound hypotension and acute right heart failure. If a patent foramen ovale is present, air can potentially cross the intraatrial septum and become a paradoxical air embolus into the systemic circulation. This risk is especially significant in sitting-position craniotomies. End-tidal CO_2, end-tidal nitrogen, transesophageal echocardiography, and precordial Doppler are sensitive indicators of venous air. In high-risk situations, a central venous catheter should be placed in the right atrium for removal of air embolism. Fortunately, neurosurgeons often use other patient positions, such as prone or lateral decubitus, to avoid such complications.

11. **Why do some patients awaken slowly after a craniotomy?**

Continuous infusion of an opioid and/or propofol in a long operation can lead to redistribution and persistent sedation because of the context sensitive half-life of these agents. Residual volatile anesthetic may contribute to delayed awakening but is less often the cause. The use of short-acting agents, which do not have a significant context sensitive half-life (i.e., agents that do not accumulate in fat), is beneficial. In patients who are slow to emerge from anesthesia, simply waiting and providing respiratory support is needed, until all residual anesthetic effects are gone. Slow awakening that persists for more than 2 hours is rarely an effect of residual anesthesia. A patient who is unresponsive for several hours after a craniotomy should be evaluated for increased ICP, embolic phenomenon, brainstem ischemia, or intracranial masses. Evaluation should be a joint effort of the neurosurgeon and anesthesiologist. In all cases, the anesthetic technique should be tailored to facilitate a rapid emergence for early testing of neurological function.

12. **What are the unique problems associated with operations for an aneurysm in the setting of subarachnoid hemorrhage (SAH)?**

- SAH: Aneurysms of the cerebral arteries are often diagnosed following SAH. Neurological impairment after SAH ranges from headache and stiff neck (Hunt-Hess grade I) to deep coma (Hunt-Hess grade V). Initial resuscitation includes observation, tight control of blood pressure (i.e., systolic BP <140 mm Hg), and support of intravascular volume. The optimal time for surgical clipping of the aneurysm is within the first few days of hemorrhage because of the risk of rebleeding. In the week following SAH, the risk of vasospasm of the vessel feeding the aneurysm markedly increases because of irritation from the breakdown of old blood. Invasive monitoring of arterial pressure is required to facilitate maintenance of hemodynamic stability and to guide volume replacement. Brain protection should include, at a minimum, the maintenance of normal oxygen delivery to brain tissue. Metabolic suppression by EEG burst suppression may be used at the time of temporary vessel clipping, but this can result in a poor outcome when accompanied by hypotension.
- Rebleeding: Approximately 30% of all intracranial aneurysms that present with SAH will rebleed if left untreated. Recall from LaPlace's law, which states that both transmural pressure and radius of the vessel increase wall tension. Therefore larger aneurysms will have a larger wall tension, predisposing to rupture and rebleeding, particularly in the setting of uncontrolled hypertension. Rebleeding of the aneurysm just before surgery (e.g., hypertension from laryngoscopy causing aneurysm rupture and rebleeding) is catastrophic. This may require the surgeon to approach the bleeding vessel blindly and may require temporarily clipping major feeding vessels.
- Vasospasm: Vasospasm is a frequent complication following SAH, is often underappreciated, and is a responsible for a large degree of neurological impairment and mortality. Vasospasm causes an ischemic stroke in the region of distribution of the aneurysmal artery. The risk of vasospasm is at its highest 7 to 10 days following

SAH but can occur anytime between 3 and 21 days. Diagnosis is by angiography is often prompted by a change in neurological status or new neurological deficit. However, vasospasm can occur with no apparent changes on neurological examination. Daily transcranial Doppler studies can be helpful in detecting vasospasm. Avoiding hypovolemia and the prophylactic treatment with nimodipine, a calcium channel blocker, for the first 21 days following a SAH, can significantly decrease the incidence of vasospasm and improve neurological outcomes. It is important to know that this finding is unique to nimodipine, as other calcium channel blockers are not interchangeable and do not provide the same level of benefit for unclear reasons.

13. Are there special anesthetic problems associated with brain tumors?

The detrimental effects of intracranial mass lesions are related to their size and location. Frontal tumors may grow to a larger size compared with other lesions, without producing neurological symptoms or increased ICP. Patients with supratentorial tumors of the motor and sensory cortical regions may have seizures, localizing neurological signs, and increased ICP. Posterior fossa masses in adults cause disturbances in gait, balance, proprioception, or cranial nerve impingement. There is a penumbra around all intracranial tumors where the adjacent brain loses autoregulatory function. Thus on induction of anesthesia, regional blood flow in these areas may increase in response to aggressive fluid replacement or increased systolic blood pressure. Following resection, this penumbra may respond to reperfusion with swelling and edema, leading to intracranial hypertension. Posterior fossa tumors cause unique problems. These tumors are often small but may surround complex vascular channels of the basilar, posterior communicating, and cerebellar arteries. Simple dissection of a brainstem tumor can cause unpredictable disturbances of heart rate and rhythm or blood pressure when nerve roots are retracted. The surgical approach to the posterior fossa often involves awkward positioning, from sitting to lateral to prone to park bench. These positions require careful attention to the position of the endotracheal tube to avoid inadvertent extubation or endobronchial migration. The plan for anesthesia must also allow for intraoperative neuromonitoring, such as auditory-evoked potentials, somatosensory-evoked potentials, or motor-evoked potentials if indicated.

14. In what instances are craniotomies done on awake patients?

The most common indication for an awake craniotomy is to place a deep brain stimulator (DBS) for the treatment of Parkinson disease and other movement disorders. Indications for DBS placement are expanding and may include some psychiatric conditions, such as obsessive-compulsive disorder. Other situations that warrant an awake craniotomy is for tumor resection when the tumor is adjacent to, or within, eloquent tissue. Specifically, tumors in areas near the motor strip and language centers are difficult to resect. Neurosurgeons may need to resect tissue, based on neurological examination in real time. This technique allows for maximal tumor resection, while minimizing permanent neurological dysfunction.

15. What are the considerations for an awake craniotomy?

Anesthetic goals should be discussed with the neurosurgeon. Once a plan is determined, the most important aspect of patient care is to provide information to the patient on what to expect for the procedure. Understandably, patients often have high anxiety and providing information on what to expect during surgery can ease anxiety. Depending upon the situation and surgeon preference, a craniotomy may range from no anesthetic agents at all to selective deep sedation during portions of the operation, which do not require active patient participation. For example, sedation may be provided to make the patient comfortable for urinary catheter and arterial catheter placement. If sedative agents are administered, strong preference should include short-acting agents to allow patient participation, with neurological testing. Once tumor resection and neurological testing is complete, sedation can be resumed until the end of the procedure. Blood pressure control can be difficult in awake patients and a plan for both short-acting and long-acting antihypertensive agents is necessary.

16. What are other anesthetic concerns during a craniotomy?

- Transsphenoidal surgery, although not technically a craniotomy, may involve manipulation of ventilation to raise the arterial partial pressure of carbon dioxide and ICP to force the pituitary into a more easily visualized position.
- Decompressive craniotomy is a common surgical treatment for medical refractory intracranial hypertension. In patients undergoing an emergent craniotomy, it is crucial to maximize medical management to lower ICP (control systolic blood pressure, administered hyperosmolar agents, etc.), reverse coagulopathy if necessary, and if brain herniation is imminent, hyperventilation strategies should be used. Intracranial hypertension may progress to involve brainstem compression and subsequent ischemia. This response, particularly when it involves the medulla, is known as the *Cushing reflex*, which is the classic triad of systemic hypertension, bradycardia, and irregular respiration. Hypertension in this setting is thought to be a protective reflex to maintain cerebral perfusion and should not be reflexively treated. Studies show that tachycardia, and not necessarily bradycardia, often occurs with impaired cerebral perfusion. Thus hypertension, coupled with either bradycardia or tachycardia, may indicate impaired cerebral perfusion.
- Craniotomies in pediatric patients are rare. The pathology that is most common in the pediatric group is the posterior fossa tumor, particularly cerebellar astrocytoma. Positioning, cranial nerve root stimulation, and venous air embolus are concerns during posterior fossa resections in children.

KEY POINTS: CRANIOTOMY

1. Maintain a mean arterial pressure of at least 60 mm Hg, but preferably 70 mm Hg or higher to ensure adequate CBF provided the ICP is normal.
2. Patients with profound mental status changes often require little or no sedation before inducing general anesthesia.
3. Although TIVA has theoretical benefits favoring cerebral perfusion compared with inhalation agents (i.e., does not blunt autoregulation), studies thus far fail to show better outcomes with TIVA versus inhalation agents.
4. Modern anesthetics (i.e., sevoflurane) used at clinical doses ($\sim$1 MAC) does not significantly blunt cerebral autoregulation.
5. Ensure adequate depth of anesthesia before laryngoscopy and head pinning to avoid abrupt increases in ICP.
6. Rapid emergence from anesthesia facilitates early testing of neurological function.
7. Judicious fluid administration with isotonic crystalloid will minimize cerebral edema and ICP fluctuations.
8. Avoid abrupt increases in systemic blood pressure before aneurysm clip placement.
9. Cerebral ischemia because of vasospasm can be exacerbated by hypotension.
10. Medical management of vasospasm include avoiding hypovolemia, permissive hypertension, and nimodipine.
11. If the patient is in a head-up position, venous air embolism risk justifies the use of a right atrial central venous catheter to remove an air embolism.
12. The Cushing reflex is the classic triad of systemic hypertension, bradycardia, and irregular respiration. It implies medullary ischemia and is often because of brainstem compression because of brain herniation.
13. Impaired cerebral perfusion is often associated with hypertension and may occur with either bradycardia or tachycardia. The classic Cushing reflex will not always be apparent in all cases of impaired cerebral perfusion.

Suggested Readings

Avitsian R, Schubert A. Anesthetic considerations for intraoperative management of cerebrovascular disease in neurovascular surgical procedures. Anesthesiol Clin. 2007;25:441–463.

Drummond JC, Patel PM, Lemkuil BP. Anesthesia for neurologic surgery. In: Miller RD, ed. Miller's Anesthesia. 8th ed. Philadelphia, PA: Elsevier Saunders; 2015.

Pasternak JJ, Lanier WL. Neuroanesthesiology update. J Neurosurg Anesth. 2018;30:106–145.

Rozet I, Vavilala MS. Risks and benefits of patient positioning during neurosurgical care. Anesthesiol Clin. 2007;25:631–653.

CHAPTER 66

SHOULDER OPERATIONS

Mitchell Fingerman, MD, Joseph Schoenfeldt, MD

1. **What types of orthopedic surgical operations are performed on the shoulder?**
   The types of shoulder operations that are commonly performed include: arthroscopy for shoulder debridement, impingement syndrome, SLAP repair (superior labrum anterior and posterior), shoulder dislocation, and frozen shoulder, as well as rotator cuff repair, acromioclavicular joint repair, and shoulder replacement.

2. **Describe the innervation of the shoulder joint.**
   The shoulder joint, also known as the *glenohumeral joint*, is a ball and socket joint with multiple sources of innervation. The brachial plexus supplies the bulk of the joint's innervation, with the superficial cervical plexus innervating the skin mostly superior to the joint. The glenohumeral joint is primarily supplied by the axillary nerve inferiorly and the suprascapular nerve superiorly. In addition to the glenohumeral joint, the suprascapular nerve also provides sensory innervation to the acromioclavicular joint. The musculocutaneous and subscapular nerves also supply innervation to the joint, but their contribution is much less and has high variability among individuals. Most of the skin surrounding the shoulder joint receives sensory innervation by branches of the axillary nerve.

3. **How is an interscalene block performed? Between which muscles does it place local anesthetics?**
   The most common regional technique performed for shoulder operations is the interscalene block. Historically, interscalene blocks have been placed by palpation of surface anatomy or with nerve stimulators. However, with the advent of new technology, ultrasound guidance has become the standard technique. This not only minimizes the risk of damage to a highly vascularized and innervated region of the neck, but also facilitates confirmation of local anesthetic injection within close proximity of the brachial plexus.

   To perform the block under ultrasound guidance, the probe is placed transversely on the neck at roughly the level of the cricoid cartilage. Deep and lateral to the sternocleidomastoid is the anterior scalene muscle and more lateral still is the middle scalene muscle. Between the anterior and middle scalene muscles courses the brachial plexus. The brachial plexus at this point often appears on ultrasound as three circles, but there is variability depending on patient anatomy and physician technique. Regardless of the exact visualization, the target remains the same: the roots of C5, C6, and C7 and the upper and middle trunks they become. If identification of the brachial plexus between the scalene muscles proves challenging, the ultrasound probe can be brought down to the supraclavicular fossa to the level of the divisions. Here, the brachial plexus can be reliably identified lateral to the subclavian artery and then traced back cephalad to the truncal level. Once identified, the needle is introduced lateral to the probe and guided medially toward the plexus. Typically, 20 to 30 mL of local anesthetic is then injected around the trunks, with spread confirmed by the ultrasound visualization.

4. **Caution should be used when performing an interscalene block in patients with severe respiratory disease. Why?**
   In almost all interscalene blocks, the ipsilateral phrenic nerve is inadvertently blocked by the spread of local anesthetics. This results in hemidiaphragmatic paresis and a subsequent decrease in respiratory function. In the healthy patient, this is usually clinically insignificant and often goes unnoticed. However, if a patient has diminished respiratory function at baseline, this loss of diaphragmatic excursion may result into respiratory distress. The risks and benefits of an interscalene approach should be assessed before placing a block in a patient with significant respiratory disease and a more distal approach to the brachial plexus should be considered.

5. **What is Horner syndrome?**
   Horner syndrome is a collection of signs resulting from inhibition of the cervical sympathetic trunk. Notable signs include ipsilateral ptosis (drooping eyelid), miosis (pupillary constriction), and anhidrosis (diminished sweating). There are multiple etiologies of Horner syndrome, one of which is inhibition of the cervical sympathetic trunk by local anesthetics. Following interscalene and supraclavicular blocks, the local anesthetic can migrate medially from the brachial plexus toward the cervical ganglion, resulting in an unintended Horner syndrome. Should this occur following a block, patients should be offered reassurance for this common side effect and instructed to follow-up if it does not resolve in time.

6. **Why might a patient's voice become hoarse after an interscalene nerve block?**
   During an interscalene block, local anesthetic is injected around the brachial plexus at the level of the C5, C6, and C7 roots. This local anesthetic may spread medially toward the recurrent laryngeal nerve. This results in hoarseness in 10% to 20% of interscalene blocks; however, the incidence may be higher on the right side than the left. In patients with preexisting injury to the contralateral recurrent laryngeal nerve, laryngeal obstruction via bilateral vocal cord paralysis may be a rare but catastrophic complication.

7. **What serious risks are associated with the interscalene approach to a brachial plexus block?**
   As mentioned earlier, the phrenic nerve is almost always blocked with the interscalene approach, resulting in respiratory distress in certain patients with limited respiratory reserve at baseline. Respiratory distress can also arise from a pneumothorax if the needle is directed too caudally; however, this is a rare complication. Intravascular injection can occur as the brachial plexus runs laterally to the internal jugular vein and carotid artery and often just superficial to the vertebral artery. This is why aspiration before injection, as well as incremental dosing is crucial. Inadvertent intraarterial injection may result in seizures. Although extremely rare, local anesthetic may be injected in the neuraxial region (either epidural, subdural, or subarachnoid) if visualization of the needle is incomplete and the tip is introduced deeper than expected. As with all peripheral nerve blocks, there does exist a small chance of local anesthetic toxicity and direct nerve damage.

8. **If an interscalene nerve block is contraindicated in a patient undergoing shoulder surgery, what other block can be offered for postoperative pain control?**
   An interscalene nerve block may be contraindicated in a patient with significant respiratory disease or risk of respiratory distress. In these cases, a suprascapular nerve block may be performed to anesthetize the shoulder, while removing the risk of phrenic nerve inhibition. Although the suprascapular nerve block will not anesthetize the same large distribution as an interscalene brachial plexus block, it will block the nerve with the largest contribution to the shoulder joint. In addition, several studies report equal analgesic efficacy of the suprascapular nerve block for shoulder surgery, while decreasing the chance of hemidiaphragmatic paresis.

9. **How is the suprascapular nerve block performed?**
   The suprascapular nerve descends from the brachial plexus to run along the superior aspect of the scapular spine before innervating the shoulder joint. It is the main sensory contributor to the posterior and superior aspect of the shoulder (including the glenohumeral and acromioclavicular joints), and it provides motor function for external shoulder rotation. To block it, one draws a line along the scapular spine, bisects it, and then makes a mark 1 cm cephalad and 1 cm lateral to this point. A needle is then inserted here and directed caudally, until contacting the scapular spine. Ultrasound guidance may be used to confirm direction toward the suprascapular notch and to confirm placement deep to the supraspinatus muscle. Once the needle tip is positioned appropriately, 10 mL of local anesthetic is injected for a single shot block.

10. **If surgery is being performed on the distal arm, which nerve will likely be insufficiently anesthetized by an interscalene block?**
    The interscalene nerve block typically spares the ulnar nerve, which innervates the medial arm distal to the elbow. For an interscalene block, local anesthetic is deposited near the upper and middle trunks of C5, C6, and C7. The ulnar nerve is a branch of the medial cord, which is supplied by the C8 and T1 roots (lower trunk). It is therefore not adequately anesthetized by most interscalene blocks. A more elegant and reliable way to anesthetize the ulnar nerve is to block it distally at the level of the mid-forearm (medial to the ulnar artery).

11. **Following a successful interscalene block, a patient has just had a total shoulder replacement. They are now in postanesthesia care unit complaining of axillary pain. What is the likely cause?**
    This is because of pain from the territory covered by the intercostobrachial nerve. The intercostobrachial nerve provides cutaneous innervation of the medial aspect of the proximal arm and the anterior axilla. It is the lateral cutaneous branch of the second intercostal nerve. It is also an important nerve to block in the prevention of tourniquet pain for more distal upper extremity surgeries.

12. **How is the intercostobrachial nerve block performed?**
    The intercostobrachial nerve starts as the ventral ramus of T2 and passes through the serratus anterior muscle at the midaxillary line before innervating the skin of the anterior axilla and the medial aspect of the proximal arm. Because the nerve provides cutaneous sensation, it runs very superficially within the arm. To block the intercostobrachial nerve, a patient's upper extremity is abducted, the axilla properly cleaned, and local anesthetic is injected subcutaneously along the axillary crease. A two-inch needle can be superficially inserted to its hub and 5 to 10 mL of local anesthetic can be deposited, as it is withdrawn. This technique minimizes the number of passes required for adequate spread and decreases the associated risk of vascular and neurological injury.

13. **Describe the beach chair position.**
    The beach chair position is a variant of the sitting position that is frequently used for shoulder surgeries. To place a patient in beach chair position, begin in the supine position and put the table in slight Trendelenburg (head tilted down) using the bed controls. Then raise the back up, flexing the hips between 30 and 90 degrees, and angle the legs down to create a bend in the knee that removes tension from the sciatic nerve. The head is secured in a neutral position by

either a cushioned mask or a strap across the forehead. Lastly, the nonoperative arm is elevated in an armboard and the operative shoulder is moved to the edge of the table for easy surgical access. The resulting position resembles the relaxed position of someone resting in a beach or barber chair (another name for this position).

14. Describe the advantages of the beach chair position for shoulder arthroscopies.
The primary advantages of the beach chair position are improved surgical access to the shoulder joint and ease of conversion from arthroscopic to open if necessary. Because the operative shoulder is brought beyond the edge of the table, the joint can be approached both anteriorly and posteriorly. The upright position also decreases arterial and venous pressures in the shoulder, thus optimizing the surgical field by decreasing bleeding.

15. What are some disadvantages to the beach chair position?
The elevated back of the beach chair position results in the patient's head resting above the level of the heart. One consequence of this is a potential for decreased arterial pressure and cerebral perfusion. Gravity decreases arterial pressure by 7.7 mm Hg for every 10 cm above the heart, and the Circle of Willis may be 30 cm above the heart, once finally positioned. Combined with decreased preload because of pooling of blood in the lower extremities and general anesthesia's impairment of cerebral autoregulation, intraoperative cerebral hypoperfusion becomes a serious concern. Precautions used to prevent cerebral hypoperfusion include: judicious preloading with intravenous fluids, maintaining cerebral blood pressures within 20% of baseline values, placing an arterial line in high-risk patients, and understanding that blood pressure cuffs placed on extremities may provide readings that misrepresent true blood pressures at the level of the brain.
   With the surgical site also being above the level of the heart, this can decrease venous pressures and encourage the entrapment of air within the vasculature. Although relatively large volumes of air may be required to induce right heart strain in healthy patients, even small amounts of air may result in catastrophic neurological deficits if a patent foramen ovale allows air to embolize to the left heart and then the brain. If venous air embolism is suspected, ask the surgeon to flood the field in water, take the patient out of the head-up position, and consider a transesophageal echocardiogram for assessment of air in the superior vena cava, heart, and pulmonary arteries.

16. What is another way to monitor a patient's cerebral perfusion aside from systemic blood pressure?
Cerebral oximetry is a technology that allows for measurement of tissue oxygenation within a particular region of the brain. Regional cerebral oxygenation is measured by placing noninvasive monitors on the patient's head that simultaneously project and receive near-infrared light. Based on the absorption of different light spectrums by the tissue, cerebral oximetry calculates an approximation of tissue oxygenation. Cerebral oximetry provides continuous monitoring of brain perfusion and may offer an early alert to a dangerous drop below baseline.

17. What are some considerations for head placement in the beach chair position?
Special attention must be paid to the positioning of the head in a neutral position to prevent several complications. Inadvertent rotation or lateral flexion of the neck may place traction on the cervical or brachial plexuses, resulting in neuropraxia. Pressure on the face can also cause damage to nerves. The chin should always remain at least 2 cm from the chest to avoid excessive flexion of the neck. Excessive flexion of the neck can compress large veins, preventing blood return from the head and, catastrophically, can compress microvasculature of the spinal cord, resulting in neurologic injury.

18. What is an alternative to beach chair position for shoulder surgery?
The lateral decubitus position is an alternative position for shoulder surgeries. The patient is placed laterally (on their side) with the operative shoulder on top. The operative arm is then placed in traction connected to a tower above the patient. This position also provides adequate access to the shoulder joint and removes the relative risk of cerebral hypoperfusion and venous air embolism, associated with the beach chair position.

19. Discuss the systemic risks associated with methyl methacrylate cement.
Orthopedic surgeries sometimes use methyl methacrylate cement (MMC) to secure hardware to bone or to create beads impregnated with antibiotics that can be left in the surgical field. Placement of MMC can be associated with hypotension, hypoxia, and bronchoconstriction. Therefore confirming adequate fluid status and increasing the fraction of inspired oxygen may be prudent before MMC injection. It has been theorized that the MMC monomer acts as a direct vasodilator within the bloodstream, but the greater concern may be for embolization. The cement itself may embolize, or the act of injecting it may pressurize bone components (marrow, fat, or air) into the vascular system. This may result in the rare but catastrophic complications of right heart strain, hemodynamic collapse, and even death. Notably, MMC may also pose an occupational threat if routinely handled. Average air concentrations of less than 100 parts per million are recommended if exposure is anticipated to be longer than 8 hours.

KEY POINTS: SHOULDER OPERATIONS

1. The shoulder is primarily supplied by the axillary nerve inferiorly and the suprascapular nerve superiorly, both of which can be anesthetized by an interscalene block.
2. Complications of the interscalene block include: ipsilateral phrenic nerve block, resulting in hemidiaphragmatic paralysis, Horner syndrome, unilateral recurrent laryngeal nerve paralysis, pneumothorax, inadvertent neuraxial injection, and accidental intravascular injection.
3. Isolated suprascapular nerve block may be performed to anesthetize the shoulder while removing the risk of phrenic nerve inhibition.
4. Advantages of beach chair position include improved surgical access to the shoulder and improved surgical visualization because of decreased bleeding. Disadvantages include risk of cerebral hypoperfusion, venous air embolism, and neurological injury, associated with malposition of the head.

SUGGESTED READINGS

Auyong D, Hanson N, Joseph R, et al. Comparison of anterior suprascapular, supraclavicular, and interscalene nerve block approaches for major outpatient arthroscopic shoulder surgery: a randomized, double-blind, noninferiority trial. Anesthesiology. 2018;129(1):47–57.
Barash P. Clinical Anesthesia. 7th ed. Philadelphia, PA: Wolters Kluwer Health/Lippincott Williams & Wilkins; 2013.
Hadzic A. Hadzic's Textbook of Regional Anesthesia and Acute Pain Management. McGraw-Hill Education; 2017.
Laflam A, Joshi B, Brady K, et al. Shoulder surgery in the beach chair position is associated with diminished cerebral autoregulation but no differences in postoperative cognition or brain injury biomarker levels compared with supine positioning: The Anesthesia Patient Safety Foundation Beach Chair Study. Anesth Analg. 2015;120(1):176–185.
Miller R, Pardo M. Basics of Anesthesia: Expert Consult. Elsevier Health Sciences, 2011.
Peebles DJ, Ellis RH, Stride SDK. Cardiovascular effects of methylmethacrylate cement. Br Med J. 1972;1(5796):349–351.
Picton P, Dering A, Alexander A, et al. Influence of ventilation strategies and anesthetic techniques on regional cerebral oximetry in the beach chair position: a prospective interventional study with a randomized comparison of two anesthetics. Anesthesiology. 2015;123 (4):765–774.

CHAPTER 67

ELECTROCONVULSIVE THERAPY

Alma N. Juels, MD, Aaron Murray, MD

1. **What are the major indications for electroconvulsive therapy treatment?**
   In the United States, electroconvulsive therapy (ECT) is used mainly to help treat patients with severe major depressive disorder, largely as a secondary treatment, after one or more trials of psychotropic medications have failed. ECT treatment can be the primary treatment when the clinical situation demands urgent symptomatic improvement. Some studies have shown ECT to be more effective than antidepressant medications alone, in treating the psychotic subtype of depression. Outside of the United States, ECT is also used commonly for the treatment of schizophrenia. ECT has also been shown to help other mental conditions as well, such as severe mania, catatonia, agitation, and aggression in people with dementia and possibly parkinsonism.

2. **What are the downsides of antidepressant psychotropical medication?**
   Although antidepressant medications are effective for many patients, the rate of response to the first agent administered can be as low as 50%. The elderly may not be able to tolerate antidepressants because of the many side effects associated with these medications. In addition, certain neuronal changes in the elderly can decrease the response to these medications.

3. **What are the proposed mechanisms by which ECT is effective?**
   During ECT, a small amount of electrical current is passed through the brain, resulting in a seizure and possible subsequent neurochemical changes. The reason these actions relieve severe depression and other psychiatric disorders remains unclear. There are four main theories of ECT's mechanism of action:
   1. The monoamine neurotransmitter theory: The monoamine neurotransmitter theory suggests that ECT works by increasing dopamine, serotonin, and adrenergic, and possibly gamma-aminobutyric acid and glutamate, neurotransmission.
   2. The neuroendocrine theory: The neuroendocrine theory suggests that ECT induces a release of hypothalamic or pituitary hormones, including prolactin, thyroid-stimulating hormone, adrenocorticotropic hormone, and endorphins. It is hypothesized that the release of these hormones results in the treatment's antidepressant effect.
   3. The anticonvulsant theory: The anticonvulsant theory proposes that ECT's beneficial effects are a result of the anticonvulsant nature of the treatment. Evidence for this theory includes the observations that seizure threshold rises, and seizure duration decreases, over a course of ECT treatment.
   4. The neurotrophic theory: The neurotrophic theory proposes that ECT's mechanism of action is by inducing neurogenesis and increasing neurotrophic signaling in the brain.

4. **Has ECT always been considered a good treatment for depression?**
   ECT was first used as a treatment for psychiatric disorders in the 1930s. However, complications, such as fractures and cognitive impairment, raised serious concerns. If not dangerous (insulin was used originally to cause a hypoglycemic seizure), it was barbaric (no anesthetic agents or muscle relaxants were used). Its use declined when antidepressant medications were introduced. However, in recent decades, further research and pharmacological advances have led to a renewed interest in the role of ECT.

5. **How safe is ECT?**
   ECT treatment is given to approximately 100,000 people each year. Interestingly, it appears to have less morbidity and mortality than with many antidepressant medications. Because of this strong safety record, patients with significant comorbidities are often candidates for ECT.

6. **What is the physiological response to ECT?**
   ECT has a dramatic effect on blood pressure and heart rate. Between the stimulus and onset of seizure, bradycardia, premature atrial or ventricular contractions, and even asystole may result, often lasting for several seconds because of the increase in vagal tone. After the seizure subsides, tachycardia and hypertension usually occur secondary to a catecholamine surge. The duration of tachycardia tends to correlate with seizure duration, as measured by electroencephalography (EEG), while hypertension often persists and requires therapy.
   During the seizure, an acute increase in cerebral blood flow and an associated increase in intracranial pressure (ICP) can occur. In addition, increases in adrenocorticotropic hormone, cortisol, epinephrine, vasopressin, prolactin, and growth hormone can be noted. Intraocular pressure and intragastric pressure may also transiently increase.

7. **Which patients are at increased risk for complications with ECT?**
There are no absolute contraindications for ECT. However, ECT should be used cautiously, if at all, when the effects on cerebral blood flow, ICP, heart rate, and blood pressure may prove problematic to the patient because of the presence of coexisting disease. Thus patients with cerebral space-occupying lesions or cerebrovascular disease are at increased risk. However, patients with a known intracranial lesion who have normal neurological examinations and minimal or no edema or mass effect on neuroimaging have safely undergone ECT. Consultation with neurology or neurosurgery is recommended for any patients with intracranial masses or vascular lesions before undergoing ECT. Similarly, patients with unstable cardiac disease, including uncompensated congestive heart failure, severe valvular disease, unstable angina, recent myocardial infarction, and uncontrolled hypertension are all at increased risk of complications. Patients with pheochromocytoma should not receive ECT because of the large amounts of catecholamines that may be released into the circulation during treatment. Patients with recent stroke should delay ECT treatment for at least 1 month. Of note, ECT has been used safely in persons with cardiac pacemakers or implantable cardiodefibrillators and during pregnancy.

8. **Describe the preoperative evaluation necessary before commencing ECT treatment?**
A standard preoperative anesthetic history must be taken, identifying medications, allergies, and prior adverse anesthetic events. The significant comorbidities discussed in Question 7 should be identified and the stability of these conditions assessed. A prior history of response to ECT (both symptomatically and physiologically) is valuable. A physical examination is also important. Remember to include an assessment of the patient's teeth and mouth, because the ECT stimulus will result in brief, yet intense masseter contraction. There are no absolute requirements for laboratory testing. The decision to order laboratory tests should be based on the stability of the patient's comorbidities and medication regimen. A pregnancy test in women of childbearing age is also reasonable.
    ECT is equivalent to a low-risk procedure (the short duration of anesthesia, the absence of significant fluid shifts, and the relatively low rate of major cardiac complications), as defined in the 2014 clinical guidelines issued by the American College of Cardiology and the American Heart Association for the perioperative care of patients undergoing noncardiac surgery. In patients with no active cardiac conditions (e.g., decompensated congestive heart failure, unstable angina, significant arrhythmias, or valvular disease), noninvasive cardiac testing is not indicated, and practitioners can proceed with risk-factor adjustment, as appropriate. Patients with active cardiac conditions can safely complete full courses of ECT once these conditions are stable. Optimal medical therapy in preparation for ECT is advised to minimize risk during and after treatment, although the patient's psychiatric condition may not allow this. In general, the patient's medications should be continued.

9. **What are the anesthetic medications most commonly used during ECT?**
Before induction of anesthesia, anticholinergic medications may be administered to lessen the effects of the initial parasympathetic discharge. They also provide antisialagogue properties. The medication most commonly used is glycopyrrolate, 0.2 to 0.4 mg intravenously. In addition, if the patient is taking benzodiazepines, flumazenil will be given immediately before the procedure to reverse the effects of the benzodiazepines and hence normalize the seizure threshold.
    Methohexital is the most common anesthetic induction agent used because it has a rapid onset, short duration of action, low cardiac toxicity, and, most importantly, minimal anticonvulsant properties. Side effects include hypotension, myoclonus, and pain with injection. A typical dose of methohexital is 0.75 to 1 mg/kg.
    In patients with left ventricular dysfunction, etomidate is an effective induction agent alternative, because it has minimal effects on myocardial contractility and cardiac output. Etomidate also may enhance seizure duration in patients who have had prior ECT, but whose seizure durations were thought inadequate to achieve a therapeutic effect. Side effects include pain on injection, nausea and vomiting, and delays in return of cognitive function. A typical dose of etomidate is 0.15 to 0.3 mg/kg.
    Propofol has a rapid onset and short duration of action and allows cognitive function to return quickly. Although propofol use is associated with shorter seizure duration, research suggests that there is no difference in outcome when compared with methohexital. A typical dose of propofol is 0.75 to 1 mg/kg.
    Although ketamine has been used in ECT, the EEG seizure duration is decreased compared with methohexital. In addition, ketamine increases ICP and myocardial oxygen consumption. Although ketamine is not currently an agent of choice for ECT, ongoing studies are examining a potential synergistic effect between ketamine and ECT for rapid relief of depression.
    The short-acting opioid remifentanil has been used as an adjunct during induction, because of its anesthetic-sparing effects. It provides a stable anesthetic when swings in heart rate and blood pressure are undesirable and it has no effect on seizure duration. Potent volatile anesthetics offer no advantage over intravenous agents, with the possible exception of late in pregnancy, during which time ECT has been noted on occasion to produce titanic uterine contractions. Intravenous lidocaine raises the seizure threshold and should be avoided in before ECT.

10. **Describe the technique of ECT, including appropriate monitoring.**
Commonly a psychiatrist, anesthesiologist, and nurse attend the patient. An intravenous line is established, and routine monitors, including electrocardiogram, intermittent blood pressure, and pulse oximetry are placed. On rare occasions, predicated on the patient's comorbidities, arterial cannulation and continuous monitoring may be required. The psychiatrist places EEG leads to measure the cortical seizure, and an additional blood pressure cuff is placed on a leg.

This second cuff will be inflated before administering muscle relaxants so that the muscles distal to it are isolated from the circulation, allowing the duration of motor seizure to be measured after initiating the ECT stimulus. Before inducing anesthesia, the patient is preoxygenated for a number of minutes with 100% oxygen by nasal cannula, face mask or ambubag.

After anesthetic induction, the blood pressure cuff on the leg is inflated and acts as a tourniquet. The patient is hyperventilated by bag mask ventilation to lower seizure threshold. Typically, the short-acting depolarizing muscle relaxant succinylcholine (0.5–1.5 mg/kg) is administered. Rocuronium, an intermediate acting nondepolarizing muscle relaxant, and sugammadex to reverse the rocuronium, is being used as an alternative to succinylcholine and has been shown to potentially allow for a longer seizure duration.

Before administering the electroconvulsive stimulus, a compressible mouth guard protector is inserted to protect the patient's teeth, lips, and tongue from injury during the associated masseter contraction. On rare occasions, based on clinical circumstances, the patient is intubated.

During the seizure, the patient receives positive-pressure ventilation with 100% oxygen, typically via bag mask, until spontaneous ventilation returns and the patient awakens. Monitoring continues in the postanesthetic care unit, until the patient is oriented and meets discharge criteria.

Occasionally, the patient is confused or complains of a headache; benzodiazepines, opioids, and ketorolac are all appropriate treatments for these problems.

Finally, it is common over a course of therapy that anesthetic medication selection or dosages require modification. These adjustments are made based on review of prior records and whether the patient experienced a seizure of therapeutic duration.

11. What additional medications are used to address hypertension and tachycardia?

The cardioselective β-adrenergic blocker, esmolol, is sometimes given by either bolus or infusion to blunt the sympathetic response of ECT. One must be careful because β blockers may reduce seizure duration. Better choices to attenuate the increase in blood pressure and provide coronary vasodilation are nitroglycerin (3 mcg/kg) intravenous, given 2 minutes before ECT, or 2% nitroglycerin ointment applied 45 minutes before ECT. For persistent hypertension, the mixed α- and β-adrenergic blocker, labetalol or hydralazine, is frequently administered.

12. What is the optimal seizure duration?

ECT-induced seizure activity lasting from 25 to 50 seconds is believed to produce the best response. Patients experiencing an initial seizure lasting less than 15 seconds or greater than 180 seconds have been found to achieve less favorable responses to ECT.

13. What can be done to prolong a seizure of inadequate duration? What about terminating a prolonged seizure?

Etomidate is the induction drug of choice in patients experiencing inadequate seizure activity.

The proconvulsant caffeine (500 mg) can be administered when the seizure duration during prior electroconvulsive treatments has been deemed suboptimal. Aminophylline has also been used for this purpose. Prolonged ECT-induced seizures can be terminated with a benzodiazepine or propofol bolus (40–80 mg).

14. How many ECT treatments are usually necessary?

ECT is administered as a therapeutic course. The total number of treatments needed varies from patient to patient. For depression, the typical range is 6 to 12 treatments. In successful cases, initial clinical improvement is usually evident after 3 to 5 treatments. In the United States, ECT is typically administered 3 times a week. In other countries, a twice-a-week schedule is more common. Evidence suggests that outcomes are comparable between the two schedules, and that a 3 times per-week schedule may produce results more swiftly but with more cognitive deficits.

15. What are some of the adverse effects of ECT?

Some common adverse side effects are headache (including precipitation of migraine headaches), musculoskeletal pain, jaw pain and worsening of temporomandibular joint issues, nausea, fatigue, and possible injury to the teeth and tongue if a bite block is not properly placed. Ketorolac can be given before treatments to alleviate muscle pain, headaches, and jaw pain. Occasionally, narcotics are given. Infrequent but serious complications include cardiac issues and emergence delirium. In patients with preexisting heart disease, an ECT can precipitate cardiac arrhythmias and cardiac ischemia. Emergence delirium is characterized by restless agitation, aimless repetitive movements, grasping at objects in view, or restless attempts to remove the monitors and intravenous line. It usually lasts from 10 to 45 minutes or more after the seizure and usually responds to benzodiazepines.

An induced seizure lasting longer than 2 or 3 minutes is considered prolonged and can result in increased cognitive deficits.

Prolonged apnea is said to occur if it takes longer than 5 minutes to regain spontaneous ventilation after ECT treatment. This may be caused by a pseudocholinesterase deficiency, resulting in prolonged succinylcholine activity.

Anterograde amnesia may occur immediately after ECT treatment and tends to resolve within an hour. Retrograde amnesia, on the other hand, can be much more debilitating. It is the most common persistent adverse effect of ECT, and is usually seen in elderly patients and in those with preexisting cognitive impairment. Use of unipolar ECT has been shown to cause less memory loss than bipolar ECT.

Memory loss of events several months or even years in the past can occur. Usually retrograde amnesia improves during the first few months after ECT, although many patients have incomplete recovery. To help improve memory, it is recommended that patients be mentally stimulated. Have them read, ask questions, stay up to date on current events, and even play games that stimulate thinking. Because of this potential for acute memory loss, it is recommended that patients postpone making any major decisions for up to 2 weeks after an ECT treatment. In addition, one should not be driving or operating any large machinery during this recovery period.

16. **Is ECT curative?**
More than 70% of depressed people who receive this treatment respond favorably, making it the most effective treatment for severe depression. However, a permanent cure is extremely rare. Maintenance therapy with occasional (weekly or monthly) ECT treatments, in combination with antidepressant pharmacotherapy decreases the relapse rate, but more effective strategies for relapse prevention in mood disorders continue to be urgently needed.

KEY POINTS: ELECTROCONVULSIVE THERAPY

1. ECT treatment is recommended for patients with severe major depressive disorder, psychotic subtypes of depression, possibly schizophrenia, and in patients who cannot tolerate the side effects of, or are treatment-refractory to, antidepressant medications.
2. Typical physiological responses to ECT include transient parasympathetic discharge resulting in bradyarrhythmias, followed by a sympathetic stimulus, resulting in hypertension and tachycardia. Increases in cerebral blood flow and ICP are also noted.
3. Methohexital is the most common induction agent used during ECT because it has minimal anticonvulsant properties, a rapid onset, short duration of action, and low cardiac toxicity.
4. Succinylcholine is the most common muscle relaxant used during ECT because of its short duration of action.

SUGGESTED READINGS

American Psychiatric Association Work Group on Major Depressive Disorder. Practice Guideline for the Treatment of Patients With Major Depressive Disorder. 3rd ed. Available at: http://psychiatryonline.org/guidelines.aspx. 2010.
Dawkins K. Refinement in ECT Techniques. Psychiatric Times. Available at: http://www.psychiatrictimes.com/electroconvulsive-therapy/refinements-ect-techniques. 2013.
Goodman WK. Electroconvulsive therapy in the spotlight. N Engl J Med. 2011;364(19):1785–1787.
Keller CH, Greenberg RM, Murrough JW, et al. ECT in treatment-resistant depression. Am J Psychiatry. 2012;169:1238–1244.
Narayan VB, Kumar JM. Review of anaesthetic management for electroconvulsive therapy. Anaesth Clin Pharmacol. 2008;24:259–276.
Tess AV, Smetana GW. Medical evaluation of patients undergoing electroconvulsive therapy. N Engl J Med. 2009;360(14):1437–1444.
Weiner RD, Prudic J. Electroconvulsive therapy in the United States: how often is it used? Biol. Psychiatry. 2013;73(2):105–106.

FUNDAMENTALS OF REGIONAL ANESTHESIA

Katie Yang, MD, Erin Gibbons, MD

1. **What are the indications and contraindications for regional anesthesia?**
   Peripheral nerve blocks can provide surgical anesthesia and/or intra- and postoperative analgesia for upper and lower limb, thoracic, abdominal, breast, and head and neck surgeries. Common surgeries performed with nerve blocks include various orthopedic procedures, amputations, thoracotomies, laparotomies, arteriovenous fistula creations/revisions, and mastectomies. Contraindications for peripheral nerve block include patient refusal, sepsis/bacteremia, infection at injection site, preexisting neuropathy, and coagulopathy.

2. **Name the advantages and disadvantages of peripheral nerve blockade versus general anesthesia when used as the primary anesthetic technique?**
   Regional techniques are especially helpful in cases for which general anesthesia is undesirable; for example, patients with anticipated difficult airway or severe cardiopulmonary disease could avoid pulmonary complications or hemodynamic instability by undergoing procedures under regional block. In addition, the opioid-sparing effects of nerve blocks are particularly useful for perioperative pain control in patients with obstructive sleep apnea, severe postoperative nausea and vomiting, chronic opioid therapy, opioid abuse history, or allergies to analgesics. Local anesthetic injection also causes vasodilation at the block site, which can aid in perfusion of flaps or extremities with compromised perfusion.

   Procedures performed under regional block require patient cooperation, so this technique may be unsuitable for children or patients with high anxiety, developmental delay, altered mental status, or dementia. Patients may report inadequate sensory loss just before surgical incision, which can be because of either incomplete nerve block or insufficient time between block and incision. Another disadvantage of performing procedures under regional anesthesia is that preoperative blocks may prove inflexible if intraoperative findings change the surgeon's approach to include areas not covered by the block. For these reasons, regional blocks are often performed in conjunction with general anesthesia, instead of being the primary anesthetic technique.

3. **What are the different methods for providing regional anesthesia?**
   Peripheral nerve blocks can be performed as a single injection or as a continuous infusion via indwelling catheter. Similarly, neuraxial blockade may be performed as an injection into the subarachnoid space (spinal anesthesia) or as a continuous infusion into the epidural space. Another method of delivery is IV regional anesthesia (also known as *Bier block*), in which local anesthetic is injected intravenously into an extremity in the presence of an inflated tourniquet.

4. **Describe the technique for performing a Bier block.**
   To perform a Bier block, an IV is placed in the operative extremity. After elevating the extremity and exsanguinating the limb (through the application of a compression bandage), a double tourniquet is inflated, and lidocaine ($\leq$3 mg/kg) is injected into the operative extremity, IV. The extremity is then lowered, the IV removed, and the surgical procedure can proceed, while the patient breathes spontaneously with or without sedation. This type of block is typically used for procedures lasting 30 to 45 minutes, as longer procedures are generally limited by tourniquet pain.

5. **What different techniques are used for performing peripheral nerve blocks?**
   Most peripheral nerve blocks today are performed using ultrasound guidance, as this technology allows direct visualization of local anesthetic spread around neural structures or between muscle and/or fascial layers. Nerve stimulation is an older technique that can be used alone or in conjunction with ultrasound, especially when anatomic structures are difficult to identify on ultrasound. Finally, some blocks can be performed using anatomic landmarks alone or via subcutaneous infiltration, resulting in a field block.

6. **Describe the ultrasound guided nerve block technique and its advantages/disadvantages.**
   Ultrasound-guided nerve blocks are performed using ultrasound images to guide needle advancement and local anesthetic injection around neural structures. They may be performed using an in-plane (IP) or out-of-plane (OP) approach. Using the IP approach, the needle is advanced in the plane of the ultrasound beam, such that the entire shaft of the needle can be visualized. In contrast, the needle is advanced perpendicular to the ultrasound beam during the OP approach. This approach still allows for visualization of local anesthetic spread, but only a cross section of the needle, will be seen (Fig. 68.1). In general, the IP approach is preferred because it shows the entire trajectory of the needle and more easily allows for avoidance of important structures, such as blood vessels, pleura, nerves, and so on. However, the OP approach can be useful because of its shorter and more direct path to the nerve.

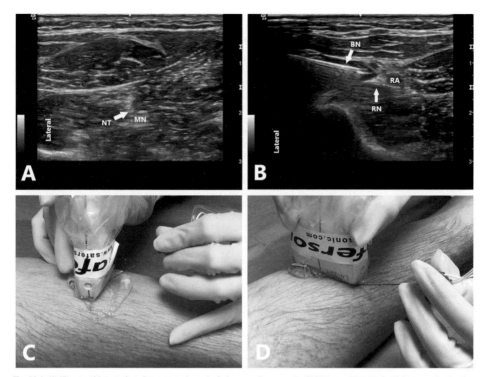

Fig. 68.1 (A) Ultrasound image of median nerve using out-of-plane needle approach. (B) Ultrasound image of radial nerve using in-plane needle approach. (C) Out-of-plane needle approach. (D) In-plane needle approach. *BN*, Block needle; *MN*, median nerve; *NT*, needle tip; *RA*, radial artery; *RN*, radial nerve.

Use of ultrasound allows for better visualization of anatomic structures, which has been shown to decrease the incidence of certain complications. With ultrasound it is possible to visualize blood vessels, thus allowing for a needle trajectory that decreases the risk of bleeding and hematoma formation. It also allows for visualization of the pleura, greatly reducing the risk of pneumothorax risk of supraclavicular block. Ultrasound is also useful in identifying anatomical variations that might limit the effectiveness of a given block technique; for example, it is possible to see muscles or blood vessels that split the target plexus and might prevent complete spread of local anesthetic. Lastly, it is possible to see the nerves themselves, ensuring that all neural structures are surrounded by local anesthetic and small branches are not missed. The major disadvantage to using ultrasound is that it requires specialized and expensive equipment that may not be available in all locations.

7. **Describe the nerve stimulator technique and its advantages/disadvantages.**
   For this technique, a nerve stimulator device emits an electrical stimulus through an insulated block needle. The stimulus is generally short (0.05–1 ms) and repetitive (1–2 Hz), and the needle is advanced until muscle twitching and/or paresthesias, specific for the targeted nerve, are elicited. The intensity of the stimulus is then decreased until the twitching or paresthesia disappears. Continued response presence at low amplitudes signifies close proximity of the needle to the nerve. However, if a response is still elicited at an intensity of 0.3 mA, the needle is likely intraneural and should be withdrawn slightly before injecting local anesthetic. Note that muscle twitching tends to disappear once even small amounts of local anesthetic have been injected, and in some patients, twitching may not appear at all, even with excellent needle positioning.

   Although the ability to elicit the appropriate muscle twitching response provides good confirmation of needle tip location, lack of visualization presents several challenges. Among these, are the possibility of unintentional nerve trauma and inability to identify variant anatomy. Also twitching can occur with direct muscle stimulation, which may be misidentified as nerve stimulation. For these reasons, the nerve stimulator technique is most often used in conjunction with ultrasound, and is of particular use in cases of difficult ultrasound visualization.

8. **What are the different types of sonographic resolution?**
   There are three types of resolution in sonographic imaging: axial, lateral, and temporal. Axial resolution relates to the number of planes along the axis of the ultrasound beam and is dependent upon pulse wavelength and the number of cycles per pulse. Lateral resolution describes the clarity between two adjacent structures visualized

simultaneously and located the same distance from the probe. Lateral resolution improves as the wave frequency increases and the ultrasound beam width decreases. Temporal resolution relates to dynamic structures, such as pulsating vessels. This type of resolution improves with increased ultrasound frame rate.

9. **What are some ways to improve visualization under ultrasound?**
   To optimize nerve visualization, first select an ultrasound probe of appropriate frequency. Superficial structures, such as ankle nerves are best visualized with a high frequency probe (10–13 MHz), medium-depth structures, such as the popliteal sciatic nerve, are best visualized with a medium frequency probe (6–10 MHz) and deep structures, such as the subgluteal sciatic nerve, are best visualized with a low frequency probe (2–5 MHz). Next, ensure that the ultrasound picture is set to an appropriate depth to locate the target nerve. Make sure to confirm the orientation of the probe and to apply sufficient gel. Adjustment of gain changes the brightness of the screen and adjustment of time-gain compensation can improve image quality by reducing artifact, secondary to ultrasound attenuation. Finally, Doppler ultrasound can be used to identify pulsating blood vessels or to identify spread of local anesthetic during injection.

   To optimize IP needle visualization under ultrasound, ensure that the needle is aligned with the plane of the ultrasound beam. If only part of the needle shaft is visualized, it is likely misaligned with the beam. Do not advance the needle until the tip is clearly visualized. Changing the tilt of the ultrasound probe may also aid in visualizing the needle. Remember that the steeper the angle of the needle, the more difficult it is to visualize on ultrasound; for this reason, it may be beneficial to puncture the skin farther away from the probe, if possible, to reach deeper structures. Echogenic needles also tend to be easier to visualize.

10. **What structures form the boundaries of the paravertebral space?**
    The superior costotransverse ligament forms the posterior border of the paravertebral space. The anterolateral border is formed by the parietal pleura and the vertebral bodies and intervertebral disks form its medial border. The paravertebral space houses the thoracic spinal nerves and the sympathetic trunk.

11. **What are the muscles of the anterolateral abdomen from superficial to deep? What is their innervation? What blocks target this area?**
    From superficial to deep, the muscle layers of the abdomen consist of the external oblique, internal oblique, and the transverse abdominis muscles. They are innervated by the anterior rami of T7–L1. The transverse abdominus plane block, ilioinguinal, iliohypogastric, and quadratus lumborum blocks target this area.

12. **What levels of spinal cord form the brachial plexus and what are its different subdivisions? What blocks target this area?**
    The brachial plexus is formed from the C5–T1 nerve roots. The subdivisions of the brachial plexus consist of: roots (C5–T1), trunks (upper, middle, and lower), divisions (anterior and posterior), cords (posterior, medial, and lateral), and branches (median, ulnar, radial, musculocutaneous, and axillary nerves). Blocks that target this area include the interscalene, supraclavicular, and infraclavicular brachial plexus nerve blocks, as well as axillary, and various forearm nerve blocks.

13. **From what nerve roots does the lumbar plexus arise and what are its branches? Which blocks target this area?**
    The lumbar plexus is formed from the T12–L4 nerve roots. It branches into the ilioinguinal, iliohypogastric, genitofemoral, lateral femoral cutaneous, femoral, and obturator nerves. You can target this area with a lumbar plexus, femoral, and fascia iliaca blocks.

14. **Along with the lumbar plexus, what other nerve provides innervation to the lower extremity? What are its nerve roots and branches? What approaches can be used to target this nerve?**
    The sciatic nerve innervates the majority of the lower extremity, excluding the anterior thigh and the medial calf, which is innervated by the lumbar plexus. It arises from the L4–S3 nerve roots and branches into the tibial and the common peroneal nerves. This nerve can be blocked proximally (anterior, transgluteal, subgluteal) or at the popliteal fossa. Its branches can also be blocked at the ankle.

15. **Describe the cutaneous innervation of the ankle.**
    The ankle is innervated by five nerves: tibial, saphenous, deep peroneal, superficial peroneal, and sural. Of these, only the saphenous arises from the femoral nerve—the other four all arise from the sciatic nerve. The tibial nerve (and its branches, the calcaneal nerve and medial and lateral plantar nerves) innervates most of the heel and plantar surface of the foot. The saphenous nerve innervates the medial aspect of the lower leg and ankle. Although the superficial peroneal nerve innervates most of the dorsum of the foot, the deep peroneal nerve only innervates a small area at the webspace between the great and second toes. The sural nerve innervates the lateral ankle.

16. **What kinds of complications can result from regional anesthesia?**
    Complications of regional anesthesia include bleeding, infection, intravascular or intraneural injection, leading to LAST or nerve damage, respectively, allergic reactions, damage to adjacent structures, and block failure. Interscalene and supraclavicular blocks are commonly associated with phrenic nerve involvement, leading to ipsilateral diaphragmatic paresis, sympathetic chain involvement, leading to ipsilateral Horner syndrome, and recurrent laryngeal nerve

involvement, leading to hoarseness. Subarachnoid or epidural injection and pneumothorax are other possible complications of these blocks.

17. **What are some ways to decrease the risk of complications?**

    To avoid complications, use sterile technique, ensure the patient is on appropriate monitors, and inject local anesthetic in small increments ($\leq$5 cc, at a rate of no more than 1 cc/s), aspirating before each injection. Also it is reasonable to allow for one complete circulation time (about 15–30 seconds) after injecting 10 cc to assess for signs/symptoms of systemic toxicity. Stop injecting and withdraw the needle slightly if the patient reports sharp pain or paresthesias. For ultrasound-guided blocks, do not advance your needle unless the tip is visualized. For nerve stimulator blocks, do not inject local anesthetic if a twitch response is obtained below 0.3 mA, as this response likely indicates that the tip of the needle is intraneural. Continuously monitor your patient closely for changes in hemodynamics or mental status.

18. **What are some commonly used local anesthetics?**

    Local anesthetics can be categorized by duration of action: short, intermediate, or long. 2-Chloroprocaine is a widely used short-acting local anesthetic with a duration of action lasting 1.5 to 2 hours. A unique feature of this drug is its rapid metabolism by plasma cholinesterases, which allows for administration of high concentrations (2%–3%), with very little risk of toxicity.

    Commonly used intermediate-acting local anesthetics include lidocaine (1–3 hours) and mepivacaine (3–5 hours). Although these two drugs are only intermediate-lasting local anesthetics, many practitioners find them more useful than longer lasting drugs. Note, epinephrine is frequently added to extend the block duration of lidocaine.

    Ropivacaine and bupivacaine are commonly used for blocks requiring longer duration. These drugs have a slower onset of action (15–30 minutes), but can provide analgesia for much longer (6–30 hours). Bupivacaine has higher cardiotoxicity and causes more motor blockade than ropivacaine, but does provide slightly longer duration of action.

19. **Which medications are commonly added to local anesthetics for regional anesthesia? What purpose do they serve?**

    Several different additives have been described for regional blocks, although more studies are needed to determine the efficacy of many of them. Vasoconstrictors, such as epinephrine, are commonly added to local anesthetics to lengthen duration of block and decrease systemic absorption. The tachycardia and hypertension effects of epinephrine can also indicate intravascular injection. Another common additive is sodium bicarbonate, which alkalinizes the pH of the local anesthetic solution and decreases time to block onset. Clonidine is an alpha-2 agonist that has been demonstrated to possess analgesic properties. When combined with local anesthetics, it may improve block quality and prolong duration. Other medications thought to prolong block duration include dexamethasone and dexmedetomidine.

20. **What characteristics of a local anesthetic affect its onset of action? Potency? What factors influence duration of action?**

    A local anesthetic's onset of action depends on its pK_a—the closer to the body's pH, the quicker the onset (Table 68.1). This phenomenon relates to the fact that local anesthetics must first cross the lipid membrane in their unprotonated basic (nonionized) form before binding sodium channels in their protonated (ionized) form. For this reason, sodium bicarbonate is sometimes added to local anesthetics before injection to increase the amount of nonionized form and decrease the onset of action.

    Local anesthetic potency correlates with lipid solubility. Lipid soluble local anesthetics that are able to easily traverse the lipid membrane require lower concentrations to achieve the same effect as less lipid soluble drugs.

    Factors determining a block's duration of action include type of local anesthetic and presence/absence of a vasoconstrictor. Greater lipid solubility and protein binding can also contribute to longer duration of action. Certain local anesthetics have short durations of action (45–90 minutes), while others have medium (90–180 minutes) and long durations of action (4–30 hours) (see Table 68.1). Vasoconstrictors, such as epinephrine, may be added to local anesthetics (which themselves have vasodilating properties) to keep the anesthetic localized to the tissue surrounding the target nerve.

Table 68.1 Commonly Used Local Anesthetics			
LOCAL ANESTHETIC	**pK$_a$**	**ONSET (min)**	**DURATION (h)**
3% 2-chloroprocaine	8.7	10–15	1–2
2% Lidocaine	7.8	10–20	3–5
1.5% Mepivacaine	7.6	10–20	3–5
0.5% Ropivacaine	8.1	15–30	6–24
0.5% Bupivacaine	8.1	15–30	6–30

21. **What is LAST? Describe the signs and symptoms.**
LAST can result from perineural injection of large doses of local anesthetic, as well as from accidental intravascular, intrathecal, or epidural injection. The central nervous system (CNS) and cardiovascular system are most affected by LAST. CNS signs classically precede cardiovascular signs, although this sequence may be reversed, especially with rapid injection or bupivacaine use. CNS disturbances generally consist of an excitatory phase, followed by a depressive phase. The excitatory phase is characterized by tinnitus, circumoral numbness, lightheadedness, altered mental status, tremors, and tonic-clonic seizures. The subsequent depressive phase may feature respiratory depression, coma, and respiratory arrest. Cardiovascular effects from LAST include hypotension (because of vasodilation), conduction disturbances, ventricular arrhythmias, and direct myocardial depression, up to and including cardiac arrest. Of note, although lidocaine is generally regarded as being less likely to lead to systemic toxicity than bupivacaine or ropivacaine, there are many case reports in the literature reporting LAST because of lidocaine.

22. **How would you treat a patient exhibiting signs of LAST?**
Remember that cardiac arrest in the setting of LAST is treated differently than cardiac arrest from other causes. The American Society of Regional Anesthesia and Pain Medicine (ASRA) recommends the following treatment algorithm according to their 2017 updated guidelines:
- Immediately discontinue administration of all local anesthetics.
- Call for help and a LAST rescue kit. Alert cardiopulmonary bypass team.
- Ventilate with 100% oxygen, placing advanced airway if necessary.
- Treat seizures with benzodiazepines. Consider lipid emulsion therapy promptly at the first sign of a severe LAST event. Note that propofol is not an adequate alternative to lipid emulsion therapy and can cause profound hypotension in an already hemodynamically unstable patient.
- Treat hypotension and bradycardia. Start cardiopulmonary resuscitation if patient becomes pulseless.
- Continue monitoring 4 to 6 hours after a cardiovascular event or at least 2 hours after a limited CNS event.
- Epinephrine boluses should be reduced to 1 mcg/kg (or lower).
- Avoid lidocaine, vasopressin, calcium channel blockers, and beta blockers.

23. **What is the proper dosing of intravenous lipid emulsion for LAST?**
Patients heavier than 70 kg should be administered 100 mL lipid emulsion 20% over 2 to 3 minutes, followed by an infusion of 200 to 250 mL over 15 to 20 minutes. Patients less than 70 kg should receive a 1.5 mL/kg bolus, followed by an infusion of 0.25 mL/kg/min ideal body weight.
If after the discussed treatment the patient remains unstable, rebolus at the same dose as described earlier 1 to 2 times and double the infusion rate. Per ASRA guidelines, the dosing measurements need not be exact, although they should not exceed the maximum dose of 12 mL/kg.

KEY POINTS: FUNDAMENTALS OF REGIONAL ANESTHESIA

- Regional anesthesia is beneficial for patients in whom general anesthesia should be avoided or in whom pain may be difficult to control, including patients with severe cardiopulmonary disease, obstructive sleep apnea, postoperative nausea and vomiting, chronic pain, and substance abuse.
- Methods of delivering regional anesthesia include peripheral nerve single injections or catheters, intravenous (IV) regional techniques, or neuraxial blockade.
- Peripheral nerves can be localized using ultrasound, nerve stimulator, elicited paresthesias, or landmark techniques.
- Complications from nerve blocks include bleeding, infection, intravascular or intraneural injection, allergic reactions, local anesthetic systemic toxicity (LAST), and damage to adjacent structures.

SUGGESTED READINGS

Gauss A, Tugtekin I, Georgieff M, et al. Incidence of clinically symptomatic pneumothorax in ultrasound-guided infraclavicular and supraclavicular brachial plexus block. Anaesthesia. 2014;69:327–336.
Hadzic A, ed. Hadzic's Textbook of Regional Anesthesia and Acute Pain Management. 2nd ed. New York: McGraw-Hill, 2017:81–335.
Neal J, Woodward C, Harrison K. The American Society of Regional Anesthesia and Pain Medicine checklist for managing local anesthetic systemic toxicity: 2017 version. Reg Anesth Pain Med. 2018;43:150–153.
NYSORA. The New York School of Regional Anesthesia. Available at: https://www.nysora.com.
USRA. Ultrasound for Regional Anesthesia. Available at: https://www.usra.ca

CHAPTER 69

PERIPHERAL NERVE AND TRUNK BLOCKS

Christopher P. Davis, MD, Ryan Guffey, MD

1. **Why would you perform a peripheral nerve block?**
   Nerve blocks are generally performed for two major indications: anesthesia or analgesia. An anesthetic peripheral nerve block may allow a patient to avoid general anesthesia and periprocedural pain medication. This can be very helpful for patients with risk factors, such as a difficult airway or intolerance to general anesthesia. Analgesic blocks are similar but do not have adequate density or coverage to enable avoidance of general anesthesia. The primary benefit to an analgesic block is to avoid postoperative opioids and their associated side effects, thus improving postoperative pain scores, increasing patient satisfaction, decreasing nausea, and decreasing the likelihood a patient requires postoperative admission for pain control.

2. **Which patients are not good candidates for a peripheral nerve block?**
   Nerve blocks can be associated with postoperative nerve damage. It is important to minimize this risk by only offering blocks to patients that are low risk for this complication. The most common reason to avoid offering a patient a nerve block is anticoagulation. If a patient has an intrinsic or pharmacological coagulopathy, there is an increased risk of hematoma formation and subsequent nerve damage. The American Society of Regional Anesthesia antithrombotic therapy guidelines, updated in April 2018, are very helpful for deciding who is an appropriate candidate. Also a peripheral neuropathy, such as symptomatic spinal stenosis or Guillain-Barré, may increase the risk. Alternatively, a successful nerve block after a traumatic injury can mask diagnosis of a compartment syndrome, delaying critical treatment. Lastly, if a patient has a systemic infection, placement of a nerve catheter can result in a perineural abscess.

3. **What are the most common nerve blocks of the upper extremity?**
   Most upper extremity nerve blocks involve blocking the brachial plexus at different anatomic locations. The blocks of the upper extremity are named for their anatomic correlation for probe position or needle insertion. Interscalene, supraclavicular, infraclavicular, and axillary are the most common brachial plexus blocks. With increased use of ultrasound, the supraclavicular block has become the mainstay for procedures below the shoulder. Individualized radial, median, and ulnar nerve blocks can be performed under ultrasound guidance to offer analgesia to the hand and fingers, while allowing for continued gross motor function.

4. **How do you decide which brachial plexus block is most suitable for various procedures on the upper extremity?**
   The interscalene brachial plexus block is most suitable for procedures on the shoulder, distal clavicle, and proximal humerus. This is discussed separately in chapter 66. Supraclavicular, infraclavicular, and axillary brachial plexus blocks are detailed in Table 69.1.

5. **What are the anatomic landmarks and basic technique for the supraclavicular, infraclavicular, and axillary brachial plexus blocks?**
   The supraclavicular nerve block is typically performed in the semi-sitting position, with the head turned to the opposite side. Reaching the arm to the ipsilateral lower extremity and externally rotating the shoulder helps depress the clavicle and increase space for the ultrasound probe. The needle is advanced from lateral to medial and local anesthetic is deposited, surrounding the divisions of the brachial plexus, lateral to the subclavian artery. Care must be taken to avoid any traversing arteries, as widespread variations in anatomy exist in the supraclavicular region.

   The infraclavicular nerve block is a deep block that has the added benefits of avoiding phrenic nerve paralysis and accommodation of peripheral nerve catheters. The patient is positioned supine and the arm is positioned either at the patient's side or above the head to elevate the clavicle and increase room for the ultrasound probe. The probe is oriented cephalad to caudad at the level of the coracoid process. The needle is advanced, until it is at approximately the 6 o'clock position of the axillary artery, and local anesthetic is deposited. This block provides coverage of all three cords of the brachial plexus with one injection. Note, it is important to achieve U shaped spread to both sides of the artery to avoid sparing of the medial or lateral cords.

   The axillary nerve block is performed with the patient's arm is abducted to approximately 90 degrees. The transducer is placed along the medial aspect of the arm in the axilla and the needle is traversed from cephalad to caudad to the 6 o'clock position of the axillary artery. Multiple injections are often required to achieve circumferential spread to anesthetize the median, ulnar, and radial nerves. A separate needle insertion point to anesthetize the musculocutaneous nerve is often required to ensure adequate distal forearm coverage.

Table 69.1 Brachial Plexus Nerve Blocks for Upper Extremity Surgery

BRACHIAL PLEXUS BLOCK	NEURAL DISTRIBUTION	LIMITATIONS
Supraclavicular	Anesthesia from below the deltoid to the fingers. Can be effective for shoulder surgery depending on technique.	Approximately 50% chance of phrenic nerve blockade Increased risk of pneumothorax Ultrasound guidance advised
Infraclavicular	Anesthesia from the mid-humerus to the fingers	Can be more technically challenging because of steep approach required
Axillary	Anesthesia from the mid-humerus to the fingers	Frequently spares musculocutaneous nerve, requiring it to be blocked separately Requires patient to abduct arm

6. **What are the specific risks of the supraclavicular, infraclavicular, and axillary brachial plexus blocks?**
The supraclavicular nerve block has an increased risk of pneumothorax compared with the infraclavicular and axillary approaches because of the block site's close proximity to the pleura. This incidence remains very low with use of ultrasound guidance, provided you have excellent needle tip visualization. Care must also be taken to avoid intravascular injection, not only in the subclavian artery, but in surrounding vessels, such as the dorsal scapular and suprascapular arteries as well. The infraclavicular nerve block carries an increased risk of intravascular injection. Target site depth and steep angle of insertion result in more difficult needle visualization, making aspiration before every injection especially important to ensure that the tip is not in the axillary artery or adjacent vein. Note that at lower depths, it can be more difficult to visualize small arteries and veins. The axillary nerve block is thought to have the least amount of risk comparatively to the other brachial plexus blocks. Should arterial puncture occur, the axillary artery has the added benefit of being compressible because of its superficial location. This makes manual compression a viable technique for preventing hematoma formation.

7. **What do you do when a supraclavicular nerve block results in a motor block of the arm, but the patient can still feel pain in one finger?**
The most appropriate course of action is to do a neurologic examination to evaluate the motor and sensory function of the median, radial, and ulnar nerves. Most likely, there has been ulnar nerve sparing from inadequate block of the lower trunk. This most commonly occurs because of a deficiency of local anesthetic in the "corner pocket," where the lower trunk is nestled in between the first rib and the subclavian artery. A supplementary rescue block can be performed to anesthetize this area, but there is theoretical increased risk of nerve damage with the passage of a needle through already anesthetized nerves. Another option would be to block the ulnar nerve more distally.

8. **What are the most common nerve blocks of the lower extremity?**
Unlike the upper extremity, the lower extremity requires multiple injections for complete coverage. The nerves of the lower extremity are derived from the lumbar plexus (L1–L5) and the sacral plexus (L4–S3). Because of this overlap, the lower extremity is often referred to as being covered by the lumbosacral plexus. The lumbar plexus gives rise to the iliohypogastric, ilioinguinal, genitofemoral, lateral femoral cutaneous, femoral, and obturator nerves. From these, the lumbar plexus, femoral, and saphenous nerve blocks are most common. The sacral plexus gives rise to the sciatic nerve, as well as the superior and inferior gluteal nerves, pudendal nerve, and the posterior cutaneous nerve of the thigh. From these, the transgluteal sciatic, subgluteal sciatic, popliteal sciatic, and ankle blocks are most common.

9. **How do you decide which nerve block is most suitable for various procedures on the lower extremity?**
Location of the surgery, possible application of a tourniquet, and need for postoperative motor function should all be considered with each block. To achieve complete surgical anesthesia of the lower extremity, a combination of sciatic and femoral blocks will need to be performed. For example, to provide complete anesthesia of the ankle for operative fixation, both a popliteal sciatic and saphenous nerve block would need to be used. However, this particular choice would not offer analgesia for pain from a thigh tourniquet. Therefore a more proximal choice, such as a subgluteal sciatic and lumbar plexus would be necessary, if this were desired. An ankle block is effective for surgery on the toes and forefoot, but the hindfoot is usually spared.

10. **What are the anatomical landmarks and basic techniques for the blocks of the lower extremity?**
The lumbar plexus block is considered a deep block. The needle insertion point is at the area 4 to 5 cm lateral to the L4-L5 interspace, as approximated by the top of the iliac crest. The block is primarily performed with nerve

stimulator guidance, until contraction of the quadriceps muscle is elicited. The lumbar plexus is located in the body of the psoas major muscle, typically 2 cm deep to the transverse process of the lumbar spine. Depending on body habitus, the depth of needle insertion is often between 6 and 8 cm.

The femoral nerve block is a very popular block for anesthesia of the anterolateral thigh and the medial skin below the knee. With ultrasound guidance, the nerve can be well visualized 1 cm lateral to the femoral artery, deep to the fascia iliaca, and superficial to the iliopsoas muscle. The saphenous nerve, the largest cutaneous branch of the femoral, is located more distal in the lower extremity, and is often blocked deep to the sartorius muscle, inside the adductor canal, next to the superficial femoral artery.

The proximal sciatic nerve is found deep to the gluteus maximus, in between the ischial tuberosity and greater trochanter of the femur. As described earlier, there are many variations to blocking this nerve, but the subgluteal approach is often less technically challenging and easiest to visualize by ultrasound because of its location over the thin tail of the gluteus maximus. In the popliteal region, the sciatic nerve has a variable branchpoint into the common peroneal and tibial nerves. Under ultrasound guidance, the sciatic nerve can be found posterior to the femur and posterolateral to the popliteal artery. The muscle borders of the nerve include the semitendinosus and semimembranosus medially and the biceps femoris laterally.

11. **What are the specific risks of nerve blocks to the lower extremity?**
    Risks of nerve blocks to the lower extremity include nerve injury, intravascular injection, infection, and damage to surrounding structures. Nerve injury is a rare and not completely understood phenomenon. Preexisting neuropathy is more common in the lower extremities, placing these nerves at an increased risk for nerve damage from intraneural injection, ischemia, or toxicity from local anesthetics. Furthermore, blocks, such as the lumbar plexus block, pose increased and unique risks because of the depth of the block and its proximity to several vulnerable structures. Cases of aortic perforation with retroperitoneal hematoma, intrathecal injection and even bowel perforation have been reported with this block.

12. **What is the difference between a plane block and a peripheral nerve block?**
    In contrast with a standard peripheral nerve block, a plane block involves anatomy where no distinct nerve needs to be identified. With the increased use of ultrasound, new block techniques have been discovered that involve the infiltration of local anesthetic, in particular fascial planes, where various nerves are known to traverse. This technique has given rise to numerous new blocks that offer analgesia to the abdomen, chest, and trunk. These blocks typically require a higher volume of local anesthetic to be effective, as compared with standard peripheral nerve blocks. Because the individual nerves are either small or not present at the location of injection, the risk of direct nerve damage from the needle is reduced.

13. **What truncal nerve blocks are appropriate for thoracic, breast, and abdominal surgery?**
    The thoracic paravertebral block involves depositing local anesthetic in the paravertebral space where the thoracic spinal nerves and sympathetic trunk reside. Injection here results in three to seven dermatomes of unilateral anesthesia to the abdomen or chest wall surrounding the insertion point, making it a good choice for smaller thoracic, abdominal, or breast surgeries.

    The transversus abdominis plane (TAP) block is indicated for lower abdominal surgeries, such as hysterectomy or hernia repair. Local anesthetic is deposited in the fascial plane, between the internal oblique and transversus abdominis muscles. With some variations in anatomy, the anterior divisions of T10–L1 and ilihypogastric and ilioinguinal nerves lie in this plane. The popular TAP block results in unilateral anesthesia of the lower anterior abdominal wall, including the groin. The upper abdomen can also be blocked using the subcostal TAP approach. Bilateral blocks can be used for midline surgeries, keeping in mind limits of local anesthetic dosing to avoid toxicity.

14. **Which nerves are blocked by the erector spinae, PECS, serratus anterior, and quadratus lumborum blocks?**
    Increased use of ultrasound has resulted in many novel truncal blocks that are on the forefront of regional anesthesia (Table 69.2).

15. **What are the specific risks of common truncal nerve blocks?**
    Paravertebral blocks have a few additional risks to the standard risks of peripheral nerve blocks. Pleural puncture and injection, resulting in pneumothorax, is possible because of the close association between the paravertebral space and the pleura. Epidural spread is also possible, which can result in unintended contralateral effects of the block and possible hemodynamic changes. A vagal reaction is also common. TAP blocks have become increasingly safe since the implementation of ultrasound. Rare serious complications are still possible, such as intraperitoneal injection and possible injury to abdominal viscera.

16. **What are the advantages and disadvantages of each truncal block?**
    The paravertebral block is very versatile in that it can be used for nearly any truncal procedure. It also provides relatively dense analgesia that can often be effective for surgical anesthesia. However, because of its location, it is higher risk than other newer truncal blocks. For breast surgery, the PECS or serratus anterior blocks are easier to perform and provide equivalent analgesia with lower potential risk. Also PECS blocks have the advantage of blocking the pectoral nerves; these are spared by other techniques.

Table 69.2 Truncal Nerve Blocks

FASCIAL PLANE BLOCK	PLANE OF INJECTION	NERVES BLOCKED	SURGICAL INDICATIONS
Erector Spinae	Between transverse process of vertebra and the erector spinae muscles	Thoracic/lumbar spinal nerves	Breast, chest, upper and lower abdominal surgery depending on injection point
PECS I	Between pectoralis major and pectoralis minor	Lateral and medial pectoral nerves.	Partial coverage for breast surgery
PECS II	Between pectoralis minor and serratus anterior	Thoracic intercostal nerves and long thoracic nerve	Breast surgery including axillary dissection
Serratus Anterior	Deep to the serratus anterior muscle	Thoracic intercostal nerves, thoracodorsal, and long thoracic nerves	Procedures of the hemi-thorax, including breast and thoracic surgery
Quadratus Lumborum	Anterolateral border of the quadratus lumborum muscle	Thoracic/lumbar spinal nerves	Upper or lower abdominal surgeries

The TAP and quadratus lumborum abdominal blocks similarly are easier to perform than the paravertebral block and are lower risk. The quadratus lumborum block has the advantage of covering more dermatomes per injection relative to the TAP block. The drawbacks to the quadratus lumborum are that it cannot be performed in the supine position and is more challenging than the TAP block.

The erector spinae is a new block that can be used for all of the same indications as the paravertebral block. Because it is farther from sensitive structures, such as the spinal cord, it is lower risk for direct injury or nerve threatening hematoma. The disadvantage to the erector spinae block is that its benefits are not currently well described in the literature. It likely delivers less effective analgesia than the paravertebral block.

KEY POINTS: PERIPHERAL NERVE AND TRUNK BLOCKS

1. Nerve blocks are generally performed for two major indications: anesthesia or analgesia, and may allow a patient to avoid general anesthesia and periprocedural pain medication.
2. Most upper extremity nerve blocks involve blocking the brachial plexus at different anatomic locations and are named for their anatomic correlation for probe position or needle insertion.
3. The nerves of the lower extremity are derived from the lumbar plexus (L1–L5) and the sacral plexus (L4–S3).
4. The lumbar plexus gives rise to the iliohypogastric, ilioinguinal, genitofemoral, lateral femoral cutaneous, femoral, and obturator nerves. From these, the lumbar plexus, femoral, and saphenous nerve blocks are most common.
5. The sacral plexus gives rise to the sciatic nerve, as well as the superior and inferior gluteal nerves, pudendal nerve, and the posterior cutaneous nerve of the thigh. From these, the transgluteal sciatic, subgluteal sciatic, popliteal sciatic, and ankle blocks are most common.
6. Increased use of ultrasound has resulted in many novel truncal blocks that are on the forefront of regional anesthesia.

Suggested Readings

Abrahams MS, Horn J, Noles LM, Aziz MF. Evidence-based medicine. Reg Anesth Pain Med. 2010;35(1).
Blanco R, Parras T, Mcdonnell JG, Prats-Galino A. Serratus plane block: a novel ultrasound-guided thoracic wall nerve block. Anaesthesia. 2013;68(11):1107–1113.
Chelly JE. Peripheral Nerve Blocks A Color Atlas, 3rd ed. Philadelphia: Wolters Kluwer Health, 2009.
Horlocker TT, Vandermeulen E, Kopp SL, Gogarten W, Leffert LR, Benzon HT. Regional anesthesia in the patient receiving antithrombotic or thrombolytic therapy: American Society of Regional Anesthesia and Pain Medicine Evidence-Based Guidelines (Fourth Edition) Reg Anesth Pain Med. 2018;43(3):263–309.
Deschner B, Robards C, Xu D, Hadzic A. Lower extremity peripheral nerve blocks. In: Raj's Practical Management of Pain, 4th ed. Philadelphia, PA: Mosby Elsevier; 2008: p. 889–903.
Forero M, Adhikary SD, Lopez H, Tsui C, Chin KJ. The erector spinae plane block. Reg Anesth Pain Med. 2016;41(5):621–627.
Hadzic A. Hadzic's Peripheral Nerve Blocks and Anatomy for Ultrasound-Guided Regional Anesthesia, 2nd ed. McGraw-Hill Companies; 2004.
Macfarlane A, Brull R. Ultrasound guided supraclavicular block. NYSORA. 2009;12:6–10.
McDonnell JG, Finnerty O. Transversus abdominis plane block. Curr Opin Anaesthesiol. 2012;25(5):610–614.
Ultrasound-Guided Axillary Brachial Plexus Block. (2017, May 04). Retrieved from https://www.nysora.com/ultrasound-guided-axillary-brachial-plexus-block
Ultrasound-Guided Infraclavicular Brachial Plexus Block. (2017, May 04). Retrieved from https://www.nysora.com/ultrasound-guided-infraclavicular-brachial-plexus-block

NERVE BLOCKS FOR THE HEAD AND NECK

Chang H. Park, MD, Samuel DeMaria, Jr, MD, Adam I. Levine, MD

1. **What are the indications for regional anesthesia in head and neck operations?**

   The abundant nerve supply and reliably identifiable bony landmarks of the head and neck allow for the effective use of regional anesthesia techniques for head and neck operations. Depending on the patient and the type of surgery, regional anesthesia can be used as the primary anesthetic, or as part of a balanced anesthetic, in conjunction with monitored anesthesia care or general anesthesia. Nerve blocks provide intraoperative and postoperative analgesia, which may reduce perioperative opioid use. As enhanced recovery after surgery (ERAS) protocols have become increasingly used by hospitals for head and neck surgery, regional techniques have been incorporated in an attempt to decrease perioperative opioid consumption and to increase the speed of recovery. In addition to providing analgesia, certain regional techniques may also decrease intraoperative bleeding and thus improve intraoperative visibility for specific procedures, particularly when epinephrine is used in conjunction with local anesthetics. Regional nerve blocks can also be used to augment local anesthesia topicalization for awake intubation, to improve patient comfort and optimize intubating conditions for the clinician. Finally, regional blocks that were performed intraoperatively for analgesic purposes can be used as the sole anesthetic for emergent bedside surgical re-exploration and hemostasis, in the unexpected and catastrophic event of postoperative bleeding.

2. **What are some unique considerations for head and neck regional anesthesia compared with other regional anesthesia techniques?**

   The proximity of the surgical site to the airway necessitates that minimal oxygen supplementation and airway support be used to decrease the risk of airway fire. Thus if the anesthetic plan relies solely on regional anesthesia, close communication with the surgical team regarding the appropriateness of such a plan is required. In addition, patients should be informed and educated about the regional technique so that they have a clear understanding of the anesthetic expectations and the surgical requirements. Because deep sedation is not recommended in this setting, effective analgesia from the nerve block is critical, as is patient cooperation.

3. **What are the contraindications to head and neck nerve blocks?**

   The contraindications for head and neck nerve blocks are essentially the same as for other regional techniques. Absolute contraindications are patient refusal, localized infections or neoplasms at the site of injection, and true allergic reactions to local anesthetics. Relative contraindications include coagulopathy and other bleeding disorders, bloodstream infections, and preexisting neuropathies. Although not unique to head and neck surgeries, neoplasms, and arteriovenous malformations are common indications for head and neck operations that would preclude regional anesthesia. Hence, a thorough understanding of the specific pathology involved in the surgery is essential.

4. **What are the risks in performing head and neck regional anesthesia?**

   In addition to the usual risks of nerve blocks, such as local anesthetic toxicity and nerve damage, there exists the potential to damage surrounding structures. Depending on the block that is performed, these may include injury to the eye or even the brain. Because of the abundance of critical blood vessels that surround the head and neck region, great care must be taken to avoid intravascular injections. Therefore aspiration before injection is mandatory. A comprehensive knowledge of head and neck anatomy and of the pharmacology of local anesthetics is critical to minimize complications.

5. **Which local anesthetics are commonly used for head and neck regional techniques?**

   Local anesthetics commonly used for head and neck nerve blocks include lidocaine (1.5%–2%), mepivacaine (1.5%–2%), bupivacaine (0.25%–0.5%), and ropivacaine (0.25%–0.5%). Head and neck regional anesthesia generally does not require large volumes of local anesthesia. Thus even though more dilute solutions of local anesthetics are often recommended for postoperative analgesia to avoid significant motor blockade, this is less of an issue for head and neck operations. Instead, using concentrated local anesthetics in small volumes can improve efficacy and duration of action.

6. **Describe the relevant anatomy for head and neck regional anesthesia.**

   The trigeminal nerve (cranial nerve V) and the cervical plexus (spinal nerves C1–C4) are responsible for most of the sensory innervation to the head, face, and neck.

   The trigeminal nerve, which provides sensory and motor innervation to the face, splits from the trigeminal ganglion into three major branches: the ophthalmic nerve (V1), the maxillary nerve (V2), and the mandibular nerve (V3).

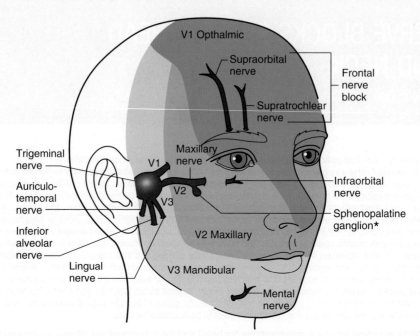

Fig. 70.1 Trigeminal nerve branches that are targets for regional blocks. *Regional blocks performed via intraoral approach.

These branches further divide into distal nerves that are often targeted for nerve blocks. One of the branches of the ophthalmic nerve that serves as a target for nerve block is the frontal nerve, which in turn splits into the supraorbital nerve and supratrochlear nerve. The maxillary nerve becomes the infraorbital nerve upon entering the infraorbital canal, and its sphenopalatine branches also comprise the sensory root of the sphenopalatine ganglion. The mandibular nerve divides into the anterior and posterior division, the latter of which becomes the inferior alveolar nerve and then lingual nerve and mental nerve. The auriculotemporal nerve also originates from the mandibular nerve (Fig. 70.1).

The cervical plexus is a network of nerves that originate from the anterior divisions of the upper four cervical nerves (C1–C4). Nerve branches, which originate from this plexus, innervate the region between the mandible to the clavicle and thus provides sensation to structures, such as the anterior and lateral neck, the jawline, the posterior head, and the posterior auricular region. The plexus lies in the posterior triangle of the neck; the rami of the cervical nerves exit the vertebral column and emerge from under the sternocleidomastoid muscle (SCM). The four cutaneous branches are innervated by roots C2 to C4. The muscular branches consist of the ansa cervicalis (C1–C3), which innervates the anterior neck muscles, and individual branches that innervate the posterolateral neck muscles.

7. Describe the various blocks that target the various branches of the trigeminal nerve.
   See Table 70.1.

8. What are the indications for a cervical plexus block?
   Because of its sensory innervation of the neck and posterior head, the cervical plexus can be blocked for perioperative analgesia and sometimes as the primary anesthetic for a variety of surgical procedures, including thyroidectomy, parathyroidectomy, carotid endarterectomy, neck dissection, lymph node biopsy, tympanomastoid surgery, otoplasty, and cochlear implantation. Both the superficial cervical plexus block and deep cervical plexus block can be performed to block the cervical plexus. The superficial cervical plexus block is performed where the nerves emerge from under the sternocleidomastoid, whereas the deep cervical plexus block is performed where the rami exit the vertebral column. Procedures performed with a midline incision (thyroidectomy and parathyroidectomy) require bilateral cervical plexus blocks, whereas one-sided operations (carotid endarterectomy) only require a unilateral block.
   The deep cervical plexus block will not be discussed in this chapter because it is technically more challenging, has higher risks compared with the superficial technique, and analgesia for most surgical operations can be managed with a superficial cervical plexus block.

Table 70.1 Branches of the Trigeminal Nerve: Targets and Indications for Regional Nerve Blocks

MAIN BRANCH	DIVISIONS	INNERVATION	INDICATIONS FOR BLOCK	METHOD
Ophthalmic (V1)	Frontal nerve → Supraorbital and Supratrochlear nerves	Upper eyelid, forehead, scalp, bridge of nose	Ophthalmological surgery, craniotomy, frontal sinus surgery, cosmetic nasal surgery	Frontal nerve block: Palpate supraorbital notch. Direct needle to medial brow. Inject 2–4 mL of LA. Leave finger on orbit to avoid injection into globe
Maxillary (V2)	Infraorbital nerve; Sphenopalatine ganglion	Cheek, upper lip, eyelid, lateral nose; Hard/soft palate, tonsils, nasal/pharynx mucosa, posterior nasal septum, paranasal sinuses, lacrimal gland	Functional endoscopic sinus surgery, surgeries involving upper lip, nose, maxilla, teeth	Infraorbital nerve block: Palpate infraorbital foramen in groove inferior to orbit rim, 3 cm from midline of face. Place needle 0.5–1 cm inferior to foramen and direct toward nerve to prevent injection into foramen. Inject 1–3 mL LA. Sphenopalatine ganglion block (transoral approach): Identify greater palatine foramen medial to gum line of 2nd or 3rd molar on the posterior portion of hard palate Advance through foramen w/ needle Inject 1.5–2 mL LA w/ epinephrine Maxillary nerve block: Insert needle below zygomatic arch, in between coronoid and condyle of mandible, until pterygoid plate reached. Withdraw needle and redirect anteriorly towards eye to enter pterygopalatine fossa. Inject 5 mL LA
Mandibular (V3)	Auriculotemporal nerve; Lingual nerve; Inferior alveolar nerve Incisive and Mental nerves	Molar/premolar teeth; Lip and chin	Procedures involving mandible, mandibular teeth, floor of mouth, lower lip, chin	Inferior alveolar nerve block: Open mouth and retract cheek. Approach from contralateral premolars. Advance needle in between coronoid notch and pterygomandibular raphe, until mandible is contacted. Redirect needle slightly posterior. Inject 4 mL LA after aspiration and 1 additional mL, while withdrawing needle Auriculotemporal nerve block: Palpate temporal artery as it crosses zygomatic arch. Infiltrate area with 2–4 mL LA using 25-gauge needle. Mental nerve block: Palpate mental foramen midway between upper and lower borders of mandible. Insert 25-gauge needle 0.5 cm deep, lateral, and superior to foramen. Inject 2–3 mL LA

LA, Local anesthetic.

9. **How do you perform a superficial cervical plexus block using anatomic landmarks?**
To perform a superficial cervical plexus block using anatomic landmarks, the posterior border of the SCM needs to be identified and demarcated. In an awake patient, this can be facilitated when the SCM contracts (i.e., ask the patient to rotate their head against the practitioner's hand placed on the contralateral forehead). Next, the mastoid process and the C6 transverse process (Chassaignac's tubercle) are identified; the midway point between these two landmarks represents the estimated location where the cervical plexus emerges along the posterior border of the SCM. Note, that the C6 transverse process is located at the level of the cricoid cartilage, which can be used as a reference point. Next, 10 to 15 mL of local anesthetic, starting at this midpoint, is injected along the posterior border of the SCM in both the caudal and cephalad directions using a "fan" like technique. While injecting local anesthetic, it is important to remain superficial below the level of the subcutaneous tissue and aspirate multiple times to avoid intravascular injection.

10. **How do you perform a superficial cervical plexus block using ultrasound?**
The superficial cervical plexus block can also be performed using ultrasound. The patient is positioned the same way as for anatomic landmark guided technique. The posterior border of the SCM is identified and referenced as a starting point for scanning, either in the transverse or longitudinal approach. The ultrasound should be moved posteriorly, until the tapering edge of the SCM is in the middle of the screen. The cervical plexus is found posterior to the SCM and lies immediately superficial to the prevertebral fascia, overlying the interscalene groove (Fig. 70.2). The plexus is usually visible as a small collection of hypoechoic nodules that is described as having a honeycomb appearance. Using either an in-plane or out-of-plane approach, 10 to 15 mL of local anesthetic is administered, following negative aspiration. Visualization of the plexus, while helpful, may not always occur and is not necessary. Visualization of local anesthetic deposited immediately deep to the SCM generally yields a reliable block, regardless if the plexus is readily visualized or not.
The potential advantages of using the ultrasound include visualizing the spread of local anesthetic in the proper plane, visualizing structures to avoid (i.e., blood vessels and phrenic nerve), and avoiding deep needle insertions. However, despite these potential advantages, studies have not definitively demonstrated a significant difference between the two techniques in terms of analgesic efficacy.

11. **What are the known complications of cervical plexus blocks?**
The risks of the superficial cervical plexus block are considered minimal because of the superficial injections along the border of the SCM. However, there are known possible complications, including infection, hematoma, and local anesthetic systemic toxicity. The deep plexus block is associated with additional complications, including vertebral artery puncture and injection, nerve root injury, local anesthetic systemic toxicity, spinal anesthesia, phrenic nerve blockade, brachial plexus injury, and pneumothorax. Phrenic nerve blockade is expected for a deep cervical plexus block, and thus bilateral deep cervical plexus blocks are likely contraindicated, particularly in patients with

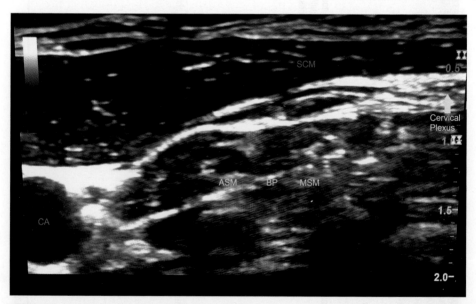

Fig. 70.2 Ultrasound image for superficial cervical plexus block. *ASM*, Anterior scalene muscle; *BP*, brachial plexus; *CA*, carotid artery; *MSM*, middle scalene muscle; *SCM*, sternocleidomastoid muscle.

pulmonary disease. Because the superficial cervical plexus block is considered equally suitable as deep cervical plexus blocks for most surgeries, some institutions now avoid deep cervical plexus blocks because of the increased risk for complications.

12. Can local anesthetics be administered via another route other than injection?

Administration of local anesthetics for head and neck procedures is not limited to nerve block injections. Local anesthetic agents can also be administered topically to provide anesthesia and analgesia, reduce patient discomfort, reduce sympathetic response, and improve conditions for the proceduralist. Local anesthetics in the form of topical sprays and viscous solutions can be administered to facilitate the passage of endoscopes for esophagogastroduodenoscopies or awake intubation. Laryngotracheal topical anesthesia (LTA) can be sprayed into the trachea just before endotracheal intubation to decrease the sympathetic response to intubation and to reduce the incidence of coughing during emergence of anesthesia. As an alternative to LTA in certain situations, such as awake intubation, the cricothyroid membrane can be punctured with a small needle to directly spray local anesthetic in the larynx and trachea (see recurrent laryngeal nerve later).

13. How can regional anesthetic techniques be used for difficult airway situations?

Airway topicalization with a local anesthetic is an essential component of preparing a patient for an awake intubation. However, topicalization effectiveness may be variable, depending on patient cooperation and pathologies not amenable for topicalization. Regional nerve blocks can provide reliable analgesia and anesthesia to augment topicalization.

The superior laryngeal nerve, a branch from the vagus nerve that innervates the base of tongue, arytenoids, and posterior surface of the epiglottis, can be blocked to reduce the cough and gag reflex to increase patient comfort and improve intubating conditions. The nerve is blocked at its internal branch at the level of the thyrohyoid membrane. The hyoid bone is palpated to identify the cornu of the hyoid bone, and 2 to 3 mL of local anesthetic is injected bilaterally, immediately inferior to the cornu, after negative aspiration.

The recurrent laryngeal nerve, another branch of the vagus nerve that innervates the glottis and trachea, can be blocked to ease the passage of the endotracheal tube into the trachea. The translaryngeal approach to blocking the recurrent laryngeal nerve is performed by advancing a small-gauge needle (attached to a syringe containing local anesthetic) through the cricothyroid membrane. Correct needle tip position is confirmed once air is aspirated into the syringe. Immediately thereafter, 4 to 5 mL of local anesthetic is injected and dispersed, as the patient coughs in response to the injection. Alternatively, the recurrent laryngeal nerve can be blocked by direct topicalization using a "spray as you go" approach during the fiberoptic intubation. This involves threading an epidural catheter through the working channel of the bronchoscope, and the tip of the catheter is advanced intermittently to spray local anesthetic throughout the passage of the bronchoscope in the airway.

KEY POINTS

1. Regional anesthesia for head and neck operations can be used as the primary anesthetic technique and/or for postoperative analgesia.
2. Use of concentrated local anesthesia is recommended to improve efficacy and duration as muscle weakness is less of a concern for head and neck regional anesthesia compared with neuraxial and peripheral nerve blocks.
3. Because of the risk of airway fire during many head and neck operations, close communication with the surgeon and patient is important when an anesthetic plan involves a combination of regional nerve block and minimal sedation.
4. A comprehensive knowledge of head and neck anatomy and of the pharmacology of local anesthetics is critical in safely and effectively performing these blocks.
5. The abundance of critical blood vessels that surround the head and neck, as well as the proximity of the brain and the globe, provides unique challenges to performing regional anesthesia in this region.

SUGGESTED READINGS

Hadzic A, ed. Hadzic's Peripheral Nerve Blocks and Anatomy for Ultrasound-Guided Regional Anesthesia. 2nd ed. New York: McGraw-Hill; 2012.
Jourdy DN, Kacker A. Regional anesthesia for office-based procedures in otorhinolaryngology. Anesthesiol Clin. 2010;28:457–468.
Kanakaraj M, Shanmugasundaram N, Chandramohan M, et al. Regional anesthesia in faciomaxillary and oral surgery. J Pharm Bioallied Sci. 2012;4:S264–S269.
Levine AI, DeMaria Jr S. Regional anesthesia. In: Taub et al., editors. Ferraro's Fundamentals of Maxillofacial Surgery. 2nd ed. New York: Springer; 2015:77–90.
Levine AI, Govindaraj S, DeMaria S, eds. Anesthesiology and Otolaryngology. 1st ed. New York: Springer; 2013.

CHAPTER 71

NEURAXIAL ANESTHESIA AND ANALGESIA

Rachel Kacmar, MD, Jason Papazian, MD

1. **What are the different kinds of neuraxial anesthesia?**
   - Epidural anesthesia refers to injection of anesthetics or analgesics into the epidural space at either the lumbar or thoracic level.
   - Caudal anesthesia refers to injection into the sacral hiatus (see Question 11).
   - Spinal anesthesia, spinal block, subarachnoid block, and intrathecal block are all terms used interchangeably to describe injection into the intrathecal space.

2. **Differentiate neuraxial analgesia and anesthesia? When might analgesia be preferred?**
   Anesthesia implies an intense sensory and motor blockade, which is necessary to perform a surgical procedure. It is usually obtained by using the highest available concentration of local anesthetic (e.g., 2% lidocaine or 3% chloroprocaine). Analgesia implies sensory blockade only, usually for postoperative pain management or labor analgesia, and may be achieved with dilute local anesthetic, epidural opioids, or a combination of the two.

3. **List the advantages of neuraxial (epidural or intrathecal) anesthesia over general anesthesia?**
   - The metabolic stress response to surgery and anesthesia is reduced.
   - Significant blood loss reduction by comparison with general anesthesia with certain surgeries. Cesarean section and major lower extremity orthopedic procedures are the best examples.
   - Decreased incidence of venous thromboembolic complications.
   - Pulmonary compromise is likely reduced.
   - Airway manipulation and loss of airway protection is usually avoided, adding benefit in patients with potentially difficult airways, severe reactive airway disease, and patients at risk for aspiration.
   - Mental status remains intact, unless the patient is otherwise sedated.
   - Total systemic dose of drug(s) is markedly decreased.
   - Motor blockade from spinal avoids the need for muscle relaxant medications for surgical manipulation. Subsequent reversal medications are also unnecessary.
   - Markedly lower incidence of anesthesia-induced postoperative nausea and vomiting (presuming hypotension is treated effectively).
   - Markedly improved pain control with minimal or no systemic opioids using either low-dose intrathecal morphine and/or continuous epidural anesthesia in either the lumbar or thoracic region, as indicated.

4. **Differentiate between a spinal and an epidural anesthetic.**
   A spinal anesthetic is performed by puncturing the dura and injecting a small amount of local anesthetic directly into the cerebrospinal fluid (CSF), producing a rapid, dense, and predictable neural blockade. An epidural anesthetic requires a 10-fold increase in dose of local anesthetic to fill the epidural space and penetrate the nerve coverings. The block onset is slower and often less dense, and the anesthesia produced tends to be segmental (i.e., a band of anesthesia is produced, extending upward and downward from the injection site). The degree of segmental spread depends largely on the volume of local anesthetic injected. For example, a 5-mL volume may produce only a narrow band of anesthesia covering three to five dermatomes, whereas a 20-mL volume may produce anesthesia from the upper thoracic to sacral dermatomes. Placement of an epidural anesthetic requires a larger needle, often includes a continuous catheter technique, and has a subtle endpoint for locating the space. The epidural space is located by following the feel of the ligaments, as they are passed through until there is loss of resistance, whereas the subarachnoid space is definitively identified by CSF flow from the needle following dural puncture.

5. **List the advantages of spinal anesthesia over epidural anesthesia?**
   - Often quicker onset time from injection to adequate surgical blockade.
   - More predictable block density, particularly regarding motor blockade.
   - Less risk for block "patchiness" and/or unilateral block.
   - Epidural anesthesia has no definitive confirmatory endpoint during placement, as opposed to observing CSF in the spinal needle during subarachnoid block.
   - Lower volume of local anesthetic required essentially eliminates the risk of local anesthetic systemic toxicity (LAST).

6. **What are some disadvantages of (single-shot) spinal anesthesia over catheter-based epidural anesthesia?**
   - More immediate and dramatic hemodynamic changes often observed.
   - Not easily titratable.
   - With rare exception, no ability to provide continued neuraxial analgesia beyond initial dose. (Very rarely, intrathecal catheters are used.)
   - No ability to augment intensity or increase duration of blockade if inadequate.
   - Block level or dermatomal window cannot be augmented or modified once set, as it can be using a continuous epidural technique.

7. **Describe how one would assess a patient before performing a neuraxial anesthetic.**
   In addition to the normal preoperative evaluation, the following specific items should be assessed before performing neuraxial anesthesia:
   - History
     - Previous back injury or surgery
     - Neurological symptoms or history of neurological disease (e.g., diabetic neuropathy, multiple sclerosis)
     - Bleeding tendencies or diseases associated with coagulopathy (e.g., preeclampsia)
     - Anticoagulation or antiplatelet medication (current or recent, including aspirin)
     - Prior regional anesthesia and any associated problems
   - Physical Examination
     - Brief neurological examination for strength and sensation
     - Back examination for landmarks and potential anatomic abnormalities (scoliosis) or pathology (infection at the site of placement)
     - Cardiovascular examination, specifically for murmurs, indications of right or left heart failure, etc.
   - Surgery Specific
     - Expected duration
     - Expected blood loss
     - Positioning required
     - Need for muscle relaxation
     - Surgeon's preferences (and potential discussion of risks and benefits with surgeon)
   - General Information
     - The patient should be given a detailed explanation of the procedure, risks, benefits, and options (including block failure and possible conversion to other modes of anesthesia/analgesia)
     - Discuss if the patient desires sedation and how much
   - Laboratory Tests
     - Not globally required unless medical history or medications indicate possible coagulation disorder
   - Imaging
     - Magnetic resonance imaging and/or computed tomography (CT) are not necessary except in case-by-case instances, in patients with specific intracranial or spinal abnormalities

8. **Where is the epidural space? Describe the relevant anatomy.**
   - The epidural space lies just outside and envelops the dural sac containing the spinal cord and CSF. As the epidural needle enters the midline of the back between the bony spinous processes, it passes through:
   - From superficial to deep: skin, subcutaneous fat, supraspinous ligament, interspinous ligament, ligamentum flavum, epidural space.
   - Deep to the epidural space lies the spinal meninges and CSF. The epidural space has its widest point (5 mm) at L2. In addition to the traversing nerve roots, it contains fat, lymphatics, and an extensive venous plexus (Batson plexus). The epidural space wraps 360 degrees around the dural membrane. Superiorly, the space extends to the foramen magnum, where the dura is fused to the base of the skull. Caudally, it ends at the sacral hiatus. The most anterior boundary of the epidural space is the posterior longitudinal ligament, situated along the posterior surface of the vertebral bodies. The epidural space can be entered in the cervical, thoracic, lumbar, or sacral regions to provide anesthesia. In pediatric patients, the caudal epidural approach is commonly used.

9. **Describe the technique for performing a lumbar epidural anesthetic.**
   - Ensure that resuscitation equipment is immediately available: oxygen, equipment for positive-pressure ventilation and intubation, and vasoactive medications to treat blood pressure changes.
   - Monitor the patient with at least a pulse oximeter and blood pressure cuff.
   - Place a well-running intravenous (IV) line and consider an appropriate coload of fluid to counteract hypotension after sympathetic blockade.
   - The patient may be sitting or lying laterally. The spinous processes should be aligned in the same vertical or horizontal plane and maximally flexed. Administer sedation as appropriate.
   - For lumbar epidural placement, visualize a line between the iliac crests to locate the L4 spinous process. Palpate the L2–L3, L3–L4, and L4–L5 interspaces and choose either the widest or the closest to the desired anesthetic level. For abdominal or thoracic surgeries, catheter insertion site should reflect the desired dermatomal coverage.

- The anesthesiologist or anesthesia provider must wear a hat, mask, and sterile gloves and remove all jewelry, including watches. The patient should wear a hat. Any additional providers or family members should wear a hat and mask. The site should be prepped/draped.
- A skin wheal is made with local anesthetic at the desired insertion site. The epidural needle is most often inserted in the midline. Once initial resistance from ligaments is felt, remove the needle stylet and attach a syringe with 3 to 4 mL of air or saline. When the barrel of the syringe is tapped, it should feel firm and bounce back, while the tip of the needle is in the ligament.
- Advance several millimeters at a time, tapping the syringe intermittently. The ability to recognize the feel of various layers of ligament comes with experience. Ligamentum flavum is often described as leathery, gritty, or producing a marked increase in resistance. This is the last layer before the epidural space.
- As the needle passes through ligamentum flavum and enters the epidural space, there is often a pop or give, and the air or fluid in the syringe injects easily; this marks the loss of resistance.
- While one hand grasps the hub of the epidural needle to brace it, the other threads the catheter about 5 cm into the epidural space (5 cm past the tip of the needle).
- The epidural needle is withdrawn carefully so as not to dislodge the catheter. After attaching the injector port to the catheter, it is aspirated for blood or CSF; if negative, a test dose may be given. The catheter is then secured in place.

10. What is the paramedian technique for epidural catheter placement? When is it useful?
    - Paramedian epidural placement starts by identifying the spinous process at the desired interspace level and using local anesthetic to create a skin wheal 1 to 2 fingerbreadths lateral to this point.
    - Insert the epidural needle through the wheal perpendicular to the patient's skin, until the transverse process of the vertebra is encountered.
    - Walk the epidural needle off the transverse process, moving superiorly and medially (about 15–30 degrees, angulation—do not cross midline), until the needle is engaged in the ligamentum flavum.
    - Attach a friction-free syringe and advance until loss of resistance is achieved.
    - This approach is useful at high thoracic levels (above $\approx$ T9–T10), where the spinous processes are acutely angled downward. It can also be advantageous when the spaces between spinous processes are small, such as in patients with limited mobility who cannot "open" their spaces (i.e., provide relative lumbar or thoracic kyphotic bend).

11. How is caudal anesthesia related to epidural anesthesia? When is it used?
    Caudal anesthesia is a form of epidural anesthesia in which the injection is made at the sacral hiatus (S5). Because the dural sac normally ends at S2, accidental spinal injection is rare. Although the caudal approach to the epidural space provides dense sacral and lower lumbar levels of block, its use in adults is limited by the following:
    - Highly variable sacral anatomy
    - Calcification/ossification of the sacral ligaments
    - Risk of injection into a venous plexus
    - Difficulty in maintaining sterility if a catheter is used
    Caudal anesthesia is used primarily in children (whose anatomy is predictable) to provide postoperative analgesia after herniorrhaphy or perineal procedures. A catheter can be inserted for long-term use if desired.

12. What is a combined spinal-epidural anesthetic or dural-puncture epidural? What are the advantages and disadvantages of these?
    A dural-puncture epidural (DPE) is performed by passing a long spinal needle through an epidural needle that has been placed into the epidural space. In this way the dura is punctured and CSF in the spinal needle acts as a confirmation of placement of the epidural needle adjacent to the dura (i.e., "epidural") and in the midline of the space. A combined spinal-epidural (CSE) is the same technique, but additionally when CSF is confirmed in the spinal needle, a dose of local anesthetic with or without adjuvants (e.g., small dose of opioid) is deposited in the subarachnoid space. In this case, onset of block is markedly faster. In either case, the spinal needle is removed after confirmation/injection and the epidural catheter is then placed. Either technique combines the advantages of both spinal and epidural anesthesia and both techniques result in a more reliable epidural catheter. Note that these techniques can only be performed in the lumbar area (below L1–L2 in adults, below L3 in children) because of risk of spinal cord entry at higher levels.

13. What physiological changes should be expected after successful initiation of an epidural anesthetic?
    - Decrease in blood pressure: Detailed discussion in question 22.
    - Changes in heart rate: Tachycardia may occur as cardiac output increases to compensate for the drop in systemic vascular resistance. Bradycardia may also occur and is discussed in question 23.
    - Ventilatory changes: In normal patients, ventilation is maintained as long as the diaphragm is not impaired (phrenic nerve: C3–C5), but patients may become subjectively dyspneic, as they become unable to feel their intercostal muscles. Patients who are dependent on the accessory muscles of respiration may experience significant respiratory distress with sedation. Note that the ability to cough and protect the airway may be lost even if ventilation is adequate. Upper extremity weakness or speech changes are signs of an evolving high block and the possibility of impending ventilatory failure.

- Bladder distention: Sympathetic blockade and loss of sensation may result in bladder atony and require catheterization. Typically, minimal with epidural placement above T9, but patients should be monitored for urinary retention.
- Change in thermoregulation: See question 28.
- Neuroendocrine changes: Neural blockade above T8 blocks sympathetic afferents to the adrenal medulla, inhibiting the neural component of the stress response. Note that this may result in better glucose regulation in some diabetic patients.

14. What are the usual doses of common local anesthetics used in epidural anesthesia?
    - See Table 71.1.

15. What anatomic structures are trespassed when attempting to enter the intrathecal space?
    From superficial to deep, the structures include: skin, subcutaneous/adipose tissue, supraspinous ligament, interspinous ligament, ligamentum flavum, dura mater, and arachnoid membrane. Note that the dura mater and arachnoid are not trespassed in successful epidural placement.

16. What boney structures might be encountered while attempting to enter the intrathecal space?
    Shallow osseous tissue is likely spinous process, which may be walked-off above or below to obtain access to the subarachnoid space. Deep osseous tissue tends to be vertebral lamina alerting the provider that they are off midline and need to redirect.

17. Where are the principal sites of effect of spinal local anesthetics?
    The principal sites of effect are sodium channels in the spinal nerve roots and the spinal cord itself. Resulting in part from anatomic variation of nerve roots and rootlets impacting the spread of injected medications in the CSF, there is typically a slight difference in the level of motor and sensory blockade.

18. What factors determine the termination of effect of spinal anesthesia?
    Dissociation of the local anesthetic from nerve sodium channels and resorption of the agent from the CSF into the systemic circulation limits duration.

19. Describe the factors involved in distribution (and extent) of spinal blockade.
    - Patient characteristics including height, position, intraabdominal pressure, anatomic configuration of the spinal canal, and pregnancy all impact the extent of spinal blockade. There is great interindividual variation in lumbosacral CSF volume; magnetic resonance imaging has shown volumes ranging from 28 to 81 mL. Lumbar CSF volumes correlate well with height and regression of blockade. With the exception of an inverse relation with weight, no external physical measurement reliably estimates lumbar CSF volumes. Note, CSF volumes are also reduced in pregnancy.
    - The total injected milligram dose (not the volume and/or concentration) of local anesthetic is important.
    - The baricity of the local anesthetic solution is important. Baricity is defined by the ratio of the density of the local anesthetic solution to the density of CSF. A solution with a ratio greater than 1 is hyperbaric and tends to sink with gravity within the CSF. An isobaric solution has a baricity of 1 and tends to remain in the immediate area of injection. A ratio of less than 1 is a hypobaric solution, which rises in the CSF. Patient position during and after intrathecal injection and vertebral column curvature (specifically lordosis and kyphosis) influence distribution in relation to baricity of injectate.

Table 71.1 Local Anesthetic Dosing for Spinal Anesthesia

	Suggested Doses (mg)			Duration of Effect (Minutes)	
USUAL CONCENTRATION	LOWER EXTREMITIES AND PERINEUM	LOWER ABDOMEN	UPPER ABDOMEN	WITHOUT EPINEPHRINE	WITH EPINEPHRINE
Lidocaine 5% in dextrose	25–50	50–75	75–100	60–75	75–90
Bupivacaine 0.75% in dextrose	5–10	12–14	12–18	90–120	100–150
Ropivacaine 0.25%–1%	8–12	12–16	16–18	90–120	90–120
Tetracaine 1% in dextrose	4–8	8–12	10–16	90–120	120–240
Ropivacaine 0.5% in dextrose	8–12	12–16	16–18	80–110	—
Levobupivacaine 0.5%	8–10	10–15	12–20	90–120	100–150

20. **At what lumbar levels should a spinal anesthetic be administered?**
    The selected level should be below L1 in an adult, and L3 in a child, to avoid needle trauma to the spinal cord. As an anatomic landmark, the L3–L4 interspace is thought to be located at the line intersecting the top of the iliac crests. In reality, this is highly unpredictable of exact level entered and anesthesia providers are often 1 to 2 levels off the estimated level.

21. **What are common doses and dosing regimens for spinal anesthesia?**
    - See Table 71.2.

22. **What are the most common complications of neuraxial anesthesia?**
    Common complications include hypotension, pruritis (from intrathecal narcotics), nausea and vomiting (often secondary to hypotension) and postdural puncture headache (PDPH). Rare but more ominous complications include nerve injury, cauda equina syndrome, meningitis, high/total spinal anesthesia, and spinal hematoma/abscess formation. Particular issues associated with these complications are discussed subsequently.

    LAST may occur with intravascular injection of a large total dose of local anesthetic. This can be prevented by ensuring negative aspiration, using epinephrine as an additive (the development of tachycardia may indicate intravascular injection), and by incremental dosing. This complication is essentially impossible in spinal anesthesia, given the very small doses of local anesthetic required.

23. **Discuss neuraxial associated hypotension. What are the causes, considerations, treatments, and safe practices?**
    Arterial pressure decreases and venous capacitance increases predictably with sympatholysis. The ultimate impact of this on cardiac output and stroke volume depends on baseline fluid status, cardiac function, and patient positioning. Heart rate may increase or decrease, depending on multiple factors.

    Hypotension occurs in many cases (especially when a higher thoracic anesthetic level is achieved), and can be mitigated with vasopressor infusion (e.g., phenylephrine). Fluid preloading does not predictably reduce the incidence of spinal-induced hypotension and should be used with caution in patients who are at high risk of cardiopulmonary compromise. However, hypovolemic patients with signs of hemodynamic compromise should be resuscitated before instituting spinal anesthesia. Colloid or crystalloid preload are equivalent options in this situation. Hypovolemia, age greater than 40 years, sensory level greater than T5, baseline systolic blood pressure below 120 mm Hg, and performance of the block at or above L3–L4, all increase the incidence of hypotension.

    Hypotension (and possibly decreased cerebral blood flow) may be responsible for nausea and vomiting observed with Spinal anesthetic block (SAB). Trendelenburg position shortly after intrathecal injection may raise the level of

Table 71.2 Local Anesthetics Used in Epidural Anesthesia for Surgical Procedures

ANESTHETIC	CLASS	CONCENTRATION (%)	ONSET	DURATION	MAXIMAL DOSE WITH EPINEPHRINE	COMMENTS
Chloroprocaine	Ester	3	Rapid	45 min	15 mg/kg	Rapid metabolism, least toxic, intense sensory and motor block
Lidocaine	Amide	2	Immediate	60–90 min	7 mg/kg	Intense sensory and motor block
Bupivacaine	Amide	0.75[a], 0.5, 0.25[b]	Slow	2–3 h	3 mg/kg	Most cardiotoxic; motor < sensory block
Ropivacaine	Amide	0.75	Slow	2–3 h	3 mg/kg	Less cardiotoxic than bupivacaine; most expensive

[a]Not available for obstetric use.
[b]May not always produce adequate surgical anesthesia.

blockade with hyperbaric spinal anesthesia and should be used with caution. Indeed, all position changes should consider the baricity of the injectate and time since onset. Strategies to create a unilateral block, such as hyperbaric injection, followed by immediately laying the patient with their surgical side down, may decrease the hypotension associated with SAB.

24. **What are the etiologies and risk factors for neuraxial associated bradycardia?**
    Bradycardia may occur secondary to unopposed vagal tone from a high sympathectomy, blockade of the cardioaccelerator fibers (T1–T4), and/or the Bezold-Jarisch or reverse Bainbridge reflexes (slowing of the heart rate secondary to a decrease in venous return). Patients with underlying increased vagal tone (children and adults with resting heart rates <60 bpm) are at increased risk. Bradycardia is often well tolerated but may be treated with anticholinergic agents (glycopyrrolate or atropine) or β-adrenergic agonists, such as ephedrine, as needed. Rarely is epinephrine required, and if needed would signal a likely undiagnosed and/or severe cardiac condition.

25. **Review the clinical features of "high" and "total" neuraxial anesthesia.**
    Acute onset nausea and or agitation, likely associated with significant hypotension, may alert the provider to impending high or total spinal. Other signs of high spinal may include bradycardia, dysphonia, dyspnea, and progressive upper extremity numbness and weakness.

    Total spinal anesthesia results from either local anesthetic depression of the cervical spinal cord and brainstem, or more likely, hypoperfusion of the respiratory center in the brainstem, leading to apnea and loss of consciousness. Readiness for airway manipulation and hemodynamic support can prevent more serious complications (cardiopulmonary arrest) in this setting. Although the patient should receive sedation once ventilation is instituted and hemodynamics stabilize, airway securement should not be delayed and patients do not require induction agents in these instances (in fact the additive hypotension from these agents may be harmful). The effects of total spinal anesthesia usually resolve, as would be predicted by local anesthetic duration, and, unless otherwise contraindicated, the patient can be extubated once they meet criteria.

26. **If a patient has an arrest with a neuraxial anesthetic in place, should resuscitative measures differ from standard advanced cardiac life support protocols?**
    Overall incidence of cardiac arrest associated with SAB or epidural is very low. With loss of consciousness and respiratory arrest, ventilation, oxygenation, and airway protection are the immediate considerations. Advanced cardiac life support algorithm standards should be followed and patient factors should be considered at the discretion of the anesthesia care team.

27. **Discuss the clinical features of a PDPH. What are the treatment options?**
    A PDPH is a potentially severe headache that develops after dural puncture, presumably secondary to intracranial hypotension from the egress of CSF through the defect in the dura. This results in a pressure differential within the cranium and thus traction on the meninges, intracranial vessels and cranial nerves, as well as cerebral hyperemia, all of which are painful. Time to headache onset is widely variable (minutes vs. hours vs. days) and is likely dependent on many factors.

    PDPHs are characteristically worse in an upright position and improved in the recumbent position. Aside from a positional nature, these headaches tend to vary widely in intensity from mild to intense, localized to the frontal and/or occipital region, and are often associated with neck pain. Positional neck pain may even occur in isolation. Signs of cranial nerve stretch (e.g., diplopia) warn of likely medical need for treatment by epidural blood patch (EBP).

    More serious but rare complications of PDPH include cranial neuropathies (e.g., diplopia, hearing loss), subdural hematoma, dural venous thrombosis, and chronic persistent headache. Concern for cranial neuropathy should prompt consideration for early EBP.

    Risk factors for PDPH include history of PDPH, female sex, younger age (<40 years), nonobese, pregnancy, labor, multiple dural entries, larger bore needles (>24-G), and use of cutting-edge needle (Quincke).

    Proposed preventative measures include Cosyntropin administration and leaving a spinal catheter in place in the event of accidental dural puncture during lumbar epidural placement. Oral analgesics and cerebral vasoconstrictors produce only transient and partial symptomatic relief. EBP remains the gold-standard treatment. Contraindications to EBP are similar to those of other neuraxial methods (discussed later). Studies regarding the effectiveness of sphenopalatine ganglion block as a treatment for PDPH are underway.

    In a patient with a postpartum headache, it is important to rule out preeclampsia, severe range hypertension, or central nervous system maladies as a cause of the symptoms before diagnosing PDPH, especially if there are no obvious risk factors present. A patient that has failed treatment with blood patch (especially twice) requires careful workup and possible referral for imaging and/or neurology/neurosurgery consultation.

28. **Discuss the risk of neurological injury after neuraxial anesthesia.**
    Direct trauma to nerve fibers may occur and may be heralded by a paresthesia, for which the spinal needle should be redirected. Rarely does this result in injury to the nerve. If pain occurs on injection, the provider should immediately stop and withdraw/redirect the needle.

    Neuraxial hematoma formation from epidural venous bleeding (from direct trauma or coagulopathy) or abscess formation is suggested by persistent focal neurological deficits, significantly delayed block resolution, or severe back pain. Early recognition and management are imperative to avoid permanent neurological sequelae in these settings. This is especially true in patients receiving anticoagulation in the setting of recent neuraxial procedure.

Lastly, adhesive arachnoiditis has been reported and is presumably caused by injection of an irritant (i.e., blood during EBP) into the subarachnoid space.

29. **What is the effect of neuraxial anesthesia on temperature regulation?**
Hypothermia is a risk because patients become vasodilated below the level of sensory blockade and cannot shiver in response to decreases in body temperature. Curiously, patients may not perceive cold because the vasodilated extremities feel warm. In addition, hypothermia may not be detected by the clinician because core temperature monitoring is not widely practiced in patients receiving regional anesthesia. If desired, such monitoring could be done via tympanic membrane thermometer. Patients receiving regional anesthetics should be actively warmed, using heated forced air devices and fluid warmers, and measures to limit heat loss should be taken. Remember that a shivering response above the level of blockade, if it were to occur, may be exaggerated and can increase oxygen consumption.

30. **What are contraindications to neuraxial anesthesia?**
- Absolute contraindications include local infection at the planned insertion site, untreated or inadequately treated septicemia, severe hypovolemia accompanied by hemodynamic instability, and patient refusal or noncooperation.
- Relative contraindications include coagulopathy, severe stenotic valvular disease, intracranial hypertension, existing neurological disease (e.g., degenerative or demyelinating neurological disease, such as multiple sclerosis), and sepsis. These conditions must prompt a risks and benefits analysis of neuraxial versus other anesthetic options.

31. **Review the current recommendations for administering neuraxial anesthesia to patients with altered coagulation caused by medications.**
The American Society of Regional Anesthesia and Pain Medicine (ASRA) and Society of Obstetric Anesthesia and Perinatology (SOAP) have defined many risks of regional anesthesia in the patient on anticoagulants and antiplatelet medications. Key points include:
- Patients on thrombolytic/fibrinolytic therapy should not receive neuraxial anesthesia except in the most extreme circumstances. Patients who have had regional anesthesia before such therapy has been instituted should receive frequent serial neurological checks.
- Warfarin should be stopped 4 to 5 days before the planned procedure, and prothrombin time/international normalized ratio should be obtained before procedure.
- Newer oral anticoagulants (e.g., dabigatran, apixaban, and rivaroxaban) typically require discontinuation of at least 72 hours before neuraxial manipulation.
- Bridging doses of unfractionated heparin (UFH) or low-molecular-weight heparin (LMWH) may be necessary during the time oral anticoagulants are held. We recommend accessing the ASRA and SOAP guidelines in the literature (see suggested reading) for specifics regarding these medications and neuraxial timing.
- Concurrent administration of medications that affect bleeding by different mechanisms (e.g., antiplatelet drugs, aspirin, heparin) complicates the decision to perform regional anesthesia; therefore decisions must be individualized. Patients taking only nonsteroidal antiinflammatory drugs (NSAIDS) alone can safely have either single-shot or catheter regional anesthetics.
- Thrombocytopenia and an altered coagulation cascade are likely contraindications to regional anesthesia.

32. **Should spinal (or epidural) anesthesia be performed when UFH has been administered?**
Historically, the subcutaneous administration of UFH for thromboprophylaxis (e.g., 5000 units subcutaneous [SC] 2–3 times [bid-tid]) has not been a contraindication. Newer recommendations suggest waiting 4–6 hours after administration and to check for normalization of coagulation status (partial thromboplastic time, PTT) before performing the neuraxial technique. It is also suggested that the next heparin dose be held for 1 hour after the block is placed. When larger prophylactic doses (7500–10,000 units SC BID) of UFH are administered, waiting 12 hours and checking a PTT is recommended.

For therapeutic heparin doses (>20,000 units total daily dose), it is suggested to wait 24 hours and recheck coagulation status (PTT). Note that IV heparin likely clears more predictably, so waiting 4 to 6 hours with proven PTT normalization is considered adequate regardless of dose administered. Obviously, if PTT is not normalized to an acceptable level waiting more time is warranted.

ASRA recently published new recommendations regarding neuraxial procedures in the setting of anticoagulation, which serves as an excellent resource for considerations regarding specific medications. Note that there are no specific data to guide decision making should a bloody or traumatic tap occur.

33. **Should spinal (or epidural) anesthesia be performed when enoxaparin has been administered?**
The timing of the neuraxial procedure and LMWH dosing is extremely important. Needle placement should occur at least 12 hours after a prophylactic LMWH dose (e.g., 40 mg enoxaparin daily), and 24 hours when the patient is receiving any other LMWH dosing regimen.

In older patients or those with impaired renal function, an anti-Xa level can be assessed, although no evidence exists regarding how to use these data if any residual anti-Xa activity remains.

34. Discuss the use of neuraxial opioids.

Opioids produce intense visceral analgesia and may prolong sensory blockade, without affecting motor or sympathetic nervous system function. The major sites of action are the opiate receptors within the second and third laminae of the substantia gelatinosa in the dorsal horn of the spinal cord. Lipophilic agents, such as fentanyl and sufentanil, have a more localized effect than do hydrophilic opioids, such as morphine. Fentanyl and sufentanil have a rapid onset of action and an effective duration greater than 6 hours. Morphine lasts 6 to 24 hours with a more gradual onset. Side effects of neuraxial opioids include respiratory depression (which may occur late with hydrophilic agents), nausea, vomiting, pruritus, and urinary retention. However, these effects are expected to be milder compared with systemic opioid administration. Opioid antagonists or agonist/antagonists can lessen adverse effects, but should be used cautiously, if given in large doses, as they may also reverse analgesia.

Total opioid dose required with neuraxial administration is significantly lower than with systemic administration for equipotent analgesia. Furthermore, intrathecal administration requires markedly lower dosing for equivalent analgesia when compared with epidural analgesia. Lastly, neuraxial (especially spinal) opioid administration may be an excellent analgesic option for analgesia in a patient unable to tolerate neuraxial local anesthesia.

35. Discuss transient neurological syndrome.

Common findings of transient neurological syndrome (TNS) include pain or dysesthesias in the buttocks, radiating to the dorsolateral aspect of the thighs and calves. The pain has been alternately described as sharp and lancinating or dull, aching, cramping, or burning. Usually symptoms improve with activity, worsen at night, and respond to NSAIDS. The pain is moderate to severe in at least 70% of patients with TNS and diminishes over time, resolving spontaneously within a week in about 90% of those affected. It is extremely rare for pain to continue beyond 2 weeks. It is significant to note that no objective neurological findings are encountered on physical examination of patients experiencing TNS.

TNS has typically been associated with the use of spinal lidocaine, and its incidence, although variable, is about 15%. TNS has been observed with both 5% hyperbaric and 2% isobaric lidocaine and there is no association with the presence of dextrose, opioids, epinephrine, or the baricity or osmolarity of the solution. Risk factors include lithotomy position and ambulatory surgery patients. Gender, weight, age, needle type, difficult block and paresthesias during block placement do not appear to impact risk for TNS. Interestingly, pregnancy may protect against lidocaine-associated TNS.

36. Because lidocaine is associated with TNS, what would be an appropriate local anesthetic for an ambulatory procedure?

Bupivacaine at 5- to 7.5-mg will achieve a peak sensory block in the mid-to-low thoracic region with a duration of about 2 hours. Motor blockade will last about 1 hour. Time to discharge may not be appreciably different with this technique than if lidocaine were used, but doses greater than 10 mg may result in delays in voiding and likely a delay in discharge. Bladder ultrasound has been used to identify patients requiring catheterization.

Spinal lidocaine is commonly used for obstetric procedures (e.g., for cervical cerclage) because of this patient population's low risk of TNS and improved time to discharge.

37. How does one choose which local anesthetic to use?

The choice of local anesthetic is usually based on the onset, duration, safety profile, and any special clinical characteristics of the patient and surgical procedure (see Tables 71.1 and 71.2).

38. Why is epinephrine sometimes combined with the local anesthetic? Should it be included in all cases?

Epinephrine is often added to local anesthetic solutions in a concentration of 5 mcg/mL (1:200,000) or less. There are several benefits to this practice:

- Local α_1 receptor-mediated vasoconstriction reduces uptake into the bloodstream, delaying local anesthetic metabolism reducing the risk of toxicity.
- Central α_2 activity likely produces improved analgesia and block quality.
- It helps to identify intravascular injection when used as the marker (i.e., tachycardia) in a test dose or aliquot dosing. Note that addition of epinephrine should consider the potential consequences of intravascular injection, for example, tachycardia in a patient with severe coronary disease may be harmful.

39. Why can some patients with epidural blockade move around and even walk, whereas others have a dense motor block?

Preserving motor function is especially important in postoperative and laboring patients. The degree of motor block can be decreased by lowering the concentration of local anesthetic and by choosing a local anesthetic with favorable sensory: motor dissociation. As local anesthetic concentration decreases, the intensity of the block decreases, and fewer motor nerves are affected. Sensory block can be augmented by the addition of epidural opioids if desired. Depending on surgical site, the rate of infusion can also be adjusted to avoid motor blockade of the lower extremities, while still providing analgesia. Bupivacaine and ropivacaine provide relatively less motor block for a given amount of sensory block (so-called *sensory:motor dissociation*). This property accounts for much of their popularity in obstetric anesthesia. A common epidural infusion for postoperative pain is 0.08% to 0.1% bupivacaine with 2 to 5 mcg/mL fentanyl.

40. **How do you determine the level of anesthesia needed for different types of surgeries?**
   To provide adequate surgical blockade with a neuraxial anesthetic, it is necessary to know the innervation of the structures involved in the procedure. For example, a transurethral resection of the prostate requires a T8 level because the bladder is innervated by T8 through its embryological origins. A laparotomy, such as a cesarean delivery requires a T4 level to cover peritoneal innervation. Testing the sensory level can be achieved using a pin-prick or ice test. Level of anesthesia is generally tested before incision (e.g., with Alis clamping on the abdomen before cesarean incision).

41. **What is a segmental block? When is it used?**
   Epidural anesthesia is segmental (i.e., it has an upper and lower level). The block is most intense near the site of catheter insertion and diminishes with distance. The needle and catheter should be placed as close to the site of surgery as possible (e.g., a thoracic injection is used for chest surgery, whereas a mid-lumbar injection is used for hip surgery).

42. **What are some examples of reasons to place a neuraxial anesthetic other than surgical or labor pain?**
   - Patients with rib fractures have been found to have a survival benefit because of improved pulmonary mechanics with neuraxial analgesia.
   - Surgeons performing vascular access procedures.
   - Neuraxial anesthesia (especially SAB) nearly eliminates the possibility of dysautonomia in patients with a history of high spinal cord injury.
   - Although there is no proven cardiovascular or neurological benefit, patients undergoing high-risk procedures may remain awake with a neuraxial technique, thus allowing the potential for earlier recognition of major complications, such as stroke or myocardial infarction.

43. **How do you determine the amount of local anesthetic solution used for different procedures when using epidural anesthesia/analgesia? What factors affect spread in the epidural space?**
   The extent of epidural blockade is determined primarily by the volume of local anesthetic administered; more dermatomes are blocked by more milliliters of local anesthetic. To achieve a T4 level from a lumbar epidural catheter, 20 to 30 mL of solution is required. Other factors that may affect spread in the epidural space include:
   - Age: older patients require less local anesthetic
   - Pregnancy: requires approximately 30% less
   - Obesity: may or may not require less; unpredictable dosing
   - Height: taller patients may require more
   - Altered spinal anatomy (scoliosis/ kyphosis): may have patchy block; may require more or less

44. **Can continuous spinal anesthesia be performed?**
   Yes. Continuous spinal anesthesia is a technique that is regaining popularity. In the early 1990s, many cases of cauda equina syndrome were noted after inappropriate dosing of spinal microcatheters. It appeared that the lack of turbulence associated with injecting through microcatheters led to a pooling of local anesthetic caudad to the lumbar lordotic curve, along with associated repeated and inappropriate dosing of local anesthetics.
   Continuous spinal anesthesia is safe and effective using 18- to 22-G epidural needles and catheters (and improved, specially designed kits). The incidence of hypotension is less, as is the need to rescue with vasopressors. This technique allows for titration of local anesthetics to effect and has been successfully used in elderly patients, patients with aortic stenosis, and trauma patients.

45. **Why is it becoming increasingly common to either perform surgeries under neuraxial anesthesia or to combine both epidural and general anesthesia? How does this relate to Enhanced Recovery After Surgery protocols?**
   Enhanced recovery after surgery (ERAS) involves combining more evidenced based and goal-directed preoperative, intraoperative, and postoperative care to improve outcomes in all types of perioperative patients. ERAS protocols have been developed at the institutional and societal/national level for orthopedic, general surgery, and obstetric patients among many others.
   Core to these protocols are improved multimodal analgesia and anesthesia techniques and a goal of minimizing systemic opioid administration. To this point, patients receiving functional neuraxial analgesia often require no systemic opioid administration. Lastly, surgical patients with epidurals in place will have an acute pain service provider to round on them at least daily, widening the anesthesiologist's role in the perioperative window and potentially improving patient care.

46. **How should the anesthesiologist assess a patient postoperatively after an epidural or spinal anesthetic?**
   - Satisfaction with the anesthetic: Was there anything that the patient thought should/could have been done differently? Assess patient satisfaction and try to correct any misunderstandings.
   - Regression of sensory and motor block: Is there any residual blockade? Can the patient ambulate? Does the patient have any problem with bowel or bladder function? Any of these complaints requires a thorough neurological examination to localize the deficit. Although the complaint is usually caused by residual local anesthetic or nerve compression during the surgical procedure (which often resolves with time), in rare instances

further evaluation may be needed. Depending on the pattern and severity of the neurological dysfunction, a formal neurology consultation, electromyogram, or CT may be needed to rule out pathology in the epidural space (such as hematoma).

- Complaints of back pain: Examine the site for bruising, redness, or swelling.
- Complaints of headache: If an accidental dural puncture occurred, the patient should be followed for several days; such headaches can appear up to 1 week later.
- Adequacy of postoperative pain relief: Was pain control acceptable at rest and with movement?
- Presence of side effects: Did any side effects of epidural medications (e.g., itching, nausea) require treatment?

KEY POINTS: NEURAXIAL ANESTHESIA

1. Neuraxial anesthesia is associated with a decreased minimal alveolar concentration, and patients who have received a spinal anesthetic may be more sensitive to other sedative medications.
2. Patients require close monitoring, with the potential for aggressive fluid resuscitation and vasopressor support, when surgical blockade via spinal injection is performed because of the onset of dense sympathectomy.
3. Following dural puncture, patients should be observed for PDPH, and if PDPH is diagnosed, EBP is the gold standard of treatment.
4. Suspect TNS in a patient who received a lidocaine spinal anesthetic and has complaints of pain in buttocks and dorsal lower extremities. Note that there are no objective neurological findings with this syndrome and treatment should start with NSAIDS.
5. Epidural anesthesia is segmental (i.e., it has an upper and a lower level). The block is most intense near the site of catheter or needle insertion and diminishes with distance.
6. A key feature of ERAS protocols is use of regional anesthesia, including the use of neuraxial anesthesia/analgesia.

Websites

American Society of Regional Anesthesia and Pain Medicine: http://www.asra.com
LipidRescue™ Resuscitation: www.lipidrescue.org
New York Society of Regional Anesthesia: http://www.nysora.com
Enhanced Recovery After Surgery Society: http://www.erassociety.org

---

SUGGESTED READINGS

D'Angelo R, Smiley RM, Riley ET, et al. Serious complications related to obstetric anesthesia: the Serious Complication Repository Project of the Society for Obstetric Anesthesia and Perinatology. Anesthesiology. 2014;120(6):1505–1512.

Horlocker TT, Vandermeuelen E, Kopp SL, et al. Regional anesthesia in the patient receiving antithrombotic or thrombolytic therapy: American Society of Regional Anesthesia and Pain Medicine Evidence-Based Guidelines (Fourth Edition). Reg Anesth Pain Med. 2018;43(3):263–309.

Kwak KH. Postdural puncture headache. Korean J Anesthesiol. 2017;70(2):136–143.

Liu SS, McDonald SB. Current issues in spinal anesthesia. Anesthesiology. 2001;94(5):888–906.

Ljungqvist O, Scott M, Fearon KC. Enhanced recovery after surgery: a review. JAMA Surg. 2017;152(3):292–298.

Norris MC, Neuraxial Anesthesia. In: Barash PG, et al., ed. Clinical Anesthesia. 8th ed. Philadelphia: Lippincott Williams & Wilkins; 2013.

Wink J, Veering BT, Aarts L, et al. Effects of thoracic epidural anesthesia on neuronal cardiac regulation and cardiac function. Anesthesiology. 2019;130:472–491.

Zaric D, Christiansen C, Pace NL, et al. Transient neurologic symptoms after spinal anesthesia with lidocaine versus other local anesthetics: a systematic review of randomized, controlled trials. Anesth Analg. 2005;100(6):1811–1816.

CHAPTER 72

ACUTE PAIN MANAGEMENT

Robert G. Saldana, BA, Eugene Hsu, MD, MBA

1. **Define acute pain.**

   Pain is defined as "an unpleasant sensory and emotional experience associated with actual or potential tissue damage, or described in terms of such damage." Acute pain refers to pain of short duration (<3 months), usually associated with a known cause, such as surgery, trauma, or an acute illness. Acute pain differs from chronic pain because its cause is usually known, it is usually temporary, and it usually resolves as part of the natural history of healing.

2. **Is pain a vital sign?**

   No, pain is a symptom (subjective) not a vital sign (objective). The "pain as the fifth vital sign" campaign, initiated by the American Pain Society in 1996, has been implicated in contributing to the current United States opioid epidemic. All major national societies in the United States, including the American Medical Association, the American College of Surgeons, the Joint Commission, the American Academy of Family Physicians, and the Centers for Medicare and Medicaid Services no longer support the initiative in treating pain as a vital sign.

3. **How is pain assessed?**

   Because pain is influenced by a number of both sensory and emotional factors, there is no single objective physiological measurement for pain. Changes in vital signs, such as an increase in blood pressure, respiratory rate, or heart rate may be indicative, but they often correlate poorly with the degree of pain without other measurements for pain.

   The magnitude of pain and the response to treatment is often monitored using the numeric rating scale (most common in adults), the visual analogue scale, or the face rating scale (most common in pediatrics). The numeric rating scale uses numbers from 0 (no pain) through 10 (maximal pain) in patients who are capable of verbally reporting their pain. A scale of 10 faces, ranging from very happy to very sad, can be used with young children (Fig. 72.1). The child points to the face matching the way he or she feels.

   It is important to avoid overemphasis on a one-dimensional scale in assessing pain. Studies show that the numeric pain score, particularly when implemented as the "fifth vital sign," may contribute to overprescribing opioids and evidence shows that it does not lead to better pain control. Further, studies have also shown an increased incidence of opioid-related adverse drug reactions (e.g., oversedation, respiratory events), following implementation of numeric pain scores. Therefore it is important to not rely on numeric pain scores in isolation but to also assess pain using functional impairment and treatment goals. For example, after abdominal surgery a goal may be for the patient to breathe without excessive pain or is the patient's pain control sufficient so they can sleep or walk to the bathroom.

4. **What medications are useful in treating acute pain?**

   The World Health Organization analgesic ladder for treating cancer pain provides a useful approach in treating acute pain (Fig. 72.2). Mild pain should be treated with nonopioid analgesics, such as nonsteroidal antiinflammatory drugs (NSAIDs) or acetaminophen. However, such drugs have an analgesic ceiling, where, above a certain dose, no further analgesia is expected. Moderate pain should be treated with the addition of a mild opioid (e.g., tramadol or codeine), while continuing nonopioid analgesic medications (e.g., acetaminophen). Severe pain should be treated with a strong opioid, such as morphine, oxycodone, or hydromorphone because such opioids have no analgesic ceiling. Some opioids may include a nonopioid adjunct, such as acetaminophen, which limits the amount these combination agents can be given within a 24-hour period to prevent acetaminophen toxicity. Although intravenous (IV) agents may have a faster onset than oral medications, oral agents are preferred whenever possible because they are cheaper and can provide the same level of pain control. Table 72.1 lists the IV and oral equivalent doses of common opioids. By the time the patient is eating and ready for discharge, opioid-acetaminophen agents or NSAIDs are often adequate.

5. **Do all forms of pain respond equally to opioids?**

   Not all forms of pain respond equally to the same medication. Opioid analgesics are helpful in controlling somatic (well localized) or visceral (poorly localized) pain. Although bone pain can partially be treated with opioids, other agents, such as NSAIDs, bisphosphonates, and steroids are more effective in treating this form of pain. Neuropathic pain, often described as pain with a burning, hyperesthetic quality, responds to a diverse group of drugs, including antidepressants, anticonvulsants, muscle relaxants (baclofen), IV infusions, such as lidocaine and ketamine, and α-adrenergic agonists (clonidine). Note, that many of these medications may also be useful as an adjuvant in treating somatic or visceral pain. Drugs that control pain by different mechanisms may be synergistic when used together (such as NSAIDs, acetaminophen, and opioids). Another option, for mild to moderate pain, is to use topical agents, such as patches impregnated with lidocaine (Lidoderm®) or diclofenac (Flector®). For example, applying a lidocaine patch to the lower back can be particularly helpful in lower back pain, as it delivers a high dose of lidocaine at a specific site but

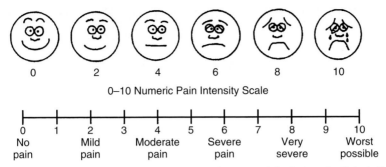

0–10 Numeric Pain Intensity Scale

0	1	2	3	4	5	6	7	8	9	10
No pain		Mild pain		Moderate pain		Severe pain		Very severe		Worst possible

Fig. 72.1 Pain scales for children and adults. (From Wong D, Whaley L. Clinical manual of pediatric nursing. St. Louis: Mosby; 1990.)

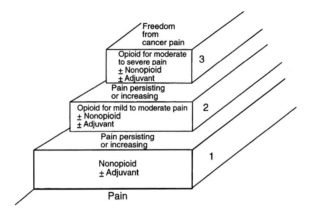

Fig. 72.2 World Health Organization analgesic ladder.

Table 72.1 Equianalgesic Doses			
	Equianalgesic Doses		
ANALGESIC	**PARENTERAL (MG)**	**ORAL (MG)**	**DOSE INTERVAL (HOURS)**
Opioid Agonist			
Morphine	10	30	3–6
Slow-release morphine	—	30	8–12
Hydromorphone (Dilaudid®)	1.5	7.5	3–5
Fentanyl (Sublimaze®)	0.1	—	0.5–1
Transdermal fentanyl (Duragesic®)	12 mcg transdermal patch	—	72
Methadone (Dolophine®)	10	20	4–6
Oxymorphone (Opana®)	1	10	3–6
Oxymorphone extended release (Opana® ER)		10	12
Oxycodone		30	3–6
Codeine	130	200	3–6
Hydrocodone		30	3–4

Continued on following page

Table 72.1 Equianalgesic Doses *(Continued)*

	Equianalgesic Doses		
ANALGESIC	PARENTERAL (MG)	ORAL (MG)	DOSE INTERVAL (HOURS)
Agonist–Antagonist/Partial Agonist			
Nalbuphine (Nubain®)	10	—	3–6
Buprenorphine (Butrans®)	5–10 mcg transdermal patch		
	Oral Drugs Approximately Equianalgesic to Aspirin (650 mg)		
Codeine	50 mg	Propoxyphene	65 mg
Hydrocodone	5 mg	Acetaminophen	650 mg
Meperidine	50 mg	Ibuprofen	200 mg
Oxycodone	5 mg	Naproxen	275 mg

limits systemic toxicity from taking oral medications (e.g., liver toxicity from acetaminophen or kidney injury from NSAIDs).

6. What are the risks of tolerance, dependence, and addiction for opioid medications in the treatment of pain?

Opioid tolerance is a state in which a higher dose is required to achieve the same analgesic effect and may occur in patients treated long term with opioids.

Opioid dependence typically refers to physical dependence on opioids to prevent withdrawal symptoms (nausea, agitation, anxiety, cramping). This may occur in patients taking opioids in as little as several weeks. Opioid withdrawal can be minimized by slowly tapering the medication over time to prevent acute withdrawal.

Addiction is classified as a pathological condition characterized by psychological, not physiological dependence, such as uncontrollable cravings, compulsion, continued use despite harm to self. Neither physical dependence nor tolerance indicates addiction. The psychological dependence seen with addiction is characterized by a compulsive behavior pattern involved in acquiring opioids for nonmedical purposes (e.g., euphoria), as opposed to pain relief. Note that patients who are inadequately treated may seem to be drug seeking because they repeatedly request opioids and are concerned with the timing of their next dose. Such *pseudo addiction* may mimic addictive behavior, but this is caused by inadequate pain treatment not addiction.

7. Does prescribing opioids for patients in pain lead to an increase in addiction?

The American Pain Society (and other related associations) claimed in the "pain as the fifth vital sign" campaign that there was no high-quality evidence of increased opioid addiction in patients with chronic pain who received opioids. It is worth noting that these associations, as well as physicians and organizations, such as the World Health Organization, took the view that the standard of care at that time was overly conservative when it came to prescribing opioids for noncancer pain, leaving patients with undertreated pain in the hospital setting. However well-intentioned, this view was not based on sufficient evidence. Before the "pain as a the fifth vital sign" campaign, the addiction overlap between heroin and prescription opioids was uncoupled because the vast majority of heroin addiction was not related to the prescription of opioids. However, the relationship between heroin and prescription opioids is now ubiquitous and has exponentially grown since the advent of this campaign in the 1990s. Studies now indicate over 80% of new heroin users start with prescription opioids. Furthermore, studies also show that in opioid naïve patients who undergo surgery, new persistent postoperative prescription opioid use can be as high as 6.5%.

The "pain as the fifth vital sign" campaign has been implicated in contributing to the United States opioid epidemic, leading to several lawsuits against pharmaceutical companies and other organizations, including the American Pain Society. Consequently, multiple pharmaceutical executives have pleaded guilty for their role in contributing to the opioid epidemic and the American Pain Society has now declared bankruptcy. Many pharmaceutical companies subsidized the "pain as the fifth vital sign" campaign in proclaiming their opioids were less addictive and less subject to abuse, particularly when prescribed for noncancer pain. Specifically, OxyContin® was released in 1996, the same year the campaign was introduced by the American Pain Society.

8. How should opioids be given?

Oral administration is usually the easiest and least expensive. Prescribing medications on a strict schedule (e.g., oxycodone-acetaminophen tablets every 4 hours) is more effective compared with an as needed (PRN) schedule. Studies show that a PRN schedule may only provide 25% of the maximal possible daily dose of opioids, despite the patient's repeated requests. If a patient cannot take a medication orally, opioids can be administered intramuscularly, IV (including patient-controlled analgesia [PCA] pumps), subcutaneously, rectally, transdermally, epidurally, intrathecally, and through buccal mucosa. Because PCA pumps are safe and effective, they are often used when the patient cannot take oral medication. The total daily PCA dose is helpful when converting to an appropriate daily oral opioid dose (see Table 72.1).

9. **Discuss the differences between opioids.**
   Morphine has an active, renally excreted metabolite (morphine-6-glucuronide) that is analgesic and has a longer half-life than its parent compound. In patients with decreased renal function, the accumulation of morphine-6-glucuronide may lead to increased side effects, including an increased risk of respiratory depression. Fentanyl acts more rapidly than morphine or hydromorphone, is 100 times more potent than morphine, is euphoric, and has no active metabolites. It is a safer choice for patients with impaired renal or liver function. Hydromorphone is also euphoric, is 5 times as potent as morphine, and has no active metabolites. Methadone can be given IV or by mouth (PO); however, the dose should be decreased to half the PO dose when given IV. Methadone is more potent than morphine, but potency varies—between 2 and 10 times as potent—depending on opioid history. Although the blood level of methadone is stable for 24 hours, the analgesic dose needs to be given every 6 to 12 hours. Methadone is also unique in that it has N-methyl-D-aspartate (NMDA) antagonism properties (similar to ketamine) and is associated with QT prolongation. Oxymorphone is a newer opioid that is 3 to 10 times more potent than morphine, is euphoric, and has no active metabolites. Tapentadol is a new oral opioid drug approved for moderate to severe acute pain that is half as potent as morphine. Tapentadol is a combination of an opioid binding drug with a norepinephrine reuptake inhibitor. Codeine is less widely used as a primary analgesic, because studies show that metabolism varies greatly because of genetic factors and may be too slowly metabolized to provide effective analgesia for 10% of patients.

   In a hospital setting, the recommended practice is to schedule pain medications for the first 1 to 2 days for acute pain (e.g., surgical related pain) and then transition to a PRN schedule. Assessment should continue by pain score and function (able to breathe or sleep without pain, etc.) to determine appropriate dosing. In an outpatient setting, 1 day of scheduled pain medications is reasonable before transitioning to a PRN dosing schedule.

10. **How should the approach differ in treating acute pain in a patient with chronic pain?**
    Managing acute on chronic pain will often require a higher opioid dose compared with an opioid naïve patient. These patients should continue to receive their baseline opioid dose to treat their chronic pain in addition to the opioids used to treat their acute pain. Treatment should primarily focus on multimodal analgesia, in addition to consideration of nonpharmacological interventions. For example, in the preoperative period, patients should receive a dose of gabapentin or pregabalin, in addition to a dose of acetaminophen. After surgery, multimodal analgesia (gabapentinoids, acetaminophen, NSAIDs, etc.) should be continued and adjuvant medications, such as ketamine, duloxetine, clonidine, and steroids may be considered. Regional anesthesia techniques should be used whenever possible, ideally with the placement of a catheter to deliver a continuous local anesthetic infusion. Pumps are also available for regional anesthesia when patients are discharged home, which can deliver a fixed dose of local anesthetic through a catheter for several days.

11. **How should a PCA pump be set?**
    Morphine, hydromorphone, and fentanyl are the most commonly used opioids in PCA pumps. If connected to an epidural as a patient-controlled epidural analgesia, a combination of local anesthetic and opioid is common. Next, decide if the pump will deliver a continuous (basal) dose and the patient-controlled demand dose. Finally, decide how often the pump should deliver medications (i.e., the lockout period). Chronic pain patients with acute pain should, in general, receive their baseline opioid dose as a basal dose if they need a PCA.

12. **How do neuraxial opioids work?**
    Opioid receptors are present in levels I and II of the substantia gelatinosa of the dorsal horn. Opiates given either intrathecally or epidurally bind to these receptors. A 300-mg oral dose of morphine is equal to 100 mg of IV morphine, which is equal to 10 mg of epidural morphine, which is equal to 1 mg of intrathecal morphine.

    Neuraxial morphine is hydrophilic, spreads throughout the spinal fluid, lasts 12 to 24 hours, and can be associated with delayed respiratory depression. Hydromorphone is somewhat lipophilic, spreads over 8 to 10 dermatomes, and lasts 8 to 10 hours. Fentanyl is very lipophilic, spreads over five dermatomes, and lasts 2 to 3 hours.

13. **How do agonist–antagonists and partial agonists differ from other opioids, such as morphine?**
    There are several opioid receptors in the central nervous system: μ-, δ-, and κ-opioid receptors. Most opioids are primarily μ-agonists with various degrees of δ and κ receptor agonism, depending upon the opioid (hydromorphone, oxycodone, fentanyl, etc.). Agonist–antagonists, such as nalbuphine are μ antagonists and κ agonists. Because κ receptor agonism has mild analgesic properties, nalbuphine can reverse opioid overdose, while still providing some analgesia, unlike naloxone. This is most clinically relevant in the postoperative clinical context when treating iatrogenic opioid overdose, whereas naloxone is more appropriate when treating life-threatening opioid overdose (e.g., heroin overdose). Naloxone may be used to reverse iatrogenic opioid overdose in the perioperative period, but it is less forgiving than nalbuphine and requires judicious administration when used in this context. Suboxone is a sublingual medication containing buprenorphine (partial μ agonist) and naloxone (μ antagonist) and is generally used for patients with a history of opioid abuse. Its benefit is that naloxone is poorly absorbed if taken PO, but if injected, naloxone antagonizes the effect of buprenorphine. Further, buprenorphine is a partial μ agonist, with a ceiling effect reducing the risk of respiratory depression from an overdose. Buprenorphine has an extremely high affinity for the μ receptor and

can be administered to reverse opioid overdose in an emergent situation when naloxone is not available. However, this can be problematic in the perioperative setting as buprenorphine binds to the μ receptor with a greater affinity than other opioids.

14. **What is chronic postoperative pain syndrome?**
Chronic postoperative pain syndrome (CPPS) refers to patients who continue to have significant pain for at least 3 months after surgery. Studies show that 10% to 50% of patients may develop CPPS, where the highest risk operations include the following: thoracotomies, inguinal hernia repairs, breast surgeries, cholecystectomies, and amputations. Studies show that multimodal or preventative analgesia can decrease the incidence of chronic postsurgical pain (CPSP), following high-risk operations. The most important predictive factor shown in studies for developing CPSP is persistent moderate to severe postoperative pain on postoperative day 4. Other predictive factors are the presence of pain preoperatively, repeat surgery, intraoperative nerve injury, and psychological factors.

15. **What is preventive or multimodal analgesia?**
Preventive analgesia refers to the practice of anticipating pain from surgery and using regional or neuraxial techniques in combination with synergistic medications started preoperatively and continued postoperatively to decrease the risk of CPSP. Gabanoids, steroids, opioids, NMDA antagonists (ketamine), clonidine, antidepressants, NSAIDs, and other anticonvulsants have all been used for this purpose. Typical dose ranges are given in Table 72.2. The usual combination would be a gabanoid or other anticonvulsant, acetaminophen, NSAID (if possible), opioid, ketamine, and a regional block (if possible). Even simply administering a gabanoid and acetaminophen together, immediately before surgery may help decrease the incidence of CPSP.

16. **What other techniques can be used for acute pain management?**
In addition to multimodal analgesia and regional blocks, psychological approaches have been shown to have an effect on acute pain. Studies on pain coping skills, such as breathing techniques, visualization, hypnosis, biofeedback, and cognitive–behavioral therapy have shown benefits. Acupuncture can help headaches and decrease anxiety. Treating the anxiety and depression that frequently accompany pain is also helpful.

Table 72.2 Multimodal Dosing

DRUG	STARTING DOSE	DAILY DOSE	IDEAL DURATION POSTOPERATIVELY
Gabapentin	900, 1200 mg	900, 1200 mg	8–10 days
Pregabalin	75, 50 mg bid	75, 50 mg bid	5 days
Duloxetine	60 mg	60 mg	1 day
Ketorolac	30 mg	15, 30 mg	3 days
Celebrex	200 mg	100 mg	2–4 days
Ketamine	0.2–0.5 mg/kg	100–300 mcg/kg/h	1–5 days
Clonidine	0.1 mg	0.1 mg	
Dexamethasone	0.11–0.21 mg/kg		
Dexmedetomidine	1 mcg.kg − 1	0.5 mcg.kg − 1.h − 1	1 day
NSAIDs (ibuprofen)	200–400 mg, 4–6 hours or 400, 800 mg, 3–4 times daily	Maximum: 3200 mg per day (prescription)	
Acetaminophen	325, 650 mg, 4–6 hours or 1000 mg, 3–4 times daily	Maximum: 4000 mg per day	
Topical lidocaine	5% patch (700 mg)	1–3 patches once daily, removed after 12 hours	
Ketorolac	20 mg once age ≥65 years, renal impairment, or weight <50kg: 10 mg once	10 mg q4–6 hours PRN not >40 mg/day	5 days
Tramadol	50–100 mg oral dose	50–100 mg, every 4–6 hours as needed; Maximum: 400 mg/day	

Bid, Twice a day; *NSAIDs*, nonsteroidal antiinflammatory drugs; *PRN*, as needed.

17. **Is there a role for IV infusions in acute pain management?**
Ketamine is an NMDA receptor antagonist that alters pain transmission without respiratory depression. Postoperatively, it is used as an infusion, typically 100 to 300 mcg/kg/h. Some patients may need a small dose of a benzodiazepine daily (0.25–0.5mg clonazepam) to prevent hallucinations. Hemodynamic changes are small at these doses. Antidepressant effects are seen at doses between 300 and 500 mcg/kg/h. Ketamine can decrease opioid requirements and decrease acute pain, especially in patients with chronic pain, and can easily be administered as an adjunct during surgery.

Lidocaine can also be used as an infusion: 1 to 1.5 mg/kg given as a bolus, followed by 2 mg/min. A lidocaine infusion may decrease opioid requirements and associated side effects. Lidocaine infusions have decreased efficacy compared with that of neuraxial blocks. Although there is a potential for toxicity, the doses administered are low and no serious complications have been reported in studies.

Dexmedetomidine may also be used as an additional multimodal adjunct during surgery, although further evidence is needed to determine optimal dosage. Its major risk is bradycardia.

18. **What are the common side effects of opioids? How are they treated?**
See Table 72.3.

19. **How is pediatric acute pain management different from adult acute pain management?**
Pain assessment can be more challenging in infants and small children than in adults. In addition to visual and photographic scales, caregivers may be helpful in interpreting behavioral clues. Functional scales are used in very young patients. Vital signs, activity level, and feeding can help determine adequacy of pain control. Most medications used in the adult population can be used in pediatric patients but are dosed by weight. Multimodal strategies are used early to reduce side effects; regional blocks are used whenever possible. Nurse-controlled analgesia or caregiver-controlled analgesia can be used when the child is unable to use a PCA button to request a demand bolus. Most PCA pumps are set with 75% of the daily dose scheduled and 25% available PRN, for breakthrough pain. Nonpharmacological interventions, such as distraction, play therapy, pain psychology, coping skills, and meditation are emphasized.

20. **What factors have contributed to the current opioid epidemic in the United States?**
The magnitude of the ongoing opioid epidemic affecting the United States is truly alarming, having claimed 400,000 lives since 1999, with over 130 Americans dying per day (2017 data) from an opioid overdose according to the Centers for Disease Control and Prevention (CDC). In the 1990s, a national effort to address the underassessment and undertreatment of pain culminated in the American Pain Society, the Joint Commission, and other organizations to advocate that pain should be treated as a "fifth vital sign" using the numeric pain scale. The Centers of Medicare and Medicaid followed suite by coupling payment reimbursement to patient satisfaction surveys (e.g., the Hospital Consumer Assessment of Healthcare Providers and Systems [HCAHPS]), which asked questions about pain control. This prompted a first wave of opioid-related deaths, which were correlated with the increase in opioid prescription rates, including oxycodone, hydrocodone, methadone from 1999 to time of writing. The second wave began in 2010, following an increase in heroin use and addiction, which are thought to be related to the pharmaceutical industry's efforts to curb prescription opioid abuse. The third wave of opioid-related deaths involved the increase in illicit synthetic opioids, such as fentanyl. As of 2017, deaths from synthetic opioids are the most common, followed by prescribed opioids, followed by heroin.

The initial exposure to opioids for many patients occurs with a surgery, which can lead to opioid abuse, particularly when the patient is discharged home with a liberal opioid prescription (i.e., >7 days). The CDC recommends, when discharging patients with acute pain, to only provide a 3-day supply of opioid medication and

Table 72.3 Common Side Effects of Opioid Use	
SIDE EFFECT	**TREATMENT**
Pruritus	Apply lotion to the affected area; intravenous or oral delivery of diphenhydramine (25–50 mg); in severe cases, use an opioid antagonist (i.e., naloxone) or agonist–antagonist (i.e., nalbuphine, 5 mg every 6 hours)
Constipation	Use of OTC laxatives for mild to moderate cases; use of methylnaltraxone for severe constipation: 12 mg SC qDay or 450 mg PO qDay in morning
Nausea/vomiting	Decrease opioid dose. Consider nalbuphine, clonidine, and antiemetics, such as ondansetron 4 mg intravenously
Urinary retention	Urinary Foley catheter or nalbuphine
Sedation/respiratory depression	Stop opioid temporarily and use naloxone or nalbuphine

OTC, Over the counter; *PO*, orally; *SC*, subcutaneously.

rarely should a 7-day or greater supply be required. In addition, multimodal nonopioid medications and nonpharmacological pain treatment strategies should be used whenever possible. Further, pain should no longer be used as a vital sign and all major organizations have now dropped endorsement of "pain as the fifth vital sign." To remove conflict between patient pain scores and reimbursement, patient satisfaction surveys (e.g., HCAHPS) have now removed all questions pertaining to pain control.

On June 22nd, 2018, the US House of Representatives passed H.R. 6 Substance Use-Disorder Prevention that Promotes Opioid Recovery and Treatment (SUPPORT) for Patients and Communities Act, which includes Medicaid, Medicare, and public health reforms to combat the opioid crisis by advancing treatment and recovery initiatives and funding, improving prevention through opioid education and research of nonaddictive pain medications, and expanding guidelines to allow physician assistants and nurse practitioners to prescribe medications that treat opioid addiction and create opioid recovery centers.

21. How does good acute pain management affect outcomes?

Pain is a form of stress and produces an elevation in stress hormones and catecholamines. Good pain management results in shorter hospital stays, improved mortality rates (especially in patients with less physiological reserve), better immune function, fewer catabolism and endocrine derangements, and fewer thromboembolic complications. In addition, specific benefits may pertain to specific procedures. Patients who undergo amputation under a regional block with local anesthetic have a decreased incidence of phantom pain. Patients in whom a vascular graft is placed have a lower rate of thrombosis. Epidural analgesia can reduce the mortality rate in patients with a flail chest or rib fractures.

Recent studies have shown the value of preemptive analgesia in some surgical situations. The blockade of the pathways involved in pain transmission, before surgical stimulation, may decrease the patient's postoperative pain. Local infiltration along the site of skin incision, in patients having inguinal hernia repairs with general anesthesia, is beneficial if the infiltration is done before the skin incision. Similar results have been found for preoperative local infiltration along the laparoscopic port sites. Several studies using IV or epidural opioids in patients undergoing thoracotomies and hysterectomies have also shown a preemptive effect. Interestingly, the use of local anesthetic in spinals and epidurals, including NSAIDs, have not been shown to be preemptive. Further studies with larger patient groups are needed to provide definitive answers regarding preemptive analgesia.

KEY POINTS: ACUTE PAIN MANAGEMENT

1. Pain is a symptom (subjective) not a vital sign (objective).
2. Pain assessment should not rely solely on numeric pain scores but should include functional impairment and treatment goals (e.g., breathe or sleep without pain).
3. Acute pain can progress to chronic pain, such as in CPSP.
4. Multimodal (preventative) analgesia can decrease postoperative complications and CPSP.
5. Multimodal analgesia may include gabapentinoids, NSAIDs, ketamine, clonidine, opioids, other membrane stabilizers, steroids, antidepressants, and regional anesthesia.
6. Psychological interventions (pain coping skills) are helpful.
7. Chronic pain patients with acute pain will often require an increase to their baseline dose of opioids, although preference should be given to multimodal analgesia.

SUGGESTED READINGS

Benzon HT, Raja SN, Lui SS, et al. Essentials of Pain Medicine. 3rd ed. Philadelphia: Saunders; 2011.

Chou R, Gordon DB, de Leon-Casasola OA, et al. Management of postoperative pain: a clinical practice guideline from the American Pain Society, the American Society of Regional Anesthesia and Pain Medicine, and the American Society of Anesthesiologists' Committee on Regional Anesthesia, Executive Committee, and Administrative Council. J Pain. 2016;17(2):131–157.

Clarke H, Bonin RP, Orser BA, et al. The prevention of chronic postsurgical pain using gabapentin and pregabalin: a combined systematic review and meta-analysis, Anesth Analg. 2012;115:428–442.

Dowell D, Haegerich TM, Chou R. CDC Guideline for prescribing opioids for chronic pain United States, 2016. MMWR Recomm Rep. 2016; 65(No. RR-1):1–49.

Sun EC, Jena AB, Kao MC, et al. Incidence of and risk factors for chronic opioid use among opioid naïve patients in the perioperative period. JAMA Intern Med. 2016;176(9):1286–1293.

Vollmer TL, Robinson MJ, Risser RC, et al. A randomized, double-blind, placebo-controlled trial of duloxetine for the treatment of pain in patients with multiple sclerosis. Pain Pract. 2014;14(8):732–744.

CHAPTER 73

CHRONIC PAIN MANAGEMENT

Robert G. Saldana, BA, Eugene Hsu, MD, MBA

1. What is the definition of pain?

The International Association for the Study of Pain defines *pain* as "an unpleasant sensory and emotional experience associated with actual or potential tissue damage, or described in terms of such damage." Acute pain is associated with an identifiable cause (e.g., surgery, trauma, acute illness) and usually resolves with healing. Chronic pain is pain that occurs on at least half of all days for 3 months or more.

2. Is pain a vital sign?

No, pain is a symptom (subjective) not a vital sign (objective), see Chapter 72.

3. How is pain assessed?

Pain should be assessed by functional impairment and treatment goals. Pain should not be assessed using the one-dimensional, numeric pain scale in isolation, see Chapter 72.

4. How does normal pain perception occur?

Nociceptors are structures located at the ends of axons that are depolarized by noxious thermal, mechanical, or chemical stimuli. The distal ends of most A-δ and C fibers are nociceptors. These axons are the ones that carry nociceptive information to the dorsal root and trigeminal ganglion and enter the spinal cord via the posterior root. The A-δ fibers are myelinated, rapidly conducting sharp, stabbing, and well-localized pain. C fibers are unmyelinated and conduct dull, aching, and poorly localized pain. Once in the spinal cord, these afferent fibers synapse with cells in Rexed laminae I and V preferentially, but also in laminae II and X. Axons from the previously mentioned neurons that travel to the contralateral side of the spinal cord will eventually form the spinothalamic tract, spinoreticular tract, and spinomesencephalic tract. Axons that enter the dorsal column will form the postsynaptic dorsal column tract. These ascending nociceptive tracts will eventually synapse with superior structures, such as the periaqueductal gray, hypothalamus, and thalamus. The ventroposterolateral, ventroposteromedial, and ventroposteroinferior nuclei of the thalamus then send projections to the somatosensory cortex and cingulated cortices.

5. What is the classification of pain based on neurophysiological mechanisms?

- Nociceptive pain occurs when nociceptors are stimulated by noxious stimuli, which can be divided into somatic and visceral pain. Somatic pain often originates from trauma, burns, and ischemia and is transmitted by both A-δ (sharp, localized pain) and C fibers (dull, poorly localized pain). Visceral pain, as its name implies, originates from visceral structures. It is transmitted preferentially via C fibers (dull, poorly localized pain) and is usually produced by distention, ischemia, or spasm of hollow viscera
- Neuropathic pain is pain produced by an alteration in structure or function of the nervous system. Neuropathic pain can be divided into peripheral and central. Examples of peripheral neuropathic pain include complex regional pain syndrome (CRPS) II (causalgia), postherpetic neuralgia, diabetic neuropathy, and radicular pain from mechanical compression. Central neuropathic pain syndromes include poststroke pain, postparaplegic pain, and pain syndromes from multiple sclerosis
- Psychogenic pain is quite controversial in the sense that it is very difficult to define. One popular definition is that this pain is better described and understood in psychological rather than physical language and is pain for which an adequate physical explanation cannot be found

6. Name the most commonly used groups of medications for the treatment of chronic pain

See Table 73.1.

7. How are nerve blocks helpful in the treatment of chronic pain?

- Diagnosis: Nerve blocks can help identify the nerve site responsible for the symptoms.
- Therapy: Nerve blocks temporarily reduce pain and therefore facilitate physical therapy. Based on the response to a diagnostic block, it might be possible to determine if a neuroablation procedure is appropriate to treat a given condition.

8. What are the differences between the biomedical and the biopsychosocial model for pain?

The traditional biomedical model of pain relied on an understanding of pain nociception in which unique receptor mechanisms and pathways transmitted pain information from the periphery to the spinal cord and brain. However, this theory is limited in its ability to explain persistent chronic pain conditions, particularly the influence of psychological factors, such as emotional stress, in the reporting of pain severity in those with chronic pain syndromes. Over the last 50 years, the biopsychosocial model has emerged as the most widely accepted heuristic for chronic pain. The biopsychosocial model maintains that to fully understand a person's perception and response to pain and illness,

Table 73.1 Commonly Used Groups of Medications for Treatment of Chronic Pain

GROUP	DRUG EXAMPLES	MODE OF ACTION	POTENTIAL SIDE EFFECTS
TCAs	Amitriptyline, Nortriptyline	Norepinephrine and 5-hydroxytryptamine uptake inhibition. Descending inhibition pathway activation	Anticholinergic actions, decreased seizure threshold, cardiac dysrhythmias, weight gain
NSAIDs	Ibuprofen, Celecoxib, Aspirin	Inhibit production of prostaglandin	Gastrointestinal bleeding, platelet dysfunction, bronchospasm, coronary thrombosis
SSRIs/SNRIs	Venlafaxine, Duloxetine, Milnacipran	Inhibit serotonin, norepinephrine reuptake	Anxiety, nausea, weight loss, increases plasma TCA levels if coadministered
Anticonvulsants	Carbamazepine, Valproic acid, Gabapentin, Pregabalin	Reduce Na^+, K^+ conductance, Increase GABA activity	Blood dyscrasias, liver dysfunction, gastrointestinal symptoms, sedation, ataxia
Neuroleptics	Fluphenazine, Haloperidol	May alter perception of pain	Extrapyramidal symptoms, orthostatic hypotension
Benzodiazepines	Diazepam, Lorazepam	Reduce anxiety	Sedation, dependence, tolerance, addiction
Opioids	Morphine, Meperidine, Oxycodone, Methadone	μ-Receptor agonists	Sedation, respiratory depression, pruritis, nausea, constipation, addiction
Muscle relaxants	Baclofen, Cyclobenzaprine	Interaction with GABA receptor	Sedation, anticholinergic effects, orthostatic hypotension, conduction block
Others	Mexiletine β-Blockers Alendronate Ketamine Acetaminophen	Na-channel blocker β-receptor antagonism Inhibit bone resorption NMDA antagonist Unknown mechanism (COX-3?)	Dysrhythmias Heart failure Musculoskeletal pain Dysphoria Liver toxicity

COX, Cyclooxygenase; *GABA,* γ-aminobutyric acid; *NMDA, N*-methyl-ᴅ-Aspartate; *NSAID,* nonsteroidal antiinflammatory drug; *SNRI,* selective serotonin-norepinephrine reuptake inhibitor; *SSRI,* selective serotonin reuptake inhibitor; *TCA,* tricyclic antidepressant.

the interrelationships among biological changes, psychological status, and the sociocultural context all need to be considered.

9. How should cancer pain be treated?

Cancer pain, also termed *malignant pain*, should be treated aggressively with a multiple therapeutic approach. This should initially include pharmacological modalities with the introduction of short- and long-acting opioid preparations, including adjuvant nonopioid medications. Adjuvants should be chosen according to the symptomatology and their side-effect profile. For example, nonsteroidal antiinflammatory drugs (NSAIDs), bisphosphonates, and steroids are very useful in the treatment of bone pain from primary or metastatic disease; anticonvulsants and tricyclic antidepressants (TCAs) can be used in the treatment of neuropathic pain.

Diagnostic nerve blocks, if successful, can be followed by either chemical or radiofrequency ablation procedures. For malignancies located within the abdomen, celiac plexus chemical ablation can be attempted; for malignancies located in the pelvis, a superior hypogastric plexus block can be beneficial; and perineal pain can be treated with a ganglion impar ablation. With the introduction of sophisticated intrathecal delivery systems, neuraxial ablative procedures are becoming less popular but are still useful. As mentioned, intrathecal delivery systems and long-term epidural catheters are used to deliver opioids, local anesthetics, and other potentially beneficial drugs to the neuraxis and therefore improve the patient's condition and decrease the side effects from other medications. Finally, radiation therapy and chemotherapy can also improve pain symptoms by reducing the extent of the disease.

10. Define CRPS I and II. What nerve blocks are commonly used to treat these conditions?

CRPS stands for *complex regional pain syndrome*. It is a painful condition, usually isolated to an extremity, in which different degrees of sympathetic dysfunction can be identified. CRPS usually presents with spontaneous pain, hyperalgesia, hyperpathia, and allodynia that is not restricted to the territory of a single nerve. Sympathetic dysfunction presents as variations in regional blood flow that can cause edema and cyanosis. Localized sweating and trophic changes in the skin and nails of the affected part of the body can be seen, as the disease progresses. CRPS I (formerly known as *reflex sympathetic dystrophy*) can occur from minor trauma (venipuncture, carpal tunnel surgery, etc.); often no identifiable cause is found. CRPS II (formerly called *causalgia*), however, is caused by identifiable nerve injury. Approximately 90% of CRPS is because of CRPS I. Sympathetic blocks are very useful because they can facilitate physical therapy and help the patient regain some function in the affected extremity. Upper-extremity sympathetic denervation is accomplished by blocking the stellate ganglion; for lower-extremity sympathetic block, a lumbar sympathetic block is performed.

11. How is neuropathic pain treated?

Medical management that includes anticonvulsants and TCAs have shown to improve symptomatology. Methadone, because of its N-methyl-D-aspartate receptor antagonism, is probably the most useful opioid in the treatment of neuropathic pain. Other agents, such as clonidine and mexiletine, have also been used successfully. Injection of local anesthetics and steroids has a role in the treatment of isolated peripheral neuropathies. The introduction of peripheral and spinal cord stimulators is now an accepted therapy for very complex problems, such as postlaminectomy pain syndromes and CRPS types I and II.

12. Define myofascial pain syndrome

Myofascial pain syndrome is a group of muscle disorders characterized by hypersensitive areas called *trigger points* that can occur in more than one muscle group. When trigger points are mechanically stimulated, they are painful and refer pain to an area called the *reference zone*. This reference zone does not correlate with any dermatome or peripheral nerve innervation area.

13. Define fibromyalgia

Fibromyalgia is a chronic pain condition characterized by widespread musculoskeletal pain, aches, stiffness, soft-tissue tenderness, general fatigue, and sleep disturbances. The most common sites of pain include the neck, back, shoulders, pelvic girdle, and hands, but any body part can be involved. Fibromyalgia patients experience a range of symptoms of varying intensities that wax and wane over time.

14. How is fibromyalgia managed?

New research shows that fibromyalgia likely has a central nervous system component. This theory helps explain the widespread nature of the patients' symptoms and its association with sleep disturbances. Pregabalin, duloxetine, milnacipran are the only US Food and Drug Administration–approved medications for the management of fibromyalgia. In a randomized, double-blinded, placebo-controlled study, monotherapy with pregabalin showed statistically significant benefit in mean pain scores and overall patient perceived improvement of symptoms. Cardiovascular exercise and management of underlying depression is also important in treating this patient population.

15. What is opioid-induced hyperalgesia?

Opioid-induced hyperalgesia is a condition in which chronic exposure to opioids leads to a paradoxical response of heightened sensitivity to painful stimuli. Note, that this problem is likely an "area under the curve" problem, as it can also be seen in the perioperative setting when extremely high dose opioids are administered for a relatively short period of time.

16. List the etiologies of lower back pain

Lower back pain can arise from multiple anatomic structures located in the lower back; such as the following:
- Muscle strain in the paravertebral muscles or quadratus lumborum
- Injury to the posterior elements of the vertebral column, such as the facet joints and ligamentous structures
- Injury to the anterior elements, such as vertebral compression fractures
- Damage or age-related degeneration of the outer, anulus fibrosus of the intervertebral disc, leading to a "herniated disk"
- Vertebral canal and foraminal stenosis, which can cause myelopathy or radiculopathy, respectively
- Sacroiliac joint dysfunction

17. What is the rationale behind the use of epidural steroids in the treatment of radicular symptoms associated with a herniated disk?

Radiculopathy is pain that is present as a result of either mechanical or chemical (most of the time both) irritation of a nerve root and can lead to pain and edema of the same nerve. The site where this usually occurs is the neural foramen. Local injection of steroids will decrease the amount of time needed to recover from an acute episode of sciatica by four mechanisms:
1. Decreasing the inflammation of the nerve root because of the antiinflammatory properties of the steroids
2. Dilution of chemical irritants coming from a ruptured disc
3. Nerve membrane stabilizers
4. Inhibiting action of phospholipase A2

18. **Explain the gate-control theory of pain**

    In 1965 Melzack and Wall proposed that the substantia gelatinosa in the spinal cord was the primary gate in the transmission of noxious and nonnoxious stimulus to the central nervous system. The theory states that the pain gate is opened by signals from the slower nerve fibers that transmit pain (A-δ and C fibers) and closed when transmitting signals from the faster myelinated fibers, such as with tactile touch (A-β fibers). For example, rubbing your foot after stubbing your toe can reduce pain symptoms. The medical application of the gate-control theory of pain is demonstrated with transcutaneous electrical nerve stimulation devices and spinal and peripheral nerve stimulators, which reduce pain symptoms.

19. **Name some indications for the use of spinal cord stimulators**

    The most common indication for the use of spinal cord stimulation in the United States is in the treatment of postlaminectomy pain syndrome aka *failed back surgery syndrome*. Other indications include the treatment of refractory CRPS, arachnoiditis, noncardiac chest pain, peripheral vascular disease, and neuropathic pain.

20. **What are the most common medications used for intrathecal delivery via implantable delivery systems?**

    The most common medication used in the implantable delivery systems are opioids, specifically morphine and hydromorphone. Local anesthetics are usually used in combination with an opioid for the treatment of cancer pain. Baclofen may be used for the treatment of spasticity and painful muscle contractions. Clonidine may be used for the treatment of neuropathic pain. Recent studies have explored the potential for the use of ketamine, neostigmine, and calcium channel blockers.

21. **What are the limitations of opioids when prescribed for chronic, noncancer pain? In what clinical setting are opioid medications particularly helpful?**

    Opioid medications may be effective initially, in part, because they have no "analgesic ceiling" compared with nonopioid medications. However, studies show that after 3 months, patients report similar pain scores compared with nonopioid medications. This is largely because of two reasons: (1) opioid tolerance develops quickly (in as little as several weeks), and (2) opioid-induced hyperalgesia. Further, studies show that opioid medications compared with nonopioid medications, when used for chronic, noncancer pain, are associated with an increase in overall mortality because of unintentional overdose and cardiovascular death.

    This is not to imply that opioid medications should never be used for chronic, noncancer pain, but that their risks and benefits should strongly be considered when prescribing these medications. Further, opioids are particularly helpful in managing cancer pain, hospice patients, comfort care in dying intensive care unit patients, and in the intraoperative setting.

22. **What factors have contributed to the current opioid epidemic in the United States?**

    The magnitude of the ongoing opioid epidemic affecting the United States is truly alarming having claimed 400,000 lives since 1999 with over 130 Americans dying per day (2017 data) from an opioid overdose according to the Centers for Disease Control and Prevention. In the 1990s, a national effort to address the underassessment and undertreatment of pain culminated in the American Pain Society, The Joint Commission, and other organizations to advocate that pain should be treated as a "fifth vital sign," using the numeric pain scale. The Centers of Medicare and Medicaid followed suite by coupling payment reimbursement to patient satisfaction surveys (e.g., the Hospital Consumer Assessment of Healthcare Providers and Systems), which asked questions about pain control. This prompted a first wave of opioid related deaths, which were correlated with the increase in opioid prescription rates, including oxycodone, hydrocodone, methadone from 1999 to time of writing. The second wave began in 2010, following an increase in heroin use and addiction, which are thought to be related to the pharmaceutical industry's efforts to curb prescription opioid abuse. The third wave of opioid related deaths involved the increase in illicit synthetic opioids, such as fentanyl. As of 2017, deaths from synthetic opioids are the most common, followed by prescribed opioids, followed by heroin.

    On June 22nd, 2018, the US House of Representatives passed H.R. 6 Substance Use-Disorder Prevention that Promotes Opioid Recovery and Treatment (SUPPORT) for Patients and Communities Act, which includes Medicaid, Medicare, and public health reforms to combat the opioid crisis by advancing treatment and recovery initiatives and funding, improving prevention through opioid education and research of nonaddictive pain medications, and expanding guidelines to allow physician assistants and nurse practitioners to prescribe medications that treat opioid addiction and create opioid recovery centers.

23. **How can pain physicians uniquely address the opioid epidemic?**

    Physicians with specialized training in pain management have several unique skills to address the opioid epidemic. Although not a comprehensive list, these skills include:

    - Knowledge and experience managing acute perioperative pain, particularly with the use of multimodal analgesia to minimize opioid requirements (see Chapter 72).
    - Knowledge and experience in multidisciplinary pain management using interventional pain procedures, physical therapy, rehabilitation, and psychological methods to reduce the necessity of opioids, while improving functional status and providing pain relief.

- Knowledge and experience in the diagnosis and treatment of neuropathic pain, which typically does not respond well to opioid mediations.
- For interventional pain specialists, knowledge and experience managing pain using interventional therapies, such as epidural steroid injections, radiofrequency ablation, and neurostimulation.

KEY POINTS: CHRONIC PAIN MANAGEMENT

1. Chronic pain is best treated using multiple therapeutic modalities. These include physical therapy, psychological support, pharmacological management, and the rational use of more invasive procedures, such as nerve blocks and implantable devices.
2. Patients suffering from cancer pain often exhibit complex symptomatology that includes various forms of nociceptive and neuropathic pain.
3. In patients suffering from chronic pain, a comprehensive multidisciplinary approach addressing biological, psychological, and social factors should be addressed if any meaningful recovery is to be achieved.
4. Neuropathic pain is usually less responsive to opioids than pain originating from nociceptors.
5. The cause of the United States opioid epidemic is multifactorial. Causes include the "pain as the fifth vital sign" campaign, patient surveys that coupled reimbursement with pain control, misalignment of incentives for pharmaceutical companies, and insufficient safety data in expanding the use of opioid medications to chronic, noncancer pain patients.

Website
International Association for the Study of Pain: http://www.iasp-pain.org

---

SUGGESTED READINGS

Cameron T. Safety and efficacy of spinal cord stimulation for the treatment of chronic pain: a 20-year literature review. J Neurosurg. 2004;100(3 Suppl):254–267.

Dowell D, Haegerich TM, Chou R. CDC guideline for prescribing opioids for chronic pain—United States, 2016. JAMA. 2016;315(15):1624–1645.

Gatchel RJ, Peng YB, Peters ML, et al. The biopsychosocial approach to chronic pain: scientific advances and future directions. Psychol Bull. 2007;133(4):581.

Mackey S. National Pain Strategy Task Force: the strategic plan for the IOM Pain Report. Pain Med. 2014;15(7):1070–1071.

Mease PJ, Russell IJ, Arnold LM, et al. A randomized, double-blind, placebo-controlled, phase III trial of pregabalin in the treatment of patients with fibromyalgia. J Rheumatol. 2008;35:502–514.

Melzack R, Wall P. Pain mechanism: a new theory. Science. 1965;150:971.

Vranken JH, van der Vegt MH, Kal JE, et al. Treatment of neuropathic cancer pain with continuous intrathecal administration of S + ketamine. Acta Anesthesiol Scand. 2004;48:249–252.

INDEX

Note: Page numbers followed by *f* indicate figures, *t* indicate tables, and *b* indicate boxes.